Interdisciplinary Approaches to Altering Neurodevelopmental Disorders

Tanu Wadhera
Dr. B. R. Ambedkar National Institute of Technology, Jalandhar, India

Deepti Kakkar
Dr. B. R. Ambedkar National Institute of Technology, Jalandhar, India

A volume in the Advances in Medical Diagnosis, Treatment, and Care (AMDTC) Book Series

IGI Global
DISSEMINATOR OF KNOWLEDGE

Published in the United States of America by
IGI Global
Medical Information Science Reference (an imprint of IGI Global)
701 E. Chocolate Avenue
Hershey PA, USA 17033
Tel: 717-533-8845
Fax: 717-533-8661
E-mail: cust@igi-global.com
Web site: http://www.igi-global.com

Library of Congress Cataloging-in-Publication Data

Names: Wadhera, Tanu, 1991- editor. | Kakkar, Deepti, 1982- editor.
Title: Interdisciplinary approaches to altering neurodevelopmental disorders / Tanu Wadhera and Deepti Kakkar, editors.
Description: Hershey, PA : Medical Information Science Reference, [2020] | Includes bibliographical references and index. | Summary: ""This book explores interdisciplinary approaches to diagnostic, assessment, support, and intervention schemes for neurodevelopmental disorders"--Provided by publisher"-- Provided by publisher.
Identifiers: LCCN 2019047149 (print) | LCCN 2019047150 (ebook) | ISBN 9781799830696 (hardcover) | ISBN 9781799830702 (ebook)
Subjects: MESH: Neurodevelopmental Disorders--therapy | Neurodevelopmental Disorders--diagnosis | Education, Special--methods | Self-Help Devices
Classification: LCC RC349.8 (print) | LCC RC349.8 (ebook) | NLM WS 350.7 | DDC 616.8/046--dc23
LC record available at https://lccn.loc.gov/2019047149
LC ebook record available at https://lccn.loc.gov/2019047150

This book is published in the IGI Global book series Advances in Medical Diagnosis, Treatment, and Care (AMDTC) (ISSN: 2475-6628; eISSN: 2475-6636)

British Cataloguing in Publication Data
A Cataloguing in Publication record for this book is available from the British Library.

For electronic access to this publication, please contact: eresources@igi-global.com.

Advances in Medical Diagnosis, Treatment, and Care (AMDTC) Book Series

ISSN:2475-6628
EISSN:2475-6636

Mission

Advancements in medicine have prolonged the life expectancy of individuals all over the world. Once life-threatening conditions have become significantly easier to treat and even cure in many cases. Continued research in the medical field will further improve the quality of life, longevity, and wellbeing of individuals.

The **Advances in Medical Diagnosis, Treatment, and Care (AMDTC)** book series seeks to highlight publications on innovative treatment methodologies, diagnosis tools and techniques, and best practices for patient care. Comprised of comprehensive resources aimed to assist professionals in the medical field apply the latest innovations in the identification and management of medical conditions as well as patient care and interaction, the books within the AMDTC series are relevant to the research and practical needs of medical practitioners, researchers, students, and hospital administrators.

Coverage

- Emergency Medicine
- Medical Procedures
- Medical Testing
- Patient Interaction
- Disease Management
- Cancer Treatment
- Alternative Medicine
- Diagnostic Medicine
- Experimental Medicine
- Critical Care

IGI Global is currently accepting manuscripts for publication within this series. To submit a proposal for a volume in this series, please contact our Acquisition Editors at Acquisitions@igi-global.com or visit: http://www.igi-global.com/publish/.

The Advances in Medical Diagnosis, Treatment, and Care (AMDTC) Book Series (ISSN 2475-6628) is published by IGI Global, 701 E. Chocolate Avenue, Hershey, PA 17033-1240, USA, www.igi-global.com. This series is composed of titles available for purchase individually; each title is edited to be contextually exclusive from any other title within the series. For pricing and ordering information please visit http://www.igi-global.com/book-series/advances-medical-diagnosis-treatment-care/129618. Postmaster: Send all address changes to above address.

Titles in this Series

For a list of additional titles in this series, please visit:
http://www.igi-global.com/book-series/advances-medical-diagnosis-treatment-care/129618

Role of Nutrition in Providing Pro-/Anti-Inflammatory Balance Emerging Research and Opportunities
Uğur Günşen (Bandırma Onyedi Eylül University, Turkey) and Ramazan Mert Atan (Bandırma Onyedi Eylül University, Trkey)
Medical Information Science Reference • © 2020 • 214pp • H/C (ISBN: 9781799835943) • US $235.00

Handbook of Research on Prenatal, Postnatal, and Early Childhood Development
Neriman Aral (Ankara University, Turkey)
Medical Information Science Reference • © 2020 • 470pp • H/C (ISBN: 9781799829522) • US $365.00

Ethnomedicinal Plant Use and Practice in Traditional Medicine
Akash (Gurukul Kangri University, India) Navneet (Gurukul Kangri University, India) and B.S. Bhandari (Garhwal University, India)
Medical Information Science Reference • © 2020 • 380pp • H/C (ISBN: 9781799813200) • US $295.00

Ethnopharmacological Investigation of Indian Spices
Neha Mishra (Sam Higginbottom University of Agriculture, Technology, and Sciences, India)
Medical Information Science Reference • © 2020 • 335pp • H/C (ISBN: 9781799825241) • US $295.00

Advanced Pharmacological Uses of Medicinal Plants and Natural Products
Ajeet Singh (National Dairy Research Institute, India) Padam Singh (Vaccine and Infectious Disease Research Centre, Translational Health Science and Technology Institute, India) and Navneet Bithel (Gurukul Kangri University, India)
Medical Information Science Reference • © 2020 • 442pp • H/C (ISBN: 9781799820949) • US $425.00

Quality Control of Cellular Protein in Neurodegenerative Disorders
Md. Sahab Uddin (Southeast University, Bangladesh) and Ghulam Md. Ashraf (King Abdulaziz University, Saudi Arabia)
Medical Information Science Reference • © 2020 • 515pp • H/C (ISBN: 9781799813170) • US $295.00

Multidimensional Perspectives and Global Analysis of Universal Health Coverage
Yeter Demir Uslu (Istanbul Medipol University, Turkey) Hasan Dinçer (Istanbul Medipol University, Turkey) and Serhat Yüksel (İstanbul Medipol University, Turkey)
Medical Information Science Reference • © 2020 • 499pp • H/C (ISBN: 9781799823292) • US $265.00

IGI Global
DISSEMINATOR OF KNOWLEDGE

701 East Chocolate Avenue, Hershey, PA 17033, USA
Tel: 717-533-8845 x100 • Fax: 717-533-8661
E-Mail: cust@igi-global.com • www.igi-global.com

Table of Contents

Detailed Table of Contents

Inclusion is the latest buzzword in the world of disability. Each society claims itself as inclusive and understanding. The families of persons with special needs, who go through the confusion associated with diagnoses, treatments, therapy and rehabilitation for their loved ones describe the journey as not easy and definitely not inclusive. The case studies presented here are eye openers regarding discrimination and problematic conditions faced by these families which need to be addressed by society as a whole in order to achieve true inclusivity.

Autism spectrum disorder is well known disorder that has its onset in early childhood and is characterized by persistent deficits in social communication/social interaction and restricted, repetitive patterns of behavior, interests, or activities. Evaluation and treatment involve multidisciplinary approach. Outcome is not always favorable and most affected children continue to face challenges in social, academic, and occupational domains of life even as adults. This chapter on autism spectrum disorder (ASD) describes clinical presentation, diagnosis and treatment through a case study of a young child.

This chapter essentially outlines the difficulties and possibilities of residential planning for Autistic Adults in India. It also stresses on the need to conduct research in future planning and devise solutions for the huge population rapidly transitioning into adulthood. In addition to this, dimensions like upbringing of an autistic child, inclusion initiatives, employment opportunities are discussed. Expectations and research directions to make the lives of care-givers easier and to ascertain and solve their support needs are mentioned. In a way, this chapter is a small attempt to address the question of many parents. "What after us?" Views expressed in the chapter are Author's experience as a sibling having a younger brother

This chapter is a review of eye tracking technology. This chapter includes all the work done in the past for the evolution of the field and different technologies developed for tracking eye movements. This chapter gives a detailed hierarchy of the development in the field and also various applications of eye gaze tracking in different areas of technology. The chapter concludes with the significance of this technology and the future scope in the development of the field.

The biggest problem with this Neurodevelopmental disorders (NDDs) is that there is no known cure for it, we can only enhance their skills by using technology and different rehabilitation schemes. The present studies provide good evidence of the children with NDDs and their parent& satisfaction with technological intervention. However, findings should be interpreted with caution, more studies are important for better understanding of the Microsoft Kinect based games effects on NDDs patients in general. Author has described broad studies and work done using Microsoft Kinect and other assistive technologies in intervening the social and behavioral impairment in children with NDDs.

The chapter communicates on yoga as an integrative complementary system for mind-body medicine. The method of application of yoga targets specified system, organ, tissue, or cells. Regular and rhythmic repetition of appropriate yoga practice stimulates the firing of various sensory and motor neurons in the brain, which in-turn rewire new neural pathways. Hence yoga therapy improves cognitive function, sensory-motor coordination, ability to comprehend and follow instructions in children with neurodevelopmental disorder.

This chapter is based on the belief of education as a human right for all students, including the special

Preface

Interdisciplinary Approaches to Altering Neurodevelopmental Disorders serves as a vital platform for clinical psychologists, special educators and counselors, therapists, academicians and researchers seeking advanced knowledge, learning and practice in developing an individual-centric ASD detection and intervention approaches. The tremendous advances across multiple disciplines have provided the ideology to catering the individual-specific demands. The goal is to design different approaches by understanding the basic demands of every affected individual. The present book features research on topics such as clinical manifestation, neural connectivity, therapies, diversity in technological methodologies adopted from educational, medical and industrial professionals to highlight the disorder demands and spread awareness globally. The objective of the book is to bring forward the ideology as well as contribution of different units in a single phase. The book has been dissected majorly into three sections:

- Description of disorder nature and condition or experience of persons with disabilities with a focus on the attitude of society. Attention on the real-life problems from the viewpoint of transition into adulthood, which includes work, education, vocational and residential facility.
- Implicit improvement with a focus on the therapies such as yoga and learning methods such as special education. Explicit improvement by embedding technology into existing techniques such as brain-computer interface and design thinking to boost as well as monitor the implicit improvement. Assistance of technological tools such as eye tracker, games, or Augmentative and Alternative Communication methods to support and enhance the routine needs or life skills based on the feedback of the affected individuals.
- Focus on recent brain mapping techniques and computational models based on more efficient and accurate approaches, such as machine learning, deep learning, and artificial intelligence to demonstrating early detection and improvement in disorder condition.

The significance of the book is to cater the techniques with a focus on different stages which include early diagnosis, routine development and intervention of the disordered individuals. Through this book we are demonstrating feasibility of different technological approaches which can be implemented in the future to assess the results and provide feedback accordingly. The perspective of different persons (researchers, academicians, doctors, etc.) and domains has been brought together in framing neurodevelopmental disorders. Thus, the professionals from different domains should find this book handy and gainful. The book will also be beneficial to the parents in providing more detailed information about the disorder and intervention schemes.

The book begins by defining the prevailing neurodevelopmental disorders which include intellectual disability, autism, epilepsy, motor and attention deficit hyperactivity disorders that are prevailing at a very high rate in India (nearly 12%). Also, this chapter demonstrated the attitude of the society towards the disordered individuals through different case studies. The personal experiences of persons with disabilities, their family and siblings have been encountered, along with, the list of the solutions. An introduction to the revolutionary advances in diagnostic tools which promise early identification and growing intervention approaches which alter the abnormal developmental trajectory has also been provided. In the second chapter, the clinical team has presented a case study to highlight the disorder occurrence, common and rare symptoms, and missed or delayed diagnosis. The chapter has also discussed a diagnostic criterion based on DSM-V and therapeutic aspects with a focus on ASD. The third chapter focused on challenge of transition to adulthood in the life of disordered individuals. The real life difficulties are described in the domain of work, recreational activities, education, vocational and residential arrangements. The issues of rehabilitation centers w.r.t Indian scene are addressed with a solution to revitalize these centers for bringing more life into the prevention and intervention options. Different life skills trainings, employment opportunities and other initiatives have been discussed for the future planning of the affected individuals. In the fourth chapter, an outline of the assistive technology-based interventions provided using mobile apps, games or robots and its outcomes on ASD, Intellectual Disability (ID) and Developmental Disability (DD) affected individual's participation, mood and social validation is provided by reviewing 18 studies involving 155 participants. The fifth and sixth chapter has briefed the principles, methods, and key features of Augmentative and Alternative Communication (AAC) systems involving switches, visual displays, apps, eye tracking systems and pointing devices to support the individuals with ASD and cerebral palsy (CP) by using their residual functional abilities. The seventh chapter has summarized the research in the expansion and technology based techniques, especially eye-tracker, and its applications in assisting disordered individuals. It provided a detailed background and continuous improvement in the field of tracking systems aiming to enhance the social interaction and attention in the learning strategies. The chapter has also listed some limitations that need to be worked upon to boost practical feasibility of eye-trackers. In this vein, eighth chapter has proposed that simple gamification is the fundamental solution for reducing the disorder traits and temporary complexities without the need of any educator or trainer. The idea of customization of games has been disseminated to cater the specific needs of the disordered individuals.

In the next phase, the emerging trends and unexplored areas have been ventured such as role of yoga, special education and design thinking in providing the solution to disorder problems by integrating the needs/requirements of disabled people. The ninth chapter has provided the impact the yoga therapy over the development of body functions and central nervous system in individuals with cognitive disabilities. The tenth chapter has recommended the inclusion of education for the individuals suffering from ADHD (Attention Deficit Hyperactivity Disorder), autism and other disorders. The ideology of classroom instructional plans and Content through Action (CAT) method is provided to teach the students with various disabilities. In the eleventh chapter, the idea that individual-centric approaches based on design thinking plays a key role in developing an interface between participants and technology. It majorly emphasizes on the point that technological assistive tools should be developed in conjunction with individuals concern, needs and demands. The twelevth chapter has described brain computer interface (BCI) from a therapeutic viewpoint in clinical settings for neurodevelopmental disorders.

Recent research based on machine learning and artificial intelligence approaches promise more improved, accurate and efficient diagnosis as well as the intervention of the disorder. The thirteenth chapter has brought the most advanced algorithms which can learn from patterns and predict the disordered individuals and if implemented, these algorithms can assist the early and efficient detection of Neurodevelopmental disorders. The fourteenth chapter aims to bridge the gap between neurodevelopmental disorder diagnosis and computer vision. The chapter proposed a convolutional neural network–based model for ASD identification through video recordings which captures motion of individuals under constrained scenarios. The fifteenth chapter has focused on the comparative analysis of state-of-the-art techniques employing machine and deep learning methodologies in neuroimaging techniques. The chapter has also described the challenges in the existing diagnosis process. The sixteenth chapter has addressed evidence from existing techniques and recent studies in the context of computational approaches for detecting neurodevelopmental disorders. The chapter has also listed the limitations and challenges in the current practices and future research directions. Last chapter has provided the application of Bigdata analysis in identifying different neurodevelopmental disorders. The chapter has proposed a data lake-based engine for faster data analysis and management while analyzing ASD. Thus, our book managed to provide ample theoretical knowledge about novel methodologies and ideologies that can complement the existing techniques by providing numerous solutions and approaches to translate such ideas into real possibilities.

A big thanks to all the authors for putting in their ideas, contribution and throughout support in creating the book. Finally, thanks to all the reviewers for providing the comments which helped in giving a shape to the book.

Introduction

Generally, there are three stages in the life of the disabled individuals; first is the early diagnosis and intervention stage; second is the education and third is the transition to adulthood stage. In India, the growing cases have raised the concern and a lot of efforts are put into the first two stages. However, the third stage is not in the priority list. Moreover, the first two stages are also in a developing mode due to non-uniformity in the disorder nature. Therefore, our book has taken an initiative to bring forward all the three stages together with individual-centric approaches to altering neurodevelopmental disorders. The present book believes that with the maturity in disorder definition, the diagnostic techniques are also becoming sophisticated and the researchers from different fields are combining their expertise to address the disorder at an early age. The concept of integrating the ideas from different domains; including clinicians, researchers, industrialists, academicians, doctors, educators and psychologists makes this book different from other published books in this domain.

Chapter 1
Attitudes of Society Towards People With Neurodevelopmental Disorders:
Problems and Solutions

Pallavi Khanna
National Institute of Technology, Jalandhar, India

ABSTRACT

Social acceptance and inclusion of people with neuro-developmental disorders is challenging. Though each human being is unique, the world population can be segregated into two groups: neuro-typical and neuro-diverse people who have conditions such as autism spectrum disorder, cerebral palsy, learning disabilities, ADHD, and several others. The neuro-typical population claims to be accepting of the neuro-diverse population, but some case studies show that it may sadly not be true. Life can be bewildering and confusing for a person with disabilities. Dealing with so many aspects can be daunting and frustrating for them and their families. Social attitude is a significant factor as the Pwd navigates the harsh world of discrimination and social abandonment and faces barriers where support, guidance, and services are required. Many go through painful journeys and come out stronger and wiser, but bitter as well. Others have had better support. This chapter is a collection of experiences of some Pwd and their families and a list of solutions to the different challenges they encounter.

INTRODUCTION

The census of 2011 states that around 2.68 cr people in India have one or another kind of disability, which is roughly around 2.21% of the population. Being a developing country, there is not much available in terms of services for diagnosis, treatment, care, education or rehabilitation for Pwds. According to a report, the country needs around 13,000 psychiatrists to achieve a ratio of 1: 8000 to 10,000 psychiatrist patient ratio. However, currently, the figure is 3,500 which puts the ratio at 1 psychiatrist per 2 lakh people. Similarly, for clinical psychologists, the need is 20,000, but only 1000 psychologists

DOI: 10.4018/978-1-7998-3069-6.ch001

are available. Psychiatric Social Workers are only 900 where the requirement is 35000, and Psychiatric nurses are only 1500, where the need is 30,000. In all, the mental health workforce in India stands at around 7000 where the need is for 55,000 professionals (Adjorlu, Høeg, Mangano, & Serafin, 2017). The attitudes of the general public in India towards those with disability range from apathy, ignorance, pity and sympathy, to charity and benevolence. However, there is a huge lacking in the spirit of equality and inclusivity in its true sense. The Pwd Act 2016 does help to bring about some justice with regards to education opportunities and employment, but this is just a small beginning towards bridging the gap between the neuro-diverse population and the neuro-typicals (Bone et al., 2016). At the end, the disability rights activists still have to scream to be heard….. They are just demanding what is rightfully theirs, and are not mere recipients of doles and charity. As is rightly said by the WHO, ' Disability is thus not just a health problem. It is a complex phenomenon, reflecting the interaction between features of a person's body and features of the society, in which he or she lives. Overcoming the difficulties faced by people with disabilities requires interventions to remove environmental and social barriers'.

BACKGROUND

An attitude can be defined as an internal affective orientation that explains the actions of a person. Attitudes have many components namely: cognitive (consciously held belief or opinion); affective (emotional tone or feeling), evaluative (positive or negative); and conative (disposition for action). Neuro developmental disorders are a group of conditions with onset in the development period. The disorders typically manifest early in development, often before the child enters grade school and are characterized by developmental deficits that produce impairments of personal, social, academic, or occupational functioning (Bosl, Tierney, Tager-Flusberg, & Nelson, 2011). The range of developmental deficits varies from very specific limitations of learning or control of executive functions to global impairments of social skills or intelligence. The neurodevelopmental disorders frequently co-occur; for example, individual with autism spectrum disorder often have intellectual disability (intellectual developmental disorder), and many children with attention-deficit/hyperactivity disorder (ADHD) also have a specific learning disorder.

Bringing up children with Neuro Developmental Disorders in India (Ali & Bhaskar, 2016) is an extremely challenging task. It is definitely an uphill task, especially for parents, it is so because the Indian society lacks a positive approach towards individuals with disability. People with NDD are viewed as abnormal and labeled as insane by their colleagues and peers. Although not everyone in society has a biased perception of them, many people have covert sympathy and kind-hearted approach towards people with NDD. Some people develop fear for such people as they had no prior exposure towards such people & they simply do not fit with the view they have of people they would like to interact with socially. Children with NDD are very prone to bullying and fighting by their classmates and this becomes a routine part of their childhood for they appear odd among others in level of intelligence & social skills.

Schools and other institutions plainly refuse to accept them as they don't want to take the responsibility of the people who are not likely to get well anytime soon and they see them as a disturbance (Chaddad, Desrosiers, Hassan, & Tanougast, 2017) to their school and the educational environment for other children. Another reason is that most schools lack the necessary infrastructure such as ramps and toilets, as well as training, knowledge, awareness or resources to adopt inclusivity. Most schools do not employ special educators. Also instances have been seen where a child with NDD is not able to adjust in the school environment and may need extra attention, empathy and understanding, especially if the behavior is hyperactive and the child has certain sensory issues.

In most families in India, mothers are the only single point of support to their children and who despite serious criticism from society, parents and even from their spouse, stick in their endeavor to train and educate their children (Didehbani, Allen, Kandalaft, Krawczyk, & Chapman, 2016). Mothers are victims of taunts such as they are wasting their time on their child. Mostly, the mother is blamed for the child's neurological disorder for no apparent cause or reason. Even when it comes to attending social functions like weddings and parties, there are some parents who will take their special child (American Psychiatric Association, 1980) out to attend the party while some may feel ashamed to do so. Visits to the super market, community park, temple, theatre or other public places become challenges for parents because there are no support structures available for them. It is worthwhile to mention here that an NGO has only recently tied up with a retail brand to allow autistic children to shop once a week in the supermarket in a quiet and subdued environment, where the lights would be dimmed, there would be no blaring announcements, and there are volunteers to assist them in making their purchases. The constant advocacy and activism are helping albeit slowly to bring about some acceptance and change (Chaddad, Desrosiers, Hassan, & Tanougast, 2017).

The directives given by the CBSE for children with special needs to get accommodations in exams makes it mandatory for the children who need a scribe, or extra time, or a reader, to get an evaluation from a government hospital. Most government hospitals do not have tests to assess Specific Learning Disability, or Autism. In cases of ADHD, where the learning disability is secondary, the child is refused a diagnosis of LD, and thus does not receive help from the CBSE board. Parents and children suffer due to these loopholes and have to drop out of the regular school system (Clifford, Young, & Williamson, 2007).

The social attitudes in the form of apathy and neglect can be understood better with the help of the two case studies (American Psychiatric Association, 1980). The first is written by a person with disability and the second by a parent. The third case study is of an organization dealing with persons with autism and their experiences with social attitudes (Coben, 2006).

CASE STUDY 1

This is an account of a person with cerebral palsy, male, aged 39 years, who is an icon and motivational speaker. He is currently pursuing a Phd in Disability Management, is an MA in Social Work, has pursued Law at Masters level, and is the recipient of many State and National awards.

There have been many incidents in my life where I've had to face indifferent attitudes of different persons as well as authorities to reach the stage I'm presently in.

The attitude of my mohalla (locality) residents when I was an infant and when my condition became known to all, I became an object of pity for them. Not only me, but my parents were also doled out lots of sympathy. They would address me as *bechara* which means' poor thing' and discouraged my parents from sending me to school. In school, as I grew older, I had to face the problem of getting a writer for my middle as well as Matric exam. The attitude of Punjab School Education Board staff members was very indifferent and unhelpful. Before each exam, my parents would have to take me to Mohali which is the city where the main office of the Punjab Education Board was, to show them my disability and ensuing handicap. The story was no better when I went to study in a college to pursue higher education. I was advised to do graduation through IGNOU as in their opinion it would be difficult for me to study in regular classes. However, I was adamant to study as a regular student in the college. I was permitted to get admission but I was not allowed to go to the classroom by scooter with my father. At that time I did not use a wheelchair and walked with the help of a walker. I was asked to reach my classes from the main gate with the help of a walker which was very difficult because it would have taken 1 hour to reach my class room. But later when I met the principal and told him about my difficulty I was allowed to reach the classroom with the help of my father's scooter.

During my graduation exams, I was refused a writer and extra time by the Guru Nanak Dev University. I had to represent my case through the then Education Minister and also personally met the vice chancellor who then permitted me extra time and a writer.

Later when I was appearing in LLB exams, I was refused extra time by GNDU evening Law College, Jalandhar. During the annual exam my answer sheet was snatched by the supervisor. She told me that she or her staff could not wait for one hour extra for me. After I complained to GNDU authorities, an enquiry was held into the matter by the university. However, during the enquiry I was compelled to withdraw my complaint by the Principal.

When I applied for PCs judicial I was refused a writer by Punjab Public Service Commission Patiala. When my father met the secretary Punjab PPSC, he told my father that if I could not write in the exam then how could I become a judge. Then I had to take up the matter with chief Commissioner for the persons with disability New Delhi who decided in my favor and directed PPSC and social security Punjab to allow me a writer. However, the irony of the situation was that this whole incident annoyed the secretary so much that he ordered to give a student of 10th class who could not write English properly to me as scribe. My problems which seemed endless at that time, were to go beyond the academic concerns to health concerns.

I met with an accident and suffered a fracture in my ribs for which I received treatment from a well-known Orthopedic doctor for 8 months. My misfortune knew no bounds when despite treatment, I didn't recover. Then I contacted a renowned doctor specializing in treatment of cerebral palsy to understand the reason of not healing. The doctor advised to get some tests, and after the results he diagnosed the reason and changed the medicines I was on.

He prescribed some medicines which were not available in my hometown Jalandhar. Doctors in my hometown were not supportive of me approaching another specialist from a different city. They wanted to give me a substitute medicine, which I had been advised against taking by the specialist. Caught in this tussle between treating doctors, and worried about my failing health, I slipped into depression. I had to get treatment from many physicians after that. Once, when I consulted a Neurologist he asked my parents if I was mentally retarded. My parents told him about my qualifications and asked him how a mentally challenged child could get so many degrees including post graduation degrees, and told him that I had CP without mental retardation. Such questions were being thrown constantly at us, and caused me much pain and anguish. Dealing with insensitivity and apathy was the norm for my family and me.

When I was to be given the National Award during December 2016 I was asked to travel to New Delhi by train. I explained to the authorities that to board a train was very difficult for me because my wheelchair could not be loaded in the train. However, they told me that as per prevailing rules I could not be allowed to travel by taxi or own car and could be paid rail fare only if I travelled by train. Anyway I boarded the train with the help of 5 persons and faced so many problems while getting down at New Delhi.

During October 2017, as I was coming back from Mumbai after getting champion award from Adapt Foundation, by an Air India flight, I was asked to pay rupees 1180 as wheelchair charges to get priority otherwise I would have to stand in queue. My father approached the Air India authorities and told them that senior citizens and disabled persons had the right to have a separate queue. It was however, refused. After long arguments and a warning to them that they would be sued if our flight was missed, only then they allowed us priority. Then I highlighted the matter through social media and only after that, the CEO of Air India apologized for the inconvenience caused to us.

CASE STUDY 2

The second case study which highlights the challenges and anxieties faced by an unsuspecting family, is of a mother of a 20-year-old autistic child. She has expressed her trials and tribulations in this write up.

Any disability, physical or neurological, causes suffering to the individual who bears it. Neuro-developmental disabilities have the maximum deleterious effect not only on the individual who has it but also on the family members, especially, parents and siblings.

My tryst with a neuro-developmental disability namely autism started when my son reached the age of one year. I was a young energetic woman performing my roles as any other typical Indian woman would do, as a mother, wife, daughter in law and career woman all rolled into one. I was bubbling with life, with my spirits always very high. It seemed somewhat strange when I saw that my son could not even stand without support and he did not even utter a single meaningful word. On the other hand the children of his peer group could easily attain these simple milestones at the same age. But as you all know, disbelief in the Indian society is rampant and I also fell prey to the notions of our elders that he will be able to make it, some children are 'slow' and also that they 'overtake' their counterparts eventually and so on and so forth.

But thankfully, this 'sham' denial period didn't last long .After about two months of his first birthday, my husband and I realized that something was amiss about our son's milestones. This was in the year 2000 when the real trials and tribulations of my life began. After consulting many doctors in Punjab, we reached Sir Ganga Ram Hospital, New Delhi where a reputed pediatric neurologist diagnosed my son under the Autistic spectrum disorder. It was a term

that was new to me and very little hope was given by the concerned doctor. What to talk about knowledge and awareness in the general public, even the medical professionals at that time were not very well aware about this condition . After listening to the neurologist, my whole world came crashing down. In due course, we decided to consult a doctor in Mumbai who turned out to be a very gentle and sensitive pediatric neurologist who gave us some hope, and a path to pursue. He recommended that we should go back to Delhi and consult an organization by the name of Action for Autism (AFA). Here, I attended the mother- child program for three months along with numerous workshops and seminars which really helped me in tackling the vagaries of an autistic child. AFA is an organization engaged in dissemination of knowledge and awareness of the autism spectrum disorder and helping parents and children deal with the condition.

The prevalence of autism when my son was diagnosed was 1 in 500 Approximately and has subsequently increased over the years. The cause is not exactly known and there is no medical treatment till date that can stop or revert this condition.

My life was thrown into an unknown territory when my son began to show so many irrelevant and inappropriate behaviors; there were obsessions, there was lack of speech and communication and above all sensory issues. And amidst all this, I did not know what to do, how to help him, and how to make this better. There were myriad challenges while bringing him up all these years.

Life was not at all rosy. Indian society at large is very judgmental and rigid and close minded especially for these children. As a result we were deprived of friends and a social circle because we did not fit in to their so called norms. All I remember is rejection, bully, comments & isolation. He was admitted in primary section of a very reputed school in Jalandhar but had to face the wrath of teachers and students alike. Even we were not spared by the management which interviewed us. We were being continually harassed for some reason or the other, and so ultimately, we had to take the decision of pulling him out of that school. We got him admitted in another school where, fortunately the management was kind hearted and sensitive. They were not aware about Autism but willing to learn and help. They allowed me to come to the school and permitted me to guide the concerned teachers. They learnt about behavior therapy and importance of structure while teaching and also sensitization of peers and other staff members. We had our small successes. For the very first time a resource room, an Individualized Education Plan (IEP) in a neurotypical environment of a regular school came up in Jalandhar. And then the real journey began.

School time was really turbulent. Only few supported us. Most of the people thought that my son is a spoiled brat because his condition became invisible with the passage of time. As the years passed by, with minimal support from family and friends around and society at large, my struggle of raising him up also increased proportionally. But the fight had to go on. My son who was growing up and becoming more and more aware of his condition, was also suffering along with me. Faced with continuous rejections, in the form of constant visible and invisible bullying, sneers and remarks from the society has been emotionally taxing for him.

Sometimes I feel that being a parent to a special child makes one more tenacious in leading life because the life of parents of differently abled children is starkly different from those of parents with neurotypical children. In spite of all odds, my son has reached college, still he doesn't get his due and people in general are judgmental and now he has this much sense and sensibility that these things bother him a lot and he still has his 'meltdowns 'albeit now far decreased in intensity than before.

The take home message is be realistic, do not compare them with other children even if they are having the same disorder, accept the way they are, remain calm and positive because it is a tedious and life long process. Constantly educate yourself about the condition and update yourself with the latest research and treatment options. Your approach to the child should be according to his/her strengths and limitations. Set short goals, attend regular seminars and workshops, be in touch with good special educators and parents groups involved in helping children and their families. Last but not the least, formal education is important but practical life skills training to make your child independent is really essential.

CASE STUDY 3

Experiences of an NGO working in the field of autism. Attitudes, thoughts and beliefs that influence the way PWDs are viewed or are treated.

I have encountered more than one hundred and fifty families in the last few years hailing from the state of Punjab, Haryana, Himachal Pradesh, Maharashtra and a few NRI families too. The social conditioning plays an important role in how they view their child's difficulty. We see a range of natural emotions initially starting from denial to anger and depression. The last to come is learning and acceptance but in many cases it never comes fully. This is where the upbringing and overall mental peace of the child and family is affected.

However in many cases a parent's determination overcomes even the obstacles created by the environment. I distinctly remember the case of a mother who came for training from Himachal Pradesh. She was unable to fully understand Hindi or English, being fluent only in Pahadi. It was through sheer will and persistence that she trained herself. She then consequently joined a school in her rural area and began to train those with special needs there too.

The way a diagnosis is presented to the family and consequent approach to training is also varied from glaringly incompetent to extremely supportive. For example in some cases there is an insensitive and blunt diagnosis meted out predicting a dark future. In other cases the family receives a sensitive series of sessions and guidance that encourages them for the future ensuring their perusal of necessary training.

There are certain laws that exist to ensure the education of the special needs child. Yet every educational facility/ institution has their own policies. These vary from those that believe the special needs child will have something to teach and bring to their institution, to those that would prefer to avoid admitting them in their institution on some pretext or another.

I distinctly remember a leading educational institute welcoming a child with open arms –allowing a trained shadow teacher to accompany the child to ensure his learning. This in turn immediately formed the perception of the child's peers. In fact many times they were seen to be defending the child if there was bullying or name calling. The peers even began to view the child's different mannerisms as a part of his unique personality and did not even bat an eyelid in the classroom when there were stimming behaviors.

A lot of perceptions are formed on the basis of existing fears /myths and beliefs rampant in our country. There have been cases of families denying their child's training claiming their "guru" forbade it and he will "cure" the child.

In contrast we have seen parents who openly educate those around them and the result in one case where a friend of one such family created a complete visual presentation and decided to educate their children towards the need of their special friend. The result the child grew up amidst those that completely accepted him for who he is.

We follow the west in our trends, very often picking up the trends that the special needs community is shunning there now. For example donations and working with special needs seems to be the upcoming trend. However the downside to this otherwise well meaning thought is that the voluntary work or contributions make the special needs child feel like a "charity".

In all the above instances what makes a truly inclusive society is education and awareness. These help in the extinction of fears, myths and dangerous or detrimental practices.

The Many 'Barriers' Faced by Families Who Have a Member Belonging to The Neurodiverse Population

The road ahead for children with neuro developmental disabilities and their families is not an easy one. The many barriers faced by them, tangible or attitudinal makes it a very challenging and rough ride for them. The discrimination and lack of facility and resources plague them at every stage.

Lack of Resources

There are very few hospitals and trained professionals like doctors and psychologists who can help the families at the time of assessment, diagnosis, and intervention. Most children especially in the case of invisible disabilities like dyslexia go without assessment and help (Ekinci, Arman, Işık, Bez, & Berkem,

2010). Children with ADHD are not included in the list of children with disabilities needing special accommodations to be included in the education system by the CBSE board, despite the fact that their ability to learn, read, write, comprehend and spell is severely affected. Similarly children with borderline IQ, find themselves not included in the education system, and have to opt for National open school which does not modify syllabus suitably enough for children with borderline intellectual deficit. There are no support groups or places where families can reach out and seek help for the emotional, educational and practical needs of children. There are few schools to help in the training and education of the children and many children stay at home without training and education for most parts of their lives or are home tutored. Again, there is no systematic vocational training available or employment opportunities available for the population of individuals with disability.

Lack of Awareness

The lack of awareness about disabilities by people who are not in touch with them is a significant factor contributing towards the discrimination meted out to individuals with disability. There is a huge stigma towards mental illness and this reflects in the attitude towards people with disabilities as well. A common person would not know the difference between a psychotic illness and an intellectual disability, using the terminology of insane for both (Fan, Wade, Key, Warren, & Sarkar, 2018). It is actually treated like a communicable disease which needs to keep the persons with disability away from the mainstream. As far as literature and use of terminology goes, there have been many changes. From the use of morons, imbeciles and idiots, and then mental retardation to person with intellectual deficit, the terminology has seen a change towards wider ranging and more acceptable definitions of the disabled. They are also referred to as differently abled and people with special needs. The PM. of the country Mr Narendra Modi called persons with special needs as *divyang,* meaning (divine body) instead of *viklang* (disabled). However, this actually hasn't translated into acceptance amongst the general public, or made the situation any better for families of children with disabilities.

What's After Us? The Dilemma for Parents

The concept of assisted community living hasn't taken off too much in India, especially for persons with disabilities, who have to be dependent always on family members. India traditionally being a close-knit society, encouraging large and joint family systems, find caring for their children relatively easier than western societies. However, the dilemma for many parents and families is the question- What after us? I personally know many parents who did not opt for another child after the birth of their child with disability, removing the option of sibling protection and support for their child. Social support and insurance may barely cover any aspect of future independent living by the child. This then needs to be an aspect of concern for the governmental and non-governmental organizations working in disability.

Medical Care: A Concern for the Disabled

Medical and health care for the disabled becomes a huge concern for the family. For example, one parent shared with me that dental care was an issue as no dentist was willing to spend the time and effort with the children who because of sensory issues did not cooperate much during treatment. Similar attitudes are found among doctors and clinicians who are not fully equipped or prepared to deal with autistic patients.

Marriage, Sexuality and Relationships

Many persons with disabilities find themselves without much of a social life, and friends. They do not get the chance to love or get into long term meaningful relationships. Given their limited communication skills and social anxiety, they find themselves withdrawn and isolated and ultimately may not find people to get close to them socially. Sexual needs of persons with disability is a grey area too, and probably rarely addressed. Similarly, sexual abuse is a lurking threat always, given the vulnerable status of this population.

The Solutions

Autism and other neuro developmental disorders need to be viewed as normal, and attempts made at normalizing need to be stopped. The difference between teaching them to function independently and maximize their potentials versus viewing them as patients needing treatment is the basis of the normalizing process. The acceptance of a diagnosis of autism or any other NDD, while being difficult for a parent, nevertheless needs to be approached differently than a diagnosis of a chronic or terminal disease is in the present. I have encountered scores of parents who have not been counseled properly and correctly, and as a result begin to view the condition as a treatable or non treatable disease. Similarly, many parents live in denial and don't go for therapy and intervention for fear of social stigma and lack of acceptance. I have also met parents who have no idea how to handle the hyperactivity and meltdowns and are struggling to deal in unknown territory. Counseling and family support groups are thereby the need of the hour. The facilities for diagnosis, assessment, therapy, education and vocational training are needed at every stage. Parents need to equip themselves with knowledge of how to help their child and deal with demands of each stage of the child's life. For this they must be actively involved in parents associations and groups formed for the support and well-being of their child and families. Schools must necessarily be equipped with resource rooms and special educators must be mandatorily hired in each school. Teachers must be well versed with screening and identification of conditions like dyslexia, ADHD, and autism and know how to deal with them. Now- a- days the B-ed curriculum does include certain screening tools and information on different learning disabilities, and awareness is better than before. The lack of intention to truly adopt inclusive education in mindsets of school administrators and policy makers is the only barrier.

Assisted living in communities providing conducive environment to the disabled with all facilities including health and medical facilities is a need to be urgently addressed. In Jalandhar, Punjab, some NGOs have come together to do the needful to provide housing to the children with disabilities at subsidized costs. Transportation is another concern which needs to be explored. Most importantly, gainful and satisfactory employment is a right to be given to the individuals with disability. The charity approach will all but help in increasing the gap between the persons with and without disability, not allowing them to live with the dignity they well deserve. Community living must also provide solutions to the loneliness and social isolation felt by individuals with disability. Insurance is an area which has been addressed by the government but still more needs to be done. Reservations for jobs and in colleges are also present and have helped empower many persons, thereby bringing about social justice and equality.

CONCLUSION

The eventual learning that we need to carry home is that life with a special needs child is not a cakewalk (Heinsfeld et al.,2018). It is an uncertain and unsure path, wrought with stress and anxiety. The need of the hour is to have systems well in place so that help is extended to the child and the family whenever needed. Myths need to be dispelled and the media needs to help in making the community aware of various conditions among the neuro-diverse population. The persons with disability need respect, love and normalcy. This is the only way inclusivity will be real instead of the false face it has in society today.

To conclude there are several myths in the minds of people at large regarding children or adults with NDD. People need to accept persons with NDD as worthy & equal part of the society in terms of opportunities and respect. Concerned family members especially mothers have been seen as adopting bold & daring roles in taking care of their NDD child despite criticism from larger sections of society which is really commendable.

ACKNOWLEDGMENT

I am extremely grateful to Dr Mala Walia, Ms Anjali Dada from the NGO SOCH, and Mr Vivek Joshi for sharing their stories for this chapter. I am grateful to Mr Amarjit Singh Anand, a disability activist and President, Punjab State Federation of Parents of PwIDD along with many other offices he holds, for being a sounding board and discussing issues of PwD with me.

REFERENCES

Adjorlu, A., Høeg, E. R., Mangano, L., & Serafin, S. (2017, October). Daily Living Skills Training in Virtual Reality to Help Children with Autism Spectrum Disorder in a Real Shopping Scenario. In *Mixed and Augmented Reality (ISMAR-Adjunct), 2017 IEEE International Symposium on* (pp. 294-302). IEEE. 10.1109/ISMAR-Adjunct.2017.93

Ali, Z., & Bhaskar, S. B. (2016). Basic statistical tools in research and data analysis. *Indian Journal of Anaesthesia*, *60*(9), 662. doi:10.4103/0019-5049.190623 PMID:27729694

American Psychiatric Association. (1980). Diagnostic and Statistical Manual of Mental Disorders, 3rd Edition (DSM-III). Washington, DC: American Psychiatric Association.

Bone, D., Bishop, S. L., Black, M. P., Goodwin, M. S., Lord, C., & Narayanan, S. S. (2016). Use of machine learning to improve autism screening and diagnostic instruments: Effectiveness, efficiency, and multi-instrument fusion. *Journal of Child Psychology and Psychiatry, and Allied Disciplines*, *57*(8), 927–937. doi:10.1111/jcpp.12559 PMID:27090613

Bosl, W., Tierney, A., Tager-Flusberg, H., & Nelson, C. (2011). EEG complexity as a biomarker for autism spectrum disorder risk. *BMC Medicine*, *9*(1), 18. doi:10.1186/1741-7015-9-18 PMID:21342500

Chaddad, A., Desrosiers, C., Hassan, L., & Tanougast, C. (2017). Hippocampus and amygdala radiomic biomarkers for the study of autism spectrum disorder. *BMC Neuroscience, 18*(1), 52. doi:10.118612868-017-0373-0 PMID:28821235

Chaddad, A., Desrosiers, C., Hassan, L., & Tanougast, C. (2017). Hippocampus and amygdala radiomic biomarkers for the study of autism spectrum disorder. *BMC Neuroscience, 18*(1), 52. doi:10.118612868-017-0373-0 PMID:28821235

Clifford, S., Young, R., & Williamson, P. (2007). Assessing the early characteristics of autistic disorder using video analysis. *Journal of Autism and Developmental Disorders, 37*(2), 301–313. doi:10.100710803-006-0160-8 PMID:17031450

Coben, R. (2006, October). *Hemoencephalography for autistic spectrum disorder.* In The14th Annual Conference of the International Society for Neuronal Regulation, Atlanta, GA.

Didehbani, N., Allen, T., Kandalaft, M., Krawczyk, D., & Chapman, S. (2016). Virtual reality social cognition training for children with high functioning autism. *Computers in Human Behavior, 62*, 703–711. doi:10.1016/j.chb.2016.04.033

Didehbani, N., Allen, T., Kandalaft, M., Krawczyk, D., & Chapman, S. (2016). Virtual reality social cognition training for children with high functioning autism. *Computers in Human Behavior, 62*, 703–711. doi:10.1016/j.chb.2016.04.033

Ekinci, O., Arman, A. R., Işık, U., Bez, Y., & Berkem, M. (2010). EEG abnormalities and epilepsy in autistic spectrum disorders: Clinical and familial correlates. *Epilepsy & Behavior, 17*(2), 178–182. doi:10.1016/j.yebeh.2009.11.014 PMID:20042370

Fan, J., Wade, J. W., Key, A. P., Warren, Z. E., & Sarkar, N. (2018). EEG-based affect and workload recognition in a virtual driving environment for ASD intervention. *IEEE Transactions on Biomedical Engineering, 65*(1), 43–51. doi:10.1109/TBME.2017.2693157 PMID:28422647

Grynszpan, O., & Nadel, J. (2015). An eye-tracking method to reveal the link between gazing patterns and pragmatic abilities in high functioning autism spectrum disorders. *Frontiers in Human Neuroscience, 8*, 1067. doi:10.3389/fnhum.2014.01067 PMID:25642182

Heinsfeld, A. S., Franco, A. R., Craddock, R. C., Buchweitz, A., & Meneguzzi, F. (2018). Identification of autism spectrum disorder using deep learning and the ABIDE dataset. *NeuroImage. Clinical, 17*, 16–23. doi:10.1016/j.nicl.2017.08.017 PMID:29034163

Höfer, J., Hoffmann, F., & Bachmann, C. (2017). Use of complementary and alternative medicine in children and adolescents with autism spectrum disorder: A systematic review. *Autism, 21*(4), 387–402. doi:10.1177/1362361316646559 PMID:27231337

Ibrahim, S., Djemal, R., & Alsuwailem, A. (2018). Electroencephalography (EEG) signal processing for epilepsy and autism spectrum disorder diagnosis. *Biocybernetics and Biomedical Engineering, 38*(1), 16–26. doi:10.1016/j.bbe.2017.08.006

Jaime, M., McMahon, C. M., Davidson, B. C., Newell, L. C., Mundy, P. C., & Henderson, H. A. (2016). Brief report: Reduced temporal-central EEG alpha coherence during joint attention perception in adolescents with autism spectrum disorder. *Journal of Autism and Developmental Disorders*, *46*(4), 1477–1489. doi:10.100710803-015-2667-3 PMID:26659813

Jamal, W., Das, S., Oprescu, I. A., Maharatna, K., Apicella, F., & Sicca, F. (2014). Classification of autism spectrum disorder using supervised learning of brain connectivity measures extracted from synchrostates. *Journal of Neural Engineering*, *11*(4), 046019. doi:10.1088/1741-2560/11/4/046019 PMID:24981017

Katuwal, G. J., Cahill, N. D., Baum, S. A., & Michael, A. M. (2015). The predictive power of structural MRI in Autism diagnosis. In *Engineering in Medicine and Biology Society (EMBC), 2015 37th Annual International Conference of the IE.* 10.1109/EMBC.2015.7319338

Chapter 2
A Case Study in Autism Spectrum Disorder

Jatinder Goraya
Dayanand Medical College and Hospital, India

ABSTRACT

Autism spectrum disorder is a common neurodevelopmental disorder with onset during early life but with life-long implications for the affected person. The term is now broader and all-inclusive and represents the whole spectrum of disorders previously classified under autism and related disorders such as Asperger syndrome. Incidence of autism spectrum disorder appears to be rising, related in part to increase in awareness and recognition by the parents and the healthcare providers. Autism spectrum disorder is most often diagnosed using DSM-V criteria. These diagnostic criteria include persistent deficits in social communication/social interaction and restricted, repetitive patterns of behaviour, interests, or activities. Treatment requires a multidisciplinary team incorporating pediatricians, therapists, social workers, special education teachers, etc. to optimize the outcomes. A case study is presented to highlight the diagnostic and therapeutic aspects of autism spectrum disorder.

INTRODUCTION

Autism spectrum disorder (ASD) is a common but serious neurodevelopmental disorder of communication and social deficits, and unusual repetitive sensory-motor behaviours. Previously known as autism, pervasive developmental disorder, the terminology of autism spectrum disorder has evolved. Autism spectrum disorder is an umbrella term used now to represent spectrum of heterogenous disorders with severity spectrum ranging from mild to severe and affecting several aspects of life of the individuals with this disorder (American Psychiatric Association, 2013). Subtypes previously classified as pervasive developmental disorder not specified otherwise and Asperger syndrome are now included in this new terminology of autism spectrum disorder.

First description of infantile autism in English literature is attributed to Leo Kanner (Kanner, 1943), who in 1943 described 11 children with impaired social interaction, atypical language development and abnormal repetitive behaviors such as hand flapping, or body rocking. Asperger syndrome, now consid-

DOI: 10.4018/978-1-7998-3069-6.ch002

ered a part of autism spectrum disorder (DSM-V) was described in 1944 by Hans Asperger (Asperger, 1944). These children had good verbal skills but were otherwise quite similar to children with autism in social and other behaviors. It was not until 1980s that autism as a clinical entity started gaining adequate attention of the scientific community.

Onset of symptoms suggesting deficits in social and communication skills during early childhood, often during infancy. It is not infrequent for parents to report normal development in their child during first 12-15 months followed by loss of language and social skills, which may appear to be heralded (or at least that is what many parents think), by a common intercurrent childhood illness. Later in the course, children may remain stable, show worsening or may show some improvement.

Clinicians, researchers, parents and lay public have become increasingly concerned about the rise in prevalence of autism spectrum disorder over a period of time. Global prevalence of autism spectrum disorder has been estimated at about 1%, and 1.5% in developed countries (Lord, Elasabbagh, Baird &Veenstra-Vanderweele, 2018; Lyall et al. 2017). Prevalence of autism spectrum disorder determined in the 2010 Autism and Developmental Disabilities (ADDM) cohort was 1 in 68, being a little more common in the white than the other racial groups (Hviid, Hansen, Frisch, & Melbye, 2019). Even in developing countries, the prevalence of autism spectrum disorder has risen in recent years, attributed at least partially to enhanced awareness among general public, teachers, and health care providers (Dalwai et al., 2017).

Despite its common occurrence, the diagnosis is often missed or delayed. The therapeutic interventions have largely remained empirical. Genetic factors are increasingly being implicated in causation, but role of environmental factors has not been entirely discounted (Lord et al., 2018; Howes, Rogdaki, Findon, Wichers, & Charman 2018). Although, autism spectrum disorder has onset during early life, the affected individuals continue to experience its consequences in social, academic and occupation settings throughout the life span. Various aspects of autism spectrum disorder will be highlighted through a case study followed by review of its relevant clinical, diagnostic and therapeutic aspects.

Case Study

MM is a 2.5 year-old-boy whose parents are concerned that he has not developed age-appropriate language skills. He is accompanied by his mother, father and grandparents. He doesn't speak any meaningful words on his own though keeps on uttering non-meaningful words and phrases. He also repeats whatever is said to him. He does not use any words to communicates his needs for such as food or toileting. He does not point at objects of his interest, and instead will hold his mother's hand and point it (mother's hand) to the object. If he needs water, he will hold mothers hand and guide her to refrigerator and then give her the bottle of water to pour it in glass. He does not look at the objects pointed at by mothers or other family members. He does not makes eye contact and appears shy. Parents say he does not respond to his name when called. In fact, deafness was suspected at some point of time, and formal testing revealed that he had normal hearing. He however, does come running to watch his favourite television programme whenever he hears that program is switched on the TV. He has liking for only certain TV program, and will watch only that program. Any attempt to change the program is met with resistance and tantrums like crying, rolling on floor with leg thrashing and even hitting his head against floor. He also likes only certain foods and resents when any other food is offered. He wants the same plate and spoon every time he has his meals. He also sits at the same chair placed at a particular side of the dining table. He seems to be always lost in himself, and world around him does not seem to exist. He will appear engaged in same repetitive plays like lining up toy cars, or repeatedly rotating their wheels. When not busy with his toys, he walks or runs around excessively in the house. Parents have to watch him constantly as he has tried to run out of house if gate is open.

He does not interact with other children of his age. He does not enjoy showing or sharing his toys with other children. He does not know how to play with other kids. He either follows other kids in activity be it playing or running, and sometimes pushes them. He tries to hold them or hug them forcefully.

He does not know body parts, though parents have tried aggressively to teach him.

He is also scared of heights and does not enjoy slides or swings. Any attempt to have him try these things provoked vigorous cry and agitation. Similarly, loud noises such as car horn, cooker whistle, or even loud music results in resentful cries and clinging to parents. Parents find it difficult to take him out-doors to visit relatives, shopping malls, music concerts, cinema hall, wedding halls. He does not like to be touched, held or hugged.

Parents are also concerned that when frustrated he often hits himself on his head or slaps himself. He even bites his hand or fingers, and grinds his teeth. When irritated he scratches and bites others. Parents noticed that he does not react much to pain and received vaccination without much fuss.

He is not toilet trained and is generally constipated. He wets and soils himself. Attempts to toilet training have met with no success. He enjoys splashing water while taking bath.

Parents have observed repetitive motor behavior. He often likes to go in circles around the furniture. When sitting idles, he rocks back and forth. Hand flapping is another activity he enjoys especially when he is happy or frustrated. When running he often tiptoes.

His sleep is also disturbed. It is difficult to put him to sleep, and he wakes up frequently during sleep at times sometimes accompanied by crying.

He is the second child of non-consanguineous parents. His father is 39 years-old and mother 37. He was born full-term and delivered vaginally. He weighed 3.2 kg at birth and there were no adverse events during pregnancy, delivery and in the period immediately after delivery. He was sent home on third day. He was exclusively breast-fed for 4 months and received all his vaccinations. He has an elder year-old sister who is developmentally normal and has no health issues. There is no family history of similar illness, any other neurodevelopmental disorders, or epilepsy.

Initial development was apparently normal. He sat at 7 months crawled at 9 months and was walking by 12 months. According to parents, he smiled at 2 months, laughed at 4 months and babbling started at 9 months. There were non-specific utterances like papa, mama, baba etc. at 12 months but speech did not progress after that. Though parents were worried, grandparents re-assured them. Parents waited till 18 months when a formal hearing test was done which showed normal results. Parents were again reassured.

He had one seizure with fever when he was 14-months-old. He has been otherwise well and has had no major illnesses other than some episodes of diarrhea and usual cough and colds.

He is a picky eater and feeding him is a major task. Forced feeding has been tried but often resulted in vomiting. As a result, his weight gain has been suboptimal.

Examination

Physical examination was non-revealing, in particularly he had no abnormal facies or any other features suggesting dysmorphism. His head size was a little on larger side. Skin examination was unremarkable for any neurocutaneous stigmata. Neurological examination revealed behavioural phenotype characteristic of autism spectrum disorder. He did not sit on chair or in mothers lap and continued to wander in the clinic trying to fiddle with various objects. He tried to open the drawers of the table. He did not respond to his name or follow simple instructions. For example, he was asked to sit on chair and not touch things, but he did not seem to listen. When parents tried to restrain him, he became irritable. He did not make any eye contact with the examiner, nor did he point to when asked about his body parts and objects around him. He did not allow to be touched during examination. He constantly snapped his fingers and sometimes flapped his hands. Tip-toeing was noticed when he walked.

Diagnosis

The child's primary care paediatrician suspected autistic spectrum disorder, and referred him to a centre with expertise in evaluation and diagnosis of autism. Child MM was evaluated by a team comprising pediatric neurologist, child psychologist, speech and language pathologist and occupation therapist. Child's symptoms and his observed behaviour, were consistent with the diagnosis of autism spectrum disorder as put forth in the latest version of the Diagnostic and Statistical Manual version 5 (APA, 2013) published in 2013 by American Psychiatric Association (Table 1).

The DSM-V also provides for defining severity of autism spectrum disorder based on the impact of symptoms on the adaptive functioning of the affected individual (Table 2). Diagnosis of autism spectrum disorder is to be made on the basis both of parental interview and direct observation of the affected child. DSM-V does not require all the symptoms of autism spectrum disorder to be present at the same time but should have occurred at some point of time during the natural course of the disorder.

Several screening and diagnostic tools based on standardized self-reports, parent, teacher reports, and direct observation measures are available to identify individuals who are in need of further evaluation Examples include Modified-Checklist for Autism in Toddlers (M-CHAT), Social Communication Questionnaire (SCQ), Childhood Autism Spectrum Test (CAST), Autism Spectrum Screening Questionnaire (ASSQ), Autism Diagnostic Interview -Revised (ADI-R), The Autism Diagnostic Observation Schedule (ADOS), Childhood Autism rating Scale (CARS) (Filipek et al., 2000; Howes et al., 2018; Johnson & Myers, 2007; Lord et al., 2018; Myers & Johnson, 2007, Zwaigenbaum et al., 2015a, Zwaigenbaum et al., 2015b).

Children suspected to have autism spectrum disorder or those who are risk for autism spectrum disorder should be assessed by a multidisciplinary team with expertise in the evaluation of autism spectrum disorder. Assessment to identify underlying disorder such as inborn errors of metabolism, fragile X syndrome may require genetic consultation. Presence of epilepsy calls for expert neurological evaluation. The child was referred to a geneticist for evaluation for possible genetic causes. Karyotype, Fragile X testing, and chromosomal microarrays returned normal. Results of newborn screening at birth were reviewed and found to be within normal limits.

Causation of Autism Spectrum Disorder

Various genetic and environmental factors have been implicated in the etiology of autism spectrum disorder but despite being a common neurodevelopmental disorder, the exact cause underlying autism spectrum disorder remains unknown in majority of the cases. Only in minority of the cases, a clear cause, mostly genetic disorder is identified.

Table 1. DSM-V Criteria for the diagnosis of autism spectrum disorder

A. Persistent deficits in social communication and social interaction across multiple contexts as manifested by- • Deficits in social-emotional reciprocity (eg, abnormal social approach and failure of normal back-forth conversion; or reduced sharing of interests, emotions, or affect, or failure to initiate or respond to social interactions) • Deficits in non-verbal communication behaviors (eg, poorly integrated verbal and non-verbal communication, abnormality in eye contact and body language, or deficits in understanding and use of gestures) • Deficits in developing, maintaining, and understanding relationships (eg, difficulties adjusting behavior to suit various social contexts; or difficulties in sharing imaginative play or making friends) **B. Restricted, repetitive patterns of behavior, interests, or activities, as manifested by** • Stereotyped or repetitive motor movements, use of objects, or speech (eg, simple motor stereotypies, lining up toys, or flipping objects, echolalia, idiosyncratic phrases) • Insistence on sameness, inflexible adherence to routines, or ritualized patterns of verbal and non-verbal behavior (eg, extreme distress at small changes, difficulties with transitions, or rigid thinking patterns, greeting rituals, need to take same route, or eat same food every day, sitting at the same seat/chair) • Highly restricted, fixated interests that are abnormal in intensity or focus (eg, strong attachment to or preoccupation with unusual objects, excessively circumscribed interests) • Hyperreactivity or hyporeactivity to sensory input, or unusual intersts in sensory aspects of the environment (eg, apparent indifference to pain or temperature, adverse responses to specific sounds or textures, excessive smelling or touching of objects, visual fascination with lights) Specify current severity: Severity is based on social communication impairment and restricted, repetitive patterns of behaviour (see table 2) C. Symptoms must be present in the early developmental period (but might not become fully manifest until social demands exceed capacities, or might be masked by learned strategies in later life) D. Symptoms must cause clinically significant impairment in social, occupational, or other areas of current functioning E. These disturbances are not better explained by intellectual disability (intellectual developmental disorder) or global developmental delay. Intellectual disability and autism spectrum disorder frequently co-occur; to make comorbid diagnoses of autism spectrum disorder and intellectual disability, social communication should be below that expected for general developmental level. Notes: • Individuals with a well-established diagnosis of autistic disorder, Asperger syndrome, or pervasive developmental disorder not otherwise specified should be given the diagnosis of autism spectrum disorder. Individuals who have marked deficits in social communication, but whose symptoms do not otherwise meet criteria for autism spectrum disorder, should be evaluated for social (pragmatic) communication disorder • Individuals must have social communication deficits (past or present) in each of the three areas defined above • Individuals must have two of the four restricted, repetitive patterns (past or present), as defined above
Specify if: - With or without accompanying intellectual impairment - With or without accompanying language impairment - Associated with a known medical or genetic condition or environmental factor - Associated with another neurodevelopmental, mental, or behavioral disorder - With catatonia

Genetic Factors

Of the known causes identified with the development of autism spectrum disorder in children, majority have a genetic basis, and frequently have other associated neurological symptoms. These disorders include but not limited to Down Syndrome (Trisomy 21), Noonan Syndrome, Neurofibromatosis (NF-1), Turner Syndrome, Tuberous Sclerosis (TSC1 and TSC2), Fragile X syndrome, Rett Syndrome (MECP2), Phenylketonuria (PKU), Smith-Lemli-Opitz syndrome, Prader-Willi syndrome, Angelman Syndrome etc (Howes, et al., 2018; Johnson & Myers, 2007; Lord et al., 2018; Schaefer et al., 2008; Zwaigenbaum et al., 2015a; Zwaigenbaum et al., 2015b) . These cases account for not more than 10-15% of all cases of autism spectrum disorder (Howes et al., 2018). In addition, increased risk of AD has been associated with copy number of variants such as microduplications or microdeletions affecting multiple genes across multiple chromosomes. Twin studies have estimated the heritability of autism spectrum disorder between 60-90% (Ozonoff et al., 2011; Sandin, Lichtenstein, Kuja-Holkola, Larsson, & Humtman, 2014; Tick,

Bolton, Happe, Rutter, & Rijsdiik, 2016,). Boys have 3-4 times higher risk of autism spectrum disorder than girls. Risk of subsequent child being born with autism spectrum disorder after a child has been diagnosed with autism spectrum disorder varies between 7-20% (Oonoff et al., 2011; Sandin et al., 2014; Tick et al, 2016). The risk is increased even further for the third child after the birth of two children with autism spectrum disorder. With recent advances in genetic testing with chromosol microarray and whole genome sequencing, an increasing number of genes are being reported to be associated with autism spectrum disorder (Lord et al., 2018; Tick et al, 2016). Further studies are needed, but it seems likely that in future, genetic basis will be identified for majority of the children with autism spectrum disorder. Also, the mechanisms by which these genes affect the neurodevelopment remains to be elaborated but are important for developing specific therapeutic interventions. Epigenetic processes may also be involved in the risk of development of autism spectrum disorder. Epigenetic changes involve modification of histone or DNA bases. Various environmental, nutritional factors can effect epigenetic changes.

Table 2. Severity Level of autism spectrum disorder

Severity Level	Social Communication	Restricted, repetitive behaviors
Level 3 "Requiring very substantial support"	Severe deficits in verbal and nonverbal social communication skills cause severe impairments in functioning, very limited initiation of social interactions, and minimal response to social overtures from others. For example, a person with few words of intelligible speech who rarely initiates interaction and, when he or she does, makes unusual approaches to meet needs only and responds to only very direct social approaches	Inflexibility of behavior, extreme difficulty coping with change, or other restricted/repetitive behaviors markedly interfere with functioning in all spheres. Great distress/difficulty changing focus or action.
Level 2 "Requiring substantial support"	Marked deficits in verbal and nonverbal social communication skills; social impairments apparent even with supports in place; limited initiation of social interactions; and reduced or abnormal responses to social overtures from others. For example, a person who speaks simple sentences, whose interaction is limited to narrow special interests, and how has markedly odd nonverbal communication.	Inflexibility of behavior, difficulty coping with change, or other restricted/repetitive behaviors appear frequently enough to be obvious to the casual observer and interfere with functioning in a variety of contexts. Distress and/or difficulty changing focus or action.
Level 1 "Requiring support"	Without supports in place, deficits in social communication cause noticeable impairments. Difficulty initiating social interactions, and clear examples of atypical or unsuccessful response to social overtures of others. May appear to have decreased interest in social interactions. For example, a person who is able to speak in full sentences and engages in communication but whose to-and-fro conversation with others fails, and whose attempts to make friends are odd and typically unsuccessful.	Inflexibility of behavior causes significant interference with functioning in one or more contexts. Difficulty switching between activities. Problems of organization and planning hamper independence

Environmental Factors

Genetic factors do not explain all the cases of autism spectrum disorder. Several pre-natal, perinatal, and post-natal factors may adversely affect the growing brain adversely. Advanced parental (both mother and father) age, short interpregnancy period, prenatal exposure to certain infections like cytomegalovirus, or rubella, teratogenic agents like drugs (valproate, phenytoin, thalidomide, alcohol etc.), have been implicated, though the evidence remains largely empirical. Maternal diabetes may be a risk factor associated with increased risk of autism spectrum disorder. Many other maternal factors such as autoimmune diseases (presence of maternal thyro-peroxidase antibody), exposure to air pollutants, maternal nutrition and weight gain during pregnancy have been speculated to be linked to the risk of autism spectrum disorder (Howes et al., 2018; Lord et al., 2018).

Preterm birth, low birth weight, and being small or large for gestational age have been found to be associated with increased risk of autism spectrum disorder. Perinatal complications such as pre-eclampsia, intracranial haemorrhage, low APGAR score, seizures, cerebral edema are associated with increased risk of autism spectrum disorder. This calls for systematic screening of such high risk children (Howes et al., 2018; Lord et al., 2018).

In the post-natal period exposure to environmental mutagens (lead, mercury, cadmium. Nickel, etc., certain foods, infections have been speculated to increase the risk. The controversial association of measles, mumps, rubella vaccine with autism spectrum disorder, once a matter of extensive debate in scientific journals and lay press has now been discounted (Hviid et al., 2019). Similarly, a causal relationship between thimerosal in vaccines and autism spectrum disorder has been rejected. Many other theories linking environmental factors with the risk of development of autism spectrum disorder remain to be proven.

Psychobiology of Autism Spectrum Disorder

Macrocephaly (large head) reflecting early brain growth is a common findings in infants and young children with autism spectrum disorder. Later during adolescence, average brain size in autism spectrum disorder tends to be similar to typically developing children. Increased brain size may be related to disturbed synaptogenesis and synaptic pruning in the growing brain resulting in altered connectivity. Microglia may play a role in this. At cellular and molecular level, alterations in various neurotransmitter systems involving serotonin, GABA, glutamate, neuropeptide oxytocin have been implicated in the psychobiology of autism spectrum disorder. Role of maternal and post-natal immune dysregulation in the etiopathogenesis (Howes et al., 2018; Lord et al., 2018).

Co-Occurring Morbidities

It is not infrequent for individuals with autism spectrum disorder to experience additional psychiatric, neurological, and other systemic disorders that may complicate rehabilitative and therapeutic interventions as well as affect ultimate outcome.

Epilepsy

The prevalence of epilepsy in children with autism spectrum disorder varies from 7-14%. There is bimodal occurrence of epilepsy in children with autism spectrum disorder. Seizures prevalence peaks during early childhood and during adolescence. Intellectual disability and positive family history are significant risk factors for epilepsy in children with autism spectrum disorder. Electroencephalographic abnormalities are observed even in larger number of children with autism spectrum disorder (Howes et al., 2018; Lee, Smith, & Paciorkowski 2015; Lord et al., 2018; Thomas, Hovinga, Rai, & Lee, 2017).

Sensory Issues

Persons with autism spectrum disorder have problems with sensory information, though perception is not impaired. As a result their response to sensory stimuli is abnormal. Children may be hypo- or hyper-responsive to certain stimuli. They may ignores certain noises but hyper-react to others. Similarly there may be phobia to height, spinning, and other vestibular stimuli. Inappropriate response to certain stimuli including tendency to smell everything, aversion to certain foods flavours and texture renders can exaggerate feeding difficulties and contribute to failure to grow. As many as 95% children with autism spectrum disorder may have sensory processing disorders (Lord et al., 2018).

Cognitive Functions

Subnormal intellectual abilities are observed in about 3/4th children with autism spectrum disorder. This may not only compound the disabilities, it also makes treatment interventions difficult. Similarly, problems with attention, memory are frequently observed in these individuals with autism spectrum disorder. There is considerable overlap between symptoms of autism spectrum disorder and attention-deficit hyperactivity disorder. Particularly in young children, hyperactivity may be the presenting symptoms and most troublesome for parents or caregiver. Similarly attention deficits are common, and the children with autism spectrum disorder often do not respond to their names, and may not even look at the caller. As many as 20 to 70% individuals with autism spectrum disorder have symptoms of attention-deficit hyperactivity disorder with or without oppositional defiant disorder, and conduct disorder (Howes et al., 2018; Lord et al., 2018).

Other Psychiatric Disorders

Irritability, self-injurious behaviors, tantrums are very common accompaniments of autism spectrum disorder. Anxiety is commonly reported symptom in children with autism spectrum disorder and may manifest in addition to irritability with restlessness, phobias, sleep disturbances (Sivertsen, Posserud, Gillberg, Lundervold & Hysing, 2012), etc. Stereotypical or repetitive motor behaviour is hall mark of autism spectrum disorder, and a significant number of children with autism spectrum disorder may meet the criteria for obsessive-compulsive disorder (Howes et al., 2018; Lord et al., 2018).

Digestive Symptoms

Gastrointestinal problems, such as food aversion, feeding difficulties, altered bowel patterns, reflux are often reported (Gorrindo et al., 2012).

Genitourinary

Toilet training is generally an issue in children with autism spectrum disorder resulting in child-parents struggles.

Treatment

There is no cure for autism and treatment generally involves a comprehensive and multidisciplinary approach. Focus of all treatments is behavioural modification and enhance communicative skills which are necessary for effective learning. In addition, pharmacology has a role in selective group of children especially those with problematic behaviors including self-injury, hyperactivity and inattention, and epilepsy. Use of dietary therapies and alternative medicine systems will be briefly touched upon.

Psychoeducational Interventions

Individuals with autism spectrum disorder require intensive and well-structured educational services. Several model-service delivery programs have been developed and are based on applied behaviour analysis (ABA) or other such programs such as treatment and education of autistic and related communication handicapped children (TEACHH), picture exchange communication system (PECS). Details of these programs and interventions is out of scope of this chapter but cornerstone of these programs is early intervention (Howes et al., 2018; Lord et al., 2018; Oono, Honey & McConachie, 2013; Reichow, Barton, Boyd & Hume, 2012).

Pharmacology

There is no specific medication treatment for core symptoms of autism spectrum disorder. Co-occurring problem behaviors such as agitation, irritability, self-injurious and other disruptive behaviours have been found to improve with treatment with antipsychotic medications namely risperidone and aripiprazole (Kent et al., 2013; Owen et al., 2009). Sedation and weight gain are common side effects. Hyperactivity is a common symptoms of autism spectrum disorder and symptoms can be ameliorated using methylphenidate, atomoxetine, and guanfacine. Effects are, however, not as marked in children with autism spectrum disorder as they are in children with autism spectrum disorder alone (Howes et al., 2018; Lord et al., 2018; Sturman, Deckx, & van Driel, 2017).

Epilepsy occurs in a significant number of children with autism spectrum disorder and requires treatment with anticonvulsant medications as for children without autism spectrum disorder. Treatment of anxiety, mood disorders, and other co-morbidities may require specific medications (Howes et al., 2018; Lord et al., 2018).

Many non-evidence-based treatments such as chelating agents, hyperbaric oxygen are potentially toxic and should be discouraged (Howes et al., 2018; Lord et al., 2018). Anecdotally, dietary interventions such as gluten and/or casein free diets, multivitamins have been reported to improve behaviors in autism spectrum disorder. Similarly there is no evidence to recommend therapies from systems of alternative medicine (Levy & Hyman, 201s).

Child MM was placed in intensive therapeutic program that involved a occupational therapist, speech therapist and an applied behavioural analysis (ABA) specialist. Therapies were done 5 times a week, with the child spending about 30 minutes each with each therapist. When reassessed 6 months later, some progress in his social skills were noted. His eye contact had improved, and his tantrums were now more manageable. On speech front he had not made any significant progress.

Outcome

Autism spectrum disorder is a pervasive and lifelong disorder. There is no cure for autism spectrum disorder but with early and intensive treatment, outlook for this severe disorder seems to be changing. A significant number (15% or more) of individuals with autism spectrum disorder can be expected to achieve independence and self-sufficiency as adults. Still, there are gaps in understanding psychobiology, neurochemical, molecular and genetic underpinnings of the disorder and further research is required to unravel these mysteries. As, our ability to understanding and safely manipulate genetic mechanisms is evolving, future for genetic interventions in the treatment of autism spectrum disorders should be exciting.

REFERENCES

American Psychiatric Association. (2013). *Diagnostic and Statistical Manual of Mental Disorders (DSM-V)* (5th ed.). Washington, DC: American Psychiatric Association Publishing.

Asperger, H. (1944). Die "autistichen Psychopathen" im Kindersalter. *Archiv für Psychiatrie und Nervenkrankheiten, 117*(1), 76–136. doi:10.1007/BF01837709

Dalwai, S., Ahmed, S., Udani, V., Mundkar, N., Kamath, S. S., & Nair, M. K. C. for the National Consultation Meeting for developing IAP guidelines on Neuro Developmental disorders under the aegis of IAP Childhood Disability Group and the Committee on Child Development and Neurodevelopmental disorders (2017). Consensus statement of the Indian Academy of Pediatrics on evaluation and management of autism spectrum disorders. *Indian Pediatr, 54*, 385-393.

Filipek, P. A., Accardo, P. J., Ashwal, S., Baranek, G. T., Cook, E. H. Jr, Dawson, G., ... Volkmar, F. R. (2000). Practice parameter: Screening and diagnosis of autism: Report of the Quality Standards Subcommittee of the American Academy of Neurology and the Child Neurology Society. *Neurology, 55*(4), 468–479. doi:10.1212/WNL.55.4.468 PMID:10953176

Gorrindo, P., Williams, K. C., Lee, E. B., Walker, L. S., McGrew, S. G., & Levitt, P. (2012). Gastrointestinal dysfunction in autism: Parental report, clinical evaluation, and associated factors. *Autism Research, 5*(2), 101–108. doi:10.1002/aur.237 PMID:22511450

Howes, O. D., Rogdaki, M., Findon, J. L., Wichers, R. H., Charman, T., King, B. H., ... Murphy, D. G. (2018). Autism Spectrum Disorder: Consensus guidelines on assessment, treatment and research from the British Association for Psychopharmacology. *Journal of Psychopharmacology (Oxford, England), 32*(1), 3–29. doi:10.1177/0269881117741766 PMID:29237331

Hviid, A., Hansen, J. V., Frisch, M., & Melbye, M. (2019). Measles, Mumps, Rubella vaccination and autism: A nationwide cohort study. *Annals of Internal Medicine, 170*(8), 513–520. doi:10.7326/M18-2101 PMID:30831578

Johnson, C. P., & Myers, S. M. (2007). Identification and evaluation of children with autism spectrum disorders. *Pediatrics, 120*(5), 1183–1215. doi:10.1542/peds.2007-2361 PMID:17967920

Kanner, L. (1943). Autistic disturbances of affective contact. *Nervous Child, 2*, 217–250.

Kent, J. M., Kushner, S., Ning, X., Karcher, K., Ness, S., Aman, M., ... Hough, D. (2013). Risperidone dosing in children and adolescents with autism spectrum disorder: A double-blind placebo-controlled study. *Journal of Autism and Developmental Disorders*, *43*(8), 1773–1783. doi:10.100710803-012-1723-5 PMID:23212807

Lee, B. H., Smith, T., & Paciorkowski, A. R. (2015). Autism spectrum disorder and epilepsy: Disorders with a shared biology. *Epilepsy & Behavior*, *47*, 191–201. doi:10.1016/j.yebeh.2015.03.017 PMID:25900226

Levy, S. E., & Hyman, S. L. (2015). Complementary and alternative medicine treatments for children with autism spectrum disorders. *Child and Adolescent Psychiatric Clinics of North America*, *24*(1), 117–143. doi:10.1016/j.chc.2014.09.004 PMID:25455579

Lord, C., Elsabbagh, M., Baird, G., & Veenstra-Vanderweele, J. (2018). Autism Spectrum Disorder. *Lancet*, *392*(10146), 508–520. doi:10.1016/S0140-6736(18)31129-2 PMID:30078460

Lyall, K., Croen, L., Daniels, J., Fallin, M. D., Ladd-Acosta, C., Lee, B. K., ... Newschaffer, C. (2017). The changing epidemiology of Autism Spectrum Disorders. *Annual Review of Public Health*, *38*(1), 81–102. doi:10.1146/annurev-publhealth-031816-044318 PMID:28068486

Myers, S. M., & Johnson, C. P. (2007). The Council on Children with Disabilities. Management of Children with Autism Spectrum Disorders. *Pediatrics*, *120*(5), 1162–1182. doi:10.1542/peds.2007-2362 PMID:17967921

Oono, I. P., Honey, E. J., & McConachie, H. (2013). Parent-mediated early intervention for young children with autism spectrum disorders (ASD). *Cochrane Database of Systematic Reviews*, CD009774. PMID:23633377

Owen, R., Sikich, L., Marcus, R. N., Corey-Lisle, P., Manos, G., McQuade, R. D., ... Findling, R. L. (2009). Aripiprazole in the treatment of irritability and in children and adolescents with autism disorder. *Pediatrics*, *124*(6), 1533–1640. doi:10.1542/peds.2008-3782 PMID:19948625

Ozonoff, S., Young, G. S., Carter, A., Messinger, D., Yirmiya, N., Zwaigenbaum, L., ... Stone, W. L. (2011). Recurrence risk for autism spectrum disorders: A Baby Siblings Research Consortium study. *Pediatrics*, *128*, e488–e495. PMID:21844053

Reichow, B., Barton, E. E., Boyd, B. A., & Hume, K. (2012). Early intensive behavioral intervention (EIBI) for young children with autism spectrum disorders (ASD). *Cochrane Database of Systematic Reviews*, CD009260. PMID:23076956

Sandin, S., Lichtenstein, P., Kuja-Holkola, R., Larsson, H., Hultman, C. M., & Reichenberg, A. (2014). The familial risk of autism. *Journal of the American Medical Association*, *311*(17), 1770–1777. doi:10.1001/jama.2014.4144 PMID:24794370

Schaefer, G. B., & Mendelsohn, N. J.Professional Practice Guidelines Committee. (2008). Clinical genetics evaluation in identifying the etiology of autism spectrum disorders. *Genetics in Medicine*, *10*(4), 301–305. doi:10.1097/GIM.0b013e31816b5cc9 PMID:18414214

Sivertsen, B., Posserud, M.-B., Gillberg, C., Lundervold, A. J., & Hysing, M. (2012). Sleep problems in children with autism spectrum disorder. A longitudinal population-based study. *Autism*, *16*(2), 139–150. doi:10.1177/1362361311404255 PMID:21478225

Sturman, N., Deckx, L., & van Driel, M. L. (2017). Methylphenidate for children and adolescents with autism spectrum disorder. *Cochrane Database of Systematic Reviews*, CD0011144. PMID:29159857

Thomas, S., Hovinga, M. E., Rai, D., & Lee, B. K. (2017). Brief report: prevalence of co-occurring epilepsy and autism spectrum disorder: the US national Survey of Children's Health 2011-2012. *Journal of Autism and Developmental Disorders*, *47*(1), 224–229. doi:10.100710803-016-2938-7 PMID:27752862

Tick, B., Bolton, P., Happe, F., Rutter, M., & Rijsdijk, F. (2016). Heritability of autism spectrum disorders: A metanalysis of twin studies. *Journal of Child Psychology and Psychiatry, and Allied Disciplines*, *57*(5), 585–595. doi:10.1111/jcpp.12499 PMID:26709141

Zwaigenbaum, L., Bauman, M. L., Choueiri, R., Fein, D., Kasari, C., Pierce, K., ... Wetherby, A. (2015a). Early identification and intervention for autism spectrum disorder. Executive Summary. *Pediatrics*, *136*(Supplement), S1–S9. doi:10.1542/peds.2014-3667B PMID:26430167

Zwaigenbaum, L., Bauman, M. L., Stone, W. L., Yirmiya, N., Estes, A., Hansen, R. L., ... Wetherby, A. (2015b). Early identification for autism spectrum disorder: Recommendation for Practice and Research. *Pediatrics*, *136*(Supplement), S10–S40. doi:10.1542/peds.2014-3667C PMID:26430168

Chapter 3
The Adult Transition Challenge of Autistic Individuals and the Way Ahead:
A Sibling's Perspective

Piyush Mishra
https://orcid.org/0000-0002-2399-1930
National Institute of Technology, Rourkela, India

ABSTRACT

Autism is a life-long neurodevelopmental condition characterized by difficulties in social communication, restricted and repetitive behaviors, and sensory processing issues. In India, there is a huge question mark regarding autistic individuals after they transition into adulthood, more specifically in housing and work options. In this chapter, beginning from the general considerations for upbringing of an autistic individual, attention is given to the need for future planning of autistic adults, more specifically in residential options. Some of the major residential centres are described followed by projections on establishing residential facilities. Following this, examples of life skills training, employment, and inclusion initiatives taking place in India are mentioned. Finally, research directions and other expectations aimed at increasing support for parents and siblings and also improving the lives of individuals on spectrum are discussed.

INTRODUCTION

Raising a child with autism is challenging and rewarding at the same time. Challenging because parents have to march on a long journey right from diagnosis stage to search an appropriate school to find occupational therapy centers and other services, all these alongside managing finances, their own health, personal lives, social circles and looking after their neuro-typical off springs too. Rewarding in the sense that they develop greater sense of empathy and have unique perspectives and experiences, appreciating the neuro-diversity of their autistic daughter/son. Acceptance and good communication among family

DOI: 10.4018/978-1-7998-3069-6.ch003

members play a crucial role in the overall development of the autistic individual. At the same time, awareness levels and acceptance in the community also have a great impact.

In general, there are 3 stages in an autistic individual's life and her/his family members and surrounding support structure: (1) the diagnosis and early intervention, (2) schooling: either regular school or special school and (3) transition to adulthood. In India, fortunately the services and know-how in the first two stages is increasing but there is an alarming need to find solutions regarding challenges encountered in stage (3). Even in the conditions when the parents and the entire family are diligently working towards individual's development, they become worried when their daughter/son reaches 18-22 years of age. This is due to the question of "What after us?". Also after a particular stage it becomes difficult for the parents to care because even their age is increasing leading to decreasing energy levels and rise in health issues. It is also a stressful condition for siblings as they not only have to look after their affected siblings but also their ageing parents while balancing their own career, ambitions and family goals. The need to find residential solutions for adults is highlighted book titled 'Autism and the Family in Urban India' by Vaidya (2016).

The challenges encountered in stage (3) are in the domain of work options, finding vocational education and regular education sources, residential arrangements, financial security, health screenings, provision of recreational activities and a good lifestyle, guardianship and other legal aspects. While pre-planning of these activities by parent's/family's end can be very difficult but it is much better than the sudden unplanned outcomes that may affect the autistic individuals negatively. The difficulties stem from the dearth of services and even more adversely by lack of information on these. Majorly parents get too consumed in taking care of their child that they fail to realize that this very child will grow into an adult and cluelessness about the future arises when the initial hints of their incapability to provide further care becomes evident. Another important but often neglected point to be noted is that: future planning should be a combined family activity. In cases when the autistic individual has sibling(s), even they should be actively involved in making decisions. In absence of siblings, parents must form a support structure consisting of their relatives or friends or professionals, well in advance so that there will be people to look after their daughter/son after them. Lindahl et al. (2019) noted that in some cases parents identified multiple people to take care, basically distributing the caregiving activities like residential arrangements, legal aspects, health screenings, likewise.

Another big factor is inclusion. Now inclusion first starts from respecting neuro-diversity, acknowledging the fact that autistic individuals' perception is different than ours (the neurotypicals). There may be intellectual disability, there may be sensory issues and there may be kaleidoscopic situations to deal with; but it is our inadequacy if we are not able to provide them platform, give them chances to grow and more urgently, understand them the way they are. One must not try to fit them into the neuro-typical box, rather their neurodiversity should be embraced. In India, situation and fate of 'autism' is unique-on one end there are people who still haven't heard about this term at all and on other end it has a huge population of autistic adults which require urgent attention.

Author's younger brother is a non-verbal severely Autistic individual who is 23 years old now. Since the subject matter described is experiential rather than from a well-defined generalized study, the points discussed in the chapter are thus a little biased towards non-verbal, severely autistic persons. The chapter is intended to provide an overview of the present scenario and future planning which may be helpful for parents/siblings and other care-givers working for the betterment of lives of the persons on spectrum.

Following are the objectives of the chapter:

1. To discuss some general considerations in upbringing and challenges encountered as the autistic individual transitions into adolescence and adulthood.
2. To discuss future planning aspects for autistic adults.
3. To mention the employment initiatives and autism friendly initiatives towards inclusion into society.
4. To describe future activities and research required to make the lives of autistic adults and their support system better.

LITERATURE REVIEW

Lindahl et al. (2019) extracted 7 major domains of future planning of individuals with intellectual and developmental disabilities (IDD) from the parent-sibling interviews: housing, legal planning, financial planning, identification of primary caregiver(s), day to day care, medical management and transportation. Out of these the 'housing' domain emerged in every interview. All the factors in some way overlapped each other. And authors suggested that accomplishing 'identification of primary care-giver(s)' as the first step made the planning for other domains easier and definitive.

Lee, Burke & Stelter (2019) studied the parent's and sibling's perspectives regarding future planning for individuals with intellectual and developmental disabilities (IDD) by interviewing 10 parent-sibling dyads. They noted that there were discussions regarding the future but with no or little 'specificity'. They also highlighted that due to parents being the main decision-makers, the siblings may be unaware of the future planning. Parents may also not want to discuss the future planning with their unaffected off spring. There is no clarity of agreement among the family members. Siblings (unlike parents) reported the need for more communication among family members regarding future planning. Authors reported three main barriers: family related barriers (uncertainty of the future, family communication, different perspectives among family members, and siblings struggling to balance their own lives); systemic barriers (limited quality programs for adults with IDD, financial costs and system navigation); and lastly barriers for individuals with IDD (parents worried about the victimization of their off springs, thus encouraging them to stay at home for greater security). It was concluded from the study that 'definitive' rather than aspirational future planning together with 'proper family communication' is the need of the hour.

Hodapp, Sanderson, Meskis, Casale (2017) contrasted the adult sibling relationship in the general population and the state when siblings have a sister/brother with disabilities. Authors have reviewed the performance of siblings on four outcomes: (1) problems-advantages and life success; (2) life choices (marriage,children, choice of career); (3) sibling relationships and (4) sibling care-giving and anticipated care-giving. They mentioned that siblings of individuals with disabilities are vastly understudied. Some unexplored topics like care giving of ageing parents, research on the surrounding people of sibling (ex. spouse), concerns particular to a disability- broader autism phenotype in case of autistic sister/brother were also discussed. Authors highlighted the need to research the support needed by the siblings in terms of information required, financial and emotional aspects.

Swaminathan (2015) assessed the vocational skills and the transition condition in adolescents with low functioning autism in Mumbai, India. The understanding of parents, and their future expectations were also studied. Regarding the future planning most of the parents admitted that they had not thought about their child's future living options, guardianships and financial supports even though they considered these to be important. Vaidya (2016) in her book titled 'Autism and the Family in Urban India' mentioned that group homes and community living models where young adults live together are found in the west. However, these are backed by long-standing systems of social security which are lacking in India. "Group homes in the Indian context will necessarily involve a good deal of investment of time and resources (economic and social) by parents and other stakeholders. As a generation of children diagnosed with autism enter adulthood and parents age and become susceptible to disabling conditions themselves, there is an urgent need for pooling resources and efforts to create viable alternatives." (Vaidya,2016, p.179). Berua, Kaushik & Gulati (2017) also stress that there is little way of social security for autistic individuals as they move to adulthood in India. In most cases, parent driven Non-Governmental Organizations (NGOs) step in to start services for adults. Some of the adults may continue to go to special schools even in their thirties and forties, while others get engaged in sheltered workplaces managed by NGOs.

Choi & O'Brien (2019) analysed the impact of familism on future planning for Korean parents for their children with disabilities. Interviews of both the parents and the professionals were conducted. It was found that there is a strong emphasis on familial care with minimal government support which has a negative impact on planning process. 'Lack of information and database' and 'parental economic capacity' emerged as factors for low level of planning.

The chapter is broadly divided into 4 sections: (1) Some general considerations and thoughts, (2) Future Planning for Autistic Adults, (3) Life skills trainings, employment and inclusion initiatives and (4) Future expectations and research directions.

SOME GENERAL CONSIDERATIONS AND THOUGHTS

In this section, starting from the diagnosis stage, other important aspects faced by the family is highlighted. Basically, the events from birth to adulthood are described through the lens of family members. In doing so, the mental and physical health of parents is talked about, the desirable dynamics amongst the family members is mentioned. Light is thrown on the challenges in family decision making process, patience required and some other practical considerations.

Going from 0 to 1: After diagnosis, the first step is 'acceptance'. It is actually going from '0' to '1' without which one cannot progress further. Knowledge of Autism Spectrum Condition and mutual understanding among family members play a key role in this. The diagnosis should not be considered as a 'burden' as this will also influence the way in which the other family members, extended family members and friend circles will absorb the idea of autism.

Stigma: It is the social stigma associated with intellectual & developmental disabilities and also to a great extent in mental health problems which is the root cause of 'acceptance issues' in India. Due to this, parents and siblings, initially try to hide the fact that their loved one is on spectrum, they also avoid social gatherings and participation in other activities. Also, in the early years parental notions like: "My child is completely fine and nothing has happened to her/him", will only cause delay in diagnosis and early intervention thus worsening the situation further. Awareness on a very serious scale is required to tackle the issue of 'stigma' associated.

Patience: Teaching a task will require huge investment of time. This will obviously depend on the learning ability of the individual but many a times, it can be frustrating to instruct an action repeatedly and still not observe much progress. In situations like these, patience is the anti-dote. In addition to this, there may be complex behavioral issues causing huge amount of stress to the care-givers. Herein also rock solid amount of patience is required as it can sometimes take a very long time to control the challenging behavioral problems.

Schooling: Needless to mention, schooling is vital for the overall development of the individual. It is a place where the individual not only learns and explores various skills but also makes friends and interacts with various other people thus improving social skills. She/he also gets chance to participate in physical training activities and games. Depending on the severity of autism coupled with intellectual disability, an individual can either go to a special school or a regular school. Though the scenario is improving but it is still difficult to find appropriate and affordable special schools even in big cities. Regular schools either don't admit them citing absence of required infrastructure or may admit and make them discontinue due to 'inappropriate behavior'. In these cases, persons with mild autism have nowhere to go, they can neither fit in special schools nor the regular schools which must support them. Even in the cases when one attends a regular school, the issue of bullying crops up impacting the mental state of the individual negatively. Thus, awareness is needed not only for the teachers and school machinery but also for the classmates, even extending to the parents of the classmates. Only then there can be acceptance at an actual level fueling 'truly inclusive education'.

Adolescence: Transition into adolescence comes with its own set of changes. During puberty, the individuals may get disturbances in sleep cycles, may become excessively hyperactive and in some cases aggressive too, there may be self-injurious and injurious behaviors to others too. Attraction towards opposite sexes, and curiosity about their own body is seen which is normal. Since in many instances, the individuals are unable to express their feelings or may express them differently, it becomes very difficult for the parents to know the reason behind their challenging behaviors. Parents have a very tough time in managing this phase. Discussions regarding management of puberty in girls and boys should be quite open and there should be evidence based information platforms for parents on how to impart sex education to their children, in the form of workshops and online content.

Exploration: Many activities according to the cognitive level of the autistic individual have to be tried and huge investment of time is really required to figure out the interest area of the individual. These areas, say for instance, art & craft or cooking or coding or floral decorations may pave the way for their future work engagement. Schools can play a great role in this. Sometimes, it may be very easy to pin down the interest area and other times, no matter what, the child doesn't seem interested in any activity at all, the right thing to do in this case is to not stop trying, not stop looking. Even if the individual loses interest in a particular activity after some years, still a sense of doing work is developed which definitely helps in the long run.

Looking After Oneself: Care-giving causes huge amount of stress, particularly in mothers. If left unchecked, this may lead to health issues like blood pressure, hypertension, cardiac problems and also cause mental health problems like anxiety and depression. It thus becomes absolutely necessary for the family members to take care of their health. In situations of mental health issues, it is important to reach out for help and not hide it.

Connecting With Other Parents: There are parent groups or associations at many places, even in places where such groups don't exist, it is a great initiative to form one. These serve as strong support system, learning medium and information exchange hub along with recreational activities. In a broader sense, these groups can then collectively plan about the future of their daughters/sons in terms of residential planning. On the same lines, there should also be initiation of sibling-groups.

Decision Making: Moving to a new city for better medical and training services, moving to a place near the school, daily transport plans, residential mode (flat vs. independent housing), transfer issues in case of parents whose occupation is in service sector, travelling plans, etc. is only a representative list on the various facets a family has to decide upon. Owing to the support needed, in some cases siblings have to also adjust their options for higher education. Many types of adjustments also have to be made in the lifestyle and timetable of the family. A healthy communication among the family members is absolutely necessary for the overall well-being of the family.

Siblings: Out of all the family members, siblings are the ones who are in the same age bracket as the autistic individual and thus spend the longest amount of time with them right from being their playmates in the childhood to potentially becoming their guardians after parents. Acknowledging this, parents must include siblings in decision making processes regarding the future planning activities of the autistic individual. There are many considerations and effects on the siblings. For instance, siblings may prefer to attend a college or work in a place/city close to home due to care-giving responsibilities. Or there may be cases when the sibling decides to return to their hometown when their parents become incapable of providing further care to their ward with special needs. Talking about effects, in case of genetic history in the family or genetic causes, the marriability or marriage prospects of the siblings may get influenced negatively. It is of greater importance to siblings to maintain their physical and mental health in order to shoulder responsibilities. There may be cases in which parents don't wish to pass on the responsibilities to the sibling or the sibling might not be able to provide care-giving. Considering this condition and also in a general sense, formation of a 'legal trust' becomes necessary.

Health Screening Difficulties: In cases of severe behavioral challenges, it becomes difficult for a parent/care-givers to make the individual undergo basic routine checkups, blood examination, eye-tests and dental check-ups. This issue can be solved by taking help from the doctor or organizing similar check-up camps in the special school in which the individual is enrolled. Another difficulty that arises is the inability of the individual to explain the medical condition to the doctor, particularly in the case of non-verbal individuals. In this case, it is the care-giver who spends more time with the individual (generally mother) and has really understood and established a way of communication with her/him, actually understands what is going on to some extent. This point necessitates teaching the individual means to communicate her/his problems in the best possible way for others to understand.

Should You Mention Autism or Should You Not?: This point is specifically directed towards persons with mild autism. Daley, Singhal and Krishnamoorthy (2013) described an example of a 9-year old boy with a diagnosis of autism who attended a second-tier private school. This boy had clear characteristics of ASC but with no disruptive behaviors making others not notice his diagnosis. His parents intentionally withheld his diagnosis from the school because it carried 'no advantage'. The authors further mentioned their observation that schools may use this diagnosis of autism as reason for the removal of a child citing that they don't have trained staff to work with children with autism. On contrary, unlike in the United States, having a diagnosis of autism may reduce the 'availability' of services for a child in India.

Finding Services: Even in cities, parents struggle to find services like speech therapists, occupational therapists, inclusive schools, respite care facilities, residential centres, financial planning services, etc. For this Nayi Disha (www.nayi-disha.org), a Hyderabad based organization is an excellent information hub. Another upcoming information hub is Reservoir Neurodiversity (https://reservoirnow.com).

Mental Illness and Autism: A common myth associated among parents is that how can their autistic daughter/son have mental illness, say depression, when she/he doesn't understand much? Mental illness can co-exist with intellectual disability. In persons with intellectual disability and more particularly autism, it becomes very difficult to distinguish whether the abnormality seen is a behavioral defect or mental illness. Neglect, boredom, physical abuse, sexual abuse and substance abuse may worsen the situation in this case.

Environment Affects Them: Due to the sensory preferences of autistic individuals, they get affected by the surrounding spaces. Some might have particular sensitivity to smell, sound, sight, taste, temperature. What can be done best to make them comfortable taking into consideration their hyper/hypo sensitivity should be found out and accordingly alterations can be made in their environment. While this is true, the individual must also be trained gradually to adapt different types of environment.

Looking at the Strengths Instead of Weaknesses: There can undoubtedly be many so to speak 'weaknesses' or shortcomings which can be strengthened by therapies and trainings. Noting the weaknesses or things to learn is fine but at the same time noting the strengths is equally important. The primary care-givers should make a list of the strong areas of the autistic individual, things that she/he enjoys doing or activities that come easy to the individual. These areas can then be further bolstered and these may make the way for their work engagements in future.

Government Schemes: Many government information portals are launched to provide information on financial assistance for self-employment, scholarships (http://www.nhfdc.nic.in/default.aspx) ; Unique Disability ID (UDID) (http://www.swavlambancard.gov.in) ; various funding schemes for day care, respite care, housing, insurance, legal guardianship, work centres and others (http://thenationaltrust.gov.in/content/) and (http://disabilityaffairs.gov.in/content/). The website of National Institute for Empowerment of Persons with Intellectual Disabilities (NIEPID) (http://niepid.nic.in) also contains information about various schemes such as Swavlamban Group Health Insurance, posting of government employees who have intellectually disabled children, etc. . Parents/interested social groups should remain updated with the support provided from the government.

FUTURE PLANNING FOR AUTISTIC ADULTS

"At least one in every 89 children aged 2-9 has been diagnosed with autism in India, according to a study by Dr Shefali Gulati, chief of child neurology at AIIMS, Delhi (Arora et. al (2018)). That is, as many as 2.2 million Indian children and 13 million adults live with the condition" (Mohan, 2018).

There is a huge lack of information among parents of Autistic individuals regarding future planning majorly in terms of living options, possible employment or work engagements and financial security. While it is true that some of the people on spectrum can lead an independent life close to neurotypical people, but majority will require life-long support, if not support then some kind of supervision. As increasingly more and more autistic adolescents are transitioning into adulthood and at the same time parents'/care-givers' incapability to provide further care is getting evident, there is an urgent need for day-care facilities, respite care facilities as short term solutions and full-fledged residential facilities in long term. Not only this, but establishment of work centres is also a necessity.

Independency: First and foremost, the autistic individuals should be independent in carrying out daily life activities to the maximum extent possible. Basic activities like brushing, bathing, using washroom/toilet, grooming, dressing and eating should not require any assistance or minimal assistance. On a more basic level, they must also know or sense that they need to use washroom, that they are hungry and thus need something to eat. In case of severely autistic and non-verbal individuals, they must know how to communicate these basic requirements and other requirements to the care-givers. They should also know how to communicate their 'medical problems' to the best possible extent.

Concept of Community Integration: In the report 'Housing options for Adults with Autism Spectrum Disorder' by Bureau of Autism Services, Pennsylvania Department of Public Welfare (Diana T.

Myers and Associates Inc., 2010, p.11), it is described that: "Community integration is the opposite of isolation; it provides the opportunity to live in the community and be valued for one's uniqueness and abilities, like everyone else. Community integration is a right of all people and encompasses housing, employment, education, leisure/recreation, social roles, peer support, health status, citizenship, self-determination, and religion/spirituality. Community integration should result in community presence and participation of persons with disabilities similar to that of persons without disabilities."

Aspiration vs Action: As noted earlier in the background of this chapter, most of the planning related activities are aspirational rather than being definitive, action oriented. The longer the delay in switching to definitive mode, the greater the chances are of getting trapped into the unplanned outcome situation. Thus merely thinking about future planning passively or just having an idea of future planning is not sufficient, gears should be shifted towards action oriented tasks like taking guardianship, creating financial security, ensuring insurance support and healthcare management, likewise. At the same time, it is also true that there is a need for establishing 'planning services' which can assist parents in various domains, right from financial planning to the residential options and potentially creating residential setups.

The Barriers: In spite of being very well aware that one day their daughter/son has to live without them, parents are still hesitant to plan about their future. As mentioned earlier, the two most prevalent barriers are: lack of available services and financial barriers. However, there are other hurdles too. The following points are not exhaustive, extensive research work has to done to find out more barriers in Indian context.

Lack of Information: There is a huge information gap among parents regarding where to search work centres, how to set up trusts, where to find residential services, how to accomplish financial and legal planning, where to find support staff in case of independent living or residential centre, etc.

Lack of Willingness: Due to the time and energy already spent in care-giving process, many parents don't want the extra stress of future planning. Say for instance in starting a group home for individuals, may parents might face willingness issues or might not want to actively lead the process. Considering this, parents/siblings definitely need to be supported in the form of a potential future planning services. These services can not only guide the parents but also fill in the knowledge gaps due to their expertise in the related domains, as many parents might be willing but again don't necessarily possess the technical knowledge to navigate the system.

Lack of Available Services: Consider availability of work centers. Daley, Weisner & Singhal (2014) studied the daily routine of 54 Autistic Adults in Delhi and NCR region. It was found that there were no suitable work and training facilities in Delhi that were easily accessible even for adults with no disruptive behaviors. This study covered the upper middle class section of the society. This reflects a need to set up work centres, vocational-training centres where the individuals can come during day time and work. Not only their establishment is needed but also they should be accessible leading to smooth transport of individual to the centre.

Financial Barriers: There are very few autistic-specific residential centres (campus type and group home type) in India and most of them charge in the ranges which is not at all affordable for the middle-class section of society. What can be done in this case is forming a group of parents and pooling in resources to form a residential setting- even this requires a huge investment of money and time, together with knowledge of other aspects like permissions to be taken from local authorities, legal aspects and other related paperwork. Not only this, it is also a task to find trained care-givers who will be looking after the individuals.

Residential Systems: This is probably the biggest concern for the parents. Residential systems can include: independent living with supervision, group home settings or community living models, separate dedicated campuses-residential centers, sibling co-residential settings, and living at one's own home with support workers. Considering the huge diversity in ASC, one may be in a job and live independently, requiring support in the form of managing finances, purchasing groceries, medical supervision and transport facilities. On the other end, one may need a dedicated residential facility with constant supervision pursuing vocational activities, for instance. There is another dimension to this: due to less no. of group homes and campuses, basically limited options, there may be cases where the autistic adult 'might not fit in' due to some complex behavioral traits or special requirements. In situations like this, the individual and the associated family members have difficult time in planning the future residential arrangements. This can be termed as an 'internal factor' which impedes the decision making. The 'external factors' which influence selection of a residential centre are costs associated (affordability), location of the residential centre (considering community integration, accessibility to medical facilities, climatic conditions) and there might be also concerns regarding proximity to individual's home (it becomes easier for the primary care-givers to stay connected with the residential centre if the centre is closer to home). One may very well continue in her/his home with siblings or other family members but all this should be solidly planned beforehand. Also, ideally the autistic individual should be able to choose among different housing options.

Brief Description of Current Residential Systems: Herein 3 different models of residential systems in India will be discussed briefly. These cover the group homes and campus type set-ups and the list is not exhaustive, there are other centres too.

A) ARUNIMA, Dehradun: ARUNIMA (http://www.projectarunima.org) is an assisted living model for autistic adults (both girls and boys) situated within a general residential space or locality in Dehradun, Uttarakhand. Since, it is situated within the general residential space, it can use the common community facilities like gym, swimming pool, medical facilities; visit nearby shopping centres and engage in other activities just like anyone else in that locality. This closeness to homes has another benefit: the support staff required in the form of cooks, guards, housekeeping workers, drivers are easy to find and more willing to join due to location within the city instead of some far-off place. The residents are called 'friends'. On a typical day, friends go to their work/training centre at 9-9:30 am which is at a walkable distance from their residence. Therein according to groups they perform various activities. For instance, the first group goes for shopping (raw material for vocational activities, their toiletries, raw material for making bakery products, other materials), the second group gets engaged in computer education task, the third gets involved in a group activity (games) followed by dance and the fourth group having completed the art & craft tasks prepares a list for shopping to be done on next day. Friends come to their residence at 1-1:30 pm and post lunch and rest, the evening activities include household chores, walks, music sessions, physical activities, TV time, bath, dinner and sleep. The essence of ARUNIMA lies in the 'diversification' of activities. A very important point to understand is that just like neurotypical individuals get bored of carrying out a similar activity and eventually lose interest in it, in the very same way Autistic individuals too regardless of their affinity to 'sameness'. In words of the founder of ARUNIMA-Aparna Das, "Life is not just about doing VOCATIONAL ACTIVITIES but vocational activities are just a part of life." Therefore Arunima has diversified it's activities in workplace: friends go to local bakery shops to learn and then make bakery items at their workplace; nursery: they also plant saplings in beautifully decorated pots; and they also make various art & craft products like paper bags, gift bags, festival cards, decorated bottles, bookmarks, diaries, pen stands, pillow covers, earrings, stone painting products, lanterns and others. All these products are sold under the brand name 'Arukriti' at local shops and also their online website and facebook page.

B) Mid-way home, Kurukshetra: Mid-way home (http://www.midwayhome.in) is a two-floor big home for autistic adults (only boys) and other IDD adults in Kurukshetra, Haryana. It has capacity for about 50 adults. On the ground floor, apart from the academic activities section, there are specialized spaces for different activities like dance room, music room, gym, yoga, art & craft space and computer education. The first floor serves as the residence for the adults. Not only this, in the space surrounding the home, there is a separate vocational activity centre, dairy, pet therapy zone, a fish pond and a small patch of land for teaching agricultural activity. Every resident gets involved in all the activities and the centre follows a timetable for each day.

C) Autism Ashram, Hyderabad (http://www.care4autism.in/index.html): It is the largest residential centre in India, spreading across 9.5 acres in Kesavaram village near Hyderabad, Telangana. This is a campus oriented model having almost all the facilities in a picturesque location. The campus is lush green with sensory pathways, auditorium, vocational centre, music activity facilities, dance room, swimming pool, cycling tracks, exercise-oriented garden. The centre also runs a day-school, combined for both residents and non-residents. Total count of adults is 100 plus (inclusive of boys and girls, also the day scholars). There is CCTV surveillance on the campus. The campus also includes parent guest houses. The founder of Autism Ashram, Dr.A.K.Kundra is very active in spreading awareness and guiding parents for the question of what after them.

In a nutshell, the first model is that of a group home, the third- campus oriented and the second model described lies between the two. Every model has its pros and cons.

Gender Differences: Most of the work centres and residential center planning activities might exclude females citing difficulties in management and other issues. This should not be the case. What can be done to ensure their full-participation has to be researched and solved.

How can parents/social groups set up a residential facility?: There is no simple answer to this question. Due to the huge no. of diverse autistic individuals transitioning into adulthood, many residential facilities have to be started. Initiation can be done by visiting the existing residential centres, meticulously studying their model, gathering information on various aspects like their day to day activities, their financial model, mode of operation- trust or private company, how to obtain, train and retain support staff required, sustainability of the model and other aspects. There can also be collaborations with the existing centres. Also one might not want to go for building a group home or residential campus but opt for living at home with support or a group of parents (say 4 families) might wish to live together. In this case, parents should know the information regarding setting the financial, legal and other support services required. Basically a trust can be formed to look after the adults when the parents will not be there.

There is also need for respite care facilities, meaning a place where parents can send their daughter/son for a fixed no. of days in cases where parents face some kind of medical emergency, or some other work. Beginnings of residential setups can also be made in the form of respite care facility or parent relief centre till the plan of full-fledged residential centre materializes. These respite centres might operate for a fixed no. of days in a month. If done in collaboration with a special school, the respite care facility can also be operated throughout the year. The benefit of sending the individual away from home is not solely for parents but this enhances the independency of the individual and in a way acts like a simulator for actual residential centre. It is very necessary to also make the individual participate in residential summer camps (if available) so that the individual becomes accustomed to live without the supervision of parents. This is also in a way training for the external care-givers (care-givers other than parents).

There are lots of issues one might encounter while setting up a residential centre. Funding is the major issue, devotion of time by parents is another consideration. Also there may be interested parents but huge differences in what they wish for their child. It is therefore necessary to first establish a very strong and clear communication among the interested parents/social groups. Since, setting up a residential centre is a mammoth task, division of work to be done is absolutely vital. As mentioned, help can be sought from the already established centre but the group of parents should not blindly follow the existing models and actually figure out what will work in their village/town/city and also where their child will fit in. Care should also be taken regarding availability of medical help, in case something happens to the individual or in cases where the individual gets seizures.

The aforementioned is only view of the author and serious research is required in the residential systems to provide a clear picture to parents/social groups of what can be done.

The care-givers need attention too: Focus should also be on the physical and mental well-being of the external care-givers (staff of the residential centres). The physical and mental fatigue encountered can be reduced if the care-givers work in shifts.

LIFE SKILLS TRAININGS, EMPLOYMENT AND INCLUSIVE INITIATIVES

Irrespective of where the autistic individuals live, they definitely require some kind of activity, some kind of work. This work can only be to engage their time but it is much better to move towards remunerative model of employment/self-employment. Again due to huge diversity in ASC, an individual might work in open employment opportunities independently while another individual might require constant assistance in doing work. One of the vital considerations to be taken care of is the individual's interest in doing a particular job/work. Majorly it is the individual's capability and interest that should dictate the work she/he pursues and not entirely based upon her/his parent's desire that their ward should work in a particular setting or not.

Talking about vocational activities, the products developed should be utility-based, there should be a market demand for the products developed. For instance, production of office stationery materials like files, notepads, etc.; production of paper bags/jute bags/cotton bags; horticulture, and other agro-based products, likewise. According to different regions, the demands will vary and thus market research should be a component in planning vocational activities.

An individual can also work in a photocopying centre, laundry services, in small retail stores. There can also be employment in big retail chains and hospitality sector. This list can go on with various other sectors, it is upto the capability, interest of the individual, training imparted to them and understanding established amongst the employers on how to work with autistic individuals that will define the entire picture.

DAIL (NIEPID): The Department of Adult Independent Living, National Institute for Empowerment of Persons with Intellectual Disabilities, Secunderabad (http://niepid.nic.in/index.php) is the pioneer in not only establishing different trades (vocational activities) and designing workstations, but also finding jobs, training the intellectually disabled persons, collaborating with the company personnel and doing follow-up training sessions, thus holistically empowering adults with ID. The department conducts training sessions; job fairs; develops vocational assessment, guide book for transition planning from school to work.

Café/Bakery/Tiffin Services: Yash Charitable Trust (Mumbai) (https://www.yashcharitabletrust.org) runs a café and tiffin service. The Café Arpan is a glittering example of how beautifully a café can be managed by adults with autism and other developmental disabilities. Shuktara Cakes, Kolkata (https://shuktaracakes.com) is another wonderful bakery, training and employing persons with disabilities having no family. Other glorifying examples are: Café Icanflyy (http://icanflyy.com/cafe-icanflyy/) ; Sip & Bite Café, Kolkata: "This Kolkata Café has a unique offering besides cupcakes and cookies" (Think Change India, 2019) and Café Ikkayees, Kozhikode ("Three Differently-Abled youngsters welcome you with a warm smile at this Kerala restaurant", 2019); Sai Bakery, Chennai: "Sai Bakery: A Mother's sweet gift to her Autistic son and his differently abled friends" (Pareek,2015).

Together Life Skills Centre: Even after attaining therapies and schooling, the young people with autism and other intellectual disabilities may not be prepared for life. To increase their capability in carrying out daily life activities and also empower them for job-related skills, Together Life Skills Centre (https://togethersee.org) is a not-for-profit organization in Mumbai (Maharashtra) whose purpose is to prepare their students to live independently after the lifetime of parents. From grooming, kitchen work, teaching communication skills, imparting computer education to performing bakery work, and having manufacturing unit for block-printed paper bags; Together foundation is a shining step towards making the differently abled self-reliant.

The CanBridge Academy, Chennai: Most of the autistic adults have no place to go after they finish their school, keeping this in mind CanBridge academy is an initiative by parents and special educators to provide them a space to learn life skills and work skills. It is in a sense college for Autistic adults. They operate in three levels of increasing complexity. In cooking, for example, the first level includes basics like doing the dishes, making sandwiches, beverages, likewise. The second level is more involved like the students will be doing meal-prepartion work- cutting vegetables, grinding. And at level three, the individual will be actually cooking. After these stages, the individual can potentially join a professional working environment. Music sessions, dance sessions, art works, going out to buy groceries and other items, learning money sense are different ways in which the academy is helping the individuals. (The CanBridge Academy, 2019)

Another important organization working towards inclusive employment is Evoluer Solutions, Gurgaon (https://www.evoluersolutions.com).

Inclusive Initiatives: Shopping can really give a tough time to parents when they are with their autistic daughter/son due to sensory issues. But this does not mean that they should be excluded from this daily life activity. To facilitate this, Big Bazaar has launched a nationwide initiative known as 'Autism Quiet Hour'. Every Tuesday 11 am onwards, Quiet hour begins with dimmed lights, no announcements, no music, and a sensitized staff. This hour also sensitizes the general public about the persons with autism. Big Bazaar has also launched a booklet to ease shopping for persons with intellectual disabilities. The booklet is a step by step visual guide to shopping at Quiet Hour.

SPI cinemas, Chennai (https://www.spicinemas.in) organizes sensory friendly screening of movies. These screening as known as SENS. There are dimmed lights throughout the duration of the show, lowered sound levels, unrestricted movement and chatter within the screen and a longer intermission (" SENS: A Special Show for Special Minds, 2019).

There are many more examples of such initiatives, News Hook (https://newzhook.com) is an excellent source to remain updated about all the happenings around.

FUTURE EXPECTATIONS AND RESEARCH DIRECTIONS

In this section, considering the Indian scenario for Autistic Adults, suggestions for awareness camps, workshops and medical screenings are discussed. Following this, what areas need more focus in the research terrain are mentioned. All these suggestions are keeping in mind to ease the care-giving process for parents/siblings/other care-givers.

Doctor Awareness Programs: There should be awareness among general physicians on how to deal with autistic patients. Since many times it becomes difficult for a patient on spectrum to express herself/himself, the doctor must understand this with the help of primary care-givers and then carry out consultation. There can be 'doctor awareness camps' by experienced Doctors who have dealt with autistic patients.

Medical Check-Up Camps: In many cases, it becomes difficult to carry out general health check-ups like dental examinations, blood tests, ENT (Ear-Nose-Throat) check-up owing to the behavioral challenges and sensory issues among people on spectrum. Forget routine check-ups, in cases where actual blood sample evaluation is required, it still becomes difficult to do so due to difficulty in managing them and the associated anxiety. Special arrangements in regular examination labs/centres can thus simplify the process. Additionally, special check-up camps can be organized, for instance in special schools wherein with the help of school staff, it becomes easier for the doctors to examine intellectually disabled students.

Future Planning Training Programs For Parents And Siblings: While parents are aware of the fact that future planning is necessary, they mostly don't possess the energy to research on it due to lack of time and energy. In these situations, workshop on future planning should be organized. For instance, Nayi Disha, an intellectual disability information dissemination organization, recently conducted a session on financial planning for their Mumbai Chapter/group of parents. Similarly, webinars and Facebook sessions by experts can also be conducted.

Research Directions

There is a wealth of research on biological end. There is also an increase in research from engineering end in the form of early detection of autism, augmented and virtual reality, games as mobile applications and on Kinect platform, eye tracking technologies, to name a few. But there are many areas that require attention. In India, a lot of focus is required in conducting parent-sibling studies: their quality of life studies, challenges faced and support needed by them. Though parent studies exist, the sibling studies is largely missing from the literature. These studies should not just cover a particular section of society but should encompass people from all backgrounds. Also, the studies must be graduated to devise solutions and not just be an inventory of information. This kind of research can also potentially contribute in policy-making process.

The parental and sibling perception regarding future planning should be studied. There can be differences in the way parents and siblings think. Even among the parents, studies should see whether there are differences between the maternal and paternal perspectives regarding future planning.

Another area which requires huge attention as is evident from this chapter is the modelling of residential systems. From classification of the existing residential set-ups to empowering parents and other social groups to set-up residential centres, there should be research covering details of various models knitted with the financial and legal aspects. Once a replicable framework of residential systems taking into focus all the sections of society and not just the economically stronger sections, is developed, it will be a great assistance to parents/siblings/social groups interested in establishing residential facilities. In addition to this, measures to make the residential centres sustainable should also be explored.

Then comes the field of 'design for autism'. Apart from product design, it also covers designing spaces for autistic individuals, for instance designing learning spaces, designing residential spaces taking into consideration their sensory preferences and architectural aspects. There can also be 'sensory garden design'. Product design for neurodiversity is another topic having huge scope. Much attention is also needed to understand the puberty in girls and boys and help parents navigate this phase with more ease. Sex education for intellectually disabled is a vital topic which should be explored and the knowledge should reach to parents on how to make the intellectually disabled individual understand concepts like 'private space', 'hygiene', 'protection against abuse', likewise. As it has been mentioned in the chapter, there is also requirement for research in health and health related aspects for autistic adults. This covers not only the physical health status but also the mental health of autistic adults. Means to develop easy screening of health issues (health assessments) is another area.

Research should not be done in silos, rather there can be university collaborations. Even within an institute, different departments can collaborate and work together. For instance, the computer science department, industrial design department together with psychology department can develop, design and test games respectively for autistic people in the form of 'apps' or in Kinect platforms. In yet another example, departments comprising of people from mechanical, electrical and computer sciences can together work on 'Robotics for Autism'. Alternately the Design & Arts department can explore the possibilities of using 'Puppetry' in developing joint attention and other skills in autistic individuals. Universities can also play a major role in spreading awareness by building clubs for neurodiversity or using existing clubs for organizing intellectual disability awareness camps, and also actually visiting special schools and inclusive schools to understand their problems and work for solving them.

CONCLUSION

There are many places in the chapter where the word 'problem' and 'challenges' has been used extensively. These are actually the areas where there is a huge need and scope of improvement. As the population with autism and other developmental disabilities will be rising, the solutions for their future planning should also be developed at a faster pace. Definitive action oriented steps rather than 'just planning' has to be the only approach to deal with the rising demands. The dialogue of future planning should be among the siblings too. In cases where there are no siblings, a support structure must be formed. To accomplish the future planning goals, parents and siblings will require immense support in the form of information, assistance for financial and legal planning, more and more life skills and work centres and eventually residential centres. Increasing inclusive initiatives as mentioned in the chapter will motivate others to respect the neuro-diversity and give the autistic adults chance to participate in the community. Research and beyond research activities can greatly contribute to develop the knowledge and implement actionable solutions thus improving lives of people on spectrum.

REFERENCES

Arora, N. K., Nair, M. K. C., Gulati, S., Deshmukh, V., Mohapatra, A., Mishra, D., ... Murthy, G. V. S. (2018). Neurodevelopmental disorders in children aged 2–9 years: Population-based burden estimates across five regions in India. *PLoS Medicine*, *15*(7), e1002615. doi:10.1371/journal.pmed.1002615 PMID:30040859

Barua, M., Kaushik, J. S., & Gulati, S. (2017). Legal provisions, educational services and health care across the lifespan for autism spectrum disorders in India. *Indian Journal of Pediatrics*, *84*(1), 76–82. doi:10.100712098-016-2261-5 PMID:27917445

Choi, C., & O'Brien, M. (2019). The impact of familism on future care planning for Korean parents caring for their children living with disabilities. *Asia Pacific Journal of Social Work and Development*, 1–14.

Daley, T. C., Singhal, N., & Krishnamurthy, V. (2013). Ethical considerations in conducting research on autism spectrum disorders in low and middle income countries. *Journal of Autism and Developmental Disorders*, *43*(9), 2002–2014. doi:10.100710803-012-1750-2 PMID:23283629

Daley, T. C., Weisner, T., & Singhal, N. (2014). Adults with autism in India: A mixed-method approach to make meaning of daily routines. *Social Science & Medicine*, *116*, 142–149. doi:10.1016/j.socscimed.2014.06.052 PMID:24998867

Hodapp, R. M., Sanderson, K. A., Meskis, S. A., & Casale, E. G. (2017). Adult siblings of persons with intellectual disabilities: Past, present, and future. *International Review of Research in Developmental Disabilities*, *53*, 163–202. doi:10.1016/bs.irrdd.2017.08.001

Inuth. (2019). *Three Differently-Abled youngsters welcome you with a warm smile at this Kerala restaurant.* Retrieved October 5, 2019 from https://m.dailyhunt.in/news/india/english/inuth-epaper-inuth/three+differently+abled+youngsters+welcome+you+with+a+warm+smile+at+this+kerala+restaurant-newsid-112330821

Lee, C. E., Burke, M. M., & Stelter, C. R. (2019). Exploring the Perspectives of Parents and Siblings Toward Future Planning for Individuals With Intellectual and Developmental Disabilities. *Intellectual and Developmental Disabilities*, *57*(3), 198–211. doi:10.1352/1934-9556-57.3.198 PMID:31120401

Lindahl, J., Stollon, N., Wu, K., Liang, A., Changolkar, S., Steinway, C., ... Jan, S. (2019). Domains of planning for future long-term care of adults with intellectual and developmental disabilities: Parent and sibling perspectives. *Journal of Applied Research in Intellectual Disabilities*, jar.12600. doi:10.1111/jar.12600 PMID:31012229

Mohan Shriya. (2018). *A bridge to planet Autism.* Retrieved October 5, 2019 from https://www.thehindubusinessline.com/blink/cover/a-bridge-to-planet-autism/article23772834.ece

Myers, T. (2010). *Housing options for Adults with Autism Spectrum Disorder.* Bureau of Autism Services, Pennsylvania Department of Public Welfare. Retrieved October 5, 2019 from http://www.dhs.pa.gov/cs/groups/webcontent/documents/report/p_012904.pdf

News Hook. (2018). *SENS: A special show for special minds.* Retrieved October 5, 2019 from https://newzhook.com/story/19420

Pareekh. (2015). *Sai Bakery: A Mother's sweet gift to her Autistic son and his differently abled friends*. Retrieved October 5, 2019 from https://www.thebetterindia.com/22773/sai-bakery-chennai-adults-with-special-needs/

Swaminathan, A. (2015). Transition Planning in adolescents with Low Functioning Autism. *The Indian Journal of Occupational Therapy*, *47*(3), 67–71.

Think Change India. (2019). *This Kolkata Café has a unique offering besides cupcakes and cookies*. Retrieved October 5, 2019 from https://yourstory.com/socialstory/2019/05/kolkata-cafe-sip-n-bite-specially-abled-team

Vaidya, S. (2016). *Autism and the family in urban India: Looking back, looking forward*. Springer. doi:10.1007/978-81-322-3607-8

KEY TERMS AND DEFINITIONS

Autism: Autism is a life-long neurodevelopmental condition characterized by difficulties in social communication, restricted & repetitive behaviors and sensory processing issues.

Neuro-Diversity: It is a concept where neurological differences are respected as any other difference. It means that there are differences in brain, and workings of brain, and thus conditions like Autism are not 'abnormal'. Neuro-diverse people perceive the world differently from neuro-typical people.

Residential Facility: A facility where the autistic individual lives after the death of parents or when the parents become incapable of providing further care. The residential facility can be independent living, sibling co-residential systems, in the form of group homes, or in the form of campus-oriented systems.

Respite Care: Temporary care unit for persons with disabilities so that their usual caregivers can attend any medical emergency or other works or simply getting relieved from the care-giving process for a few days.

Chapter 4
Enhancing Life Skills of Children and Adolescents With Autism Spectrum Disorder and Intellectual Disabilities Through Technological Supports:
A Selective Overview

Fabrizio Stasolla
https://orcid.org/0000-0003-1626-9664
University Giustino Fortunato of Benevento, Italy

Anna Passaro
University Giustino Fortunato of Benevento, Italy

ABSTRACT

This chapter provides the reader with the newest empirical contributions available on the use of assistive technology-based interventions aimed at enhancing life skills of children and adolescents with autism spectrum disorders and developmental or intellectual disabilities. A selective overview along the last decade was carried out. Eighteen studies were reviewed, and 155 participants were involved. Five main categories of studies were identified, namely (1) emotional regulation, (2) communication skills, (3) academic performance, (4) social inclusion, and (5) challenging behavior. Results were fairly positive, although occasional failures occurred. Clinical, educational, psychological, and rehabilitative implications of the findings were critically discussed. Some useful guidelines for future research and practice were highlighted.

DOI: 10.4018/978-1-7998-3069-6.ch004

INTRODUCTION

Children and adolescents diagnosed with autism spectrum disorders (ASD), may be frequently socially, communicatively, and emotionally impaired. They may present stereotypic and tantrum behaviors, self-injuries, isolation, passivity, and withdrawal. Learning difficulties and lack of positive interactions with their surrounding world and/or environment are usually embedded. Furthermore, individuals with ASD may have few adaptive responses available in their own behavioral repertoire and fail to constructively engage while dealing with functional activities of daily life accordingly. Because they are commonly unable of positively participate in occupational tasks once enrolled in everyday life (e.g., community, medical rehabilitative and/or medical centers, school classroom), their social desirability, image, and status are significantly hampered, implying deleterious outcomes on their quality of life (Chen, Leader, Sung, & Leahy, 2015; Felce & Perry, 1995; Konst & Matson, 2014; Matson & Sturmey, 2011; Stasolla, Damiani, & Caffò, 2014; Stasolla, Perilli, & Damiani, 2014). Additionally, students with ASD may be affected by intellectual disabilities (ID). Either they evince low, moderate, or significant ID and developmental delays (DD), they continuously depend on caregivers' aid. Because their clinical conditions are relevantly compromised, the challenging behaviors above described may negatively interfere with daily regular functioning (e.g., monitoring and management of executive functions, emotional regulation, academic achievements, inclusion in daily contexts). Moreover, ASD and ID population may pose serious problems to conventional interventions (e.g., stimulation sessions and speech therapies). Thus, the self-determination and independence of children with ASD and DD may be relevantly compromised (Matson & Jang, 2014; Politte, Howe, Nowinski, Palumbo, & McDougle, 2015; Sanchack & Thomas, 2016). One way to tackle the aforementioned issues is to resort on assistive technology-based (AT) interventions (Lancioni & Singh, 2014; Lancioni, Sigafoos, O'Reilly, & Singh, 2012; Smith, Atmatzidis, Capogreco, Lloyd-Randolfi, Seman, 2017; Stasolla, Boccasini, & Perilli, 2017).

For example, a child with ASD and ID may be included in a microswitch cluster technology-based intervention for occupational activities. Thus, the participant may be constructively engaged in a functional task as sorting objects in a container while the mouthing behavior is progressively reduced. The dual simultaneous objective of improving a positive behavior and reducing the challenging response is pursued through the microswitch cluster technology (i.e., two optic sensors fixed in a container available in front of the child and on the child's chin in an adapted frame respectively constitute the cluster, see Stasolla, Perilli et al., 2017).

Furthermore, a participant with ASD and ID may be introduced and taught to learning activities administrated through cardboards or a touch screen support. The support preference was assessed in a choice evaluation and quantitative analysis was performed on items concerning both communicative skills and challenging behavior (Brunero, Venerosi, Chiarotti, & Arduino, 2019). Moreover, a student who attended the primary school and was aged of 7.5 year with a diagnosis of moderate intellectual impairment with communication delays was exposed to a two-part six-week study with a starting twenty-one days suitability training followed by a twenty-one days longitudinal effectiveness training. Both training included the implementation of a socio-emotional program, twice per day, with an assistive smart-glasses-based technology. Educators filled pre-intervention and post-intervention *Aberrant Behavior Checklist* (ABC) at the beginning of the suitability training and weekly during the effectiveness training. Primary data evidenced enhancements in the ABC sub-scales (Vahabzadeh et al., 2018).

The above described programs may: (a) have positive outcomes on participants' happiness, (b) decrease relevantly caregivers' s burden, (c) corroborate the integration of children and adolescents with

ASD in daily settings, and (d) be corroborated by external raters who have either a personal or a professional experience in the field through social ratings (e.g., caregivers and support teachers, or parents of children with learning difficulties) (Lancioni, O'Reilly, et al., 2006; Lancioni, Singh, et al., 2006; Stasolla, Caffò, et al., 2015).

In light of the above, the first objective of this contribution is to support the reader with a selective review of the newest evidence-based studies available on this specific topic. The second goal of the chapter is to outline the outcomes of the AT-based interventions on participants' quality of life (i.e., indices of happiness), active involvement (i.e., positive participation) and external rating (i.e., social validation). The third aim of the chapter is to underline advantageous and disadvantageous features of the retained empirical contributions. Lastly, the current review will critically argue on the rehabilitative consequences of the selective overview, emphasizing meaningful directions for both practice and research within this specific framework.

BACKGROUND

AT encompasses any piece, device, equipment or tool capable of enhancing independence and self-determination among children and adolescents with relevant DD. That is, by using an AT-based strategy, a person with ASD and ID will be enabled of self-manage the environmental events. Based on learning evidence (i.e., close and firm link between a behavioral response and environmental consequences), a participant with ASD and DD may learn the awareness of his/her own behavioral responses and use it for functional purposes (e.g., get a beverage whenever needed) independently (Alabbas & Miller, 2019; Bhat, Acharya, Adeli, Bairy, & Adeli, 2014; Stasolla, Perilli, & Boccasini, 2016). Consequently, both families and caregivers' burden may be notably reduced (Bozkurt, Uysal, & Duzkaya, 2019; Rogge & Janssen, 2019).

A basic form of AT is represented by microswitches (i.e., electronic tools ensuring persons with multiple disabilities with the autonomous getting to a short delivery of favorable stimuli). For example, a child with ASD and ID may enhance occupational activities and reduce hand/objects mouthing through a microswitch-cluster technology (Stasolla et al., 2017). Next to this goal, one may envisage aided-alternative and augmentative communication approaches (e.g., vocal output communication aids or speech generating devices) to improve the participant's social interaction with one or more caregivers (Gilroy, Leader, & McCleery, 2018). New technologies have recently generate a growing number of high technology-based devices combined to computer applications aimed at enhancing the participation of children and adolescents with ASD and ID (Johnston, Egermann, & Kearney, 2018; Koumpouros & Kafazis, 2019). Additionally, serious games finalized at improving both emotional regulation and social inclusion have been considered (Grossard et al., 2017; Lau, Smit, Fleming, & Riper, 2017; Tsikinas &. Xinogalos, 2018). In fact, emotional regulation, executive functions, academic tasks, functional and/or occupational activities, social inclusion are the crucial targeted behaviors among ASD population (Elmquist, Simacek, Dimian, & Reichle, 2019; Light et al., 2019; Schlosser & Koul, 2015).

According to the above, we attempted to present an overview of the contributions available on the use of AT-based interventions to improve life skills of children and adolescents with ASD and ID since we feel that a categorization on this specific topic was warranted. Because a wide range of AT devices or equipments have been currently used, our effort was to summarize and organize the retained studies keeping in mind the targeted behaviors (i.e., see the criterion stated in the following section).

METHOD

ASD, AT, DD, ID, quality of life, rehabilitative interventions, inclusion, academic performance, challenging behaviors, emotional regulation, executive functions, on-task behavior, and caregivers burden were merged in Scopus as keywords. A manual search was also performed as completion. The eligible criteria were (a) an AT-based program implemented, (b) children and adolescents enrolled as participants (i.e., from birth up to 19 years old) with ASD and ID, (c) English language of the study, (d) publication year along the last decade (i.e., 2010 - 2019 as time interval) as including criteria. Excluding criteria were (a) theoretical contribution, (b) book chapter, (c) conference paper, (d) an adult with ASD as participant (i.e., 20 year of age or oldest), (e) review paper, and other neuro-developmental disorders than ASD (e.g., ADHD and/or cerebral palsy) because their consideration would exceed the objective of the current overview. A selection of studies was retained accordingly. The empirical contributions were summarized according the targeted behaviors. Five basic groups were recognized, namely (a) emotional regulation, (b) communication skills, (c) academic performance, (d) social inclusion, and (e) challenging behavior. A concise description of each reviewed study was provided. A synoptic table with the contributors of the retained studies, the quantitative of the enrolled participants, their ages, the AT strategy implemented, and the effects was additionally included as further information. Overall, 18 studies were reviewed and 155 participants were involved.

SELECTIVE OVERVIEW

The reviewed studies, were summarized according to their functional goals (i.e., emotional regulation, communication skills, academic performance, social inclusion, and challenging behavior) and listed in table 1.

Emotional Regulation

One of the most common targeted behavior among ASD population is emotional regulation. In fact, children with ASD are frequently described as unable to manage their emotional responses. Beside aggression and tantrum behaviors, they may exhibit withdrawal and specific incapacities of integration among their peers because they are not positively occupied (Sturm, Peppe, & Ploog, 2016). AT-based interventions are usually focused on promoting constructive engagement of children with ASD and ID, regulating their social emotions, and facilitating their positive participation in daily settings (Bhat, Acharya, Adeli, Bairy, & Adeli, 2014). Four contributions were reviewed in this group with 57 individuals enrolled (Fage et al., 2019; Lahiri, Warren, & Sarkar, 2011; Torrado, Gomez, & Montoro, 2017; Tsangouri, Li, Zhu, Abtahi, & Ro, 2018).

Fage et al. (2019) exposed three groups of participants (i.e., adolescents who were aged between 14 and 15 years with ASD, ID, and a control group) to an AAC-based application delivered through a tablet dedicated to improve the self-management of emotional behaviors in an inclusive school setting. The technology relied on evidence-based emotional management programs reported by educators and parents through an active participatory design. Feasibility performance as well as academic performance (i.e., emotion-management effects) were evaluated. Results demonstrated that the technology was suitable, effective, and favorably implemented in the school setting. Additionally, participants with ASD were capable of regulating their emotions by their own using the AT-device. Social responses and learning associated with characteristics of ASD were adequately regulated.

Table 1. Reviewed studies grouped according their category and listed in alphabetic order

Authors	Participants	Ages	Category	AT device	Outcomes
Arthanat et al. (2013)	4	4	Academic	IPAD	Four positive
Borsos & Gyori (2017)	13	4-5	Inclusion	Serious Game	All positive
Copple et al. (2015)	3	4	Communication	SGD	Three positive
David et al. (in press)	5	3-5	Communication	Robot	One negative
Fage et al. (2018)	30	6-8	Inclusion	Mobile App	Three negative
Fage et al. (2019)	14	14-15	Emotional	Tablet	All positive
Flores et al. (2014)	10	3-11	Communication	IPAD	Two negative
Ganz et al. (2015)	1	5	Communication	VOCA	One positive
Hughes & Yakubova (2016)	10	7-10	Challenging	Video-based	All positive
Lahiri et al. (2011)	6	14-16	Emotional	Virtual Reality	Six positive
Mohan et al. (2019)	1	4	Communication	Assisted platform	One positive
Sigafoos et al. (2013)	2	4-5	Challenging	IPAD-SGD	Two positive
Stasolla et al. (2014)	3	8-10	Challenging	Microswitches	Three positive
Stasolla et al. (2016)	3	8-10	Academic	Tablet	Three positive
Stasolla et al. (2017)	6	6-10	Challenging	Microswitches	Six positive
Torrado et al. (2017)	2	10	Emotional	Smart-watch	Two positive
Tsangouri et al. (2018)	1	9	Emotional	Interactive platform	One positive
Valadao et al. (2016)	5	7-8	Inclusion	Robot	Five positive

Lahiri, Warren, and Sarkar (2011) examined a new virtual reality-based system (i.e., virtual reality-based interactions) with gaze-sensitive positive behavior technology (VIGART) with six adolescents who were diagnosed with ASD and moderate ID, aimed at enhancing emotional regulation and executive functions. Data emphasized the acceptability and the usefulness of VIGART. Results indicated the potential and the validity of the new technology based on the improvements in behavioral viewing and modifications in relevant eye physiological indexes of the participants while interacting with the technology itself.

Torrado, Gomez, and Montoro (2017) carried out an experiment with two children who were aged of 10 years, diagnosed with ASD, and evidenced a various emblematic repertoire of emotional abnormalities. Specifically, a smart-watch technology that implemented a large interval of self-management methodologies and inferred outcome patterns from physiological data and movement was adopted, contingently with meaningful tool for smart-phones that was to be implemented by educators or parents to support the use of the strategies in a profitable mode. Both participants learned to use suitable useers-tailored emotional self-regulation approaches by means of the technology, improving from the majority of mild stress events and modulate tantrum behaviors in the nine days of the experiment conducted in the school setting.

Tsangouri, Li, Zhu, Abtahi, and Ro (2018) fostered the emotional facial recognition and the appropriate emotional responding of a child with autism who were aged of 9 years through an interactive technology that used deep learning to record customer's facial outcome from a wearable technological aid and assisted the participant in acquiring the meaning of facial expressions and understand how to produce them. Empirical data underlined the effectiveness of the platform and outlined its validity to promote facial expressions recognition.

Communication Skills

A critical issue for children and adolescents with ASD and DD or ID is represented by the communication skills. Because they are communicatively impaired, individuals with autism are unable to profitably communicate their daily needs. Thus, AT-based strategies with both low and/or high levels of technology complexity such as the *picture exchange communication system* (PECS) by Bondy and Frost (2001) and the vocal output communication aid (VOCA) (Sigafoos et al., 2004) are focused on the improvement of the participants' options of selecting their needs (e.g., leisure solution). Otherwise, one may envisage their systematic comparability and evaluate the participants' preferences (Beck, Stoner, Bock, & Parton, 2008; Bock, Stoner, Beck, Hanley, & Prochnow, 2005). Lately, the upgrading of new (high) technological equipments outline the adoption of new speech generating devices (SGD) (Kagohara et al., 2013; Rispoli, Franco, Van der Meer, Lang, & Camargo, 2010; Van der Meer & Rispoli, 2010; Van der Meer, Sigafoos, O'Reilly, & Lancioni, 2011). That is, I-Pad, I-Pod, personal computers and tablets have been positively implemented with ASD and/or ID participants. That is, at least one may state that AT-based programs increase the autonomy of the enrolled participants in those interventions (Waddington, 2018). Five contributions were retained in this section with 22 participants included (Copple, Koul, Banda, & Frye, 2015; David, Costescu, Matu, Sventagotai, & Dobrean, *in press*; Flores et al., 2014; Ganz, Hong, Goodwyn, Kite, & Gilliland, 2015; Mohan, Kunnath, Philip, Mohan, & Thampi, 2019).

For instance, Copple, Koul, Banda, and Frye (2015) evaluated the implementation of a SGD for learning opprtunities of three pre-school participants with risk of autism. That is, the intervention was conducted through a multiple baseline design across participants (Barlow, Nock, & Hersen, 2009) and assessed if the children were capable of the independent access to an object following a video-modeling program. Furthermore, the intervention was aimed at considering if the children involved were successfully capable of extend their acquisition across settings. Data emphasized that all participants learned that ability and generalized it. Accordingly, the intervention was suitable to enhance communication among non-verbal individuals.

David, Costescu, Matu, Sventagotai, & Dobrean (*in press*) presented five single-subject interventions with participants who were diagnosed with ASD aged between 3 and 5 years. Each participant received 20 trials (i.e., 8 robot-enhanced trials, that is robot-enhanced intervention, 8 standard human-trial, and 4 trials with the program which was more effective of both), aimed at assessing the efficacy of a robot-fostered training on turn-taking capacities. The goal was to clarify to what level social robot could enhance turn-taking capacities and if this group of program produced similar or better advantages than typical program. Both strategies were equally effective. Nevertheless, in the robot-mediated options, participants appeared to see their partners as more engaged and involved than their human partner, because they were more directed at the robotic partner.

Flores et al. (2014) investigated literacy-based behavioral interventions to increase interactive comprehension and varied the behavior of participants with ASD and DD. Additionally, the Picture Exchange Communication System (i.e., PECS) was implemented to facilitate communication, evoke structure, and change response for the same participants. The contribution considered literacy-based behavioral program by using an Apple IPAD as an AT device to deliver social stories and literacy access opportunities to students who were aged between 3 and 11 years enrolled in an extended intervention. Results revealed that the AT device was effective for improving communication skills of the included participants.

Ganz, Hong, Goodwyn, Kite and Gilliland (2015) carried out an AT-based program, which used a tablet with a voice output for increasing the receptive communicative skills of interpreting photos by a participant estimated with ASD. The child was a preschool little boy with few intelligible verbal language. The investigation was conducted according to a multi-baseline design across words. Results evidenced a partial enhancement for the enrolled participant in the reception for two of the three retained words.

Mohan, Kunnath, Philip, Mohan, and Thampi (2019) discussed the use of a person-centered clinical strategy finalized at the application of an assisted communication program to prevent negative outcomes derived from severe communication deficits of a 4-year child with ASD and ID. The initial assessment outlined basic rudimental communication skills with significant dysfunctions at oral, olfactory, and tactile levels. Stereotypic behaviors were also observed, combined to a complete dependence on caregiver's assistance. Following a customer-tailored picture-based communication intervention the mother was used as communicator facilitator. This approach was no more embedded in the intervention program because the participant' s performance was low as well as the mother's level of acceptance of picture-based intervention. A favorable choice option for printed material was registered. Consequently, supplementary monitoring was tailored on adopting a computerized system as a part of an alternative augmentative communication strategy (AAC), which was taught along few months. A remarkable improvement was finally observed in the child's communication skills.

Academic Performance

A further relevant group is undoubtedly represented by the enhancement of academic performance. In fact, individuals with ASD and ID may experience relevant difficulties within school settings because their learning process is impaired with negative outcomes on their academic achievements. AT-based strategies may be effective for their support, with beneficial consequences on the class management because those strategies may facilitate their independence and self-determination while pursuing the academic goals (Nicolaidis, Kripke, & Raymaker, 2014; Sigafoos et al., 2019: Smith, Atmatzidis, Capogreco, Lloyd-Randolfi, & Seman, 2017). Nevertheless, only two contributions were reviewed within this section with seven participants enrolled (Arthanat, Kurtin, & Knotak, 2013; Stasolla et al., 2016).

Arthanat, Kurtin, and Knotak (2013) evaluated the application of the Apple IPAD for teaching purposes to four participants with ASD and DD. A single-case design was implemented to demonstrate the participation of the children's performance when taught with their standard computer at baseline, and at the introduction of the IPAD (i.e. intervention phase). A six-component participation test was evaluated to determine the number of the measures of the participants during the trials. Graphical inspection revealed no differences between the conditions for three participants. Conversely, the fourth participant showed a significant higher level of participation in the IPAD condition. Individual modifications were recorded for each participant on on-task behavior, task engagement, and goal oriented behavior with the implementation of the IPAD. Although academic performance improved during training, its adoption seemed not to be sufficiently justified over the computer and vice-versa for positively completing academic activities in participants with autism and DD.

Stasolla et al. (2016) exposed three participants with ASD and mild ID, who were aged between 8 and 10 years, to a computerized tablet-based intervention with an adapted software in a school setting. The program was aimed at improving the academic trend through a multi-step strategy, which was expected to increase the participants' on-task behavior. Additionally, the generalization process at participants' home, and the reduction of the repetitive behaviors (i.e., hand clapping, washing, and voice noises) were monitored. Finally, a social rating including 48 teachers was conducted. Data showed an increased academic performance and an improvement of the on-task behavior of all the participants, who reduced their stereotyped responses. Moreover, they extended their acquisition once it was transferred into their homes. External teachers favorably rated the implementation of an AT-based program.

Social Inclusion

A critical concern which involves caregivers, clinicians, practitioners, and researchers is surely the social inclusion of individuals with ASD and DD. The positive management of individuals with autism in daily settings is systematically warranted and highly recommended. The specific purpose may be pursued through AT-based interventions because this specific approach is focused on the enhancement of positive participation and constructive engagement in students with ASD and DD. Within this framework serious games may play a central role since they promote social interactions among peers. Computer-based process through serious games is emphasized as highly promising for fostering social inclusion of people with ASD and ID (Tsikinas & Xinogalos, 2018). Three studies were included in this section (Borsos & Gyori, 2017; Fage et al., 2018; Valadao et al., 2016), with 48 participants included.

Borsos and Gyori (2017) carried out an exploratory investigation of emotional recognition adopting an available facial expression computerized system with an adapted software, from the context of a serious game for evaluation objectives. Data, assessed on comparative analysis of two matched groups of kindergarten-age participants (i.e., thirteen participants with ASD and thirteen typically developed participants) emphasized that the technology could recognize autism-specific emotion expression characteristics, and had a specific function in AT-based strategies and affective diagnosis.

Fage et al. (2018) exposed 50 participants (i.e., thirty with ASD, of which twenty with ID) to a set of wearable applications which embedded both assistive and cognitive rehabilitation systems to enhance first class inclusion of students with autism. The applications were examined in a 3-month program in both home and school settings. Positive outcomes on social dependent variables and measures were considered. Data evidenced that the experimental group with ASD enhanced the socio-cognitive skills in school setting. Both groups improved their socio-cognitive functioning.

Valadao et al. (2016) recruited 5 children who attended the primary school (i.e., their ages ranged between 7 and 8 years) with ASD for promoting the inclusion and social interaction through a customer-tailored robot with a special costume and a monitor enabling the access to multimedia contents. The interaction between the robot and the participants was evaluated. A mediator controlled the robot's movement in an environment for the interactive training. Dependent variables were eye gazing, touching the robot, and imitating the mediator. The relationship was analyzed through the *Goal Attainment Scale* and Likert scale. The experimental group doubled the control group in terms of performance while interacting with the robot. Additionally, ASD children looked away and followed the mediator similarly to the control group and evidenced extra social skills (i.e., both verbal and non-verbal skills).

Challenging Behavior

A final section is dedicated to the challenging behavior. Challenging behaviors are broadly described as deleterious behaviors because commonly have negative effects on the everyday normal functioning of individuals with ASD and DD (Hutchins & Prelock, 2014; Walton & Ingersoll, 2015). Stereotyped and repetitive behaviors such as hand/clapping, washing or mouthing are usually included, added to hyperactivity, impulsivity, drooling, incorrect postural movements and/or psychological problems such as passivity, anxiety, isolation, and withdrawal (Jones, Gliga, Bedford, Charman, & Johnson, 2014). AT-based programs focused on cognitive-behavioral approaches are generally finalized at pursuing the dual objective of enhancing a positive behavior and decreasing the challenging response (Matson, 2012). Within this section 4 contributions were reviewed with 21 participants included (Huges & Yakubova, 2016; Sigafoos et al., 2013; Stasolla et al., 2014, 2017).

Huges and Yakubova (2016) implemented a video-based intervention (VBI) for teaching academic skills and reducing challenging behavior of ten participants with ASD and ID. VBI enabled the participants with social skills, communication and functional behaviors, and self-help skills. VBI allowed options to automatically provide tailored, pertinent and prerecorded instructions. Handled tools such as smart-phones and tablets made the VBI manageable for students with autism. The VBI successfully taught adaptive skills and decreased challenging behaviors of the participants involved.

Sigafoos et al. (2013) exposed two non-verbal participants with ASD to an AAC-based program with a VOCA device to request the continuation to play. Moreover, a challenging behavior such as disruptive response was also measured. The investigation was carried out according to a non-concurrent multiple baseline design across participants. Data evidenced that both participants learned the functional use of the AAC device for asking the continuation to play and decreased, at the same time the disruptive behavior (i.e., aggression). That is, both boys substututed the challenging behavior (with an adaptive (i.e., functional) use of the AAC device (i.e., IPAD) for requesting the continuation to play.

Stasolla et al. (2014) examined the use of a microswitch-cluster technology (i.e., electronic sensors enabling people with multiple disabilities to independently access to positive stimulation through a system unit control) in three children with ASD and ID within home setting. Specifically, the cluster provided the boys with the dual rehabilitative goal of increasing an adaptive behavior (i.e., manipulating an object) through a wobble microswitch (i.e., a ball fixed in front of the participant) that should be pulled, pushed or moved side way to be activated) and decreasing the challenging behavior of objects/hand mouthing recorded through an optic sensor fixed on participants' chin with an adaptive frame. Both sensors (i.e., wobble and optic sensors) represented the cluster. The study was conducted according to an ABB^1AB^1 experimental design, where A indicated baselines, B the intervention aimed at increasing the adaptive behavior irrespective of the challenging response, and B^1 the cluster phases, where the adaptive behaviors were positively reinforced only if it occurred with the absence of the challenging behaviors. Intervals with indices of happiness (i.e., smiling, laughing, energized body movements with or without vocalizations) as outcome measure of the positive mood were additionally considered. Data evidenced that all participants relevantly enhanced their performance (i.e., increased adaptive responses and indices of happiness and decreased challenging behaviors) during both cluster phases compared to baselines.

Stasolla et al. (2017) generalized the implementation of a microswitch-cluster technology to six children with ASD and severe to profound ID for functional activities. The first objective of the study was to increase the adaptive responding (i.e., sorting an object) and simultaneously reduce mouthing as a challenging behavior. The second goal was to evaluate its effects on the participants' indices of happiness. The third aim was to carry out a 3-month follow-up. Finally, a social rating assessment invcluding 60 external raters was collected. Data emphasized an increased functional activity and a reduced challenging behavior for all the participants enrolled, who maintained their performance over the time. Social raters positively considered the use of such technology.

DISCUSSION

Data were fairly encouraging, although few failures occurred (4%). AT-based interventions were effective and suitable at promoting independence and self-determination along the life skills of individuals diagnosed with ASD and ID. Their emotional control was adequately regulated. Their academic tasks were successfully achieved. Their communication abilities and social inclusion in daily settings were fostered. Their challenging behaviors were meaningfully reduced because they were constructively engaged and positively occupied. Whenever available, data demonstrated that the implemented interventions were both clinically and socially valid. The participants enjoyed the sessions and were favorably involved. Data were supported by previous findings (Chen, Leader, Sung, & Leahy, 2015; Koumpouros & Kafazis, 2019; Schlosser & Koul, 2015; Smith, Atmatzidis, Capogreco, Lloyd-Randolfi, & Seman, 2017) and suggested the following considerations.

Identifying a suitable AT-based program may have different effects for different individuals. For instance, depending on their levels of either intellectual or motor capacities, one may rely on the automatic access to positive stimulation (i.e., for participants with ASD and severe to profound DD and ID). Else, one may consider a combined microswitch and VOCA-based intervention for those individuals who are dealing with the choice options between the automatic access to positive stimulation and asking for the social contact with a caregiver (Lancioni et al., 2009). Screening the environmental consequences that the individual can receive directly through microswitch activations and/or the VOCA, which mediated the social contacts represents a crucial issue. The selection of stimuli is commonly conducted through both indirect and direct procedures, such as through informal interviews with parents, staff and caregivers, and stimulus preference screening strategy, or empirical observations of the individuals within their daily life contexts and settings (Crawford & Schuster, 1993). Two preliminary suggestions could easily ameliorate the chance of success, namely (a) the selection and implementation of more than one stimulus so as to prevent satiation and saturation risks, and (b) protraction of the screening preferences over the time as to ensure that the environmental events are related to the person's current agreements (Kennedy, 2005). Otherwise, one could apply a microswitch-cluster technology for reaching the dual objective of enhancing an adaptive response and decreasing a challenging behavior, as detailed in the study conducted by Stasolla et al. (2014).

As further opportunity, one may recommend the enhancement of both expressive and receptive communication skills with a more sophisticated equipment (i.e., high technology) such as an I-Pad, I-Pod, a personal computer, and/or a tablet. That is, by implementing various options offered by the AT tool, a child with ASD may communicate their needs (e.g., leisure option) autonomously and access to them alone or with the mediation of an educator (Stasolla, Caffò, Picucci, & Bosco, 2013). Furthermore, one may envisage a high technology-based device (e.g., virtual reality, smart-phone) for fostering positive behaviors (e.g., as reminder and/or providing both visual and verbal istructions to profitably achieve complex tasks through a task analysis procedure) (Lancioni et al., 2014). The detailed above promising findings may have positive consequences on indices of happiness of the enrolled participants as dependent variable and outcome of their quality of life (Felce & Perry, 1995). Moreover, those rehabilitative interventions may be formally endorsed by external raters (e.g., psychologists, parents, practitioners, educators) involved within social validation procedures as to corroborate both social and clinical efficacy of the programs (Caffò et al., 2014; Perilli et al., 2013a, 2013b). Lastly, the inclusion individuals with ASD was relevantly enhanced in school settings with beneficial effects on the class management (Ismaili & Ibrahimi, 2017; Stasolla, Caffò, et al., 2017; Stasolla, Perilli, et al., 2017). The data were further confirmed by previous contributions (Campbell & Mears, 2009; Reber, 2009; Spence-Cochran & Pearl, 2012; Tsui, Feil-Seifer, Mataric, & Yanco, 2009) and recommended the following considerations.

First, assistive technology-based programs and cognitive-behavioural interventions may be considered as significant and crucial psychological and practical options helpful for fostering independence, positive participation, constructive engagement and direct involvement of individuals with ASD and DD. That is, by ensuring both children and adolescents with ASD with active interactions towards the outside world, one may emphasize their gratification, pleasure, and high motivation in choosing their environmental consequences by their own. Thus, one may claim that within this strategy individuals with ASD and DD decrease their isolation, avoiding passivity and withdrawal with beneficial effects on their quality of life. Furthermore, the above described approaches may constitute a basic modality of intervention with clinical implications for both research and practice (Lancioni & Singh, 2014; Stasolla, Damiani, et al., 2015).

Second, by fostering their communicative skills, imncreasing their social and life abilities, and reducing their challenging responses, individuals with ASD and DD are more frequently included in daily settings such as home, medical, rehabilitative and school environments, with a significant reduction of caregivers' burden (Mulroy, Robertson, Aiberti, Leonard, & Bower, 2008). That is, participants with ASD and DD will be ensured with communication opportunities, increased options of request and choice desired events, and the independent access to items automatically delivered through the technological system or with the mediation of the caregiver. Morover, by enhancing their active role, recreation and leisure options in such activities, they would decrease their need of exhibiting stereotypic or repetitive behaviors, with beneficial effects on their quality of life (Lancioni, Singh, et al., 2006). Beside their inclusion, participants with ASD and severe to profound DD would learn new adaptive responses, and would be enabled with positive and high motivating (external and/or environmental) stimulation (Lancioni et al., 2012; Lancioni & Singh, 2014).

Third, a customer-tailored intervention such as those proposed in the current overview is relevantly critical for any participant with ASD and DD. Hence, by designing an intervention with the described options strictly customized for one person and differing their suitability depending on the individual's features, it provides their feasibility for various children and adolescents with ASD and/or other DD. Moreover, often their costs are low (i.e., cheap or not expensive) and they could accordingly be implemented on a large quantity of users, emphasizing a basic modality to apply those programs in everyday ecological conditions (Lancioni, Comes, et al., 2005; Stasolla, Perilli, & Damiani, 2014; Stasolla, Damiani, & Caffò, 2014). That is, their affordability is corroborated. Indeed, their close upgrading according the complexity of the individuals depending on their features and/or clinical conditions due to their pathology is warranted (Brown, Schalock, & Brown, 2009).

Fourth, a wide number of the enrolled participants along the different reviewed contributions appreciated the sessions, with an improving of their positive mood during the intervention phases compared to baselines (i.e., for those investigations where this specific dependent variable was measured). Moreover, the individuals corrobotated their enjoyment over the time. That is, by differentiating systematically the environmental consequences as rewarding events for consolidating the adaptive responses learned by the participants, one may argue that their active role, favorable occupation, satisfaction, and fulfilment were enhanced, preventing satiation ad saturation, with encouraging consequences on their quality of life (Lancioni et al., 2005). Because the participants maintained their performance over the time, one may state that the implemented programs were efficient and useful in increasing positive mood of the individuals involved (De Pace & Stasolla, 2014).

Fifth, challenging behaviours relevantly decreased during interventions phases. Thus, by being positively occupied, highly motivated, and motivated by positive stimuli automatically provided by the technological systems contingently to the exhibition of an adaptive response, participants redirected the repetitive behaviors, spending less time while engaged with stereotypic responses. Moreover, their social image and status with their acceptance as a consequence were relevantly supported, once more with positive consequences on their quality of life (De Pace & Stasolla, 2014; Matson & Sturmey, 2011). It was not a given fact since both (i.e., adaptive responding and challenging behaviour) are never mutually exclusive.

Sixth, social validity (i.e., clinical and practical) was widely confirmed by follow-up, generalization, and/or maintenance phases and preference checks and/or social rating, whenever recorded. That is, either the enrolled participants (i.e., through preference checks) and social experts (i.e., with social assessments) corroborated the efficacy of the rehabilitative interventions implemented within the reviewed contributions. Thus, both internal (i.e., participants included) and external (i.e., social validation experts) formally corroborated the above detailed approaches (Caffò, et al., 2014; Lancioni, O'Reilly, et al., 2006).

Seventh, promising evidences and positive outcomes of an assistive technology-based intervention would largely rely on four basic elements, that is: (a) behavioural response(s) retained and requested by the participant, (b) positive stimulation screened as motivating rewarding, (c) technological options implemented, and (d) extension along the day (Lancioni et al., 2005). Regarding the first point, one should claim that the more preferable would be the one easily exhibited by the participant within his/her repertoire (i.e., exhibited without effort), produced with external prompt (i.e., physical, verbal or both combined togrther), objectively recordable, and affordably registered by the technological option (e.g., microswitch). Regarding the second point, it should be highly rewarding, motivating, and systematically differentiated within the same implemented intervention. Thus, by identifying highly motivating (i.e., pleasant) stimulation to be used as environmental consequence, one may significantly decrease the response cost for the individual (i.e., the fatigue required to produce and exhibit the adaptive behavior) and by differentiating systematically the favourable stimulation, saturation is significantly avoided. Lastly, by enlarging the interval of the time along the day and by proposing it along the week, the rehabilitative intervention may constitute a promising educational and psychological strategy, which should be systematically considered for children and adolescents with ASD and DD in daily settings. (Lancioni & Singh, 2014; Stasolla, Caffò, et al., 2015).

Eighth, their inclusion in mainstream classrooms was fostered. Thus, they successfully achieved their academic tasks through basic AT-based devices or equipments. The participants enhanced their performance and allowed a profitably management of the classes. Because their independence and self-determination were enhanced, both teachers and parents' burden was relevantly reduced, with positive consequences on their daily life. In fact, the participants with ASD were constructively engaged and positively occupied (Benssassi, Gomez, Boyd, Hayes, & Ye, 2018; Boucenna et al., 2014).

CONCLUSION

The literature overview emphasized five basic groups of contributions with different rehabilitative objectives to promote the success of children and adolescents diagnosed with ASD and DD or ID. The effects of the included interventions were widely satisfactory. However, caution was undoubtedly needed while interpreting some of these findings. Thus, questions emerged about (a) some of the outcomes (i.e., dependent measures) used to evaluate the effects of the programs and some of the evidence available about them, (b) the absence of control over the time variable evidenced along some of the contributions, and (c) the lack of direct emphasis on the participants' awareness of a constructive engagement role. Given the above detailed limits and the contingent caution mandatory to interpret part of the available literature, the need to extend the research activity seems to be necessary. Moreover, it is indeed critical to examine the retained contributions in light of (a) their size (i.e., the quantitative significance of the observed modifications in the targeted behaviors) and (b) their fidelity depending on the experimental conditions underlying the programs (Barlow, Nock, & Hersen, 2009; Kazdin, 2001; Kennedy, 2005).

Regarding the first point, one may argue that there were relevant variations among the contributions. Many of them reported statistically and functionally relevant changes in the participants' behavior, which were coded through specific scales or by means of response frequencies (Taube-Schiff, Suvak, Antony, Bieling, & McCabe, 2007). Other contributions (a) included modifications which were not strictly linked to scales or response frequencies but rather to behavioral ratings reported by professionals included in the rehabilitative strategy and other representative figures and/or (b) pointed out partial, inconclusive or negative statistical significance e on formal measures (Lancioni et al., 2012). The outcomes of the contributions using single-subject designs could be taken as more reliable and valid, since these experimental designs allow for the control over the time (history) measure (Kennedy, 2005). Quantitative significance and validity are the two basic criteria on which to evaluate the results. A supplementary criterion could be the practical and clinical significance of changes observed in terms of participants' positive participation and constructive engagement. Regarding this criterion, it might be noticed that not all the contributions assess this outcome, but it is becoming more frequent.

FUTURE RESEARCH

In light of the above, the future directions for both research and practice should look at the following framework. A first research effort could be focused on evaluating the generalization of assistive technologies, such as microswitches, I-Pad, I.Pod, VOCA, smart phones, tablets and adapted software embedded in computerized programs for other children with severe to profound developmental disabilities (e.g., post-coma patients). Those efforts should analyze the following characteristics: (a) the large literature on the practical and clinical application of this strategy in other rehabilitation trades, such as in the area of acquired or congenital pathology (e.g., rare genetic syndromes); (b) the ethical issues related to assess if the participants' legal representatives may consider the implementation of such strategy; and (c) the opportunity to emphasize methodological issues and concerns so as to recommend that the use of this strategy to any performance enhancement can be undoubtedly observed. Moreover, AT-based rehabilitative interventions should include the individual's involvement in the choice-making and his/her positive interaction with the external environment (Lancioni & Singh, 2014).

A second future direction may examine the maintenance, the generalization and settings the over time. Regarding the first point, one may envisage rehabilitative interventions in different contexts, including school, home, or community. Regarding to the second point, one may evaluate different tasks, educators, psychologists, speech therapists or physiotherapists concerned in the rehabilitative strategies. Regarding the third point, one may analyze generalization, maintenance, and/or post intervention sessions added to preference checks by participants enrolled, as systematically included within those contributions.

A third perspective may relate to the new technologies. One assess new euipments and new technological devices responding to participants' features on the one hand and to contexts' resources on the other. Recently, serious games have been commonly adopted and used for improving the positive participation, active role, and communication skills of children and adolescents with ASD and DD (Boucenna et al., 2014). Regarding participants' features, one may examine new technologies that ensure that participants can be positively occupied with minimal effort while identifying new behavioral responses and/or functional activities. Regarding the second point, one should evaluate both human and financial resources available among families and rehabilitative centers.

REFERENCES

Alabbas, N. A., & Miller, D. E. (2019). Challenges and assistive technology during typical routines: Perspectives of caregivers of children with autism spectrum disorders and other disabilities. *International Journal of Disability Development and Education*, *66*(3), 273–283. doi:10.1080/1034912X.2019.1578864

Arthanat, S., Curtin, C., & Knotak, D. (2013). Comparative observations of learning engagement by students with developmental disabilities using an iPad and computer: A pilot study. *Assistive Technology*, *25*(4), 204–213. doi:10.1080/10400435.2012.761293 PMID:24620703

Barlow, D. H., Nock, M., & Hersen, M. (2009). *Single-case experimental designs: Strategies for studying behavior change* (3rd ed.). New York: Ally & Bacon.

Beck, A. R., Stoner, J. B., Bock, S. J., & Parton, T. (2008). Comparison of PECS and the use of a VOCA: A replication. *Education and Training in Developmental Disabilities*, *43*, 198–216.

Benssassi, E. M., Gomez, J., Boyd, L. A. E., Hayes, G. R., & Ye, J. (2018). Wearable assistive technologies for autism: Opportunities and challenges. *IEEE Pervasive Computing*, *17*(2), 11–21. doi:10.1109/MPRV.2018.022511239

Bhat, S., Acharya, U. R., Adeli, H., Bairy, G. M., & Adeli, A. (2014). Autism: Cause factors, early diagnosis and therapies. *Reviews in the Neurosciences*, *25*(6), 841–850. doi:10.1515/revneuro-2014-0056 PMID:25222596

Bock, S. J., Stoner, J. B., Beck, A. R., Hanley, L., & Prochnow, J. (2005). Increasing functional communication in non-speaking preschool children: Comparison of PECS and VOCA. *Education and Training in Developmental Disabilities*, *40*, 264–278.

Borsos, Z., & Gyori, M. (2017). *Can automated facial expression analysis show differences between autism and typical functioning?* Doi:10.3233/978-1-61499-798-6-797

Boucenna, S., Narzisi, A., Tilmont, E., Muratori, F., Pioggia, G., Cohen, D., & Chetouani, M. (2014). Interactive technologies for autistic children: A review. *Cognitive Computation*, *6*(4), 722–740. doi:10.100712559-014-9276-x

Bozkurt, G., Uysal, G., & Duzkaya, D. S. (2019). Examination of care burden and stress coping styles of parents of children with autism spectrum disorder. *Journal of Pediatric Nursing, 47*, 142-147.

Brown, R. I., Schalock, R. L., & Brown, I. (2009). Quality of life: Its application to persons with intellectual disabilities and their families-introduction and overview. *Journal of Policy and Practice in Intellectual Disabilities*, *6*(1), 2–6. doi:10.1111/j.1741-1130.2008.00202.x

Brunero, F., Venerosi, A., Chiarotti, F., & Arduino, G. M. (2019). Are touch screen technologies more effective than traditional educational methods in children with autism spectrum disorders? A pilot study. *Annali dell'Istituto Superiore di Sanita*, *55*, 151–160. PMID:31264638

Caffò, A. O., Hoogeveen, F., Groenendaal, M., Perilli, V., Damen, M., Stasolla, F., ... Bosco, A. (2014). Comparing two different orientation strategies for promoting indoor traveling in people with Alzheimer's disease. *Research in Developmental Disabilities*, *35*(2), 572–580. doi:10.1016/j.ridd.2013.12.003 PMID:24380786

Campbell, J. E., & Mears, K. M. (2009). *Habilitative treatments for children with ASDs: Speech and occupational therapy, assistive technology*. doi:10.1017/CBO9780511978616.010

Chen, J. L., Leader, G., Sung, C., & Leahy, M. (2015). Trends in employment for individuals with autism spectrum disorder: A review of the research literature. *Research Journal of Autism and Developmental Disorders*, *2*(2), 115–127. doi:10.100740489-014-0041-6

Copple, K., Koul, R., Banda, D., & Frye, E. (2015). An examination of the effectiveness of video modelling intervention using a speech-generating device in preschool children at risk for autism. *Developmental Neurorehabilitation*, *18*(2), 104–112. doi:10.3109/17518423.2014.880079 PMID:24564246

Crawford, M. R., & Schuster, J. W. (1993). Using microswitches to teach toy use. *Journal of Developmental and Physical Disabilities*, *5*(4), 349–368. doi:10.1007/BF01046391

David, D. O., Costescu, C. A., Matu, S., Szentagotai, A., & Dobrean, A. (in press). Effects of a robot-enhanced intervention for children with ASD on teaching turn-taking skills. *Journal of Educational Computing Research*. doi:10.1177/0735633119830344

De Pace, C., & Stasolla, F. (2014). Promoting Environmental Control, Social Interaction, and Leisure/Academy Engagement Among People with Severe/Profound Multiple Disabilities Through Assistive Technology. In G. Kouroupetroglou (Ed.), Assistive Technologies and Computer Access for Motor Disabilities (pp. 285–319). Hershey, PA: IGI Global. doi:10.4018/978-1-4666-4438-0.ch010

Elmquist, M., Simacek, J., Dimian, A. F., & Reichle, J. (2019). Impact of aided AAC interventions on speech comprehension of children with neurodevelopmental disabilities: A critically appraised topic. *Evidence-Based Communication Assessment and Intervention*, *13*(1-2), 67–84. published online16Apr2019. doi:10.1080/17489539.2019.1598011

Fage, C., Consel, C., Etchegoyhen, K., Amestoy, A., Bouvard, M., Mazon, C., & Sauzéon, H. (2019). An emotion regulation app for school inclusion of children with ASD: Design principles and evaluation. *Computers & Education*, *131*, 1–21. doi:10.1016/j.compedu.2018.12.003

Fage, C., Consel, C. Y., Balland, E., Etchegoyhen, K., Amestoy, A., Bouvard, M., & Sauzéon, H. (2018). Tablet apps to support first school inclusion of children with autism spectrum disorders (ASD) in mainstream classrooms: A pilot study. *Frontiers in Psychology*, *9*. PMID:30405498

Felce, D., & Perry, J. (1995). Quality of life: Its definition and measurement. *Research in Developmental Disabilities*, *16*(1), 51–74. doi:10.1016/0891-4222(94)00028-8 PMID:7701092

Flores, M. M., Hill, D. A., Faciane, L. B., Edwards, M. A., Tapley, S. C., & Dowling, S. J. (2014). The apple iPad as assistive technology for story-based interventions. *Journal of Special Education Technology*, *29*(2), 27–37. doi:10.1177/016264341402900203

Ganz, J. B., Hong, E. R., Goodwyn, F., Kite, E., & Gilliland, W. (2015). Impact of PECS tablet computer app on receptive identification of pictures given a verbal stimulus. *Developmental Neurorehabilitation*, *18*(2), 82–87. doi:10.3109/17518423.2013.821539 PMID:23957298

Gilroy, S. P., Leader, G., & McCleery, J. P. (2018). A pilot community-based randomized comparison of speech generating devices and the picture exchange communication system for children diagnosed with autism spectrum disorder. *Autism Research*, *11*(12), 1701–1711. doi:10.1002/aur.2025 PMID:30475454

Grossard, C., Grynspan, O., Sylvie Serret, S., Jouen, A.-L., Bailly, K., & Cohen, D. (2017). Serious games to teach social interactions and emotions to individuals with autism spectrum disorders. *Computers & Education*, *113*, 195–211. doi:10.1016/j.compedu.2017.05.002

Hughes, E. M., & Yakubova, G. (2016). Developing handheld video intervention for students with autism spectrum disorder. *Intervention in School and Clinic*, *52*(2), 115–121. doi:10.1177/1053451216636059

Hutchins, T. L., & Prelock, P. A. (2014). Using communication to reduce challenging behaviors in individuals with autism spectrum disorders and intellectual disability. *Child and Adolescent Psychiatric Clinics of North America*, *23*(1), 41–55. doi:10.1016/j.chc.2013.07.003 PMID:24231166

Ismaili, J., & Ibrahimi, E. H. O. (2017). Mobile learning as alternative to assistive technology devices for special needs students. *Education and Information Technologies*, *22*(3), 883–899. doi:10.100710639-015-9462-9

Johnston, D., Egermann, H. W., & Kearney, G. C. (2018). Innovative Computer Technology in music based interventions for individuals with autism - Moving beyond traditional interactive music therapy techniques. *Cognitive Psychology*, *5*, 1554773.

Jones, E. J. H., Gliga, T., Bedford, R., Charman, T., & Johnson, M. H. (2014). Developmental pathways to autism: A review of prospective studies of infants at risk. *Neuroscience and Biobehavioral Reviews*, *39*, 1–33. doi:10.1016/j.neubiorev.2013.12.001 PMID:24361967

Kagohara, D., van der Meer, L., Ramdoss, S., O'Reilly, M., Lancioni, G., Davis, T. N., ... Sigafoos, J. (2013). Using iPods and iPads in teaching programs for individuals with developmental disabilities: A systematic review. *Research in Developmental Disabilities*, *34*(1), 147–156. doi:10.1016/j.ridd.2012.07.027 PMID:22940168

Kazdin, A. E. (2001). *Behavior modification in applied settings* (6th ed.). New York: Wadsworth.

Kennedy, C. (2005). *Single case designs for educational research*. New York: Allyn & Bacon.

Konst, M. J., & Matson, J. L. (2014). Temporal and diagnostic influences on the expression of comorbid psychopathology symptoms in infants and toddlers with autism spectrum disorder. *Research in Autism Spectrum Disorders*, *8*(3), 200–208. doi:10.1016/j.rasd.2013.11.009

Koumpouros, Y., & Kafazis, T. (2019). Wearable and mobile technologies in Autism Spectrum Disorder interventions: A systematic literature review. *Research in Autism Spectrum Disorders*, *66*, 101405. doi:10.1016/j.rasd.2019.05.005

Lahiri, U., Warren, Z., & Sarkar, N. (2011c). Dynamic gaze measurement with adaptive response technology in virtual reality based social communication for autism. *2011 International Conference on Virtual Rehabilitation, ICVR 2011,* 10.1109/ICVR.2011.5971840

Lancioni, G. E., Comes, M. L., Stasolla, F., Manfredi, F., O'Reilly, M. F., & Singh, N. N. (2005). A microswitch cluster to enhance arm-lifting responses without dystonic head tilting by a child with multiple disabilities. *Perceptual and Motor Skills*, *100*(3), 892–894. doi:10.2466/pms.100.3.892-894 PMID:16060461

Lancioni, G. E., O'Reilly, M. F., Singh, N. N., Groeneweg, J., Bosco, A., Tota, A., ... Pidala, S. (2006). A social validation assessment of microswitch-based programs for persons with multiple disabilities employing teacher trainees and parents as raters. *Journal of Developmental and Physical Disabilities*, *18*(4), 383–391. doi:10.100710882-006-9024-6

Lancioni, G. E., O'Reilly, M. F., Singh, N. N., Sigafoos, J., Didden, R., Oliva, D., ... Groeneweg, J. (2009). Persons with multiple disabilities accessing stimulation and requesting social contact via microswitch and VOCA devices: New research evaluation and social validation. *Research in Developmental Disabilities*, *30*(5), 1084–1094. doi:10.1016/j.ridd.2009.03.004 PMID:19361954

Lancioni, G. E., Sigafoos, J., O'Reilly, M. F., & Singh, N. N. (2012). *Assistive technology: Interventions for individuals with severe/profound and multiple disabilities*. New York: Springer.

Lancioni, G. E., & Singh, N. N. (2014). *Assistive technologies for people with diverse abilities*. New York: Springer. doi:10.1007/978-1-4899-8029-8

Lancioni, G. E., Singh, N. N., O'Reilly, M. F., Oliva, D., Smaldone, A., Tota, A., ... Groeneweg, J. (2006). Assessing the effects of stimulation versus microswitch-based programmes on indices of happiness of students with multiple disabilities. *Journal of Intellectual Disability Research*, *50*(10), 739–747. doi:10.1111/j.1365-2788.2006.00839.x PMID:16961703

Lau, H. M., Smit, J. H., Fleming, T., & Riper, H. (2017). Serious sames for mental health: Are they accessible, feasible, and effective? A systematic review and meta-analysis. *Frontiers in Psychiatry*, *7*, 209. doi:10.3389/fpsyt.2016.00209 PMID:28149281

Light, J., McNaughton, D., Beukelman, D., Fager, S. K., Melanie Fried-Okenc, M., Jakobs, T., & Jakobs, E. (2019). Challenges and opportunities in augmentative and alternative communication: Research and technology development to enhance communication and participation for individuals with complex communication needs. *Augmentative and Alternative Communication*, *35*(1), 1–12. doi:10.1080/07434618.2018.1556732 PMID:30648903

Matson, J. L., & Jang, J. (2014). Treating aggression in persons with autism spectrum disorders: A review. *Research in Developmental Disabilities*, *35*(12), 3386–3391. doi:10.1016/j.ridd.2014.08.025 PMID:25194514

Matson, J. L., & Sturmey, P. (2011). *International handbook of autism and pervasive developmental disorders*. New York: Springer. doi:10.1007/978-1-4419-8065-6

Mohan, V., Kunnath, S. K., Philip, V. S., Mohan, L. S., & Thampi, N. (2019). Capitalizing on technology for developing communication skills in autism spectrum disorder: A single case study. *Disability and Rehabilitation. Assistive Technology*, *14*(1), 75–81. doi:10.1080/17483107.2017.1413144 PMID:29241371

Mulroy, S., Robertson, L., Aiberti, K., Leonard, H., & Bower, C. (2008). The impact of having a sibling with an intellectual disability: Parental perspectives in two disorders. *Journal of Intellectual Disability Research*, *52*(3), 216–229. doi:10.1111/j.1365-2788.2007.01005.x PMID:18261021

Nicolaidis, C., Kripke, C. C., & Raymaker, D. (2014). Primary care for adults on the autism spectrum. *The Medical Clinics of North America*, *98*(5), 1169–1191. doi:10.1016/j.mcna.2014.06.011 PMID:25134878

Perilli, V., Lancioni, G. E., Hoogeveen, F., Caffó, A., Singh, N., O'Reilly, M., ... Oliva, D. (2013a). Video prompting versus other instruction strategies for persons with Alzheimer's disease. *American Journal of Alzheimer's Disease and Other Dementias*, *28*(4), 393–402. doi:10.1177/1533317513488913 PMID:23687181

Perilli, V., Lancioni, G. E., Laporta, D., Paparella, A., Caffò, A. O., Singh, N. N., ... Oliva, D. (2013b). A computer-aided telephone system to enable five persons with Alzheimer's disease to make phone calls independently. *Research in Developmental Disabilities*, *34*(6), 1991–1997. doi:10.1016/j.ridd.2013.03.016 PMID:23584179

Politte, L. C., Howe, Y., Nowinski, L., Palumbo, M., & McDougle, C. J. (2015). Evidence-Based Treatments for Autism Spectrum Disorder. *Current Treatment Options in Psychiatry*, *2*(1), 38–56. doi:10.100740501-015-0031-z

Reber, M. E. (2009). *The autism spectrum: Scientific foundations and treatment* Doi:10.1017/CBO9780511978616

Rispoli, M. J., Franco, J. H., Van Der Meer, L., Lang, R., & Camargo, S. P. H. (2010). The use of speech generating devices in communication interventions for individuals with developmental disabilities: A review of the literature. *Developmental Neurorehabilitation*, *13*(4), 276–293. doi:10.3109/17518421003636794 PMID:20629594

Rogge, N., & Janssen, J. (2019). The economic costs of autism spectrum disorder: A literature review. *Journal of Autism and Developmental Disorders, 49*(7), 2873–2900. doi:10.100710803-019-04014-z PMID:30976961

Sanchack, K. E., & Thomas, C. A. (2016). Autism spectrum disorders: Primary care principles. *American Family Physician, 94*, 972–979. PMID:28075089

Schlosser, R., & Koul, R. (2015). Speech output technologies in Interventions for individuals with autism spectrum disorders: A scoping review. *Augmentative and Alternative Communication, 31*(4), 285–309. doi:10.3109/07434618.2015.1063689 PMID:26170252

Sigafoos, J., Drasgow, E., Halle, J. W., O'reilly, M., Seely-York, S., Edrisinha, C., & Andrews, A. (2004). Teaching VOCA use as a communicative repair strategy. *Journal of Autism and Developmental Disorders, 34*(4), 411–422. doi:10.1023/B:JADD.0000037417.04356.9c PMID:15449516

Sigafoos, J., Lancioni, G. E., O'Reilly, M. F., Achmadi, D., Stevens, M., Roche, L., ... Green, V. A. (2013). Teaching two boys with autism spectrum disorders to request the continuation of toy play using an iPad®-based speech-generating device. *Research in Autism Spectrum Disorders, 7*(8), 923–930. doi:10.1016/j.rasd.2013.04.002

Sigafoos, J., O'Reilly, M. F., Ledbetter-Cho, K., Lim, N., Lancioni, G. E., & Marschik, P. B. (2019). Addressing sequelae of developmental regression associated with developmental disabilities: A systematic review of behavioral and educational intervention studies. *Neuroscience and Biobehavioral Reviews, 96*, 56–71. doi:10.1016/j.neubiorev.2018.11.014 PMID:30481529

Smith, D. L., Atmatzidis, K., Capogreco, M., Lloyd-Randolfi, D., & Seman, V. (2017). Evidence-based interventions for increasing work participation for persons with various disabilities: A systematic review. *OTJR: Occupation, Participation, and Health, 37*, 3–13.

Spence-Cochran, K., & Pearl, C. (2012). *Assistive technology to support people with autism spectrum disorders.* Doi:10.4324/9780203848180

Stasolla, F., Boccasini, A., & Perilli, V. (2017). Assistive technology-based programs to support adaptive behaviors by children with autism spectrum disorders: A literature overview. In Y. Kats (Ed.), *Supporting the education of children with autism spectrum disorders* (pp. 140–159). Hershey, PA: IGI Global. doi:10.4018/978-1-5225-0816-8.ch008

Stasolla, F., Caffò, A. O., Damiani, R., Perilli, V., Di Leone, A., & Albano, V. (2015). Assistive technology-based programs to promote communication and leisure activities by three children emerged from a minimal conscious state. *Cognitive Processing, 16*(1), 69–78. doi:10.100710339-014-0625-1 PMID:25077461

Stasolla, F., Caffò, A. O., Perilli, V., Boccasini, A., Damiani, R., Albano, V., & Albano, A. (2017). Comparing self-monitoring and differential reinforcement of an alternative behavior to promote on-task behavior by three children with cerebral palsy: A pilot study. *Life Span and Disability, 20*, 63–92.

Stasolla, F., Caffò, A. O., Picucci, L., & Bosco, A. (2013). Assistive technology for promoting choice behaviors in three children with cerebral palsy and severe communication impairments. *Research in Developmental Disabilities, 34*(9), 2694–2700. doi:10.1016/j.ridd.2013.05.029 PMID:23770888

Stasolla, F., Damiani, R., & Caffò, A. O. (2014). Promoting constructive engagement by two boys with autism spectrum disorders and high functioning through behavioral interventions. *Research in Autism Spectrum Disorders*, *8*(4), 376–380. doi:10.1016/j.rasd.2013.12.020

Stasolla, F., Damiani, R., Perilli, V., D'Amico, F., Caffò, A. O., Stella, A., ... Leone, A. D. (2015). Computer and microswitch-based programs to improve academic activities by six children with cerebral palsy. *Research in Developmental Disabilities*, *45-46*, 1–13. doi:10.1016/j.ridd.2015.07.005 PMID:26196086

Stasolla, F., Perilli, V., & Boccasini, A. (2016). Assistive technologies for persons with severe-profound intellectual and developmental disabilities. In J. K. Luiselli & A. J. Fischer (Eds.), *Computer-assisted and web-based innovations in psychology, special education, and health* (pp. 287–310). New York: Springer. doi:10.1016/B978-0-12-802075-3.00011-5

Stasolla, F., Perilli, V., Boccasini, A., Caffò, A. O., Damiani, R., & Albano, V. (2016). Enhancing academic performance of three boys with autism spectrum disorders and intellectual disabilities through a computer-based program. *Life Span and Disability*, *19*, 153–183.

Stasolla, F., Perilli, V., Caffò, A. O., Boccasini, A., Stella, A., Damiani, R., ... Albano, A. (2017). Extending microswitch-cluster programs for promoting occupational activities and reducing mouthing by six children with autism spectrum disorders and intellectual disabilities. *Journal of Developmental and Physical Disabilities*, *29*(2), 307–324. doi:10.100710882-016-9525-x

Stasolla, F., Perilli, V., & Damiani, R. (2014). Self monitoring to promote on-task behavior by two high functioning boys with autism spectrum disorders and symptoms of ADHD. *Research in Autism Spectrum Disorders*, *8*(5), 472–479. doi:10.1016/j.rasd.2014.01.007

Stasolla, F., Perilli, V., Damiani, R., Caffò, A. O., Di Leone, A., Albano, V., ... Damato, C. (2014c). A microswitch-cluster program to enhance object manipulation and to reduce hand mouthing by three boys with autism spectrum disorders and intellectual disabilities. *Research in Autism Spectrum Disorders*, *9*(9), 1071–1078. doi:10.1016/j.rasd.2014.05.016

Sturm, D., Peppe, E., & Ploog, B. (2016). EMot-iCan: Design of an assessment game for emotion recognition in players with autism. *2016 IEEE International Conference on Serious Games and Applications for Health, SeGAH 2016,* 10.1109/SeGAH.2016.7586228

Taube-Schiff, M., Suvak, M. K., Antony, M. M., Bieling, P. J., & McCabe, R. E. (2007). Group cohesion in cognitive-behavioral group therapy for social phobia. *Behaviour Research and Therapy*, *45*(4), 687–698. doi:10.1016/j.brat.2006.06.004 PMID:16928359

Torrado, J. C., Gomez, J., & Montoro, G. (2017). Emotional self-regulation of individuals with autism spectrum disorders: Smartwatches for monitoring and interaction. *Sensors (Switzerland)*, *17*(6), 1359. doi:10.339017061359 PMID:28604607

Tsangouri, C., Li, W., Zhu, Z., Abtahi, F., & Ro, T. (2018). An interactive facial-expression training platform for individuals with autism spectrum disorder. *2016 IEEE MIT Undergraduate Research Technology Conference, URTC 2016,* 1-4. doi:10.1109/URTC.2016.8284067

Tsikinas, S., & Xinogalos, S. (2018). Studying the effects of computer serious games on people with intellectual disabilities or autism spectrum disorder: A systematic literature review. *Journal of Computer Assisted Learning*, *35*(1), 61–73. doi:10.1111/jcal.12311

Tsui, K. M., Feil-Seifer, D. J., Matarić, M. J., & Yanco, H. A. (2009). *Performance evaluation methods for assistive robotic technology*. Doi:10.1007/978-1-4419-0492-8_3

Vahabzadeh, A., Keshav, N. U., Abdus-Sabur, R., Huey, K., Liu, R., & Sahin, N. T. (2018). Improved socio-emotional and behavioral functioning in students with autism following school-based smartglasses intervention: Multi-stage feasibility and controlled efficacy study. *Behavioral Science*, *8*(10). doi:10.3390/bs8100085 PMID:30241313

Valadão, C. T., Goulart, C., Rivera, H., Caldeira, E., Bastos Filho, T. F., Frizera-Neto, A., & Carelli, R. (2016). Analysis of the use of a robot to improve social skills in children with autism spectrum disorder. *Revista Brasileira de Engenharia Biomédica*, *32*, 161–175.

Van der Meer, L., Sigafoos, J., O'Reilly, M. F., & Lancioni, G. E. (2011). Assessing preferences for AAC options in communication interventions for individuals with developmental disabilities: A review of the literature. *Research in Developmental Disabilities*, *32*(5), 1422–1431. doi:10.1016/j.ridd.2011.02.003 PMID:21377833

Van der Meer, L. A. J., & Rispoli, M. (2010). Communication interventions involving speech-generating devices for children with autism: A review of the literature. *Developmental Neurorehabilitation*, *13*(4), 294–306. doi:10.3109/17518421003671494 PMID:20629595

Waddington, H. (2018). Meta-analysis provides support for the use of high tech speech-generating devices for teaching a range of communication skills to children with autism spectrum disorders. *Evidence-Based Communication Assessment and Intervention*, *12*(1-2), 7–11. doi:10.1080/17489539.2018.1472903

Walton, K. M., & Ingersoll, B. R. (2015). Psychosocial adjustment and sibling relationships in siblings of children with autism spectrum disorder: Risk and protective factors. *Journal of Autism and Developmental Disorders*, *45*(9), 2764–2778. doi:10.100710803-015-2440-7 PMID:25847756

ADDITIONAL READING

American Psychiatric Association. (2013). *Diagnostic and statistical manual of mental disorders* (5th ed.). Arlington, VA: American Psychiatric Publishing.

Catania, A. C. (2012). *Learning* (5th ed.). New York: Sloan.

Horne-Moyer, H. L., Moyer, B. H., Messer, D. C., & Messer, E. S. (2014). The use of electronic games in therapy: A review with clinical implications. *Current Psychiatry Reports*, *16*(12), 520. doi:10.100711920-014-0520-6 PMID:25312026

Matson, J. L. (2009). *Applied behavior analysis for children with autism spectrum disorders*. New York: Springer. doi:10.1007/978-1-4419-0088-3

Miguel Cruz, A., Ríos Rincón, A. M., Rodríguez Dueñas, W. R., Quiroga Torres, D. A., & Bohórquez-Heredia, A. F. (2017). What does the literature say about using robots on children with disabilities? *Disability and Rehabilitation. Assistive Technology*, *12*(5), 429–440. doi:10.1080/17483107.2017.1318308 PMID:28440095

Rabbitt, S. M., Kazdin, A. E., & Scassellati, B. (2015). Integrating socially assistive robotics into mental healthcare interventions: Applications and recommendations for expanded use. *Clinical Psychology Review*, *35*, 35–46. doi:10.1016/j.cpr.2014.07.001 PMID:25462112

Tang, J. S. Y., Chen, N. T. M., Falkmer, M., Bölte, S., & Girdler, S. (2019). A systematic review and meta-analysis of social emotional computer based interventions for autistic individuals using the serious game framework. *Research in Autism Spectrum Disorders*, *66*, 101412. doi:10.1016/j.rasd.2019.101412

KEY TERMS AND DEFINITIONS

Academic Performance: Extent to which a student, a teacher or an institution has achieved their short- or long-term educational goals.

Assistive Technology: Comprehensive expression which includes any item, piece, equipment or device used to increase, maintain or improve functional capacities of persons with disabilities.

Autism Spectrum Disorders: Core of complex disorders of brain development characterized by cognitive, communicative, emotional, and social impairments.

Challenging Behavior: Abnormal behavior that compromises the person's regular functioning, and/or precludes the learning processes.

Indices of Happiness: Behavioral signs of happiness including smiling, laughing, energized body movements of persons with severe to profound developmental disabilities with or without vocalizations.

Life Skills: Psychosocial abilities for positive behaviors enabling individuals to deal efficiently in everyday life.

Quality of Life: Multi-dimensional construct including happiness, pleasure, fulfillment, satisfaction, and well-being.

Serious Games: Games designed for a primary goal other than pure entertainment.

Social Validation: Perceived social acceptance and/or formal endorsement of a rehabilitative intervention by external and expert raters.

Chapter 5
Augmentative and Alternative Communication Systems for Children With Cerebral Palsy

Yashomathi
Department of Speech-Language Pathology, All India Institute of Speech and Hearing (AIISH), Mysuru, India

Gayathri Krishnan
All India Institute of Speech and Hearing (AIISH), India

ABSTRACT

Cerebral palsy (CP) is a congenital neurological disorder of movement, muscle tone, or posture. Children with CP may also have associated sensory and motor disorders such as visual impairment, hearing loss, intellectual disability, speech-language and communication disorders, as well as swallowing-related problems. They often require long-term treatment and rehabilitation from various disciplines such as speech-language therapy, augmentative and alternative communication (AAC) therapy, physiotherapy, occupational therapy, along with medical/surgical line of treatment. Augmentative and alternative communication (AAC) therapy approaches focus on providing the individual with communication methods using residual functional abilities. This chapter aims at briefing the reader on the principles, methods, and key features of AAC communication systems such as switches, pointing devices, visual displays, virtual and modified keyboards, AAC devices with digitized speech output, AAC apps and software, eye gaze systems, etc.

INTRODUCTION

Cerebral Palsy (CP) is a non-progressive, neurodevelopmental disorder that affects muscle tone, movement, motor co-ordination and body posture secondary to lesions or anomalies of the brain acquired during the pre-natal, peri-natal or post-natal period (Mutch, Leyland, & McGee, 1993). There is no one known cause for CP. However, few conditions have been identified as significant risk factors. These includes

DOI: 10.4018/978-1-7998-3069-6.ch005

low birth weight (Reddihough, 2011), birth complications such as asphyxia (Krigger, 2006), lesions or mal-development of brain structures (Krägeloh-Mann & Cans, 2009), and many genetic causes (Badawi et al., 1998). The motor disorders of cerebral palsy are often accompanied by disturbances of sensation, perception, cognition, communication, and behaviour, by epilepsy, and by secondary musculoskeletal problems (Rosenbaum et al., 2007). It is a life-long condition resulting in motoric impairment and it is reported to be the most common cause of physical disability in childhood (Krageloh-Mann & Cans, 2009).

In nearly 50% of the population with CP, professionals fail to identify one exact cause. However, they are in consensus that the most common cause of cerebral palsy is deviated brain development in embryological stages or an acquired brain lesion during or after birth. Table 1 summarizes the causes for such brain damage that potentially could result in CP.

Table 1. Common causes of Cerebral Palsy

Prenatal causes	
Cerebral Haemorrhage	It is a bleeding in a specific area of brain that is commonly seen in premature children causing CP
Infections	Intrauterine infections, high fever, UTI may be passed from mother to child in the womb. E.g. Cytomegalo-virus (CMV), measles, rubella etc
Environmental factors	Maternal exposure to toxic substance (methyl mercury, exposure to drugs, radiations, smoking, alcohol consumption by mothers, and other environmental factors) (Kondo, 2000).
Genetic/Hereditary factors	A small number of cases may be due to genetic factors (Schaefer, 2008)
Nutrition	Iron deficiency, iodine deficiency in expecting mothers.
Maternal diseases	Diabetes, hypertension, hyperthyroidism etc during pregnancy
Fertility problems	Advanced age at conception, history of infertility, recurrent fetal wastage
Other possible factors	Poor antenatal care Poor socioeconomic status
Perinatal causes	
Birth asphyxia	Lack of oxygen circulation to fetal brain induced with placental failure, drug, breech delivery, forceps delivery and maternal anoxia or maternal hypotension.
Prematurity	Child born before 38 weeks of gestation.
Abruptio placentae	Premature separation of placenta from the foetus.
Postnatal causes	
Head injuries	Fall, accidents or similar head trauma sustained during the first five years of life.
Infections	Brain infections such as Encephalitis, Meningitis in early life.
Lack of oxygen	Accidents or chocking that deprive oxygen to brain
Low birth weight	Child born with < 2.5Kg weight at birth.
APGAR score	A low health score soon after birth due to variations in activity, pulse, respiration and other health factors.

Based on the number and distribution of limb weakness, CP is topographically classified as monoplegia, diplegia, hemiplegia, paraplegia, triplegia, quadriplegia. As a disorder of muscle tone and activity, CP is also classified as spastic, flaccid, ataxic, athetoid, and mixed type. Odding, Roebroeck and Stam (2006) reported that up to 80% of those with CP have dysarthria (disorder of movement), and they are classified as non-verbal (Ratcliff & Little, 1996; Hustad, Gorton, & Lee, 2010). Children with CP experience a range of difficulties such as intellectual impairment (Blair & Watson, 2006; Odding et al., 2006; Sigurdardottir et al., 2008), epilepsy (Carlsson, Hagberg, and Olsson, 2003), hearing impairment (Reddihough, 2011), visual impairment (Himmelmann, Hagberg, & Uvebrant, 2010; Jan, Lyons, Heavennet al, 2001; Park, Myung Jin, et al, 2016, Venkateshwaran & Shevell, 2008), and sensory problems (hyposensitivity/hypersensitivity). As a result of varying degree and pattern of deficits and other associated problems, individuals with CP often show severe expressive communication disorder (Beukelman & Mirenda, 1998; Pennington, 1999; Pennington & McConachie, 1999; Krigger, 2006; Goldbart, & Marshall, 2004; Pirila et al, 2007). Pirila, van der Meere, Pentikainen, Russu-Niemi, Korpela, Kilpinen and Nieminen (2007) reported that when compared to typically developing children, children with CP are less likely to initiate conversations, they take fewer turns in conversations and they do not ask questions.

Communication is a vital part of everyone's life and it is acknowledged to be a central element needed for cognitive, emotional and social-well-being of an individual. Communication impairments have a multi-dimensional impact on the life of the child and also their caregivers. The co-occurring developmental difficulties in children with CP lead to a complex array of problems. Few research findings suggested that communication difficulty results in significantly smaller social network size, fewer possible social exchange of information, reduced level of social participations in social activities, higher levels of loneliness etc. (Andrew, Jason, & Karen, 2016; Berkman & Glass, 2000; Berkman, Glass, Brissette & Seeman, 2000; Cohen, 2004; Holt-Lunstad, Smith & Layton, 2010; Uchino, 2006). Thus, for children with CP who has difficulty, developing communication skill is a challenge but also a hope towards inclusion and integration into the society as a productive human being.

Augmentative and Alternative Communication Intervention in Children with Cerebral Palsy

Children with Cerebral Palsy experience a range of impairments in oro-motor control, cognition, language and sensation which has direct impact on communication performance. The routine participation of these children in a variety of therapeutic services such as physiotherapy, occupational therapy, and vocational therapy, and they also undergo other medical or surgical procedures in their early period of life (Palisano, Begnoche, Chiarello, Bartlett, McCoy, & Chang, 2012; McLellan, Cipparone, Giancola, Armstrong, & Bartlett, 2012). The initial focus is on promoting survival, and treating major health risks such as seizures. Communication is rarely given any priority. As speech and language problems in children with CP are not readily detectable till the second year of life, parents and professionals prioritize improving gross motor skills over communication skills. Also, the presence of motor impairment often places children with cerebral palsy at risk for not being able to communicate using speech. These children present to speech-language pathology clinics with little or no intelligible speech and are often referred to as individuals with Complex Communication Needs (CCN). Furthermore, the multitude of impairments makes it difficult for children with CP to develop adequate verbal communication with traditional speech and language therapy. Difficulties with social interaction, academics, and quality of life may subsequently arise (Falkman, Dahlgren Sandberg, & Hjelmquist, 2002) affecting their overall performance. These individuals often benefit from the provision of Augmentative and Alternative Communication (AAC) systems that help them to develop a full range of communicative functions.

Augmentative and Alternative Communication (AAC) refers to a group of methods, strategies and/or techniques that supports the use of functional and effective communication (Beukelman & Mirenda, 2005). It is an area of specialized clinical and educational practice that provides communication options and interventions for people with complex communication needs. Wilkinson and Hennig (2007) defined AAC as an area comprising of methods and technologies designed to assist or replace communication of people with speech limitation and identified four roles of AAC: a) to enhance the expressive speech of individuals who can understand language to some extent, but have difficult producing it; b) to enable the expression of a variety of communication functions across different settings with different people; c) to reduce challenging behaviour such as aggression or unwanted social behaviours; and d) to function as a bridge to later linguistic development.

Any AAC communication requires the use of symbols (any form/picture/character/mark to represent an object/idea/ parts of communication) that are accessed and transmitted to the communication partner. An effective AAC communication system require appropriate selection of symbols used, the most comfortable and sustainable method of accessing the symbol, and successful transmission of the message to communication partner for them to comprehend the message and reciprocate. These systems are broadly categorized as "unaided" or "aided" (Lloyd, Fuller, & Arvidson, 1997). Unaided AAC involves user's body to convey meaning. Examples of unaided AAC include gestures, facial expressions, and sign language. An aided AAC system requires an external aid to the person's physical body (Tonsing, Alant, & Lloyd, 2005). Examples of aided AAC system are pictures, photographs, line drawings, objects, technology-involved communication aids. The evaluation, selection, design and development of an effective AAC system is a team work and requires inter- disciplinary collaboration from speech- language pathologists, bio-medical and software engineers, occupational therapists, special educators and also the caregivers of individual with CP. It is also important that the strategies and techniques for use and troubleshooting of AAC systems are thought not only to the individual using the system but also their communication partners. The integrated use of these components supplements receptive or expressive language and social interactions (Murray & Goldbart, 2009) or provides an alternative method of communication for conveying messages effectively in individuals with CCN.

Early AAC intervention is crucial for overall communication development in children with CP. Individuals with CP constitute the largest proportion of AAC users (Murphy, Markovà, Moodie, Scott, & Boa, 1995) as a multimodal communication repertoire. For selection of the most appropriate AAC, McBride (2011) suggested that the process of selecting an appropriate AAC systems for individuals with complex communication needs (CCN) needs to consider several important factors that include thorough understanding of an individual's cognitive level, linguistic level, motoric and sensory abilities, and neurological conditions Children with CP often present with primary impairments in muscle tone (hypertonia/ hypotonia, fluctuating) with varied degree and pattern of involvement throughout the body and with inherent postural impairments (Bax, Goldstein, Rosenbaum, Leviton, & Paneth, 2005; Treviranus & Roberts, 2003). This limited motoric abilities in children with CP interfere with their ability to use their own body for unaided communication such as gestural and sign-language. Therefore, AAC intervention in CP typically focuses on supporting symbol use through no tech (Example: communication boards, picture books), low-tech (Example: adapted picture boards, sign language and walkers), and high-tech AAC communication systems (Example: electronic communication devices using synthetic or digitalized speech, micro switches to control computers, powered wheelchairs and environmental control) (Bailey, Parette, Stoner, Angell, & Carroll, 2006, DeCoste, 1997).

Research studies have indicated that access to AAC helps children with CP to acquire some of the necessary pre-linguistic skills and cognitive skills that are essential for language development (Brady, 2000; Light, Collier &Parnes, 1985; Romski & Sevcik, 1996) by helping then access a broader vocabulary, connect them to form meaningful language, and thereby helping them to become independent communicators (Pennington, 2008; Clarke & Price, 2012; Thiemann-Bourque, Brady, McGuff, Stump, & Naylor, 2016). Successful training in use of AAC communication involves various stages of progression from early pre- linguistic behaviour to symbolic representation, and technological skills. Non-symbolic communication modes such as verbal speech, unaided signs and abstract symbols are also enhanced with training (Siegel & Cress, 2002).

At present, many corporate companies are thriving to develop disability-friendly technology and techniques in order to facilitate social inclusion of people with physical and communication impairments (Galvao& Garcia, 2012). This has led to a new genre in technology and engineering known as Assistive Technology (AT), an umbrella term for any device or system that enables a person to perform a task that would otherwise be too hard to execute or that facilitates how a task can be performed (WHO, 2004). According to the concept created by Colker (1999), Cook and Polgar (2014) defines AT as "a wide range of equipment, services, strategies and practices designed and implemented to reduce the functional problems encountered by individuals with disabilities". AAC communication falls as a sub-area in Assistive Technology.

Identification, assessment of candidacy, selection, design and development of AAC communication system and training the individual with CP along with their communication partners is a team work. Given the complexity of AAC intervention, a successful intervention program requires collaborative team approach, skills, and knowledge of the team members (Beukelman&Mirenda, 2005; Bailey, Stoner, Parette& Angell, 2006). Members of the AAC team include various professionals such as Speech-Language Pathologists (SLPs), Physical therapists (PT), Occupational therapists (OT), Special educators (SpeEd), medical professionals, ophthalmologists, social workers, software engineers, psychologists and so on. Their involvement should base on prevailing evidences so that the best services are offered to individuals with complex communication needs (SIgafoos, Drasgow& Schlosser, 2003). Using evidence-based practices necessitated a constant improvement of skills and knowledge which is crucial in facilitating skills of professionals providing AAC services (Fallon & Katz).

Constraints in AAC

In order to communicate functionally using aided AAC systems, individuals with CP must be able to see the vocabulary symbol, access them and transmit the message to the communication partner. Associated sensory deficits such as visual impairment influences the arrangement and characteristics of display of symbols in the AAC communication system.

These may be a major constraint in inclusion of large vocabulary into the communication system. Difficulty in producing typical movement patterns is another main constraint in this process (Steenbergen & Gordon, 2006; Valvano & Newell, 1998) is a major constraint in accessing the symbols of AAC communication system. There is considerable variability in the motor impairments seen in individuals with CP (Barlett & Palisano, 2002; Treviranus & Roberts, 2003). The unique presentation of motor characteristics in each individual with this condition dictates the specific constraints that influence the use of an AAC communication system. It becomes crucial to establish a fit between the functional abilities of the individual with CP and the operation of AAC communication system for successful communication. Occupational therapists might work beyond the motor skill assessment and directly address the barrier to overcome the constraints. Occupational therapists strive to understand and improvise the hand functions of children with CP to facilitate better access and use of aided AAC systems for individuals with CP further helping them communicate and perform better in life. The constraints at each process of AAC communication (display, interface, and access of symbols) should be targeted in design and development of the most appropriate AAC communication device for an individual with CP. Below are the current options from which the AAC team selects the 'best fit' for AAC communication training.

Display Options

The most common electronic communication devices used by individuals with CP range from mid-tech to high-tech AAC devices. Mid-tech AAC devices comprised of static, single message communicators and multimessage communicators that re-produced pre- recorded audio/text messages that could be accessed with a single-push button, joystick, microswitch etc. Examples of such commercially available single message communicators include iTalk2™, BIG/LITTLEmack™, and Talking Brix™. Several variants of these products with step-by-step level of complexity are also available, for example the BIG/LITTLE Step-by-Step™. Some of these offer an unlimited number of output messages. Other mid-tech AAC devices such as Tobii® S32, GoTalk Series, SuperTalker™ Progressive Communicator, and the QuickTalker™ Family of Communication Devices offer multi- message communication. These devices have a static display board, and they allow for custom-made interchangeable overlays for which different pre-recorded audio messages can be played with a press on each overlay. These mid-tech AAC devices are readily available, easy to use and learn, making them suitable for young children with complex communication needs (Light & Drager, 2007).

However, with the technological advances, high-tech AAC devices have become more prevalent, as these devices allow dynamic display options, provide larger vocabulary, and permit multiple message output for limited number of inputs thereby enabling more natural and responsive communication (Judge & Friday, 2011). The market for high-tech, dynamic AAC devices were dominated by few companies (Deruyter, McNaughton, Caves, Bryen, Williams, 2007). These companies developed dedicated systems for communication (Radomski & Latham, 2008). Table 2 attempts to provide the reader with the list of commercially available high-tech AAC devices that could be considered for facilitating communication in individuals with CP.

With the mobile technology revolution, developing communication systems with the use of smart phones, tablets, iPads has become widespread (McNaughton & Light, 2013; Bradshaw, 2013; Shane, 2012; Dixon, 2011). This adaptation of mainstream hardware in the field of aided AAC has created a significant paradigm shift, as they offer several advantages that includes cost (McNaughton & Light, 2013; Bradshaw, 2013; Shane, 2012; Dixon, 2011), ease of use (McNaughton & Light, 2013; Bradshaw, 2013), availability, transportability (McNaughton & Light, 2013; Bradshaw, 2013; Shane, 2012; Dixon, 2011), and social acceptance (Light &, Drager, 2007;McNaughton & Light, 2013; Bradshaw, 2013; Hodge, 2007). These multifunctional mobile devices provide access to several mainstream phone applications such as email, text messaging and internet browsing which have become important aspects of communication today (Shane, 2012; Light & McNaughton, 2012). Because of the economic and social appeal of this mainstream mobile technology, there has been surge in the development of mobile apps in the field of AAC (McNaughton & Light, 2013; Bradshaw, 2013). Table 3 is an attempt to summarize the readers with the applications that are available for communication in individuals with complex communication needs.

Table 2. List of commercially available High-tech Augmentative and Alternative Communication (AAC) devices (released since 2008)

AAC Devices	Description	Release date
1) Tango!	Symbol-list system and text-to-speech	February 2009
2) DynaVox Xpress ™	Symbol-grid system and text-to-speech	August 2010
3) Dynavox Maestro ™	Symbol-grid system and text-to-speech	October 2010
4) Tellus 4	Text-to-speech	2010
5) ComLinkProSlate 4™	Symbol-grid system and text-to-speech	July 2011
6) ComLinkProSlate 8™	Symbol-grid system and text-to-speech	July 2011
7) ComLinkProSlate 10™	Symbol-grid system and text-to-speech	November 2012
8) ComLinkLT(3G) ™	Symbol-grid system and text-to-speech	January 2012
9) SoundPOD™	Wearable AAC device – converts ComLinkdevice or iPod/ iPad to wearable AAC device with speaker	July 2011
10) PowerBox 7	Symbol-grid system	June 2011
11) DynaWrite™2.0	Text to speech	June 2011
12) ECO2	Symbol-grid system	January 2012
13) Accent™1000, 1200	Symbol-grid system	November 2012
14) Tobii® C-Series C8, C12, C15	Symbol-grid system and text-to-speech	May 2013
15) Sahara EyeState	Tablet with built in eye gaze	June 2013
16) LightWriter® SL40	Text to speech	June 2013

Table 3. List of commercially available Augmentative and Alternative Communication (AAC) applications (released since 2008)

AAC apps	Description	Operating software
1) Talking TILES	Symbol-grid system	IOS and Android
2) Proloquo2go	Symbol-grid system and text-to-speech	IOS
3) Verbally	Text-to-speech, Access method-touch	IOS (Ipad only)
4) Sono Flex	Symbol-grid system and text-to-speech, Access method-touch	IOS, Android, Kindle Fire devices with Tobii Communicator
5) Scene & Heard	Photo story, Access method-Bluetooth switch, 'touch anywhere' scanning	IOS
6) Speech Button	Symbol-grid system, Simple vocabulary, Access method-touch	IOS
7) RocketKeys	Text-to-speech, Access method-touch	IOS and Android
8) MyTalkTools Mobile	Symbol-grid system, Access method-touch, Bluetooth switch	IOS
9) TalkRocketGo	Symbol-list system and text-to-speech	IOS and Android
10) SoundingBoard	Symbol-grid system, Access method-touch, Bluetooth switch	IOS

The high-tech assistive communication apps are available for a variety of operating platforms including windows, android, IOS (Apple Inc's mobile operating system for iPods, iPhones, and iPads) (Dixon, 2011). Unfortunately, most of these were developed without considering the typical language development process and stages (McNaughton, & Light, 2013; Light & McNaughton, 2012). They failed to reap the expected benefits, and this was attributed to mismatch between utility of the application functions and the individual's communication needs. Another constraint in use of these devices was its lack of support to connect thorough alternate access technologies. To overcome this, many AAC devices and applications with customization options have started to emerge. The customization features such as content of vocabulary, its organization, and visual appearance along with the medium of message transmission are now being made available in many of the AAC devices and applications. This flexibility allows the communication devices to be tailor-made to a specific user and thereby making it more applicable for individuals with CP with different communication needs. In addition, there is also a growing multilingual support in such AAC apps (Nakamura, Newell, Alm, Waller, 1998). Most AAC systems are symbol-based (pictures, spoken words or phrases) that are organized into grids or lists. The systems can be expanded, new words or phrases can be added and grouped topically to form communication pages as in Accent 1200, ComLinkLT 3G, PowerBox 7, Dynavox Maestro, Dynavox Xpress, Proloquo2Go,TalkRocket Go, TalkRocketGoMyVoice, Sono Flex, MyTalkTools Mobile, GoTalk Now, SoundingBoard. TalkingTILES. Tobii. The communication pages in these devices provide access to other pages that provide extensive organization, thus allowing caregivers, clinicians, and teachers to personalize the system and quickly adapt to changing communication needs of the AAC user. In addition to the vocabulary expansion, many AAC devices and applications permit the modification of visual appearance of symbols. They allow freedom to adjust the size, color and organisation of the symbols (e.g. Proloquo2Go, TalkRocket Go, Tobii C15) to make it suitable for individuals with visual acuity, visual field neglects, color blindness and other visuo-sensory impairments associated with CP. Device personalization can also be made in terms of voice output or text output.

Interface Options

Due to muscle tone and postural issues, managing the functional degrees of freedom of movement to reach the target location is of a particular concern for individuals with CP. The customization of aided AAC becomes crucial for establishing effective communication in children ith CP. This requires a strong understanding of the task constraints imposed by different selection methods/techniques. For devices that work with direct selection (alternative keyboards, touch screen) interface is through the target location. Whereas in indirect selection, input devices (e.g., standard mouse, joystick, trackball, mechanical switch etc.) require an interface that is independent of target location and activation i.e., the AAC user should first transport the effector to the input, then navigate the input device unit through the target location/activation to access the AAC device. To make this clear, for a child with CP to use a standard mouse (input device), the child has to lift his/her hand from a resting position and move his/her hand horizontally or vertically through space to contact the input device. Sometimes adaptations might be required to reach the target location on the input device to make a symbol selection. In few cases, the individual may be capable of lifting their hand from the resting position, and they may negotiate it through horizontal and longitudinal space, but may have limited degrees of freedom of movements in the x, y and z planes to make the selection. In such cases, adaptive devices such as control extenders similar to stylus and head pointers may be prescribed that can extend the range of motion of the effectors.

Access Options

For the aided communication to be effective, the user should be able to access the vocabulary within their functional abilities. Rosenbaum (2003) opined that early introduction of access solutions for children with CP can enable better communication and promote spoken language development. Using aided AAC systems with appropriate access options, dependence on communication partner for effective communication is minimized. This allows individuals with CP to become independent communicators in a variety of the social contexts (Blain, McKeever & Chau, 2010; Mumford, Lam, Wright, & Chau; 2014). However, in children with CP, access is a major barrier due to their limited range, flexibility, rate and degree of movement. Various access solutions are available, that facilitate AAC communication in individuals with CP. Any such solution consists of three main components- the access pathway, a signal processing unit and, the AAC system. The access pathway refers to the input that controls the AAC symbol selection. It can be direct (pointing, touching) or indirect (scanning, external mechanical switches). For children with CP who have some controlled movement, standard input devices such as trackballs, keyboards, mouse, joysticks, mechanical switches facilitate access to communication symbols on a communication aid or application. Few individuals may be capable of deictic gestures such as 'pointing' and devices that have capacitive and resistive touch screen technology can offer direct access to the vocabulary. In some severely impaired individuals, access solutions may be operated through switched that work with controlled intra-oral air pressure, and 'sip and puff' switches that are available commercially.

Prevailing Research Evidences

Although the number of available aided AAC devices has increased, evidences of their clinical effectiveness is only emerging. The empirical data on children with cerebral palsy and assistive technology have not been such that the results can be generalized (Carter, 2003; Clarke, McConachie, Price, & Wood, 2001; Garcia, Loureiro, Gonzales, Riveiro, & Sierra, 2011; Huang, Sugden, & Beveridge, 2009; McNaughton et al., 2008; Soto et al., 2001; Sutherland, Gillion, & Yoder, 2005). There is a clear dearth of high-quality randomized controlled trials that aim at establishing effectiveness of particular AAC interventions in children with CP. The variations in degree, distribution, type, onset, and associated deficits in the population and the complexity of AAC Communication design and development make the prevailing evidences in this science inconclusive. However, this section aim to summarize the available research findings related to AAC intervention in individuals with CP.

Though high- tech AAC usage have increased over the years, a survey revealed that low-tech AAC was still being used by approximately 50% of their population with CP (Murphy Markova, Moodie, Scott, & Boa, 1995). A major constraint in learning to use aided high-tech AAC communication by children with CP is their associated intellectual disability that slows down the process and limits the extent of effective usage. (Novac, Hines, & Goldsmith, et al., 2012; Geytenbeek, Vermeulen, & Becher et al., 2015) necessary for device usage. Therefore, active and supportive communication partners are critical for language and communicative development in children with CP and intellectual disability (Ballin, Balandin & Stancliffe, 2012; Tetzchner, Brekke, Sjothun et al., 2005).

The aided language modelling approach begins with the communication partner pointing out picture symbols on the child's communication display in conjunction to referring to real objects in the environment and providing verbal language modelling while using the AAC system (Romski, 2011; Sennott, Light, & McNaughton, 2016). Across the body of evidences, the findings have suggested an increase in overall expressive communication skills in the AAC users who were exposed to aided language modelling (Binger, 2008; Chiang, 2009; Kent-Wlash, 2015; Romnski, 2012; Sennott, 2016; Solomon Rice, 2014). Apart from expressive communication, an increase in expressive spontaneous communication and autonomous word production, these studies also reported an increase in mutli-symbolic AAC turns in individuals exposed to this approach (Binger, 2008; Chiang, 2009; Iacono, 1995; Kent-Wlash, 2015; Romnski, 2011; Sennott, 2016; Solomon Rice, 2014). Using aided communication was found to improve language to a greater extent compared to unaided alternate communication methods (Dada & Alant, 2009; Harris & Reichle, 2004; Iacono & Duncum, 1995; Iacono, 1995; Sennott, 2016; Solomon-Rice & Soto, 2014; Taylor & Iacono, 2003). Implementation of aided language stimulation with low tech static boards increased both receptive and expressive language among children with complex communication needs (Sennott, 2016; Dada & Alant, 2009; Harris & Reichle, 2004; Iacono & Duncum, 1995; Solomon-Rice & Soto, 2014; Taylor &Iacono, 2003). Similarly, in a study by Iacono (1995), a combination of high-tech aided communication using symbols of sign language was found to be more effective in eliciting expressive word productions than unaided sign language communication. Assistive devices such as micro switch-based program improved the adaptive skills of children with cerebral palsy (Stasolla, Caffo, Perilli, Damiani and D'Amico, 2019).

Studies on aided language stimulation techniques have included a variety of AAC systems including aided and non-aided modalities, static boards, structured use of picture symbols, Speech Generating Devices (SGDs), and Voice-Output Communication Aids (VOCA) (Iacono, 1995; Kent-Walsh, Binger, & Buchanan, 2015; Romski, Sevcik, Adamson, Smith, Cheslock, & Bakeman, 2011; Sennott, 2016; Solomon-Rice, 2014). A survey on 216 individuals with CP in Scotland, conducted by Murphy Markova, Moodie, Scott, and Boa (1995) revealed that among the high-tech AACs, voice output technology was most preferred for use by children with CP. With speech generating and voice output devices, partner strategies were found to be effective in facilitating communication and they provide additional communicative opportunities for the AAC user (Ballin, Balandin, & Stancliffe, 2012; Caron & Light, 2016; Gevarter & Zamora, 2018, 2018; Morin, Ganz, Gregori, Foster, Gerow, Genc-Tosun & Hong, 2018; Soto & Clarke, 2017). Few research studies have indicated positive outcome of using of high-tech speech generating devices in children with CP (Borgestig, Sandqvist, Ahlsten, Falkmer, &Hemmingsson, 2016; Clarke & Wilkinson, 2008; Ganz, Morin, Foster, Vannest, GencTosun, Gregori & Gerow, 2017; Gevarter & Zamora, 2018; Hormeyer & Renner, 2013; Roche, Lancioni & Green, 2015; Soto& Clarke, 2017). Borgestig, Sandqvist, and Ahlsten et al. (2016) found that the gaze-based assistive technology was effective in children with severe speech, language and physical impairment due to severe CP. The participants in their study learnt to use high-tech SGDs independently. Sai Aishwarya Ramani and Amudhu Sankar (2015) studied the effectiveness of learning to communicate through their SGD, named ISpeak and reported that the speech output acted as a positive reinforcement for the user. SGDs also reduce demand on the motoric activities which makes it easier to use by children with motoric impairment, including CP.

Though the future of assistive technology in language and communication rehabilitation seems promising, research studies showed that there are some hitches in its usage. Garcia, Loureiro, Gonzales, Riveiro, and Sierra (2011) reported that only 20% of their participants with CP used a communication devise. Similar proportion of usage was reported in adolescents with CP in the United Kingdom by Cockerill, Elbourne, Allen, Scrutton, Will, McNee, and Baird (2013). The Speech Generating Devices were not used by children with CP in school set up and they limited their communication to idiosyncratic gestures, facial expressions and yes/no answers (Clarke & Kirton, 2003) and this limited their social participation (Raghavendra, Olsson, Sampson, McInerney, & Connell, 2012). However, in an attempt to understand the usage of computer technology in children with CP attending school identified that it was used more frequently than mobility equipments (Borgestig et al., 2013; Hemmingsson, Gustavsson, & Townsend, 2007; Lidström, Almqvist, & Hemmingsson, 2012). Also, the aforementioned survey of Murphy Markova, Moodie, Scott, and Boa (1995) mentioned that a quarter of their population resort to AAC usage only in formal contexts.

As a member of the rehabilitation team, it is then important to understand the reason for this restriction of AAC usage in the social contexts. Soto, Muller, Hunt, and Goetz, (2001a, b) described 13 indicators of success for children who use AAC in inclusive school settings. These were (a) ownership of the students by the general educator, (b) collaborative teaming, (c) appropriate training to both the user and the communication partner (d) presence of an effective instructional assistant, (e) natural supports from classmates, (f) social interaction between the AAC user and peers, (g) academic participation by the AAC user, (h) successful use of the device, (i) supports and services in place, (j) AAC user membership and belonging, (k) classroom structure that supports the learning and participation of a heterogenous classroom, (l) philosophical support of inclusive education at the school district level, and (m) adequate classroom support. Treviranus and Roberts (2003) opined that successful communication using AAC systems results only when the AAC user is able to operate technical aspects of the AAC device. Huang, Sugden and Beveridge (2009) interviewed the perception of assistive device use in school going children with CP aged between 8 – 15 years, their mothers, and teachers. Their results suggested that the extent of usage was related to child's willingness, teachers' attitudes, mothers' support, physical environmental factors, and also the device-related features. Therefore, selecting the most apt features for the AAC communication device becomes top priority for rehabilitation team.

Stasolla, Caffo, Picucci and Bosco (2013) remarked that the customized input devices/sensors, personal computers, and screening of preferred stimuli according to a binomial criterion had positive impact on the social and education well-being of children with CP. Multimodal feedback was found to improve the speed of typing compared to its absence (Majaranta, MacKenzie, Aula, & Raiha, 2003). Such interactions with the AAC system and feedback is important for children with CP to persistently use the device for improving their function and performance (Buitrago, Bolanos & Caicedo Bravo, 2019).

Continued and unrestricted use of AAC device requires a life-long commitment, active involvement of family and peers, a supportive social environment and up-to-date information about the most recent technology options (Copley &Ziviani, 2007; Hemmingsson et al., 2007; Lidström et al., 2012; Mirenda & Mathy-Laikko, 1989). The current practice is to adopt a family centred care in early intervention and paediatric rehabilitation using AAC because proficiency in its use by communication partner is as important as the user themselves (Craddock, O'Halloran, Borthwick, & McPherson, 2006; Dunst, 2002; Hanna & Rodger, 2002; Rosenbaum et al., 1998; Trivette, Dunst, & Hamby, 1996). This approach is also welcomed by the parents and caregivers of AAC users. A One of the findings in the McNaughton et al., (2008) was that the parents often had to take the communication lead and therefore their demand to be proficient in operating the AAC device was stronger. Parental AAC communication proficient could be beneficial as they best support the child's communication attempts and strategies. Therefore, the current practices of AAC rehabilitation team include the caregiver, communication partner as well as the individual with complex communication need at all stages of design and development of the AAC system (Clarke et al., 2001; Jones & Stewart, 2004; Kent-Walsh & Light, 2003; McNaughton et al., 2008; Soto et al., 2001).

With a supportive familial and social involvement in AAC rehabilitation, the individual with CP gradually gain mastery over communication further improving confidence and self-belief (Craddock, 2006). This can have a positive impact on the user experience, further motivating them to use AAC in a variety of social context without social withdrawal. (Copley & Ziviani, 2004). Successful communication experience can motivate children with CP to use AAC in school settings rather than at home (Huang, Sugden, & Beveridge, 2009).

With communication, interaction, learning and education, the demand for improving the AAC device arise. Literacy is also one of the important factors to the use of more complex AAC systems (Bedrosian, 1999; Foley & Staples, 2003; Koppanhaver & Williams, 2010) and in children with complex communication needs, this becomes crucial. Smith, Dahlgren- Sandberg, and Larsson, (2009) opined that many children with severe speech and physical impairment fail to develop the level of literacy ability appropriate with their cognitive abilities. Therefore, inclusive education of AAC devise users is the need of the hour.

Communication requires two or more individuals who are involved in the process of sending and receiving messages. In children with cerebral palsy, the language learning and use is influenced by the motoric impairment and thus, they rely more upon their communication partners (parents, teachers, peers etc.). in any type of AAC intervention (aided/unaided), the communication partners play a crucial in providing communication opportunities which requires a guided practice. Thus, communication intervention using AAC requires communication partner training as well. However, few research studies have attempted to explore the effectiveness of parental training approaches (McConachie & Pennington, 1997; Hochstein, 2003). Few studies addressed the effectiveness of learning strategies in communication using SGDs in children with CP. Communication partner training involves teaching of partner strategies such as responsive strategy, environmental arrangements, open-ended questions, aided augmented input, behaviour chain interruption strategy (least-to-most) were emphasized.

The use of responsive strategy involves the communication partner to await, attend to and respond to the child's verbal and non-verbal behaviours (intention/unintentional) using SGDs. Few studies reported that using responsive strategy by the communication partner facilitated communication in children using SGDs (Fey et al., 2006; Hornmeyer & Renner, 2013; Engelke & Higginbotham, 2013). A study by Roche, Sigafoos, Lanciono, O'Reilly & Green (2015) found that 'environmental arrangement' strategy has been helpful for teaching those individuals who have severe physical, communicative and cognitive impairments to request for items and to initiate social communication. Asking 'open-ended' questions by the communication partner have proved to provide non-speaking children with additional opportunities to formulate linguistically complex answers using SGDs (Soto & Clarke, 2017). In addition, the use of an 'aided augmented input' (point to name symbols on SGDs during ongoing conversation) have shown positive outcomes to model language in terms of both comprehension and expression for children using SGDs (Allen, Schlosser, Brock, & Shane, 2017; O'Neill, Light & Pope, 2018).

Various strategies used for AAC communication training has also been researched upon for its effectiveness in children with CP. Among many behavioral strategies used with these children are the Behaviour Chain Interruption Strategy (BCIS) and the Least-to-Most Prompting Strategy. The BCIS is a naturalistic procedure wherein a routine is consciously interrupted by the trainer or the caregiver as a point of initiation of communication and its training. Least-to-Most prompting is an instructional strategy that provides a systematic hierarchy of prompts (cues) for the child to establish a communication task. Research has shown these to be effective in teaching to request things in individuals with cognitive impairment (Carter & Grunsell, 2001; Finke et al., 2017; Kent-Walsh, Binger & Malani, 2010).

Also, several studies have indicated that without adequate support and training to the communication partner, there is a risk of low use or even rejection of speech generating devices by the AAC user (Anderson, Balandin, & Stancliffe, 2014; Nailey, Parette, Stoner, Angell & Caroll, 2006a, McMillian, 2008; Stadskleiv, 2017; van Niekerk & Tonsing, 2015). Thus, training parents or communication partners with different AAC strategies, increased communication supports, using of AAC devices, aids and appliances can be beneficial and warrants further research.

FUTURE DIRECTIONS

Individuals with cerebral palsy pose greatest challenge in motor, sensory, language, behaviour, social, cognitive, language, communication and literacy development. There is considerable growing evidence in the field of AAC and its effectiveness in improving communication in individuals with cerebral palsy. Though the positive outcomes of AAC intervention has been documented, they are based on case studies or small group studies. Thus, there is need for research using a comprehensive AAC intervention programs that promises conclusive findings. Also, there is a drastic increase in the Individuals with Complex Communication Needs (CCN) and with the medical advances, the life span of these individuals with CCN has been increased. Thus, they require AAC services for a lifetime with changing needs across several environments. Also, there is increased awareness and acceptance of AAC by the caregivers and family members in the society and that provided adequate partner training, success of AAC intervention program can be warranted.

REFERENCES

Allen, A., Schlosser, R., Brock, K., & Shane, H. (2017). The effectiveness of aided augmented input techniques for persons with developmental disabilities: A systematic review. *Augmentative and Alternative Communication*, *33*(3), 1–11. doi:10.1080/07434618.2017.1338752 PMID:28633531

Andrew, D. P., Jason, T. N., & Karen, S. R. (2016). How does difficulty communicating affect the social relationships of older adults? An Exploration using data from a National Survey. *Journal of Communication Disorders*, *62*, 131–146. doi:10.1016/j.jcomdis.2016.06.002 PMID:27420152

Bailey, R. L., Stoner, J. B., Parette, H. P., & Angell, M. E. (2006). AAC team perceptions: Augmentative and alternative communication device use. *Education and Training in Developmental Disabilities*, *41*(2), 139.

Ballin, L., Balandin, S., & Stancliffe, R. J. (2012). The speech-generating device (SGD) mentoring program: Training adults who use an SGD to mentor. *Augmentative and Alternative Communication*, *28*(4), 254–265. doi:10.3109/07434618.2012.708880 PMID:23256857

Bax, M., Goldstein, M., Rosenbaum, P., Leviton, A., Paneth, N., Dan, B., ... Damiano, D. (2005). Proposed definition and classification of cerebral palsy, April 2005. *Developmental Medicine and Child Neurology*, *47*(8), 571–576. doi:10.1017/S001216220500112X PMID:16108461

Bedrosian, J. (1999). Efficacy research issues in AAC: Interactive storybook reading. *Augmentative and Alternative Communication, 15*(1), 45–55. doi:10.1080/07434619912331278565

Berkman, L. F., & Glass, T. (2000). Social integration, social networks, social support, and health. In L. F. Berkman & I. Kawachi (Eds.), *Social epidemiology*. Oxford, UK: Oxford University Press.

Berkman, L. F., Glass, T., Brissette, I., & Seeman, T. E. (2000). From social integration to health: Durkheim in the new millennium. *Social Science & Medicine, 51*(6), 843–857. doi:10.1016/S0277-9536(00)00065-4 PMID:10972429

Beukelman, D., & Mirenda, P. (1998). *Augmentative and alternative communication: Supporting children and adults with complex communication needs* (3rd ed.). Baltimore: Brookes.

Binger, C. (2008). Grammatical morpheme intervention issues for students who use AAC. *Perspectives on Augmentative and Alternative Communication, 17*(2), 62–68. doi:10.1044/aac17.2.62

Blain, S., McKeever, P., & Chau, T. (2010). Bedside computer access for an individual with severe and multiple disabilities: A case study. *Disability and Rehabilitation. Assistive Technology, 5*(5), 359–369. doi:10.3109/17483100903323275 PMID:20131978

Borgestig, M., Falkmer, T., & Hemmingsson, H. (2013). Improving computer usage for students with physical disabilities through a collaborative approach: A pilot study. *Scandinavian Journal of Occupational Therapy, 20*(6), 463–470. doi:10.3109/11038128.2013.837506 PMID:24041227

Borgestig, M., Sandqvist, J., Ahlsten, G., Falkmer, T., & Hemmingsson, H. (2017). Gaze- based assistive technology in daily activities in children with severe physical impairments–An intervention study. *Developmental Neurorehabilitation, 20*(3), 129–141. doi:10.3109/17518423.2015.1132281 PMID:26930111

Bradshaw, J. (2013). The use of augmentative and alternative communication apps for the iPad, iPod and iPhone: An overview of recent developments. *Tizard Learning Disability Review, 18*(1), 31–37. doi:10.1108/13595471311295996

Brady, N. (2000). Improved comprehension of object names following voice output communication aid use: Two case studies. *Augmentative and Alternative Communication, 16*(3), 197–204. doi:10.1080/07434610012331279054

Buitrago, J. A., Bolaños, A. M., & Caicedo Bravo, E. (2019). A motor learning therapeutic intervention for a child with cerebral palsy through a social assistive robot. *Disability and Rehabilitation. Assistive Technology*, 1–6. doi:10.1080/17483107.2019.1578999 PMID:30806105

Carlsson, M., Hagberg, G., & Olsson, I. (2003). Clinical and aetiological aspects of epilepsy in children with cerebral palsy. *Developmental Medicine and Child Neurology, 45*(6), 371–376. doi:10.1111/j.1469-8749.2003.tb00415.x PMID:12785437

Caron, J., & Light, J. (2016). "Social media has opened a world of 'open communication:'" Experiences of adults with cerebral palsy who use augmentative and alternative communication and social media. *Augmentative and Alternative Communication, 32*(1), 25–40. doi:10.3109/07434618.2015.1052887 PMID:26056722

Carter, M. (2003). Communicative spontaneity of children with high support needs who use augmentative and alternative communication systems II: Antecedents and effectiveness of communication. *Augmentative and Alternative Communication, 19*(3), 155–169. doi:10.1080/0743461031000112025

Carter, M., & Grunsell, J. (2001). The behaviour chain interruption strategy: A review of research and discussion of future directions. *Research and Practice for Persons with Severe Disabilities, 26*(1), 37–49. doi:10.1177/1540796919828082

Chiang, H. M. (2009). Naturalistic observations of elicited expressive communication of children with autism: An analysis of teacher instructions. *Autism, 13*(2), 165–178. doi:10.1177/1362361308098513 PMID:19261686

Clarke, H., McConachie, K., Price, P., & Wood, M. (2001). Views of young people using augmentative and alternative communication systems. *International Journal of Language & Communication Disorders, 36*(1), 107–115. doi:10.1080/13682820150217590 PMID:11221427

Clarke, M., & Kirton, A. (2003). Patterns of interaction between children with physical disabilities using augmentative and alternative communication systems and their peers. *Child Language Teaching and Therapy, 19*(2), 135–151. doi:10.1191/0265659003ct248oa

Clarke, M., & Price, K. (2012). Augmentative and alternative communication for children with cerebral palsy. *Paediatrics & Child Health, 22*(9), 367–371. doi:10.1016/j.paed.2012.03.002

Clarke, M., & Wilkinson, R. (2008). Interaction between children with cerebral palsy and their peers 2: Understanding initiated VOCA-mediated turns. *Augmentative and Alternative Communication, 24*(1), 3–15. doi:10.1080/07434610701390400 PMID:18256962

Cockerill, H., Elbourne, D., Allen, E., Scrutton, D., Will, E., McNee, A., ... Baird, G. (2014). Speech, communication and use of augmentative communication in young people with cerebral palsy: The SH & PE population study. *Child: Care, Health and Development, 40*(2), 149–157. doi:10.1111/cch.12066 PMID:23656274

Cohen, S. (2004). Social relationships and health. *The American Psychologist, 59*(8), 676–684. doi:10.1037/0003-066X.59.8.676 PMID:15554821

Colker, R. (1999). Americans with disabilities act: A windfall for defendants. *Harvard Civil Rights-Civil Liberties Law Review*, 34–99.

Cook, A. M., & Polgar, J. M. (2014). *Essentials of Assistive Technologies-E-Book*. Elsevier Health Sciences.

Copley, J., & Ziviani, J. (2004). Barriers to the use of assistive technology for children with multiple disabilities. *Occupational Therapy International, 11*(4), 229–243. doi:10.1002/oti.213 PMID:15771212

Copley, J., & Ziviani, J. (2007). Use of a team-based approach to assistive technology assessment and planning for children with multiple disabilities: A pilot study. *Assistive Technology, 19*(3), 109–127. do i:10.1080/10400435.2007.10131869 PMID:17937054

Craddock, D., O'Halloran, C., Borthwick, A., & McPherson, K. (2006). Interprofessional education in health and social care: Fashion or informed practice? *Learning in Health and Social Care, 5*(4), 220–242. doi:10.1111/j.1473-6861.2006.00135.x

Dada, S., & Alant, E. (2009). The effect of aided language stimulation on vocabulary acquisition in children with little or no functional speech. *American Journal of Speech-Language Pathology*, *18*(1), 50–64. doi:10.1044/1058-0360(2008/07-0018) PMID:19106207

DeCoste, D. C. (1997). T: programs for children who employ AAC systems due to severe speech and physical disabilities continues to present a monumental challenge to professionals. The reason is simple yet confounding: unable to speak or to manipulate pencil and paper, these children have difficulty developing and demonstrating their ability to read and write through convention. The Handbook of Augmentative and Alternative Communication, 283.

Deruyter, F., McNaughton, D., Caves, K., Bryen, D. N., & Williams, M. B. (2007). Enhancing AAC connections with the world. *Augmentative and Alternative Communication*, *23*(3), 258–270. doi:10.1080/07434610701553387 PMID:17701744

Dixon, D. (2011). The future of apps in the classroom. *ASHA Leader*, *16*(12), 30–30. doi:10.1044/leader.SCM.16122011.30

Dunst, C. J. (2002). Family-centered practices: Birth through high school. *The Journal of Special Education*, *36*(3), 141–149. doi:10.1177/00224669020360030401

Engelke, C., & Higginbotham, J. (2013). Looking to speak: On the temporality of misalignment in interaction involving an augmented communicator using eye-gaze technology. *Journal of Interactional Research in Communication Disorders*, *4*(1), 95–122. doi:10.1558/jircd.v4i1.95

Fallon, K. A., & Katz, L. A. (2008, May). Augmentative and alternative communication and literacy teams: Facing the challenges, forging ahead. *Seminars in Speech and Language*, *29*(02), 112–119. doi:10.1055-2008-1079125 PMID:18645913

Fey, M., Warren, S., Brady, N., Finestack, L., Brejin-Oja, S., Fairchild, M., ... Yoder, P. (2006). Early e.ffects of responsivity education/prelinguistic milieu teaching for children with developmental delays and their parents. *International Journal of Speech-Language Pathology*, *49*(3), 526–547. PMID:16787894

Finke, E., Davis, J., Benedict, M., Goga, L., Kelly, J., Palumbo, L., ... Waters, S. (2017). Eff ects of a least-to-most prompting procedure on multi-symbol message production in children with autism spectrum disorder who use augmentative and alternative communication. *American Journal of Speech-Language Pathology*, *26*(1), 81–98. doi:10.1044/2016_AJSLP-14-0187 PMID:28056153

Foley, B. E., & Staples, A. H. (2003). Developing augmentative and alternative communication (AAC) and literacy interventions in a supported employment setting. *Topics in Language Disorders*, *23*(4), 325–343. doi:10.1097/00011363-200310000-00007

Ganz, J. B., Morin, K. L., Foster, M. J., Vannest, K. J., Genç Tosun, D., Gregori, E. V., & Gerow, S. L. (2017). High-technology augmentative and alternative communication for individuals with intellectual and developmental disabilities and complex communication needs: A meta-analysis. *Augmentative and Alternative Communication*, *33*(4), 224–238. doi:10.1080/07434618.2017.1373855 PMID:28922953

Gevarter, C., & Zamora, C. (2018). Naturalistic speech-generating device interventions for children with complex communication needs: A systematic review of single-subject studies. *American Journal of Speech-Language Pathology*, *27*(3), 1073–1090. doi:10.1044/2018_AJSLP-17-0128 PMID:29971336

Geytenbeek, J. J., Vermeulen, R. J., Becher, J. G., & Oostrom, K. J. (2015). Comprehension of spoken language in non-speaking children with severe cerebral palsy: An explorative study on associations with motor type and disabilities. *Developmental Medicine and Child Neurology*, *57*(3), 294–300. doi:10.1111/dmcn.12619 PMID:25349105

Hanna, K., & Rodger, S. (2002). Towards family-centered practice in pediatric occupational therapy: A review of the literature on parent–therapist collaboration. *Australian Occupational Therapy Journal*, *49*(1), 14–24. doi:10.1046/j.0045-0766.2001.00273.x

Harris, M. D., & Reichle, J. (2004). The impact of aided language stimulation on symbol comprehension and production in children with moderate cognitive disabilities. *American Journal of Speech-Language Pathology*, *13*(2), 155–167. doi:10.1044/1058-0360(2004/016) PMID:15198634

Hemmingsson, H., Gustavsson, A., & Townsend, E. (2007). Students with disabilities participating in mainstream schools: Policies that promote and limit teacher and therapist cooperation. *Disability & Society*, *22*(4), 383–398. doi:10.1080/09687590701337892

Himmelmann, K., Hagberg, G., & Uvebrant, P. (2010). The changing panorama of cerebral palsy in Sweden. X. Prevalence and origin in the birth-year period 1999–2002. *Acta Paediatrica (Oslo, Norway)*, *99*(9), 1337–1343. doi:10.1111/j.1651-2227.2010.01819.x PMID:20377538

Hochstein, D. D., McDaniel, M. A., Nettleton, S., & Neufeld, K. H. (2003). The fruitfulness of a nomothetic approach to investigating AAC: Comparing 2 speech encoding schemes across cerebral palsied and nondisabled children. *American Journal of Speech-Language Pathology*, *12*(1), 110–120. doi:10.1044/1058-0360(2003/057) PMID:12680818

Hodge, S. (2007). Why is the potential of augmentative and alternative communication not being realized? Exploring the experiences of people who use communication aids. *Disability & Society*, *22*(5), 457–471. doi:10.1080/09687590701427552

Holt-Lunstad, J., Smith, T. B., & Layton, B. (n.d.). Social relationships and mortality risk: A meta-analytic review. *PLoS Medicine*, *7*(7), e1316. doi:1.1371/journal.pmed.1316

Hörmeyer, I., & Renner, G. (2013). Confirming and denying in co-construction processes: A case study of an adult with cerebral palsy and two familiar partners. *Augmentative and Alternative Communication*, *29*(3), 259–271. doi:10.3109/07434618.2013.813968 PMID:23952567

Huang, I. C., Sugden, D., & Beveridge, S. (2009). Children's perceptions of their use of assistive devices in home and school settings. *Disability and Rehabilitation. Assistive Technology*, *4*(2), 95–105. doi:10.1080/17483100802613701 PMID:19253098

Hustad, K. C., Gorton, K., & Lee, J. (2010). Classification of speech and language profiles in 4-year-old children with cerebral palsy: A prospective preliminary study. *Journal of Speech, Language, and Hearing Research: JSLHR*, *53*(6), 1496–1513. doi:10.1044/1092-4388(2010/09-0176) PMID:20643795

Iacono, T., & Duncum, J. (1995). Comparison of sign alone and in combination with an electronic communication device in early language intervention: Case study. *Augmentative and Alternative Communication*, *11*(4), 249–259. doi:10.1080/07434619512331277389

Jan, J. E., Lyons, C. J., Heaven, R. K., & Matsuba, C. (2001). Visual impairment due to a dyskinetic eye movement disorder in children with dyskinetic cerebral palsy. *Developmental Medicine and Child Neurology*, *43*(2), 108–112. doi:10.1017/S0012162201000184 PMID:11221897

Jones, J., & Stewart, H. (2004). A description of how three occupational therapists train children in using the scanning access technique. *Australian Occupational Therapy Journal*, *51*(3), 155–165. doi:10.1111/j.1440-1630.2004.00445.x

Judge, S., & Friday, M. (2011). Ambiguous keyboards for AAC. *Journal of Assistive Technologies*, *5*(4), 249–256. doi:10.1108/17549451111190650

Kent-Walsh, J., Binger, C., & Buchanan, C. (2015). Teaching children who use augmentative and alternative communication to ask inverted yes/no questions using aided modeling. *American Journal of Speech-Language Pathology*, *24*(2), 222–236. doi:10.1044/2015_AJSLP-14-0066 PMID:25650561

Kent-Walsh, J., Binger, C., & Malani, M. (2010). Teaching partners to support the communication skills of young children who use AAC: Lessons from the ImPAACT program. *Early Childhood Services (San Diego, Calif.)*, *4*(3), 210–226.

Kent-Walsh, J., & Light, J. (2003). General education teachers' experiences with inclusion of students who use augmentative and alternative communication. *Augmentative and Alternative Communication*, *19*(2), 104–124. doi:10.1080/0743461031000112043

Kondo, T., & Raff, M. (2000). Oligodendrocyte precursor cells reprogrammed to become multipotential CNS stem cells. *Science*, *289*(5485), 1754–1757. doi:10.1126cience.289.5485.1754 PMID:10976069

Koppenhaver, D., & Williams, A. (2010). A conceptual review of writing research in augmentative and alternative communication. *Augmentative and Alternative Communication*, *26*(3), 158–176. doi:10.3109/07434618.2010.505608 PMID:20874079

Krägeloh-Mann, I., & Cans, C. (2009). Cerebral palsy update. *Brain & Development*, *31*(7), 537–544. doi:10.1016/j.braindev.2009.03.009 PMID:19386453

Krigger, K. W. (2006). Cerebral palsy: An overview. *American Family Physician*, *73*(1), 91–100. PMID:16417071

Lidström, H., Almqvist, L., & Hemmingsson, H. (2012). Computer-based assistive technology device for use by children with physical disabilities: A cross-sectional study. *Disability and Rehabilitation. Assistive Technology*, *7*(4), 287–293. doi:10.3109/17483107.2011.635332 PMID:22612787

Light, J., Collier, B., & Parnes, P. (1985). Communicative interaction between young nonspeaking physically disabled children and their primary caregivers: Part II— Communicative function. *Augmentative and Alternative Communication*, *1*(3), 98–107. doi:10.1080/07434618512331273591

Light, J., & Drager, K. (2007). AAC technologies for young children with complex communication needs: State of the science and future research directions. *Augmentative and Alternative Communication*, *23*(3), 204–216. doi:10.1080/07434610701553635 PMID:17701740

Light, J., & McNaughton, D. (2012). Supporting the communication, language, and literacy development of children with complex communication needs: State of the science and future research priorities. *Assistive Technology, 24*(1), 34–44. doi:10.1080/10400435.2011.648717 PMID:22590798

Lloyd, L. L., Fuller, D. R., & Arvidson, H. H. (1997). *Augmentative and alternative communication: A handbook of principles and practices*. Allyn and Bacon.

Majaranta, P., MacKenzie, I. S., Aula, A., & Räihä, K. J. (2003, April). Auditory and visual feedback during eye typing. In *Conference on Human Factors in Computing Systems: CHI'03 extended abstracts on Human factors in computing systems* (Vol. 5, No. 10, pp. 766-767). 10.1145/765891.765979

McBride, D. (2011). AAC evaluations and new mobile technologies: Asking and answering the right questions. *Perspectives on Augmentative and Alternative Communication, 20*(1), 9–16. doi:10.1044/aac20.1.9

McConachie, H., & Pennington, L. (1997). In-service training for schools on augmentative and alternative communication. *European Journal of Disorders of Communication, 32*(s3), 277–288. doi:10.1080/13682829709177101 PMID:9474293

McLellan, A., Cipparone, C., Giancola, D., Armstrong, D., & Bartlett, D. (2012). Medical and surgical procedures experienced by young children with cerebral palsy. *Pediatric Physical Therapy, 24*(3), 268–277. doi:10.1097/PEP.0b013e31825be2f6 PMID:22735479

McNaughton, D., & Light, J. (2013). The iPad and mobile technology revolution: Benefits and challenges for individuals who require augmentative and alternative communication. *Augmentative and Alternative Communication, 29*(2), 107–116. doi:10.3109/07434618.2013.784930 PMID:23705813

McNaughton, D., Rackensperger, T., Benedek-Wood, E., Krezman, C., Williams, M. B., & Light, J. (2008). "A child needs to be given a chance to succeed": Parents of individuals who use AAC describe the benefits and challenges of learning AAC technologies. *Augmentative and Alternative Communication, 24*(1), 43–55. doi:10.1080/07434610701421007 PMID:18256963

Mirenda, P., & Mathy-Laikko, P. (1989). Augmentative and alternative communication applications for persons with severe congenital communication disorders: An introduction. *Augmentative and Alternative Communication, 5*(1), 3–13. doi:10.1080/07434618912331274916

Morin, K. L., Ganz, J. B., Gregori, E. V., Foster, M. J., Gerow, S. L., Genç-Tosun, D., & Hong, E. R. (2018). A systematic quality review of high-tech AAC interventions as an evidence-based practice. *Augmentative and Alternative Communication, 34*(2), 104–117. doi:10.1080/07434618.2018.1458900 PMID:29697288

Mumford, L., Lam, R., Wright, V., & Chau, T. (2014). An access technology delivery protocol for children with severe and multiple disabilities: A case demonstration. *Developmental Neurorehabilitation, 17*(4), 232–242. doi:10.3109/17518423.2013.776125 PMID:23869969

Murphy, J., Marková, I., Moodie, E., Scott, J., & Boa, S. (1995). Augmentative and alternative communication systems used by people with cerebral palsy in Scotland: Demographic survey. *Augmentative and Alternative Communication, 11*(1), 26–36. doi:10.1080/07434619512331277119

Murray, J., & Goldbart, J. (2009). Cognitive and language acquisition in typical and aided language learning: A review of recent evidence from an aided communication perspective. *Child Language Teaching and Therapy*, *25*(1), 31–58. doi:10.1177/0265659008098660

Mutch, L., Leyland, A., & McGee, A. (1993). Patterns of neuropsychological function in a low-birthweight population. *Developmental Medicine and Child Neurology*, *35*(11), 943–956. doi:10.1111/j.1469-8749.1993.tb11576.x PMID:8224562

Nakamura, K., Newell, A., Alm, N., & Waller, A. (1998). How do members of different language communities compose sentences with a picture-based communication system?—A cross–cultural study of picture–based sentences constructed by English and Japanese speakers. *Augmentative and Alternative Communication*, *14*(2), 71–80. doi:10.1080/07434619812331278226

Novak, I., Hines, M., Goldsmith, S., & Barclay, R. (2012). Clinical prognostic messages from a systematic review on cerebral palsy. *Pediatrics*, *130*(5), e1285–e1312. doi:10.1542/peds.2012-0924 PMID:23045562

O'Neill, T., Light, J., & Pope, L. (2018). Effects of interventions that include aided augmentative and alternative communication input on the communication of individuals with complex communication needs: A meta-analysis. *Journal of Speech, Language, and Hearing Research: JSLHR*, *61*(7), 1743–1765. doi:10.1044/2018_JSLHR-L-17-0132 PMID:29931287

Odding, E., Roebroeck, M. E., & Stam, H. J. (2006). The epidemiology of cerebral palsy: Incidence, impairments and risk factors. *Disability and Rehabilitation*, *28*(4), 183–191. doi:10.1080/09638280500158422 PMID:16467053

Palisano, R. J., Begnoche, D. M., Chiarello, L. A., Bartlett, D. J., McCoy, S. W., & Chang, H. J. (2012). Amount and focus of physical therapy and occupational therapy for young children with cerebral palsy. *Physical & Occupational Therapy in Pediatrics*, *32*(4), 368–382. doi:10.3109/01942638.2012.715620 PMID:22954372

Park, M. J., Yoo, Y. J., Chung, C. Y., & Hwang, J. M. (2016). Ocular findings in patients with spastic type cerebral palsy. *BMC Ophthalmology*, *16*(1), 195. doi:10.118612886-016-0367-1 PMID:27821110

Pennington, B. F. (2008). *Diagnosing learning disorders: A neuropsychological framework*. Guilford Press.

Pennington, L., Goldbart, J., & Marshall, J. (2004). Speech and language therapy to improve the communication skills of children with cerebral palsy. *Cochrane Database of Systematic Reviews*, (2): CD003466. PMID:15106204

Pennington, L., & Mcconachie, H. (1999). Mother-child interaction revisited: Communication with non-speaking physically disabled children. *International Journal of Language & Communication Disorders*, *34*(4), 391–416. doi:10.1080/136828299247351 PMID:10884908

Pennington, M. C. (1999). Computer-aided pronunciation pedagogy: Promise, limitations, directions. *Computer Assisted Language Learning*, *12*(5), 427–440. doi:10.1076/call.12.5.427.5693

Pirila, S., van der Meere, J., Pentikainen, T., Ruusu-Niemi, P., Korpela, R., Kilpinen, J., & Nieminen, P. (2007). Language and motor speech skills in children with cerebral palsy. *Journal of Communication Disorders*, *40*(2), 116–128. doi:10.1016/j.jcomdis.2006.06.002 PMID:16860820

Pousada García, T., Pereira Loureiro, J., Groba González, B., Nieto Riveiro, L., & Pazos Sierra, A. (2011). The use of computers and augmentative and alternative communication devices by children and young with cerebral palsy. *Assistive Technology*, *23*(3), 135–149. doi:10.1080/10400435.2011.588988

Radomski, M. V., & Latham, C. A. T. (Eds.). (2008). *Occupational therapy for physical dysfunction*. Lippincott Williams & Wilkins.

Raghavendra, P., Olsson, C., Sampson, J., Mcinerney, R., & Connell, T. (2012). School participation and social networks of children with complex communication needs, physical disabilities, and typically developing peers. *Augmentative and Alternative Communication*, *28*(1), 33–43. doi:10.3109/07434618.2011.653604 PMID:22364536

Ramani, S. A., & Sankar, A. (2016). "ISpeak"- Augmentative and Alternative Communication for children with Communication Disorders. *Sri Ramachandra Journal of Medicine*, *9*(1), 1–4.

Ratcliff, A., & Little, M. (1996). A conversation based barrier task approach to teach sight- word vocabulary to a young augmentative communication system user. *Child Language Teaching and Therapy*, *12*(2), 128–135. doi:10.1177/026565909601200203

Reddihough, D. (2011). Cerebral palsy in childhood. *Australian Family Physician*, *40*(4), 192. PMID:21597527

Roche, L., Sigafoos, J., Lancioni, G. E., O'Reilly, M. F., & Green, V. A. (2015). Microswitch technology for enabling self-determined responding in children with profound and multiple disabilities: A systematic review. *Augmentative and Alternative Communication*, *31*(3), 246–258. doi:10.3109/07434618.2015.1024888 PMID:25791421

Roche, S., & Lancioni, O. (2015). Microswitch technology for enabling self- determined responding in children with profound and multiple disabilities: A systematic review. *Augmentative and Alternative Communication*, *31*(1), 246–258. doi:10.3109/07434618.2015.1024888 PMID:25791421

Romanski, L. M. (2012). Integration of faces and vocalizations in ventral prefrontal cortex: Implications for the evolution of audiovisual speech. *Proceedings of the National Academy of Sciences of the United States of America*, *109*(Supplement 1), 10717–10724. doi:10.1073/pnas.1204335109 PMID:22723356

Romski, M., Sevcik, R. A., Adamson, L. B., Smith, A., Cheslock, M., & Bakeman, R. (2011). Parent perceptions of the language development of toddlers with developmental delays before and after participation in parent-coached language interventions. *American Journal of Speech-Language Pathology*, *20*(2), 111–118. doi:10.1044/1058-0360(2011/09-0087) PMID:21330651

Romski, M. A., & Sevcik, R. A. (1996). Breaking the speech barrier: Language development through augmented means. Brookes Publishing Company.

Rosenbaum, P. (2003). Cerebral palsy: What parents and doctors want to know. *BMJ (Clinical Research Ed.)*, *326*(7396), 970–974. doi:10.1136/bmj.326.7396.970 PMID:12727772

Rosenbaum, P., King, S., Law, M., King, G., & Evans, J. (1998). Family-centred service: A conceptual framework and research review. *Physical & Occupational Therapy in Pediatrics*, *18*(1), 1–20.

Rosenbaum, P., Paneth, N., Leviton, A., Goldstein, M., Bax, M., Damiano, D., ... Jacobsson, B. (2007). A report: The definition and classification of cerebral palsy April 2006. *Developmental Medicine and Child Neurology. Supplement, 109*, 8–14. PMID:17370477

Schaefer, G. B. (2008). Genetics considerations in cerebral palsy. *Seminars in Pediatric Neurology, 15*(1), 21–26. doi:10.1016/j.spen.2008.01.004 PMID:18342257

Sennott, S. C., Light, J. C., & McNaughton, D. (2016). AAC modeling intervention research review. *Research and Practice for Persons with Severe Disabilities, 41*(2), 101–115. doi:10.1177/1540796916638822

Shane, S. (2012). Reflections on the 2010 AMR decade award: Delivering on the promise of entrepreneurship as a field of research. *Academy of Management Review, 37*(1), 10–20. doi:10.5465/amr.2011.0078

Siegel, E. B., & Cress, C. J. (2002). Overview of the Emergence of Early AAC Behaviors: Progression from Communicative to Symbolic Skills. *Exemplary Practicies for Beginning Communicators: Implications for AAC.*

Sigafoos, J., Drasgow, E., & Schlosser, R. W. (2003). Strategies for beginning communicators. In R. W. Schlosser (Ed.), *The efficacy of augmentative and alternative communication: Toward evidence-based practice* (pp. 323–346). Boston, MA: Academic Press.

Sigurdardottir, S., Eiriksdottir, A., Gunnarsdottir, E., Meintema, M., Arnadottir, U., & Vik, T. (2008). Cognitive profile in young Icelandic children with cerebral palsy. *Developmental Medicine and Child Neurology, 50*(5), 357–362. doi:10.1111/j.1469-8749.2008.02046.x PMID:18355334

Smith, M., Sandberg, A. D., & Larsson, M. (2009). Reading and spelling in children with severe speech and physical impairments: A comparative study. *International Journal of Language & Communication Disorders, 44*(6), 864–882. doi:10.1080/13682820802389873 PMID:19105069

Solomon-Rice, P. L., & Soto, G. (2014). Facilitating vocabulary in toddlers using AAC: A preliminary study comparing focused stimulation and augmented input. *Communication Disorders Quarterly, 35*(4), 204–215. doi:10.1177/1525740114522856

Solomon-Rice, P. L., & Soto, G. (2014). Facilitating vocabulary in toddlers using AAC: A preliminary study comparing focused stimulation and augmented input. *Communication Disorders Quarterly, 35*(4), 204–215. doi:10.1177/1525740114522856

Soto, G., & Clarke, M. T. (2017). Effects of a conversation-based intervention on the linguistic skills of children with motor speech disorders who use augmentative and alternative communication. *Journal of Speech, Language, and Hearing Research, 60*(7), 1980–1998. doi:10.1044/2016_JSLHR-L-15-0246 PMID:28672283

Soto, G., Müller, E., Hunt, P., & Goetz, L. (2001). Critical issues in the inclusion of students who use augmentative and alternative communication: An educational team perspective. *Augmentative and Alternative Communication, 17*(2), 62–72. doi:10.1080/aac.17.2.62.72

Soto, G., Müller, E., Hunt, P., & Goetz, L. (2001). Professional skills for serving students who use AAC in general education classrooms. *Language, Speech, and Hearing Services in Schools, 32*(1), 51–56. doi:10.1044/0161-1461(2001/005) PMID:27764437

Stasolla, F., Caffò, A. O., Perilli, V., Boccasini, A., Damiani, R., & D'Amico, F. (2019). Assistive technology for promoting adaptive skills of children with cerebral palsy: Ten cases evaluation. *Disability and Rehabilitation. Assistive Technology, 14*(5), 489–502. doi:10.1080/17483107.2018.1467972 PMID:29732901

Stasolla, F., Caffo, A. O., Picucci, L., & Bosco, A. (2013). Assistive technology for promoting choice behaviors in three children with cerebral palsy and severe communication impairments. *Research in Developmental Disabilities, 34*(9), 2694–2700. doi:10.1016/j.ridd.2013.05.029 PMID:23770888

Steenbergen, B., & Gordon, A. M. (2006). Activity limitation in hemiplegic cerebral palsy: Evidence for disorders in motor planning. *Developmental Medicine and Child Neurology, 48*(9), 780–783. doi:10.1017/S0012162206001666 PMID:16904028

Sutherland, D. E., Gillon, G. G., & Yoder, D. E. (2005). AAC use and service provision: A survey of New Zealand speech-language therapists. *Augmentative and Alternative Communication, 21*(4), 295–307. doi:10.1080/07434610500103483

Taylor, R., & Iacono, T. (2003). AAC and scripting activities to facilitate communication and play. *Advances in Speech Language Pathology, 5*(2), 79–93. doi:10.1080/1441704051000166911 1

Thiemann-Bourque, K., Brady, N., McGuff, S., Stump, K., & Naylor, A. (2016). Picture exchange communication system and pals: A peer-mediated augmentative and alternative communication intervention for minimally verbal preschoolers with autism. *Journal of Speech, Language, and Hearing Research: JSLHR, 59*(5), 1133–1145. doi:10.1044/2016_JSLHR-L-15-0313 PMID:27679841

Tönsing, K. M., Alant, E., & Lloyd, L. L. (2005). Augmentative and alternative communication. *Augmentative and alternative communication and severe disabilities: Beyond poverty*, 30-67.

Treviranus, J., & Roberts, V. (2003). Supporting competent motor control of AAC systems. *Communicative competence for individuals who use AAC*, 199-240.

Trivette, C. M., Dunst, C. J., & Hamby, D. W. (1996). Factors associated with perceived control appraisals in a family-centered early intervention program. *Journal of Early Intervention, 20*(2), 165–178. doi:10.1177/105381519602000207

Uchino, B. N. (2006). Social support and health: A review of physiological processes potentially underlying links to disease outcomes. *Journal of Behavioral Medicine, 29*(4), 377–387. doi:10.100710865-006-9056-5 PMID:16758315

Valvano, J., & Newell, K. M. (1998). Practice of a precision isometric grip-force task by children with spastic cerebral palsy. *Developmental Medicine and Child Neurology, 40*(7), 464–473. doi:10.1111/j.1469-8749.1998.tb15397.x PMID:9698060

Venkateswaran, S., & Shevell, M. I. (2008). Comorbidities and clinical determinants of outcome in children with spastic quadriplegic cerebral palsy. *Developmental Medicine and Child Neurology, 50*(3), 216–222. doi:10.1111/j.1469-8749.2008.02033.x PMID:18248493 von Tetzchner, S., Brekke, K. M., Sjøthun, B., & Grindheim, E. (2005). Constructing preschool communities of learners that afford alternative language development. *Augmentative and Alternative Communication, 21*(2), 82–100. doi:10.1080/07434610500103541

Wilkinson, K. M., & Hennig, S. (2007). The state of research and practice in augmentative and alternative communication for children with developmental/intellectual disabilities. *Mental Retardation and Developmental Disabilities Research Reviews, 13*(1), 58–69. doi:10.1002/mrdd.20133 PMID:17326111

World Health Organization. (2004). *International statistical classification of diseases and related health problems: instruction manual* (Vol. 2). World Health Organization.

Chapter 6
Aided Augmentative and Alternative Communication (AAC) Systems for Individuals With Autism Spectrum Disorders

Yashomathi
Department of Speech-Language Pathology, All India Institute of Speech and Hearing (AIISH), Mysuru, India

ABSTRACT

Autism spectrum disorders (ASDs) are complex neuro-developmental disorders. They demonstrate pervasive deficits in social communication, restricted and repetitive behaviors, cognitive impairments, etc. Most often individuals with ASDs are often considered "non-verbal" and they require comprehensive intervention to improve their functional communication skills. Augmentative and alternative communication (AAC) was always viewed as a "last resort" for people with complex communication needs when all other interventions failed to achieve the potential benefit. However, with growing evidence, AAC has been implemented even in children with communication difficulties to augment spoken language development. Thus, this chapter aims to discuss the characteristics of ASD, to describe the need for AAC intervention in children with ASD, challenges and practices of AAC in ASD, to review implementation of aided AAC systems for children with ASD in different contexts, to indicate the gaps and future prospective in AAC intervention for people with ASDs.

INTRODUCTION

Autism Spectrum Disorders (ASD) is a neurodevelopmental disorder that begins in early childhood/ developmental period. It is a complex condition marked by a wide range of symptoms and varying degree of severity. ASD is characterised by persistent impairments in social interaction, communica-

DOI: 10.4018/978-1-7998-3069-6.ch006

tion, and restricted, repetitive, and stereotyped patterns of behaviours, interests, or activities (American Psychiatric Association [APA], 2013). Autism Spectrum Disorders (ASD) are also referred to as Pervasive Developmental Disorders (PDD) that includes a spectrum of disorders such as Autism, Asperger's syndrome, Rett's syndrome, Childhood Disintegrative Disorder (CDD), and Pervasive Developmental Disorder – Not Otherwise Specified (PDD-NoS). As per the reports of Autism Society of America, the rate of incidence of autism is increasing 10-17% per year in the US and the prevalence of autism is expected to reach 4 million people in the next decade in the United States. Also, autism is found to be four times more prevalent in males than girls in the US. However, in India, the incidence rate of autism is found to be approximately 1 in11,914 people and prevalence rate of autism is found to be 1 in 500 people (Centre for Disease Control).

Characteristics of Autism Spectrum Disorders (ASDs)

There is evidence to suggest that the diagnostic features of ASD are evident in very young children as early as 2 years of life. Studies have indicated that following are some of the early indicators of ASD:

1) Impairment in the children's language development and social relatedness noticed as early as 14 months of age (Chawarska, Paul, Klin, Hannigen, Dichtel, & Volkmar, 2007);
2) Display of significantly lesser number of joint attention and communication behaviours at 1 year of age compared to their age equivalent typically developing peers (Osterling & Dawson, 1994; Werner & Dawson, 2005);
3) Demonstrates impaired eye-contact, decreased activity level, and passivity by 12 months of age (Zwaigenbaum, Bryson, Rogers, Roberts, Brian & Szatmari, 2005);
4) Subtle differences in sensory-motor domains and social behavior (Baranek, 1999) as well as differences in the use of communicative gestures (Watson, Crais, Baranek, Dykstra, Wilson, Hammer, & Woods, 2013) observed by 9 to 12 months of age;
5) A decline from normative levels in eye fixation from 2 to 6 months of age not observed in infants who did not develop autism (Jones & Klin, 2013).

As per DSM – V criteria, children with ASD are characterized by

A. Persistent deficits in social communication and social interaction across contexts, not accounted for by general developmental delays and as manifested by the following symptoms, currently or by history:
    1) Deficits in social-emotional reciprocity, ranging for example, from abnormal social approach and failure of normal back and forth conversation; to reduced sharing of interests, emotions, or affect; to failure to initiate or respond to social interactions.
    2) Deficits in nonverbal communicative behaviours used for social interactions ranging, for example, from poorly integrated verbal and nonverbal communication; to abnormalities in eye contact and body language or deficits in understanding and use of gestures; to a total lack of facial expressions and nonverbal communication.
    3) Deficits in developing, maintaining, and understanding relationships, ranging, for example, from difficulties adjusting behaviour to suit various social context; to difficulties in sharing imaginative play or in making friends; to absence of interests in peers.

B. Restricted, repetitive patterns of behaviours, interests, or activities as manifested by at least two of the following symptoms:
   1) Stereotyped or repetitive motor movements, use of objects or speech (e.g., simple motor stereotypes, lining up of toys or flipping objects, echolalia, idiosyncratic phrases).
   2) Insistence on sameness, inflexible adherence to routines, or ritualized patterns of verbal or nonverbal behaviour (e.g., extreme distress at small changes, difficulties with transitions, rigid thinking patterns, greeting rituals, need to take same route or eat same food every day).
   3) Highly restricted, fixated interests that are abnormal in intensity or focus (e.g., string attachment to or preoccupation with unusual objects, excessively circumscribed or perseverative interests).
   4) Hypo- or hyperactivity to sensory input or unusual interest in sensory aspects of the environment (e.g., apparent indifference to pain/temperature, adverse response to specific sounds or textures, excessive smelling or touching of objects, visual fascination with lights or movement).

C. Symptoms must be present in early developmental period (but may not become fully manifest until social demands exceed limited capacities, or may be masked by learned strategies in later life).

D. Symptoms cause clinically significant impairment in social, occupational, or other important areas of current functioning.

These disturbances are not better explained by intellectual disability (intellectual developmental disorder) or global developmental delay. Intellectual disability and autism spectrum disorder frequently co-occur; to make comorbid diagnoses of autism spectrum disorder and intellectual disability, social communication should be below that expected for general developmental level. The early identification of behavioural indicators can help families to attain appropriate diagnostic referrals and also avail access to early intervention services, even before a definitive diagnosis is being made (Woods & Wetherby, 2003). Furthermore, early intervention can improve long-term outcomes for many children (Dawson & Osterling, 1997; Harris & Handleman, 2000; Landa & Kalb, 2012).

Causes of Autism Spectrum Disorders (ASDs)

Autism Spectrum Disorders (ASD) is a neurodevelopmental disorder that begins in early childhood/ developmental period. There is no known exact cause for autism spectrum disorders (ASDs). However, research findings have suggested that both genetic and environmental factors are known to cause ASDs.

1. Neurobiological factors

a) Genetic factors: research studies have identified particular genes that may increase the risk for ASDs (Campbell, Sutcliffe, Ebert, Militerni, Bravaccio et al., 2006; Arking, Cutler, Brune, Teslovich, West, et al., 2008). Some research findings (Sebat, Lakshmi, Malhotra, Troge, Lese-Martin et al., 2007; Morrow, Yoo, Flavell, Kim, Lin et al., 2008) have a contrary findings suggesting that most individuals with ASD are reported to have no family history of autism, and that some random, rare genetic mutation may likely to affect a person with autism. Fragile X syndrome is a genetic disorder and it is known to be associated with some form of intellectual disability, that may show symptoms similar to that of ASDs (Zafeiriou, Ververi & Vargiami, 2007). It is reported that 1 in 3 children with Fragile X syndrome met the diagnostic criteria for ASD and 1 in 25 children diagnosed with ASD were observed to have the gene mutation that caused Fragile X syndrome (Peterman, & Kennedy, 2003). Folstein and Rosen-Sheidley (2001) have reported that regions on chromosomes 2, 7, and 13 may contain one or more susceptible genes, particularly in the region 15q11-13[w5 w6] that is linked to cause autism.

b) Tuberous Sclerosis: This is a rare genetic disorder and it occurs in 1-4% of people with ASDs (Zafeiriou, Ververi & Vargiami, 2007; Peterman, & Kennedy, 2003, Smalley, 1998).

c) Structural and functional brain abnormalities: Problems with genetic code may result in abnormal mechanisms for brain development. This leads structural and functional abnormalities of the brain, thus leading to cognitive and neurobiological abnormalities and symptomatic behaviours (Willaims, 2012).

- Larger volumes of white matter, subtle structural changes in cell density and alignment in the limbic system (Casanova, Buxhoeveden, Switala, & Roy, 2002; Courchesne, Redcay, Morgan, & Kennedy, 2005; Hazlett, Gu, McKinstry RC et al, 2012; Petersson, Pedersen, Schalling, & Lavebratt, 1999) have been observed in individuals with ASDs.
- Decreased white matter compared to gray matter by adulthood (Volkmar, Lord, Bailey, Schultz, & Klin, 2004).
- Increased gray matter observed in the frontal and temporal lobes of the brain (Carper & Courchesne, 2005; Hazlett, Poe, Gerig, Smith, & Piven, 2006; Palmen et al., 2005).
- Anatomical and functional differences in the limbic system and cerebellum (Volkmar et al., 2004)
- Atypical activation of the amygdala and the surrounding structures in response to the social stimuli (Critchle, et al., 2000).
- Decreases neural sensitivity to dynamic gaze shifts in infancy (Elsabbagh et al., 2012).
- Preference for non-social versus social processing and hemispheric asymmetries in event-related potentials (Mccleery, Askchoomoff, Dobkins, & Carver, 2009);
- Disruptions in normative activation patterns of social neurodevelopment that contribute to a diminished attention to social stimuli (Jones, Carr, & Klin, 2008).
- Increased activation of extrastriata and parietal region areas (Koshino, Carpenter, Minshe, Cherkassky, Keller, & Just 2005) and decreased activation of frontal/prefrontal areas has been observed in individuals with ASD (Koshino, Carpenter, Minshe, Cherkassky, Keller, & Just, 2005; Silk, Rinehart, Bradshaw JL et al., 2006).

2) Environmental factors: External factors such as family medical conditions, parental age, and other demographic factors, and complications during pregnancy or birth (Myers & Johnson, 2007; Kolevzon, Gross, and Reichenberg, 2007; Lawler, Croen, Grether, and Van de Water, 2004; Daniels, Forssen Hultman, Cnattingius, Savitz, Feychting, & Sparen; 2008). A number of environmental exposure to toxins such as lead, polychlorinated biphenyls (PCBs), insecticides, automotive exhaust, hydrocarbons, and flame retardants (Landrigan, Lambertini, & Birnbaum, 2012; Shelton, Hertz-Picciotto, & Pessah, 2012). However, no specific environmental triggers have been identified. Research has indicated that it's likely that more than one environmental factor is involved in increasing the risk for ASD. There is a preliminary evidence suggesting thalidomide induced embryopathyw3 and anti-convulsants taken during pregnancy (Taylor, Miller, Lingam, Andrews, Simmons, & Stowe, 2002).
3) Vaccines: Many studies have been conducted to try to determine whether MMR vaccine has a role in causing Autism. However, research studies have ruled out link between vaccine and autism (Taylor, Miller, Lingam, Andrews, Simmons, & Stowe, 2002).

Communication Impairment in Individuals with Autism Spectrum Disorders (ASDs)

Children with ASD exhibit difficulty in developing sufficient natural speech or writing skills to meet their communication needs. Thus, they are at a substantial risk across several aspects of their development such as (a) functional communication, (b) Cognitive skills, (c) speech and language skills, (d) literacy skills, (e) social participation, (f) access to education and (g) overall quality of life. Often their communication abilities are be limited to pre-intentional communication behvaiors, such as reaching for a desired item through simple behaviours such as pointing (Yoder, McCathren, Warren & Watson, 2001).

Also, children with ASD have been found to have profound impairment in comprehending and using verbal and non-verbal communication used for social interaction (Matson, Dempsey, & LoVullo, 2009; Shriberg, Paul, McSweeny, Klin, Cohen, & Volkmar, 2001), social communication (Kuo, Orsmond, Cohn, & Coster, 2013). The degree and severity of communication disorders differ widely across the autism spectrum disorders and they are classified as 'non-verbal' or 'minimally verbal' (Tager-Flusberg & Kasari, 2013). Also, children with ASD are those who are considered to have CCN and they are likely to have associated problems such as intellectual disabilities (Hewitt et al., 2012; Luyster, Kadlec, Carter, & Tager-Flusberg, 2008), oral-motor difficulties (Gernsbacher, Sauer, Geye, Schweigert, & Goldsmith, 2008), sleeping problems (Krakowiak, Goodlin-Jones, Hertz-Picciotto, Croen, & Hansen, 2008; Johnson, Giannotti, & Cortes, 2009), seizures (Volkmar & Nelson, 1990), Fragile X syndrome (Zafeiriou, Ververi, and Vargiami, 2007), food allergies and frequent gastrointestinal (GI) problems (Kuddo & Nelson, 2003; Nikolov, et al., 2009) and symptoms of Attention Deficit Hyperactivity Disorder (ADHD) (Aman, Farmer, Hollway, & Arnold, 2008; Goldstein & Schewebach, 2004; Handen, Johnson & Lubetsky, 2000; Lovaas, 1987). This further complicates their expressive communication skills. Also, the prevalence of ASD is increasing (Baxter, Brugha, Erskine, Scheurer, Vos & Scott, 2015; Christensen, Baio, Van Naarden Brau et al., 2012) and thus, individuals with ASD are more likely to require intensive rehabilitation particularly addressing their complex communication needs. Furthermore, the communication skills in children with ASDs is limited to pre-intentional communication behaviours such as pointing, reaching for a desired item etc. and they do not develop adequate speech or writing to meet their daily communication needs. Some children with ASDs tend to develop speech, but it is often limited to unusual and echolalic utterances (Paul, 2005). There is an increased prevalence of ASDs further which, there is also increased demand for the effective educational and therapeutic intervention. Thus, they are considered candidates for Augmentative and Alternative Communication (AAC) intervention.

AAC Intervention for Individuals with Autism Spectrum Disorders (ASDs)

Children with ASDs exhibit severe speech and language disabilities and thus, AAC intervention can provide them a foundation to improve their overall communication skills. AAC intervention supplements or provides a replacement to natural speech and/or writing using aided and/or unaided strategies in individuals with little or no functional speech (Lloyd, Fuller, & Arvidson, 1997). Beukelman and Mirenda (1998) defined AAC system as 'An integrated group of components, including the symbols, aids, strategies and techniques used by an individual to enhance communication'. An AAC system is classifies as aided and/or unaided methods of communication and this includes strategies, techniques, aids and devices used to communicate (Lloyd, Fuller, & Arvidson, 1997). Unaided AAC involves user's body to convey meaning. Examples of unaided AAC include gestures, facial expressions, and sign language. An aided

AAC system requires use of an aid external to the person's physical body (Tonsing, Alant, & Lloyd, 2005). Examples of aided AAC system are pictures, photographs, line drawings, objects, aids, devices etc. With the advent in technology, many companies started to develop aids, devices, and techniques in order to help social inclusion of people with disabilities. This tremendous change in technology lead to a new field known as Assistive Technology (AT) and AAC is a sub-area of Assistive Technology (AT). Cook and Polgar (2014) defined AT according to the concept created by Colker (1999): "a wide range of equipment, services, strategies and practices designed and implemented to reduce the functional problems encountered by individuals with disabilities". As per 'Assistance for Individuals with Disabilities Act (1997), an assistive technology refers to any item, piece of equipment, or product system whether acquired commercially, off-the shelf, modified or customized, that is used to increase, maintain or improve functional capabilities of individuals with disabilities. Assistive Technology (AT) service is any service that directly assists individuals with disabilities to select, acquire and use any assistive technology based devices. AAC system/devices make use of AT which can be of low-tech, mid-tech and high-tech strategies.

Low tech strategies/low tech AAC makes use of visual support strategies and this include devices such as picture boards, alphabet boards, sign boards, dry erase board, clipboards, 3-ring binders, manila file folders, photo albums, laminated PCS/photographs, highlight tape, etc. In early 1980's, AAC practitioners began to explore the potential benefits of graphic symbols (Mirenda & Schuler, 1988). Research implied that graphic symbols were found to be effective when the intervention gaol was to teach requesting skills (Schlosser & Wendt, 2008). Also, these graphic symbols have proven to be beneficial as visual supports to perform and transit across activities. Typically, individuals with ASDs have better visual information processing than the auditory information. Temple Grandin (1995) famously has remarked that, "I think in pictures. Words are like a second language to me. When somebody speaks to me, his words are instantly translated into pictures". As individuals with ASDs process information better in visual modality compared to auditory counterpart. Visual schedules typically make use of graphic symbols such as line drawing, photographs, symbols, or text, displayed in a vertical or horizontal line representing the sequence of events/activities in a day. This assists them in understanding and preparing for transitions between activities. For example, a child is shown a photograph of bathing activity followed by a dressing activity. Furthermore, the use of visual schedules has been found to be effective for children with ASD and paved them a way in performing the activity in a day to day living (Bopp, Brown, & Mirenda, 2004). Also, appropriate use of visual schedules has resulted in significant and rapid decrease in problem behaviours in children with ASD (Bopp, Brown, & Mirenda, 2004). Other low tech aided AAC devices such as topic boards and cue cards (graphic symbols) have been proved to effective in improving understanding of verbal and non-verbal behaviour in children with ASDs (Prizant, Wetherby, Rubin, & Laurent, 2003). Ewald and Lightfoot (2001) stated that, low tech AAC such as "photos can create moments of authentic collaboration" and that these types of experiences are essential to the acquisition and application of social communication. Additional benefits such as enhancement of both creativity and imagination (Munakata & Vaidya, 2012), development of visual literacy skills (Walter, Baller, & Kuntz, 2012), and an increased ability of critical thinking (Felten, 2008) are reported with the use of photography in individuals with ASDs. Also, as these types of aided low-tech AAC systems are easily created, portable, durable and replaceable, the use of low-tech aided AAC systems were not ignored (Ganz et al., 2010). Romski and Sevcik, (2005) studied the perception of AAC users (young infants and children with CCN) for both low-tech and high-tech methods of PECS i.e., board version and computerized version of PECS. The findings suggested that the participants were comfortable with combination of both low and high-tech methods as they could choose any system based on the communication environments.

Mid-tech AAC includes use of battery-operated devices such as tape-recorders, voice recorders, overhead projectors, calculators, timers and simple voice output devices. Some of the VOCAs based on mid-tech technology that were used to augment expressive communication are "Big Mack", Voice in the Box", Cheap Talk 4, Talk Pad, "Step by Step Communicator" etc. These devices were known to develop skills with language comprehension, expressive communication skills, social skills, organizational and academic skills.

High-tech systems are those devices that require power supply & re-chargeable battery packs as they generally use lighted dynamic displays & synthesised voices. They run these AAC systems makes use of sophisticated software vocabularies, multiple voices, and are fully accessible, & can be thoroughly customised. These high-tech AAC devices makes use of operating systems that can be Windows, Android or iOS. O'Neill, Smyth, Smeaton and O'Connor, (2019) investigated the effectiveness of Assistive Technology (AT) in individuals with ASD and the findings have shown positive effects of AT in their study. Examples of high-tech AAC devices include electronic communication devices, using synthetic or digitalized speech for Augmentative and Alternative Communication (AAC), micro switches to control computers, powered wheelchairs and environmental control (Bailey, Parette, Stoner, Angell, & Carroll, 2006). Research studies have indicated that, more support for aided AAC compared to unaided AAC such as manual sign language for individual with ASD (Schlosser & Wendt, 2008).

Research studies have been attempted to compare the effectiveness across low-tech and high-tech aided AAC systems. Results of the same have demonstrated that use of both low-tech and high-tech aided AAC systems have been effective in individuals with ASD. Positive outcomes with aided communication systems such as Picture Exchange Communication System (PECS) and Speech-Generating Devices (SGDs) in individuals with ASD (Flippin, Reszka, & Watson, 2010; Ganz, Earles-Vollrath, et al., 2012; Ostryn, Wolfe, & Rusch, 2008; Preston & Carter 2009; Millar, Light, & Schlosser, 2006) have been reported in the literature. Furthermore, review of literature suggests that, the use of Assistive technology (AT) in children with autism helps to facilitate and enhance their learning abilities. AT functions as an assisting tool, acts as a language device for children with autism (Mallin, & de Carvalho, 2015). There are some assistive technology devices specifically designed for individuals with Autism Spectrum disorders (ASDs) (Table 1).

As individuals with ASDs are visual learners, technology is making visual images more accessible for individuals with ASDs, following by which computer graphics are able to capture and maintain their attention. Researchers have also suggested that most autistic individuals have high visuo-perceptual skills (Mazurek & Wenstrup, 2013) and that autistic children tend to be more receptive to learning concepts on mobile devices as these devices provide touch screen interface and also they are also easily portable. Mobile learning has been broadly used as an assistive technology for individuals with ASDs. There are some existed mobile learning apps that focuses on improving various functional skills and they are presented in table 2.

A study by Petersen, Baalsrud, Eds, and Hutchison, (2014) indicated that, the touch screen interface features of mobile devices enable individuals with ASDs with intuitive interaction, thereby improving their focus. Correspondingly, such devices help children with ASD learn concepts rapidly as they provide tangible feedback to the users (Saleh, Aljaam, Karime, & El Saddik, 2013). Dehkordi and Rias (2014) opined that children with ASD are able to learn while playing with technological devices that helps to capture their attention. Binger and Light (2006, 2007) found that aided AAC modelling had a positive effect and that pre-schooler children who used AAC were able to produce multi-symbol messages; also, results of the same showed that these children were able to learn and generalize novel vocabulary and novel contexts as well.

Table 1. List of commercially available assistive technology used in Individuals with ASDs.

Assistive Technology	Purpose
Serious Game (Helmi, Faaizah Shahbodin, & Naim Che Pee, 2012)	For therapy and education including learning and training to improve social skill, communication skill, visual motor coordination and sensory integration
Virtual Learning Environment (Volioti, Tsiatsos, Mavropoulou & Karagiannidis, 2015)	An educational intervention to overcome persistent differences in social communication and imagination throughout social stories.
Virtual Reality (Parsons, 2016)	Used as a treatment to prepare children with autism to handle real world interaction and to study how individuals with ASD behave under predefined social scenarios.
Augmented Reality (Chen, Chou & Huang, 2016)	To improve children with ASD perceptions and reactions of facial expression and emotions using video modelling storybook of nonverbal facial cues.
Mobile Learning (Lin, Su, Chao, Hsieh, & Tsai, 2016)	The use of behaviour modelling training to improve functional communication.
Edutainment (Hussain, Mkpojiogu, & Hassan, 2016)	To capture children with autism attention and to improve communication skills.

Table 2. Mobile learning apps that focuses functional skills.

Apps	Platform	Age	Functional skills
Put It Away	iPad	All age	To train daily life skills
Avakid: See Me Go Potty	Android iPad iPhone iTouch	All age	To train personal hygiene focusing in potty training through avatar -cartoon model
The Photo Cookbook Quick & Easy	iPad iPhone iTouch	All age	To improve Cognitive skills
Big Blue Box Farm	iPad iPhone iTouch	Preschool (2-5)	To assist in cognitive development, social development and motor skills through puzzle.
Computers at Work iPad App	iPad	Adolescents (13-17) Adults (18+)	To improve Computer skills in job preparation
I Get…Cooking	iPad iPhone iTouch	Children (6-12) Adolescents (13-17) Adults (18+)	To improve constructive skills through cooking game
Life Skill Winner	Android iPad iPhone iTouch	All ages	Helps to learn activities of daily living in an interactive setting.
FaceSay Social Skills Software Games	Windows	All ages	Help ASD children/adults to better recognize non-verbal cues.

Some individuals with ASDs may also have sensitivity issues to auditory stimuli and thus are better able to respond to softer sounds as well. Thus, the assistive devices such as SGDs or VOCAS requires adjusting to appropriate sound and voice levels matching the needs of the individuals. Some individuals with ASDs do have sequencing problems. Technology has made it possible to overcome this barrier by reducing the number of steps required to perform and complete the tasks or provide a visual demo of the task steps in a sequence making them overcome the sequencing errors. Individuals with ASDs also exhibits deficits and delays with fine motor skills (Bhat, Landa, & Galloway, 2011; LeBarton & Iverson, 2013) and thus they may exhibit handwriting difficulty. Thus, Assistive devices or high-tech AAC devices such as keyboard, touch screen or speech-to-text conversion apps have helped individuals with ASDs to overcome this difficulty and increase their enjoyment of learning. In general, many research studies have come to a consensus that 'high-tech AAC systems such as SGDs, computerized version of PECS, are proved to be effective AAC systems in improving speech and language skills, socio-communication skills, behaviour, and academic skills in children with ASD and other developmental disabilities (Flippin, Reszka & Watson, 2010; Ganz, Earles-Vollrath, Mason, Rispoli, Heath & Parker, 2011; Ganz, Earles-Vollrath, Heath, Parker, Rispoli, & Duran, 2012; Ganz, Davis, Lund, Goodwyn & Simpson, 2012; Ganz, Rispoli, Mason, & Hong, 2014; Preston & Carter, 2009; Hart & Banda, 2010; Kent-Walsh, Murza, Malani & Binger, 2015; Lorah, Parnell, Whitby & Hantula, 2014; Millar, Light, & Schlosser, 2016; Schlosser & Wendt, 2008; Schlosser & Koul, 2015; Still, Rehfeldt, Whelan, May Dymond, 2014; Tincani & Devis, 2011; van der Meer & Rispoli, 2010). This necessitated the high relevance of introducing AAC systems to the individuals with ASD as early as possible to attain the best outcomes (Hall, 2013).

Communication is a dynamic process in which communication partners continually influence each other. The success of communication act relies on the communication skills of each individual who are participating in the information exchange (Kent-Walsh & Mcnaughton, 2005). Children with ASDs are those who are with Complex Communication Needs (CCN), they have numerous communication partners including parents, sibling, teachers peer groups etc. who are crucial for providing communication opportunities. Also, providing support for individuals with CCN requires a skilled communication partner which requires skills and techniques that needs guided practice (Binger & Kent-Walsh, 2012). Thus, partner training is a crucial part of any quality program for individuals with ASDs. Professionals have been training the parents and teachers to be more responsive to children's communication. Majority of the research studies reported that communication partners including family members, teachers, educational assistants and other key stakeholders were able to learn strategies to promote communication using AAC systems (Douglas, 2012; Kent-Walsh, Binger & Hasham, 2010; Rosa-Lugo & Kent-Walsh, 2008; Light, Binger, Agate & Ramsay, 1999; Starble, Hutchins, Favro, Prelock, & Bitner, 2005; Stiebel, 1999). Also, there is a dearth of research studies on communication partner training. McNaughton and Light (2015) reviewed 30 years of research published in the AAC journal, and reported that 85% of AAC intervention research focused solely on the person with CCN, while only 15% addressed intervention with the communication partner. However, there are few research studies that have attempted to explore the effectiveness of parental training approaches (Beukelman & Mirenda, 2005; Cook, Tessier, Klein & Armbruster, 2000; Culp & Carlisle, 1988; Douglas, 2012; Green et al., 2010; Light, Binger, Agate, & Ramsay, 1999; Mirenda & Iacono, 2009; Nunes, 2008 & Shire & Jones, 2015). Riksen-Walraven (1978) conducted a randomized group experiment and the results showed that training mothers to use non-linguistic responses facilitated better learning in infants. Also, effective communication in preschool and school environment demands for peer group interaction by the AAC user. Thus, peer training plays a crucial role and this has received special attention perhaps because these are the environments in which children spend a significant period of time. However, few studies on peer training has been conducted and the results has shown positive outcomes in children with ASD (Beukelman & Mirenda, 2013; Therrien & Light, 2018; Thiemann-Bourque, McGuff, & Goldstein, 2017; Trottier, Kamp, & Mirenda, 2011). Thus, training parents or communication partners with different AAC strategies, increased communication supports, using of AAC devices, aids and appliances can be beneficial and warrants further research.

FUTURE DIRECTIONS

Individuals with ASDs pose greatest challenge in the social, language, cognitive behaviour, literacy, and communication development. There is a growing evidence investigating the potential benefits of AAC (aided and unaided) for individuals with Autism Spectrum Disorders (ASDs). However, the field of AAC intervention has been identified as emerging rather than established by the National Autism Centre (NAC) in the US. Though, positive outcomes of AAC intervention has been documented, most of the studies are based on case studies or small group studies. Thus, this necessitates for a comprehensive AAC intervention in individuals with ASDs. Also, this lack of empirical data has accounted for a tendency among researchers and practioners to disregard AAC intervention. Therefore, there is a need for more well-designed studies with more conclusive findings. Also, there are rising number of individuals with Complex Communication Needs (CCN), of varying ages, wide array of disabilities across several domains (motor, sensory, perceptual, cognitive and linguistic skills) and they all hail from a diverse linguistic and cultural backgrounds. Thus, individuals with CCN may require AAC services over a longer life span with changing needs over time in different environments. In addition, there is also increased awareness and acceptance of AAC among individuals with Complex Communication Needs (CCN) and thus, greater amount of research is required to determine the effectiveness of different types of AAC options with children with CCN. Also, additional research is required to explore the effectiveness of parent/communication training which has a crucial role in intervening individuals with ASDs using AAC approaches. Further, awareness about AAC intervention needs to be created among paediatrician and other medical professionals because they are the first professionals to encounter children with disabilities and that they can refer children and their families to programs that can support access to AAC and functional communication.

REFERENCES

Alper, S., & Raharinirina, S. (2006). Assistive Technology for Individuals with Disabilities: A Review and Synthesis of the Literature. *Journal of Special Education Technology, 21*(2), 47–64.

Aman, M., Farmer, C., Hollway, J., & Arnold, L. (2008). Treatment of Inattention, Overactivity, and Impulsiveness in Autism Spectrum Disorders. *Child and Adolescent Psychiatric Clinics of North America, 17*, 713–738. PMID:18775366

American Psychiatric Association. (2013). *Diagnostic and statistical manual of mental disorders* (5th ed.). Arlington, VA: American Psychiatric Publishing.

Arking, D. E., Cutler, D. J., Brune, C. W., Teslovich, T. M., West, K., Ikeda, M., & … . (2008). A common genetic variant in the neurexin superfamily member CNTNAP2 increases familial risk of autism. *American Journal of Human Genetics*, *82*, 160–164. PMID:18179894

Bailey, R. L., Parette, H. P. Jr, Stoner, J. B., Angell, M. E., & Carroll, K. (2006). Family members' perceptions of augmentative and alternative communication device use. *Language, Speech, and Hearing Services in Schools*, *37*(1), 50–60. doi:10.1044/0161- 1461(2006/006) PMID:16615749

Baranek, G. (1999). Autism during infancy: A retrospective video analysis of sensory-motor and social behaviours at 9–12 months of age. *Journal of Autism and Developmental Disorders*, *9*(29), 213–224. PMID:10425584

Baxter, A. J., Brugha, T. S., Erskine, H. E., Scheurer, R. W., Vos, T., & Scott, J. G. (2015). The epidemiology and global burden of autism spectrum disorders. *Psychological Medicine*, *45*, 601–613. PMID:25108395

Beukelman, D., & Mirenda, P. (2005). *Augmentative and alternative communication: Management of severe communication impairments* (3rd ed.). Baltimore: Brookes.

Beukelman, D., & Mirenda, P. (2013). *Augmentative and alternative communication: Supporting children and adults with complex communication needs* (4th ed.). Baltimore, MD: Brookes.

Beukelman, D. R., & Mirenda, P. (1998). *Augmentative and alternative communication: Management of severe communication disorders in children and adults* (2nd ed.). Baltimore: Paul H. Brookes.

Bhat, A., Landa, R., & Galloway, J. (2011). Current perspectives on motor functioning in infants, children, and adults with autism spectrum disorders. *Physical Therapy*, *91*, 1116–1129. PMID:21546566

Binger, C., & Kent-Walsh, J. (2012). Selecting skills to teach communication partners: Where do I start? *Perspectives on Augmentative and Alternative Communication*, *21*, 126–134.

Binger, C., & Light, J. (2006). Demographics-of-preschoolers-who-require-augmentative-and-alternativecommunication. *Language, Speech, and Hearing Services in Schools*, *37*, 200–208. PMID:16837443

Binger, C., & Light, J. (2007). The effect of aided AAC modeling on the expression of multi-symbol messages by pre-schoolers who use AAC. *Augmentative and Alternative Communication*, *23*, 30–43. doi:10.1080/07434610600807470 PMID:17364486

Bopp, K. D., Brown, K. E., & Mirenda, P. (2004). Article. *American Journal of Speech-Language Pathology*, *13*, 5–19. PMID:15101810

Campbell, D. B., Sutcliffe, J. S., Ebert, P. J., Militerni, R., Bravaccio, C., Trillo, S., & … . (2006). A genetic variant that disrupts *MET* transcription is associated with autism. *Proceedings of the National Academy of Sciences of the United States of America*, *10*, 16834–16839. PMID:17053076

Carper, R., & Courchesne, E. (2005). Localized enlargement of the frontal lobe in autism. *Biological Psychiatry*, *57*, 126–133. PMID:15652870

Casanova, M. F., Buxhoeveden, D., Switala, A., & Roy, E. (2002). Minicolumn pathology in autism. *Neurology*, *58*, 428–432. PMID:11839843

Chawarska, K., Paul, R., Klin, A., Hannigen, S., Dichtel, L. E., & Volkmar, F. (2007). Parental recognition of developmental problems in toddlers with autism spectrum disorders. *Journal of Autism and Developmental Disorders*, *37*(1), 62–72. PMID:17195921

Chen, C. H., Chou, Y., & Huang, C. Y. (2016). An Augmented-Reality-Based Concept Map to Support Mobile Learning for Science. *The Asia-Pacific Education Researcher*, *25*(4), 567–578. doi:10.100740299-016-0284-3

Christensen, D. L., Baio, J., & Van Naarden Braun, K. (2016). Prevalence and characteristics of autism spectrum disorder among children aged 8 years—autism and developmental disabilities monitoring network, 11 sites, United States, 2012. *MMWR. Surveillance Summaries*, *65*, 1–23. PMID:27031587

Cook, A. M., & Polgar, J. M. (2014). *Assistive technologies: Principles and practice* (4th ed.). St. Louis, MO: Elsevier Health Sciences.

Cook, R., Tessier, A., Klein, M., & Armbruster, V. (2000). Nurturing communication skills. In R. E. Cook, A. Tessier, & M. D. Klein (Eds.), *Adapting early childhood curricula for children in inclusive settings* (5th ed., pp. 290–339). Englewood Cliffs, NJ: Merrill.

Courchesne, E., Redcay, E., Morgan, J. T., & Kennedy, D. P. (2005). Autism at the beginning: Microstructural and growth abnormalities underlying the cognitive and behavioural phenotype of autism. *Development and Psychopathology*, *17*(3), 577–597. PMID:16262983

Critchley, H. D., Elliott, R., & Mathias, C. J. (2000). Neural activity relating to the generation and representation of galvanic skin conductance response: A functional magnetic imaging study. *The Journal of Neuroscience*, *20*, 3033–3040. PMID:10751455

Culp, D. M., & Carlisle, M. (1988). *Partners in augmentative communication training (PACT): A resource guide for interaction facilitation training for children.* Tucson: Communication Skill Builders.

Daniels, J. L., Forssen, U., Hultman, C. M., Cnattingius, S., Savitz, D. A., Feychting, M., & Sparen, P. (2008). Parental Psychiatric Disorders Associated with Autism Spectrum Disorders. *Paediatrics*, *121*, 1357–1362. PMID:18450879

Dawson, G., & Osterling, J. (1997). Early intervention in autism. In M. Guralnick (Ed.), *The effectiveness of early intervention* (pp. 307–326). Baltimore, MD: Brookes.

Dehkordi, S. R. & Riaza. M. R. (2014). *Using Mobile Game Application to Teach Children with Autism Spectrum Disorder (ASD) Multiple Cues Responding: A Pilot Study.* doi:10.1109/IUSER.2014.7002705

Douglas, S. N. (2012). Teaching para educators to support communication of individuals who use augmentative and alternative communication: A literature review. *Current Issues in Education*, *15*(1), 1–12.

Elsabbagh, M., Mercure, E., Hudry, K., Chandler, S., Pasco, G., Charman, T., … Johnson, M. H. (2012). *Infant neural sensitivity to dynamic eye gaze is associated with later emerging autism.* Academic Press.

Ewald, W., & Lightfoot, A. (2001). *I wanna take me a picture: Teaching photography and writing to children.* Boston: Beacon Press.

Felten, P. (2008). Resource review: Visual literacy. *Change Magazine,* 60-63.

Flippin, M. & Reszka, S. & Watson, L. (2010). Effectiveness of the Picture Exchange Communication System (PECS) on Communication and Speech for Children with Autism Spectrum Disorders: A Meta-Analysis. *American Journal of Speech-Language Pathology, 19,* 178-95. . doi:10.1044/1058-0360(2010/09-0022)

Folstein, S. E., & Rosen-Sheidley, B. (2001). Genetics of autism: Complex aetiology for a heterogeneous disorder. *Nature Reviews. Genetics*, *2*, 943–955. PMID:11733747

Ganz, J. B., Davis, J. L., Lund, E. M., Goodwyn, F. D., & Simpson, R. L. (2012). Meta-analysis of PECS with individuals with ASD: Investigation of targeted versus non-targeted outcomes, participant characteristics, and implementation phase. *Research in Developmental Disabilities*, *33*, 406–418. PMID:22119688

Ganz, J. B., Earles-Vollrath, T. L., Heath, A. K., Parker, R. I., Rispoli, M. J., & Duran, J. B. (2012). A meta-analysis of single case research studies on aided augmentative and alternative communication systems with individuals with autism spectrum disorders. *Journal of Autism and Developmental Disabilities*, *42*, 60–74. doi:10.100710803-011-1212-2 PMID:21380612

Ganz, J. B., Earles-Vollrath, T. L., Mason, R. A., Rispoli, M. J., Heath, A. K., & Parker, R. I. (2011). An aggregate study of single-case research involving aided AAC: Participant characteristics of individuals with autism spectrum disorders. *Research in Autism Spectrum Disorders*, *5*(4), 1500–1509. doi:10.1016/j.rasd.2011.02.011

Ganz, J. B., Lashley, E., & Rispoli, M. J. (2010). Non-responsiveness to intervention. Children with autism spectrum disorders who do not rapidly respond to communication interventions. *Developmental Neurorehabilitation*, *13*, 399–407.

Ganz, J. B., Rispoli, M. J., Mason, R. A., & Hong, E. R. (2014). Moderation of effects of AAC based on setting and types of aided AAC on outcome variables: An aggregate study of single-case research with individuals with ASD. *Developmental Neurorehabilitation*, *17*(3), 184–192. doi:10.3109/17518423.2012.748097 PMID:24102440

Gernsbacher, M. A., Sauer, E. A., Geye, H. M., Schweigert, E. K., & Goldsmith, H. H. (2008). Infant and toddler oral- and manual-motor skills predict later speech fluency in autism. *Journal of Child Psychology and Psychiatry, and Allied Disciplines*, *49*, 43–50.

Goldstein, S., & Schwebach, A. J. (2004). The comorbidity of pervasive developmental disorders and attention deficit hyperactivity disorder: Results of a fretrospective chart review. *Journal of Autism and Developmental Disorders*, *34*(3), 323–339. PMID:15264500

Grandin, T. (1995). How People with Autism Think. In E. Schopler & G. B. Mesibov (Eds.), *Learning and Cognition in Autism. Current Issues in Autism*. Boston, MA: Springer.

Green, J., Charman, T., McConachie, H., Aldred, C., Slonims, V., Howlin, P., ... Pickles, A. (2010). Parent-mediated communication-focused treatment in children with autism (PACT): A randomised controlled trial. *Lancet*, *375*(9732), 2152–2160. doi:10.1016/S0140-6736(10)60587-9 PMID:20494434

Hall, L. (2013). *Autism spectrum disorders: From theory to practice* (2nd ed.). Boston, MA: Pearson.

Handen, B. L., Johnson, C. R., & Lubetsky, M. (2000). Efficacy of methylphenidate among children with autism and symptoms of attention-deficit hyperactivity disorder. *Journal of Autism and Developmental Disorders, 30*, 245–255. PMID:11055460

Harris, S. L., & Handleman, J. S. (2000). Age and IQ at intake as predictors of placement for young children with autism: A four-to six-year follow-up. *Journal of Autism and Developmental Disorders, 30*(2), 137–142. PMID:10832778

Hart, S., & Banda, D. (2010). Picture Exchange Communication System with individuals with developmental disabilities: A meta-analysis of single subject studies. *Remedial and Special Education, 31*, 463–477.

Hazlett, H. C., Gu, H., McKinstry, R. C., Shaw, D. W. W., Botteron, K. N., Dager, S. R., & … . (2012). Brain volume findings in 6-month-old infants at high familial risk for autism. *The American Journal of Psychiatry, 169*, 601–608. PMID:22684595

Hazlett, H. C., Poe, M. D., Gerig, G., Smith, R. G., & Piven, J. (2006). *Cortical grey and white brain tissue volume in adolescents and adults with autism*. Academic Press.

Helmi Adly, M. N., Faaizah, S., & Naim, C. P. (2012). Serious Game for Autism Children: Review of Literature. *International Conference on Computer Games, Multimedia, and Allied Technology*, 647-652.

Hewitt, G., Jurk, D., Marques, F. D., Correia-Melo, C., Hardy, T., Gackowska, A., ... Passos, J. F. (2012). Telomeres are favoured targets of a persistent DNA damage response in ageing and stress-induced senescence. *Nature Communications, 28*(3), 1–9. PMID:22426229

Hussain, A., Mkpojiogu, E. O. C., & Hassan, F. (2016). Systematic review of mobile learning applications for children. *Proceedings of the 2nd International Conference on Information and Communication Technology for Transformation.* 5-7.

Individuals with Disability Education Act Amendments of 1997 (IDEA). (1997). Retrieved from http://www.congress.gov/105/plaws/publ17/PLAW-105pub17.pdf

Johnson, K. P., Giannotti, F., & Cortesi, F. (2009). Sleep patterns in autism spectrum disorders. *Child and Adolescent Psychiatric Clinics of North America, 18*, 917–928. PMID:19836696

Jones, W., Carr, K., & Klin, A. (2008). Absence of preferential looking to the eyes of approaching adults predicts level of social disability in 2-year-old toddlers with autism spectrum disorder. *Achieves of general. Psychiatry., 65*(8), 946–954. PMID:18678799

Jones, W., & Klin, A. (2013). Attention to eyes is present but in decline in 2–6-month-old infants later diagnosed with autism. *Nature, 504*, 427–431. PMID:24196715

Kent-Walsh, J., Binger, C., & Hasham, Z. (2010). Effects of parent instruction on the symbolic communication of children using augmentative and alternative communication during storybook reading. *American Journal of Speech-Language Pathology, 19*, 97–107. PMID:20181850

Kent-Walsh, J., & McNaughton, D. (2005). Communication partner instruction in AAC: Present practices and future directions. *Augmentative and Alternative Communication, 21*, 195–204.

Kent-Walsh, J., Murza, K. A., Malani, M. D., & Binger, C. (2015). Effects of communication partner instruction on the communication of individuals using AAC: A meta-analysis. *Augmentative and Alternative Communication*, *31*(4), 271–284. PMID:26059542

Kolevzon, A., Gross, R., & Reichenberg, A. (2007). Prenatal and perinatal risk factors for autism: A review and integration of findings. *Archives of Pediatrics & Adolescent Medicine*, *1*(4), 326–333. PMID:17404128

Koshino, H., Carpenter, P. A., Minshew, N. J., Cherkassky, V. L., Keller, T. A., & Just, M. A. (2005). Functional connectivity in an fMRI working memory task in high-functioning autism. *NeuroImage*, *24*(3), 810–821. PMID:15652316

Krakowiak, P., Goodlin-Jones, B., Hertz-Picciotto, I., Croen, L. A., & Hansen, R. L. (2012). Sleep problems in children with autism spectrum disorders, developmental delays, and typical development: A population-based study. *Journal of Sleep Research*, *21*(2), 231. PMID:23176607

Kuddo, T., & Nelson, K. B. (2003). How common are gastrointestinal disorders in children with autism? *Current Opinion in Pediatrics*, *15*, 339–343. PMID:12806268

Kuo, M. H., Orsmond, G. I., Coster, W. J., & Cohn, E. S. (2014). Media use among adolescents with autism spectrum disorder. *Autism*, *18*, 914–923. PMID:24142797

Landa, R. J., & Kalb, L. G. (2012). Long-term outcomes of toddlers with autism spectrum disorders exposed to short-term intervention. *Pediatrics*, *130*(2), 186–190. PMID:23118250

Landrigan, P. J., Lambertini, L., & Birnbaum, L. S. (2012). A research strategy to discover the environmental causes of autism and neurodevelopmental disabilities. *Environmental Health Perspectives*, *120*, 258–260. PMID:22543002

Lawler, C. P., Croen, L. A., Grether, J. K., & Van de Water, J. (2004). Identifying environmental contributions to autism: Provocative clues and false leads. *Mental Retardation and Developmental Disabilities Research Reviews*, *10*, 292–302. PMID:15666339

LeBarton, E., & Iverson, J. M. (2013). Fine motor skill predicts expressive language in infant siblings of children with autism. *Developmental Science*, *16*(6), 815–827. PMID:24118709

Light, J., Binger, C., Agate, T., & Ramsay, K. (1999). Teaching partner-focused questions to individuals who use augmentative and alternative communication to enhance their communicative competence. *Journal of Speech and Hearing Research*, *42*, 241–255. PMID:10025558

Lin, H. C. K., Su, S. H., Chao, C. J., Hsieh, C. Y., & Tsai, S. C. (2016). Construction of Multi-Mode Affective Learning System: Taking Affective Design as an Example. *Journal of Educational Technology & Society*, *19*(2), 132–147.

Lloyd, L. L., Fuller, D. R., & Arvidson, H. H. (1997). *Augmentative and alternative communication: A handbook of principles and practices*. Boston: Allyn & Bacon.

Lorah, E. R., Parnell, A., Whitby, P. S., & Hantula, D. (2014). A systematic review of tablet computers and portable media players as speech generating devices for individuals with autism spectrum disorder. *Journal of Autism and Developmental Disorders*, *45*, 3792–3804. doi:10.100710803-014-2314-4 PMID:25413144

Lovaas, O. I. (1987). Behavioural treatment and normal educational and intellectual functioning in young autistic children. *Journal of Consulting and Clinical Psychology*, *55*, 3–9. PMID:3571656

Luyster, R. J., Kadlec, M. B., Carter, A., & Tager-Flusberg, H. (2008). Language assessment and development in toddlers with autism spectrum disorders. *Journal of Autism and Developmental Disorders*, *38*(8), 1426–1438. PMID:18188685

Mallin, S. S. V., & de Carvalho, H. G. (2015). Assistive technology and user-centred design: Emotion as element for innovation. *Procedia Manufacturing*, *3*, 5570–5578.

Matson, L. J., Dempsey, T., & LoVullo, A. V. (2009). Characteristics of social skills for adult with intellectual disability, Autism and PDD-NOS. *Research in Autism Spectrum Disorders*, *3*, 207–213.

Mazurek, M. O., & Wenstrup, C. (2013). Television, video game and social media use among children with ASD and typically developing siblings. *Journal of Autism and Developmental Disorders*, *43*(6), 1258–1271. PMID:23001767

McCleery, J. P., Akshoomoff, N., Dobkins, K. R., & Carver, L. J. (2009). Atypical face versus object processing and hemispheric asymmetries in 10-month-old infants at risk for autism. *Biological Psychiatry*, *66*(10), 950–957. PMID:19765688

Millar, D. C., Light, J. C., & Schlosser, R. W. (2006). The impact of augmentative and alternative communication intervention on the speech production of individuals with developmental disabilities: A research review. *Journal of Speech, Language, and Hearing Research: JSLHR*, *49*, 248–264. PMID:16671842

Mirenda, P., & Iacono, T. (2009). *Autism spectrum disorders and AAC*. Baltimore: Paul H. Brookes.

Mirenda, P., & Schuler, A. L. (1988). Augmenting communication for persons with autism: Issues and strategies. *Topics in Language Disorders*, *9*, 24–43.

Morrow, E. M., Yoo, S. Y., Flavell, S. W., Kim, T. K., Lin, Y., Hill, R. S., & … . (2008). Identifying autism loci and genes by tracing recent shared ancestry. *Science*, *321*, 218–223. PMID:18621663

Munakata, M., & Vaidya, A. (2012). Encouraging creativity in mathematics and science through photography. Teaching Mathematics and Its Applications: *An International. The Journal of IMA / Islamic Medical Association of North America*, *31*(3), 121–132.

Myers, S. M., & Johnson, C. P. (2007). Management of children with autism spectrum disorders. *Pediatrics*, *120*, 1162–1182. PMID:17967921

Nikolov, R. N., Bearss, K. E., Lettinga, J., Erickson, C., Rodowski, M., Aman, M. G., … Scahill, L. (2009). Gastrointestinal symptoms in a sample of children with pervasive developmental disorders. *Journal of Autism and Developmental Disorders*, *30*, 405–413. PMID:18791817

Nunes, D. (2008). AAC interventions for autism: A research summary. *International Journal of Special Education*, *23*(2), 17–25.

O'Neill, S., Smyth, S., Smeaton, A. F., & O'Connor, N. E. (2019). Assistive technology: Understanding the needs and experiences of individuals with Autism Spectrum Disorder and/or Intellectual Disability in Ireland and the UK. *Assistive Technology: The Official Journal of RESNA*. doi:10.1080/10400435.2018.1535526

Osterling, J., & Dawson, G. (1994). Early recognition of children with autism: A study of first birthday home videotapes. *Journal of Autism and Developmental Disorders*, *24*, 247–257. PMID:8050980

Ostryn, C., Wolfe, P., & Rusch, F. (2008). A Review and Analysis of the Picture Exchange Communication System (PECS) for Individuals with Autism Spectrum Disorders Using a Paradigm of Communication Competence. *Research and Practice for Persons with Severe Disabilities*, *33*, 13–24.

Palmen, S. J., Hulshoff Pol, H. E., Kemner, C., Schnack, H. G., Durston, S., Lahuis, B. E., & .... (2005). Increased gray-matter volume in medication-naive high-functioning children with autism spectrum disorder. *Psychological Medicine*, *35*(4), 561–570. PMID:15856726

Parsons, S. (2016). Authenticity in *virtual reality* for assessment and intervention in Autism: A conceptual review. *Educational Research Review*, *19*, 138–157. doi:10.1016/j.edurev.2016.08.001

Paul, R. (2005). *Language Disorders from Infancy through Adolescence: Assessment & Intervention* (2nd ed.). Mosby, Inc.

Peterman, N. E., & Kennedy, J. (2003). Enterprise Education: Influencing Students' Perceptions of Entrepreneurship. *Entrepreneurship Theory and Practice*, *28*, 129–144.

Petersen, S., Baalsrud, J., Eds, H., & Hutchison, D. (2014). *Serious Games Development and Applications*. Springer International Publishing.

Petersson, S., Pedersen, N.L., Schalling, M., & Lavebratt, C. (1999). *Primary megalencephaly at birth and low intelligence level*. Academic Press.

Preston, D., & Carter, M. (2009). A review of the efficacy of the Picture Exchange Communication System Intervention. *Journal of Autism and Developmental Disabilities*, *39*, 1471–1486. PMID:19495952

Prizant, B. M., Wetherby, A. M., Rubin, E., & Laurent, A. C. (2003). The SCERTS Model: A Transactional, Family-Centered Approach to Enhancing Communication and Socioemotional Abilities of Children with Autism Spectrum Disorder. *Infants and Young Children*, *16*, 296–316.

Riksen-Walraven, J. M. (1978). Effects of caregiver behavior on habituation and self-efficacy in infants. *International Journal of Behavioral Development*, *1*, 105–130.

Romski, M., & Sevcik, R. (2005). Augmentative communication and early intervention: Myths and realities. *Infants and Young Children*, *18*, 174–185.

Rosa-Lugo, L. I., & Kent-Walsh, J. (2008). Effects of parent instruction on communicative turns of Latino children using augmentative and alternative communication during storybook reading. *Communication Disorders Quarterly*, *30*(1), 49–61.

Saleh, M. S., Aljaam, J. M., Karime, A., & El Saddik, A. (2013). An edutainment system for assisting qatari children with moderate intellectual and learning disability through exerting physical activities. *IEEE Global Engineering Education Conference (EDUCON),* 886–892.

Schlosser, R. W., & Koul, R. (2015). Speech Output Technologies in Interventions for Individuals with Autism Spectrum Disorders: A Scoping Review. *Augmentative and Alternative Communication, 31*(4), 1–25. PMID:26170252

Schlosser, R. W., & Wendt, O. (2008). Effects of augmentative and alternative communication intervention on speech production in children with autism: A systematic review. *American Journal of Speech-Language Pathology, 17,* 212–230. PMID:18663107

Sebat, J., Lakshmi, B., Malhotra, D., Troge, J., Lese-Martin, C., Walsh, T., & … . (2007). Strong association of *de novo* copy number mutations with autism. *Science, 316,* 445–449. PMID:17363630

Shelton, J. F., Hertz-Picciotto, I., & Pessah, I. N. (2012). Tipping the balance of autism risk: Potential mechanisms linking pesticides and autism. *Environmental Health Perspectives, 120,* 944–951. PMID:22534084

Shire, S. Y., & Jones, N. (2015). Communication partners supporting children with complex communication needs who use AAC. *Communication Disorders Quarterly, 37*(1), 3.

Shriberg, L., Paul, R., McSweeney, J., Klin, A., Cohen, D., & Volkmar, F. (2001). Speech and prosody characteristics of adolescents and adults with high functioning autism and Asperger syndrome. *Journal of Speech, Language, and Hearing Research: JSLHR, 44,* 1097–1115. PMID:11708530

Silk, T. J., Rinehart, N., Bradshaw, J. L., Tonge, B., Egan, G., O'Boyle, M. W., & Cunnington, R. (2006). Article. *The American Journal of Psychiatry, 163*(8), 1440–1443. PMID:16877661

Smalley, S. L. (1998). Autism and tuberous sclerosis. *Journal of Autism and Developmental Disorders, 28*(5), 407–414. PMID:9813776

Starble, A., Hutchins, T., Favro, M. A., Prelock, P., & Bitner, B. (2005). Family-centered intervention and satisfaction with AAC device training. *Communication Disorders Quarterly, 27*(1), 47–54.

Stiebel, D. (1999). Promoting augmentative communication during daily routines: A parent problem-solving intervention. *Journal of Positive Behavior Interventions, 1*(3), 159–169. doi:10.1177/109830079900100304

Still, K., Rehfeldt, R. A., Whelan, R., May, R., & Dymond, S. (2014). Facilitating requesting skills using high-tech augmentative and alternative communication devices with individuals with autism spectrum disorders: A systematic review. *Research in Autism Spectrum Disorders, 8*(9), 1184–1199.

Tager-Flusberg, H., & Kasari, C. (2013). Minimally verbal school-aged children with autism spectrum disorder: The neglected end of the spectrum. *Autism Research, 6,* 468–478. PMID:24124067

Taylor, B., Miller, E., Lingam, R., Andrews, N., Simmons, A., & Stowe, J. (2002). MMR vaccination and bowel problems or developmental regression in children with autism: Population study. *British Medical Journal, 324,* 393–396. PMID:11850369

Therrien, M. C. S., & Light, J. C. (2018). Promoting peer interaction for preschool children with complex communication needs and autism spectrum disorder. *American Journal of Speech-Language Pathology*, *27*, 207–221. doi:10.1044/2017_AJSLP-17-0104 PMID:29383382

Thiemann-Bourque, K. S., McGuff, S., & Goldstein, H. (2017). Training peer partners to use a speech-generating device with classmates with autism spectrum disorder: Exploring communication outcomes across preschool contexts. *Journal of Speech, Language, and Hearing Research: JSLHR*, *60*, 2648. doi:10.1044/2017_JSLHR-L-17-0049 PMID:28854313

Tincani, M., & Devis, K. (2011). Quantitative synthesis and component analysis of single- participant studies on the picture exchange communication system. *Remedial and Special Education*, *32*, 458–470. doi:10.1177/0741932510362494

Tonsing, K. M., Alant, E., & Lloyd, L. I. (2005). Intervention issues. In E. Alant & L. Lloyd (Eds.), *Augmentative and Alternative Communication and Severe Disabilities: Beyond Poverty* (pp. 30–67). London, UK: Whurr Publishers.

Trottier, N., Kamp, L., & Mirenda, P. (2011). Effects of peer-mediated instruction to teach use of speech-generating devices to students with autism in social game routines. *Augmentative and Alternative Communication*, *27*, 26–39. doi:10.3109/07434618.2010.546810 PMID:21284561

van der Meer, L. A., & Rispoli, M. (2010). Communication interventions involving speech-generating devices for children with autism: A review of the literature. *Developmental Neurorehabilitation, 13,* 294–306. 0367149413 doi:10.3109/175184210

Volioti, C., Tsiatsos, T., Mavropoulou, S., & Karagiannidis, C. (2016). VLEs, Social Stories and Children with Autism: A Prototype Implementation and Evaluation. *Education and Information Technologies*, *21*(6), 1679–1697.

Volkmar, F. R., Lord, C., Bailey, A., Schultz, R. T., & Klin, A. (2004). Autism and pervasive developmental disorders. *Journal of Child Psychology and Psychiatry, and Allied Disciplines*, *45*(1), 135–170. PMID:14959806

Volkmar, F. R., & Nelson, D. S. (1990). Seizure disorder in autism. *Journal of the American Academy of Child and Adolescent Psychiatry*, *29*, 127–129. PMID:2295565

Walter, K. O., Baller, S. L., & Kuntz, A. M. (2012). Two Approaches for Using Web Sharing and Photography Assignments to Increase Critical Thinking in the Health Sciences. *International Journal on Teaching and Learning in Higher Education*, *24*(3), 383–394.

Watson, L. R., Crais, E. R., Baranek, G. T., Dykstra, J. R., Wilson, K. P., Hammer, C. S., & Woods, J. (2013). Communicative gesture use in infants with and without autism: A retrospective home video study. *American Journal of Speech-Language Pathology*, *22*(1), 25–39. PMID:22846878

Werner, E., & Dawson, G. (2005). Validation of the phenomenon of autistic regression using home videotapes. *Archives of General Psychiatry*, *62*(8), 889–895. PMID:16061766

Williams, D. (2012). *Neurological basis for autism: Implications for speech-language pathologists.* Mini-seminar presented at the Ohio Speech-Language-Hearing Association, Columbus, OH.

Yoder, P., McCathern, R., Warren, S., & Watson, A. (2001). Important distinctions in measuring maternal responses to communication in pre-linguistic children with disabilities. *Communication Disorders Quarterly*, *22*(3), 135–147.

Zafeiriou, D. I., Ververi, A., & Vargiami, E. (2007). Childhood autism and associated comorbidities. *Brain & Development*, *29*, 257–272. PMID:17084999

Zwaigenbaum, L., Bryson, S., Rogers, T., Roberts, W., Brian, J., & Szatmari, P. (2005). Behavioural manifestations of autism in the first year of life. *International Journal of Developmental Neuroscience*, *23*(2–3), 143–152. PMID:15749241

Chapter 7
A Review on Eye Tracking Technology

Pavneet Bhatia
Dr. B. R. Ambedkar National Institute of Technology, Jalandhar, India

Arun Khosla
Dr. B. R. Ambedkar National Institute of Technology, Jalandhar, India

Gajendra Singh
Dr. B. R. Ambedkar National Institute of Technology, Jalandhar, India

ABSTRACT

In past few decades, eye tracking has evolved as an emerging technology with wide areas of applications in gaming, human-computer interaction, business research, assistive technology, automatic safety research, and many more. Eye-gaze tracking is a provocative idea in computer-vision technology. This chapter includes the recent researches, expansion, and development in the technology, techniques, and its wide-ranging applications. It gives a detailed background of technology with all the efforts done in the direction to improve the tracking system.

INTRODUCTION

Eye tracking is a process of measuring the eye movements. It is a sensor technology which enables a device to track eye activity. Psychological studies consider eye movements as a strong penetration into one's perception framing a mental picture of its' line of thinking. Gaze patterns provides an idea about how we discern what we see and visualize. Eye Tracking is a process of estimation of eye development/action whereas tracking gaze pattern is the analysis of eye following information in accordance with the head/visual scene. Generally, the incorporation of head and eye position is utilized to process the area of the look in the visual scene. Basic eye trackers report just the bearing of the look in respect to the head with head-mounted framework, cathodes, scleral coils or for a settled position of the eyeball (frameworks which require a head obsession). Such eye following frameworks are alluded as meddlesome or obtrusive

DOI: 10.4018/978-1-7998-3069-6.ch007

frameworks since some uncommon reaching gadgets are connected to the skin near the eye to get the client's look (Duchowski, 2007). Such frameworks are also called as invasive or intrusive systems. There are few frameworks which don't have any physical contact with the client. Such systems are alluded as non-meddling frameworks or remote frameworks or non- intrusive or non- invasive systems (Morimoto & Mimica, 2005). Such methods generally illuminate eye with IR light instead of using any instruments in direct contact with eye or body of the subject.

BACKGROUND

The potential and importance of eye tracking was recognized by researchers, investigators and analysts in the early 18th century. The development in the field and technology of eye tracking have been through many phases and efforts in the past many years. An attempt to track eye developments while reading was depicted by Hering and by Lamare in 1879; both utilized comparative strategies of tuning in to sounds made by withdrawals of the extraocular muscles (Wade, 2010). Photographic records and light reflections from the eyes during reading task was used by Dodge and Cline to estimate horizontal eye movements (Drewes, 2010). An idea to measure both horizontal and vertical eye developments was conceived by Jung in 1939 placing electrodes close to the eye which measure changing electric field of the eye-ball due to its movement. Such a method involving electrodes relating electric properties of eye with its movements is called Electro-Oculography (EOG). Even the magnetic properties of human eye were cashed to retrace eye developments using principle of electromagnetic induction. Scleral search coils were placed into the eye in form of a lens to monitor eye movements (Bates et al., 2005). With advancement in technology, real-time computation of eye movements was made possible using video-based frameworks known as Video-Oculography. Improvement in the innovation, compact designs, enhanced algorithms, high precision and falling prices of the systems has encouraged the usage of the technology in many fields like business research (Koller et al., 2012),marketing and advertising (Rayner, Rotello, Stewart, Keir, & Duffy, 2001), human-computer interaction(HCI) (Drewes, 2010; Goldberg, Stimson, Lewenstein, Scott, & Wichansky, 2002; Jacob, 1990; Lee & Tsai, 2010), assistive technology as if eye typing for physically disabled (Balan, Moldoveanu, Morar, & Asavei, 2013; Lupu & Ungureanu, 2013; Majaranta & Raiha, 2002) automated safety systems, drowsiness detection (Picot, Charbonnier, & Caplier, 2010), as a clinical support for iris acknowledgment (Xu, Zhang, & Ma, 2006), visual search (Greene & Rayner, 2001), psychology and neuroscience (Rayner, 1998; Snodderly, Kagan, & Gur, 2001; Vidal, Turner, Bulling, & Gellersen, 2012), evaluation of e-learning systems (Hend & Remya, 2010), Cognitive and behavioral therapy (Grillon, Riquier, Herbelin, & Thalmann, 2006).

ANATOMY OF HUMAN EYE

Human eye is a natural optical instrument used to see objects by human beings. An eye is a photosensitive organ which responds to light and pressure. In an improved view, the anatomy of eye can be perceived like a camera with picture adjustment having lens and screen system (Drewes, 2010) that helps to give a 3-D moving picture, typically hued in light. Rod and cone cells in the retina permit cognizant light recognition and vision including shading separation and the impression of profundity (Judd, 1975).

Around 10 million hues can be separated by a normal human eye and is conceivably fit for recognizing a solitary photon.

The eye isn't formed like an immaculate circle, in fact it is a melded two-section unit (the front section and the back fragment). The anterior portion is comprised of the cornea, iris and focal point. The cornea is a curved, transparent part connected to the bigger back fragment, comprised of the vitreous, choroid, retina and the external white opaque layer called the sclera. The cornea is normally around 11.5 mm in width, and 1/2 mm in thickness close to its middle. The posterior part constitutes the remaining five-sixths; its breadth is regularly around 24 mm. The cornea and sclera are associated by a region named the limbus. The iris is the pigmented round structure surrounding the pupil which controls the measure of light entering the eye. The pupil size is balanced by the iris' dilator and sphincter muscles. The basic structure of human eye is projected in Figure 1.

Figure 1. The structure of human eye
(http://www.allaboutvision.com/resources/anatomy.html)

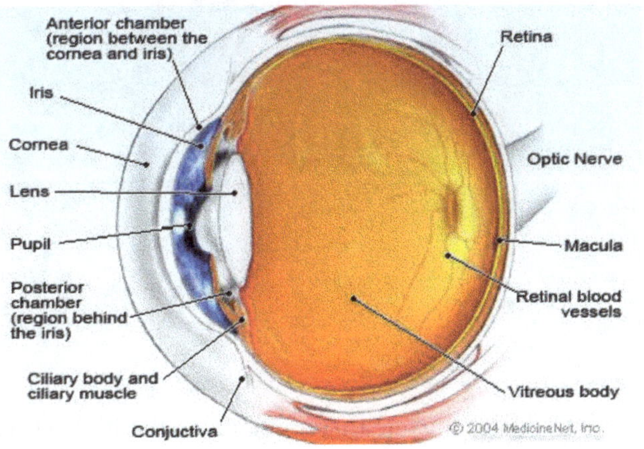

Light vitality entering through pupil is focused on the screen of eye referred as retina by a transparent structure called as eye lens. Eye lens are converging in nature. The focal point shape is reformed for close concentration (convenience) by the ciliary muscles. Photons of light falling on the light-delicate photoreceptor cells (cones and rods) of the retina are changed over into electrical signs that are transmitted to the brain by the optic nerve for further interpretation.

Blind spot, little segment of the visual field that corresponds to the space where axons of the receptor cells of retina coil together referred to as optic disk (otherwise called the optic nerve head) inside the retina. There are no photoreceptors rods or cones in this region, and, along these lines, there is no picture recognition around there. The blind side of the right eye is to the right side of the focal point of vision and similarly to the left in the left eye. It is roughly 7.5° high and 5.5° wide (MIL-STD-1472F (1999)). Blind spot cannot be seen by the open eyes as the visual fields of the two cover it. Even with one closed eye, the blind side is hardly recognized because of the capacity of the mind to "fill in" or disregard the unaccounted bit of the picture (https://www.britannica.com/science/blind-spot).

I. Eye Muscles

Developments of eye are controlled by six muscles present in eye socket. Superior oblique, superior rectus, medial rectus, lateral rectus, inferior rectus, inferior oblique control the rotation of eye as well as the movement along upside, downwards and sidewise.

Figure 2. Extraocular Muscle Anatomy
(https://www.aapos.org/terms/conditions/22)

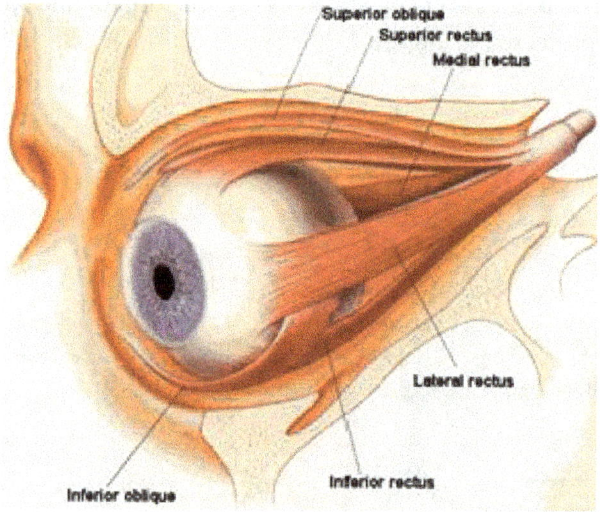

The superior rectus is an extraocular muscle that connects to the highest point of the eye responsible for the upward motion of eye. However, inferior rectus appends to the base of the eye. It controls the descending of eye. The medial rectus present to the side of the eye close to the nose controls the inward motion of eye towards the nose while the outward motion is supervised by lateral rectus. Also, the upward and downward movement of eye is regulated by inferior oblique and superior oblique respectively.

All kind of eye movements are depicted in the Figure 3 that allow the eye to elevate, depress, converge, diverge and roll. These muscles work voluntarily and involuntarily to track objects correctly for synchronous head developments.

Figure 3. Degrees of freedom for the eye (Lukander, 2003)

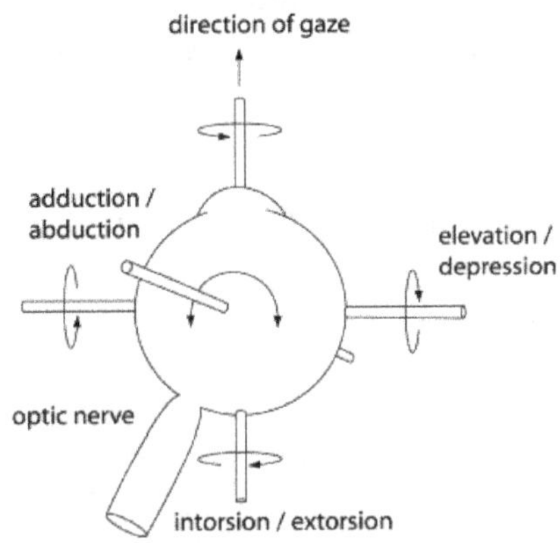

II. Field of View

The rough field of view of an eye (estimated from the obsession point, i.e., the time when one's look is coordinated) shifts by facial structures, yet is regularly 30° superior (up, constrained by the forehead), 45° nasal (restricted by the nose), 70° mediocre (down), and 100° temporal (towards the temple) (Ryan et al., 2012; Savino & Danesh-Meyer, 2012; Trattler et al., 2012). For the two eyes joined (binocular) visual field is 135° vertical and 200° horizontal.

III. Eye Movements

The two eyes enable the cerebrum to decide the depth and distance of an object, referred to as stereovision, which is an added feature of three-dimensionality to the vision. The two eyes need to point precisely enough that the image of object falls on the two retinas to invigorate stereovision. Eye developments can be comprehensively sorted into two principle classes. Stabilizing movements that endeavor to hold the eye, or rather the picture on the retina and saccadic developments that move the eye around the visual field and bring objects of enthusiasm to the zone of sharp vision. Settling/ stabilizing eye developments incorporate fixations, smooth pursuit movements, and nystagmus. Saccadic eye movements incorporate saccades and vergence developments.

Saccades

Saccades are quick and conjugate eye developments that suddenly alter the point of foveal fixation. They extend in abundancy from the little developments while reading, for instance, to the substantially bigger developments while looking around a room. The rapid eye movements striking up during sleep are also saccades. Figure 4 depicts the course of time during saccadic eye movement. After the beginning of an objective for a saccade, it requires around 200 ms for eye development to start. While this setup time, the position of the target in accordance with the fovea is computed (that is, how far the eye must move), and the difference between the initial and intended position, or "motor error", is used as a motor command regulating the eye movement in appropriate direction and distance. Saccadic eye developments are said to be ballistic as the saccade-producing framework can't react to consequent changes in the position of the target over the span of the eye movement. During this time period of 15-100 ms, if there is again some movement in the target, the saccade will miss the target, and a second saccade will be required to correct the error.

Figure 4. Time course of saccadic eye movement (Purves et al., 2001)

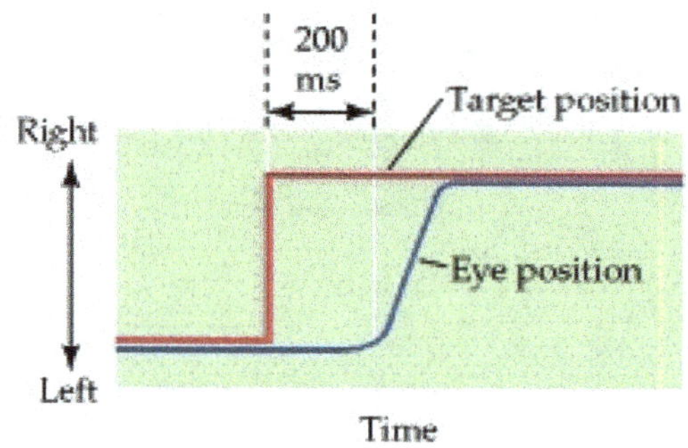

In Figure 4, target position is indicated by red line whereas blue line depicts eye position. When the target moves suddenly to the right, the eye begins to move to the new target position with a delay of around 200ms. (Purves et al., 2001). Saccade movements can achieve of peak accelerations 40000 degree/s2 and a pinnacle velocity of 400-600 degree/s, influenced by the amplitude of the saccade. Saccadic eye developments can be carried out deliberately or reflexively as a response to a visual boost, and as a restorative development related with optokinetic or vestibular development (Lukander, 2003).

Microsaccades

Many a times each second, the slow drift developments of the eyes while fixation are hindered by little quick movements. These jolt-like developments were noticed by Dodge in 1907. In most of the current examinations, they were termed as microsaccades, by Zuber, Crider, and Stark (1964) (Rolfs, 2009). Microsaccades look like general saccades in most regards aside from that they are little and happen not withstanding when we are endeavoring to focus the eyes on a specific area. Consequently, they are regularly alluded to as 'fixational saccade' Microsaccade amplitudes vary from 2 to 120 arcminutes.

Rapid Eye Movement

Rapid eye movement (REM) refers to the sleep stage during which the most distinct dreams happen. REM are quick rapid eye developments. The REM phase is also known as paradoxical sleep (PS) and sometimes desynchronized sleep because the EEG wave pattern during this course is similar to that of waking state.

Visual Fixation

Fixation or visual fixation refers to sustaining visual gaze on an object or location. The fovea is the point of clearest vision located at center of the retina where the image of the target object is focused during fixation. The eyes are not stationary during fixation but rather make ceaseless small developments, including ocular drifts and microsaccades, which are controlled by the same neuronal systems that produce bigger saccades (Krauzlis, Goffart, & Hafed, 2017).

No less than three procedures occur during fixation. Firstly, visual data is encoded. Next, the subsidiary field of the present look is inspected, to decide resulting informative areas. At last, the following next saccade is arranged (Goldberg & Kotval, 1999). These procedures occur simultaneously as depicted in Figure 5.

Figure 5. Events occurring during fixation (Goldberg & Kotval, 1999)

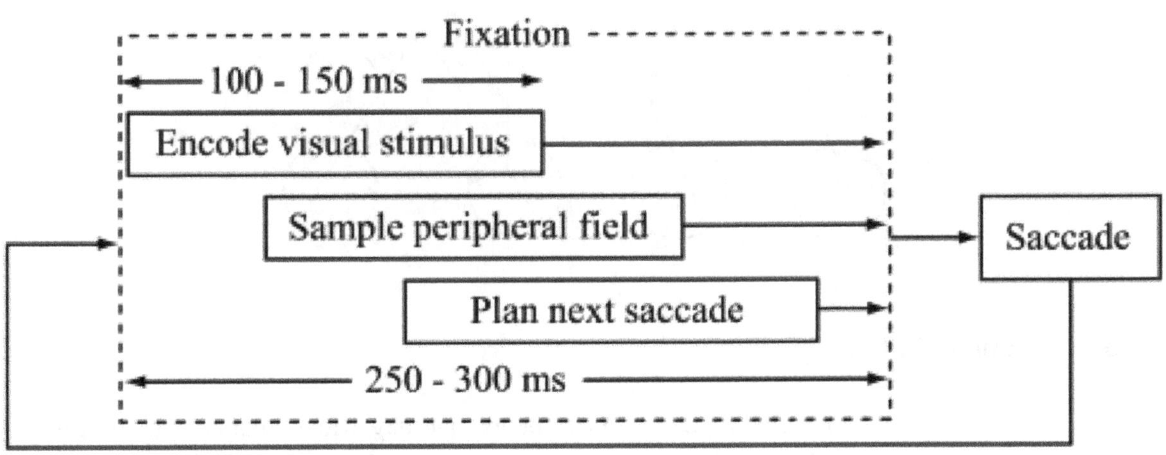

Miniature Eye Movements

During Fixation also eyes are never still, small scale developments of the eyes move the retinal picture over several foveal photoreceptors which are referred to as miniature eye movements which include tremor, drift and microsaccades. Tremor is small amplitude, high – frequency development of eye. Its amplitude is of the order of seconds of arc and frequency above flicker fusion frequency of around 90 Hz. Drift is slow random motion of eye usually treated as noise in the oculomotor system with low velocity of around 4' arc per second. Microsaccade as discussed above is rapid eye movement less than 15' of arc.

Smooth Pursuit Movements

Smooth pursuit movements are slow developments of the eye intended to keep the image of moving stimulus sharp on the retina. Such developments are under deliberate control as in the spectator can pick regardless of whether to track a moving target so is voluntary in action. Tracking a moving object with a velocity less than 5-30 degree/sec involves smooth pursuit movements and above this saccadic movements.

Vergence Movements

Vergence eye movements occur during movement of eyes in opposite direction to each other whereas *version* eye movements happen to be in same direction at the two eyes as shown in Figure 6. Both types of eye movement are binocular in nature. Vergence computes the difference in the positions of the two eyes however version is the mean position of the two eyes. For binocular vision eyes move about horizontal axis for obtaining a sharp image exactly on fovea in both eyes (Masson, Yang, & Miles, 2002). For nearby objects eyes converge towards each other, whereas for far off object divergence of eyes occurs. Cross eyed viewing occurs due to exaggerated convergence for example while concentrating on the nose. When looking at far away point, the eyes diverge till the line of sight becomes parallel.

Figure 6. Version and Vergence movements
(http://www.opt.indiana.edu)

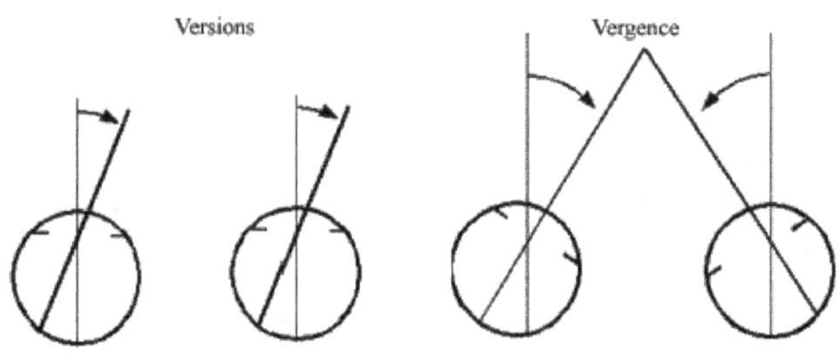

Vestibulo -Ocular Reflex

In Nystagmus eyes make uncontrolled repetitive movements that may affect balance and coordination. The vestibulo-visual reflex (VOR) is reflex action, where initiation of the vestibular framework causes eye development which is intended to settle the image on the retinal screen during motions of head by making eye movements in opposite direction. This inverse motion of eye compensates for head movements.

Optokinetic Reflex

Optokinetic nystagmus is an ordinary reflexive reaction of the eyes because of huge scale developments of the visual scene. This reflex action stabilizes the picture on the retinal screen through visual feedback. It is instigated when the whole visual sight drifts over the retina, hence triggering eye movement in same direction with a speed that limits the movement of the picture on the retinal screen.

IV. Electrical Properties of Eye

Emil du Bois-Reymond in 1848 found that the eye cornea is electrically positive with respect to retina. Human eye appears like a dipole oriented from the retina to the cornea. The micro-currents are setup from high-potential terminal to the lower one flowing through the conductive tissue as shown in the Figure 7. These corneoretinal currents range in 0.4 - 1.0 mV.

Figure 7. Eye as a dipole (Dhillon, Singla, Rekhi, &Jha, 2009)

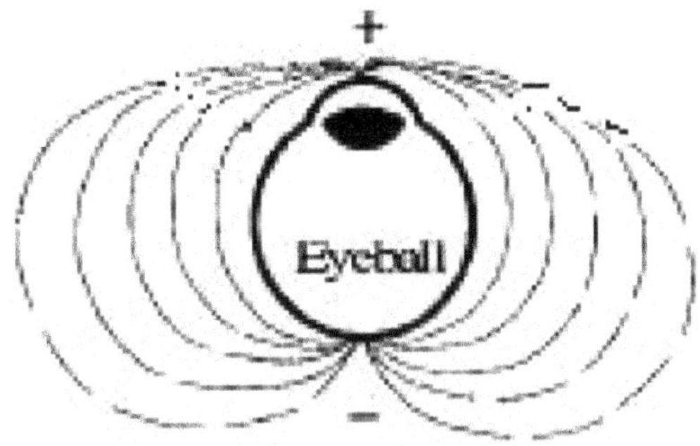

Movements in Eye result in changing potentials that can be recorded and analyzed to track developments in gaze.

METHODS OF EYE TRACKING

Oculography is a medical term referring to the technique of measuring and recording eye position, development and movement. The tracking techniques can be grouped into two categories: one estimating angular eye position relative to the head for example electro-oculography, Infrared oculography, and head mounted frameworks, and other one measuring eye position in accordance to the surroundings, table-top systems and the scleral search coil method falls in this category. The tracking method to be used generally depends on the application to be employed. For the study of oculomotor dynamics eye position relative to the head is considered more accurate and suitable however for human computer interface applications eye position with respect to the surroundings are considered for gaze point measurements. Other deciding factors are temporal and spatial accuracy, easy access, suitability for operational conditions, invasiveness, cost. Following are the most widely used technologies on which commercial trackers and systems are manufactured by leading brands:

- Electro- Oculography
- Scleral Search Coils
- Infrared-Oculography
- Video-Oculography
    - Single Camera Eye Tracker
    - Multi Camera Eye Tracker

I. Electro- Oculography

This method of recording eye movements was invented in 1934 by Fenn and Hursh. It is based on the principle of measuring changing potentials resulting from polarization and depolarization of corneoretinal dipole. The small differences in skin potential is recorded by placing electrodes/sensors around the eye and hence estimating the horizontal and vertical movements. Electro-Oculography (EOG) is sometimes also referred to as Electronystagmography (ENG) however EOG is based on DC (direct current coupling) amplification, whereas ENG is clinically acclaimed method using AC amplification generating a high pass filtered signal free from baseline drifts which are treated as noise signals. Different strategies for recording visual nystagmus, have also been marked as 'electronystagmography'.

Figure 8. Signal generation in accordance with Horizontal Eye Movement (Malmivuo & Plonsey, 1995)

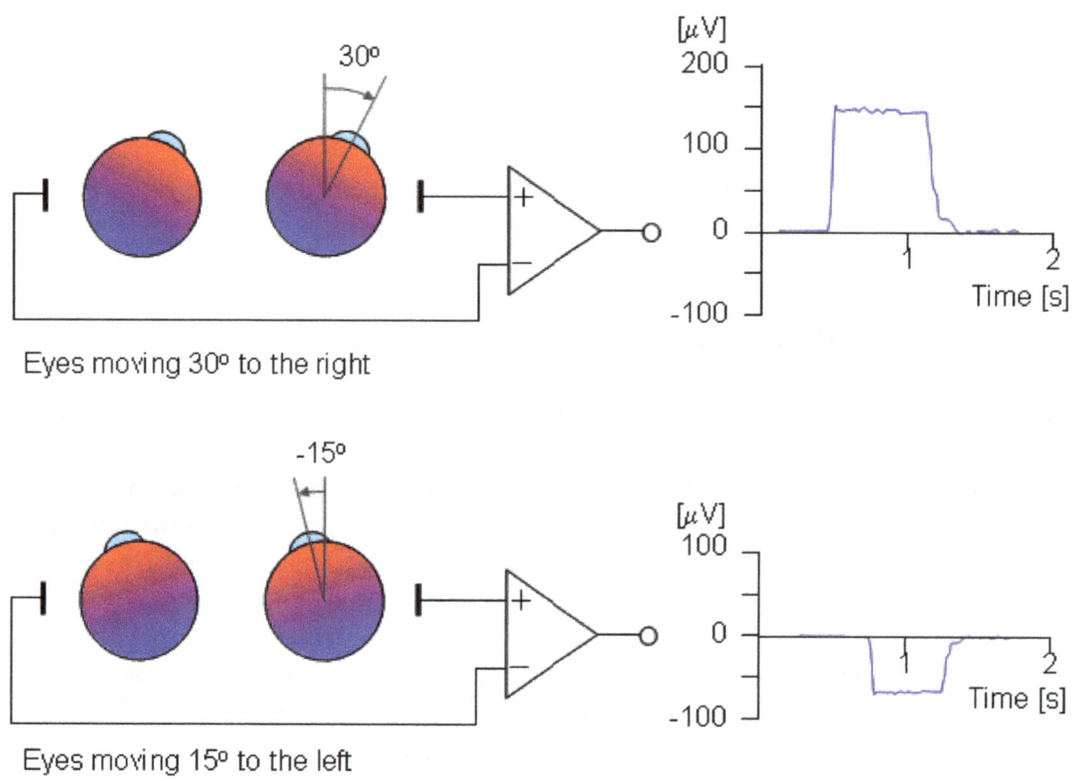

Five Electrodes are placed, for binocular horizontal recording two silver – silver chloride is placed on the external canthi of eyes (D and E) similarly for vertical accounts two electrodes are attached one above and one underneath eye (B and C) and A as reference electrode placed overhead as depicted in Figure 9 (Barea, Boquete, Mazo, & López, 2002; Heide, Koenig, Trillenberg, Kompf, & Zee, 1999). This corneo-retinal potential differs between 0.4 and 1.0 mV and is amplified via differential amplifier. A degree of eye movement can vary the corneoretinal potential around 15 – 20 μV. EOG thus obtained do have many artifacts and interfering signals such as EEG, head or eye movements, noise due to incorrect electrode placement or powerline noise due to A.C. equipment. The filtered EOG signal is obtained by using differential amplifier with high gain ranging around 1000-5000 and common mode rejection ratio of about 70-90 Hz followed by a band pass filter with passing band 0.05 to 35 Hz as shown in Figure 10. Metro Vision Systems made a project called MONEOG (http://www.metrovision.fr) based on eye tracking implementing EOG technique. Eagle Eyes from Opportunity Foundation of America also implemented EOG method for human – computer interface for physically disabled (http://www.bc.edu/eagleeyes).

Figure 9. Electrode placement in EOG (Barea, Boquete, Mazo, & López, 2002)

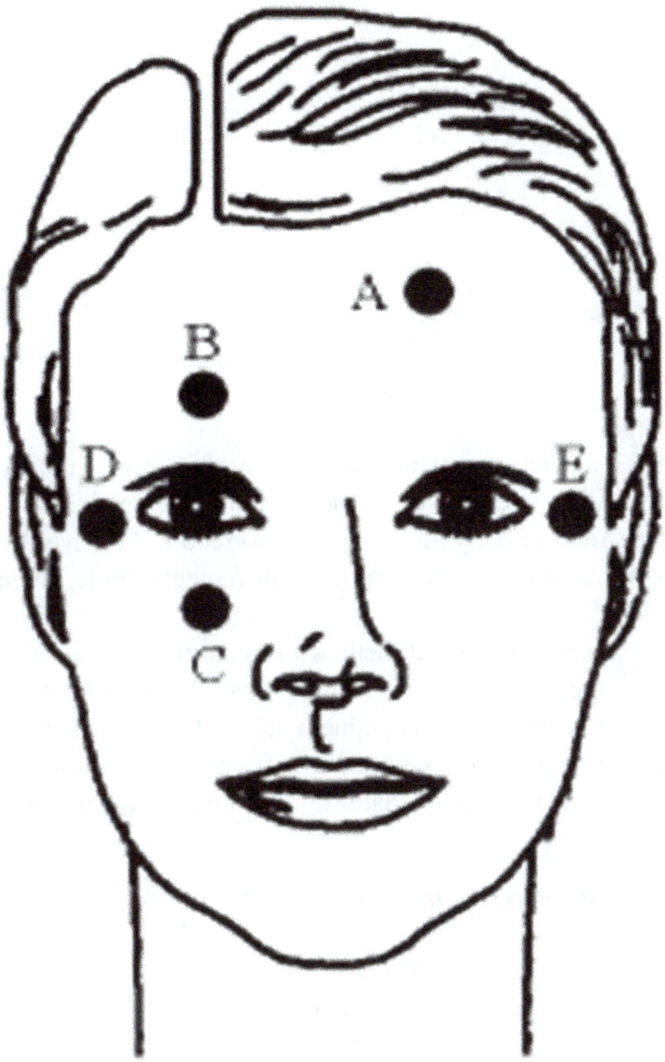

Figure 10. EOG signal generation from eye movements (Venkataramanan, Prabhat, Choudhury, Nemade, & Sahambi, 2005)

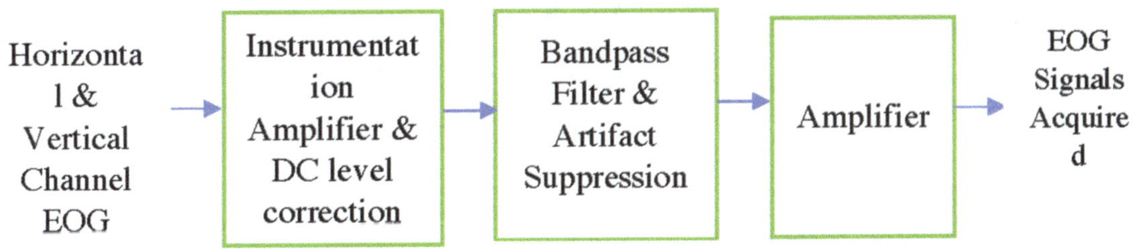

Figure 11. 2D scleral coil
(http://www.chronos-vision.de)

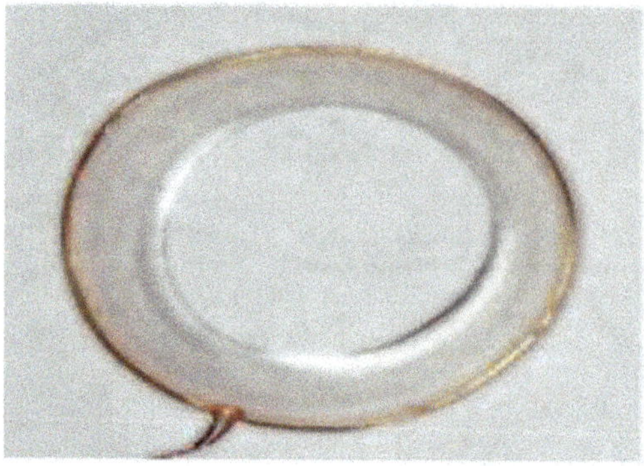

Advantages: Though it is an invasive method and requires close contact of electrodes with the subject however it is easy, cheap and trouble-free technique to record eye proceedings. The biggest advantage of this technology is wide field of view and capability to record data even when eyes are closed for example while sleeping or even while continuous head movement (Heide, Koenig, Trillenberg, Kompf, & Zee, 1999).

Disadvantages: It is not a recommended method for recording eye developments of subjects with mental disorders. Even the amplitude of corneoretinal potential is subjected to changes by varying illumination, so it is required to maintain constant ambient light. Also, EOG data is usually contaminated by electrical, electroencephalographic artifacts, baseline drifts, powerline noise, flicker noise due to changing skin resistance and electrode impedance that ask for more accurate methods for scientific purpose.

Figure 12. Principle of Scleral Search Coils (Drewes, 2010)

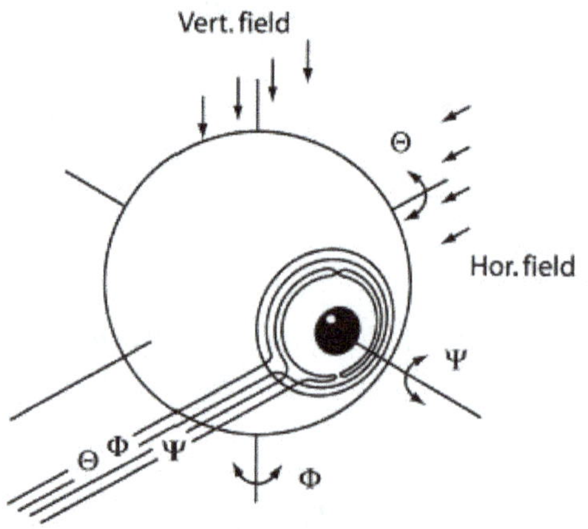

Figure 13. IROG Technique
(https://www.liverpool.ac.)

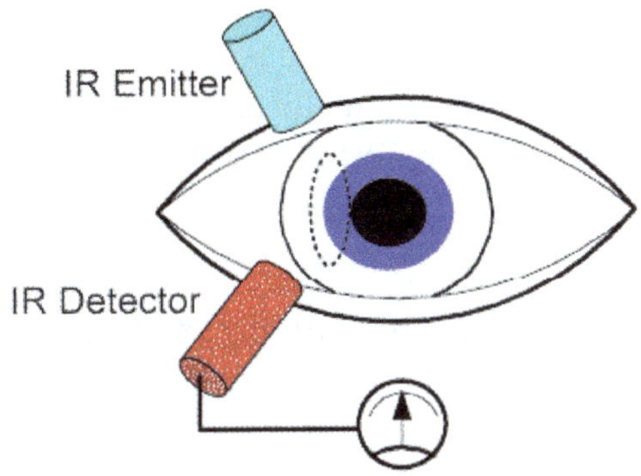

II. Scleral Search Coil Method

It is based on the principle of Faraday's electromagnetic induction which states that whenever there is a relative motion between coil and magnetic field, a potential is induced in the coil. The field is generated by placing magnetic poles on either side of head (for horizontal movement) and other set over head (for vertical movements), coil of wire is modified in form of contact lens leaving eye at temporal canthus as shown in Figure 11.

The two magnetic fields have 90° phase shift with high frequency of about 50 to 100 Hz. The induced voltage amplitude in proportion to the sine of the angle between the axes of the search coil and the magnetic field. This method has been used by Chronos Vision (http://www.chronos-vision.de) and Skalar Medical (http://www.nzbri.org/research/labs/eyelab/)

Advantages: This technique is capable of tracking fast eye movements accurately in 3D space with high temporal and spatial resolution of order of 1 or 2 min of arc. If appropriately designed, then even rotating eye movements can be recorded.

Disadvantages: This technique requires special examiner for mounting and removing ring on the anesthetized eye. Moreover, it is an invasive method which is not comfortable and may cause irritation to eyes. Also, it has high cost invested in equipment as a coil breaks easily even if handled with care and needs to be replaced after three to four sessions (Heide, Koenig, Trillenberg, Kompf, & Zee, 1999). Another restricting factor is the Helmholtz Coils which hinder the field of view. This technique has limited applications and is hardly recommended for clinical testing and Human Computer applications.

III. Infrared Oculography (IROG)

This method is based on the fact that intensity of reflected light varies for different parts of eye (much light is reflected from sclera than pupil and iris). This difference in intensity of light tracks the boundaries of ocular structures such as limbus (sclera- iris boundary) or pupil – iris boundary. This information is decoded to measure eye motion. The system setup requires IR light sources as infrared light is invisible to eye, also it is hardly affected by other light sources and photodetectors for detecting reflected light. There are three different setups which are commonly used. First, focused infrared light wave and a wide-angle photodetector measuring the reflected light; second, diffused infrared light energy and a photodetector with a limited range; third, wide angle illuminator as well as wide range photo detector. The strategies were enhanced by deploying two light sources for each eye and two photodetectors equally spaced on either side of the iris. It has high resolution of about 0.1° to 0.5° along horizontal line and temporal resolution of about 1ms. It has fair range of ±15° and ±40° for measuring horizontal eye movements. Commercially available IROG eye trackers are Intelligaze IG-30 (http://www.alea-technologies.com), EyeMax (http://www.dynavoxtech.com), EyeTech Digital Systems (http://www.eyetechds.com) and SeeTech (http://www.see-tech.de).

Figure 14. Purkinje images indicating reflection through surfaces of eye (Vidal, Turner, Bulling, & Gellersen, 2012)

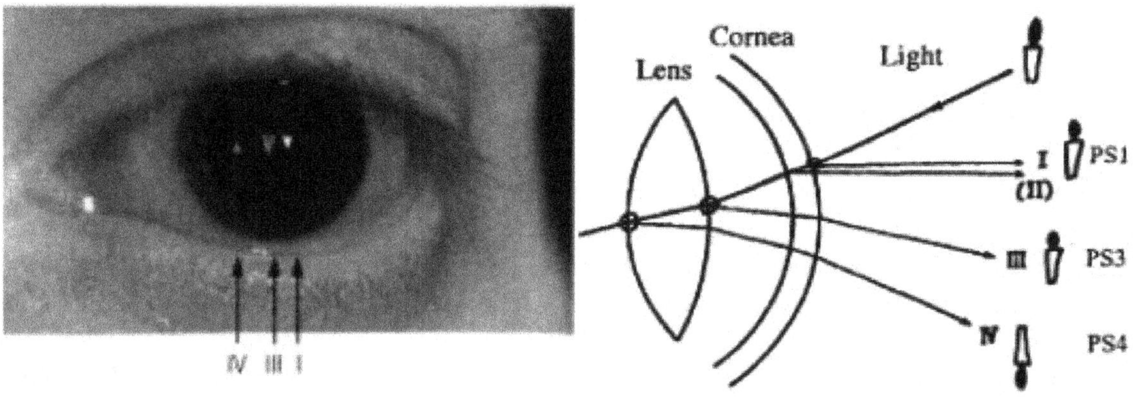

Advantages: Since it is a non- invasive method, so it doesn't cause any discomfort to the subject. Other advantage is the separate recording of the eye movements for the two eyes as may help comparing the two in case required. Also, this technique can be employed in darkness so is used to track eye developments during Magnetic Resonance Imaging (MRI).

Disadvantages: Along the vertical lines signal is obstructed due to occlusion of iris-sclera boundary because of eyelids hence vertical eye movements range in ±5° or ±8°. This method is insufficient to track torsional eye movements and even fails in case of closed eye or eye with spectacles or lens.

IV. Video Oculography (VOG)

It is the most exploited method when it comes to commercial eye tracking. VOG is broadly categorized into invasive and non-invasive system. Invasive system includes head mounted setups which estimate eye position relative to head whereas non- invasive setups are remote systems that track eye position with respect to surroundings. However, these broad categories can further be classified based on light source involved (visible light or infrared light) or number of cameras used (single camera or multi camera-based system), but the basic idea is estimating eye developments from the captured images using different analysis algorithms. The reflected light produces glint on the cornea referred to as corneal reflection which is used as reference point for estimating gaze. It is based on the principle of 'Purkinje' images which are the reflections of light from different surfaces of eye lens and cornea as shown in Figure 14.

Figure 15. Optalert glasses with infrared oculography (Balan, Moldoveanu, Morar, & Asavei, 2013)

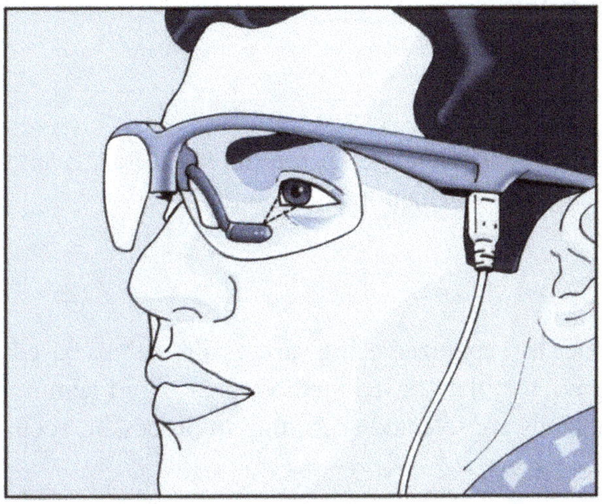

Figure 16. Steps involved in VOG (Singh & Singh, 2012)

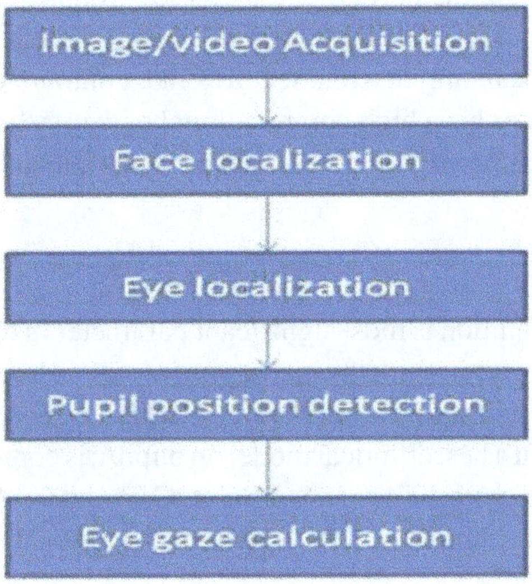

Movements are tracked according to relative motion in images. Single Camera Eye Trackers make use of only one camera and one or more light source. Many such commercial setups were launched in the market by leading brands like LC (http://www.eyegaze.com), ASL (http://www.a-s-l.com), Eyetech (http://www.eyetechds.com), Tobii (http://www.tobii.se). Multi camera eye trackers achieve high accuracy by using different camera for head position tracking to compensate for head movements and hence allow free head movements. The data from all the cameras is calibrated to optimize the eye position (Beymer & Flickner, 2003; Brolly & Mulligan, 2004; Ohno & Mukawa, 2004; Shih & Liu, 2004; Yoo & Chung, 2005; Zhang, Zhao, Ma, & Man, 2010; Zhu & Bennett, 2006). The steps involved in VOG technique are image acquisition, face recognition, eye localization, pupil position recognition and finally gaze estimation as shown in Figure 16.

Image Acquisition

Firstly images/videos are captured using single or multiple cameras. Even webcam has also been proposed by many researchers making VOG a popular technique.

Face Recognition

From the captured images, face is recognized using various algorithms based on skin color, feature based method, texture-based method, template-based method, haar based feature extraction and many more. These image processing methods are selected according to processor, accuracy, computation time and complexity.

Eye Localization

Eyes are detected in face images. There are basic two techniques for eye recognition. One approach aims to detect eye region which is itself a dominant structure. It is appearance-based estimation and is considered to be easy and stable method however it is less robust. Commonly considered methods are morphable model, gray projection model, appearance manifold, cross- ratio. The other approach is established on the grounds of localizing discrete features like contours of iris, pupil, eyelids, eyebrows etc. This abstractive approach does have high computational expenses but is reliable and more accurate. This feature-based method is less prone to variations in illumination and viewpoint.

Pupil Position Recognition

Accurate and reliable pupil recognition is most significant parameter in eye tracking. Several approaches have been developed over past few years with the increasing interest in human computer interface. Feature based algorithm searches for blackest pixels in the image which corresponds to pupil or iris. Whereas model- based algorithm tries to fit a best elliptical model on pupil/iris contour (Lupu & Ungureanu, 2013). Various algorithms reported in applications are Starburst, Cumulative distribution function algorithm, Swirski, Projection function algorithm, Pupil labs, SET, Edge analysis, Integral projection, Harris corner detection, Isophotes curvature etc.

APPLICATIONS

Eye tracking technology had lot of add on's from 1901 when the first head mounted eye tracker was built and was commercially employed in 1947 for the first time by American Air Force. With advancements in technology and research, present eye trackers have become more accessible, comforting, non-invasive, affordable, accurate, less intrusive, easy to calibrate hence have been successfully utilized in wide ranging areas. The technology is currently being exploited by psychologists, neuroscientists, human factor engineers, advertisers, marketers, designers and architects. Some prominent areas of applications are:

Psychology (cognitive neuroscience), Commercial gaze tracking (Web usability, advertising, marketing etc.), Product development (package or product design), computer usability (Websites, application evaluation etc.), Simulation (Car, ship and airplane simulators), Gaming, Learning and education (Classroom attention and distractibility), medical research and neurological disorders.

I. Eye Tracking in Assistive Technology

Advancements in eye tracking technology has evolved as boon to people with disabilities enabling them to accomplish their task with the help of eye control. A perfectly designed human computer system operating from eye movements can serve as a communication tool to disabled subjects. ASISTSYS project team proposed such a system in which request and response messages are sent via communication network as shown in Figure 17.

Figure 17. Eye Tracking in assistive technology
(http://telecom.etc.tuiasi.ro)

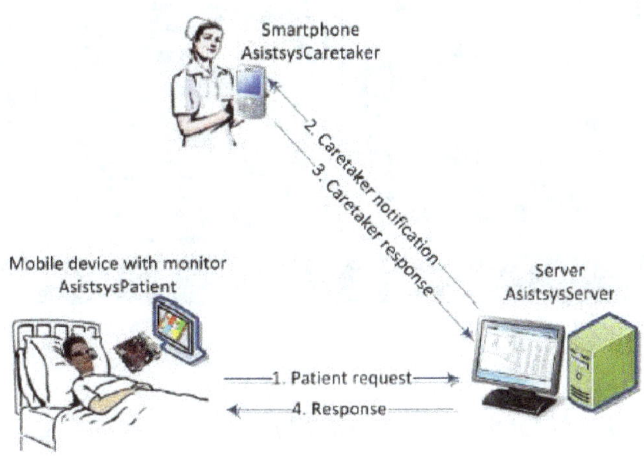

Ii. Eye Tracking in Medical Research

Eye developments give deep inside one's thought process and psychiatric condition hence eye patterns can potentially diagnose neurological disorders like Attention Deficit Hyperactivity Disorder (ADHD), Autism Spectrum Disorder (ASD), Obsessive Compulsive Disorder (OCD), Schizophrenia, Parkinson's Disease, Alzheimer's Disease, multiple sclerosis, dyslexia etc.

Iii. Eye Tracking in Market Research and Advertisement

Eye tracking technology is a powerful serving tool for market researchers and advertisers to identify consumers attention, interest and experience with product. It provides deep insight into costumers shopping behavior i.e. how they browse the aisles of store, which visual sights are ignored or noticed and purchase choices. Even eye tracking is used by brands to test the appeal of product/package design i.e. which package prototype is attractive or key brand attributes that communicate well with consumers as shown in Figure 18.

Figure 18. Eye Tracking in advertisement
(http://brandandmarket.com)

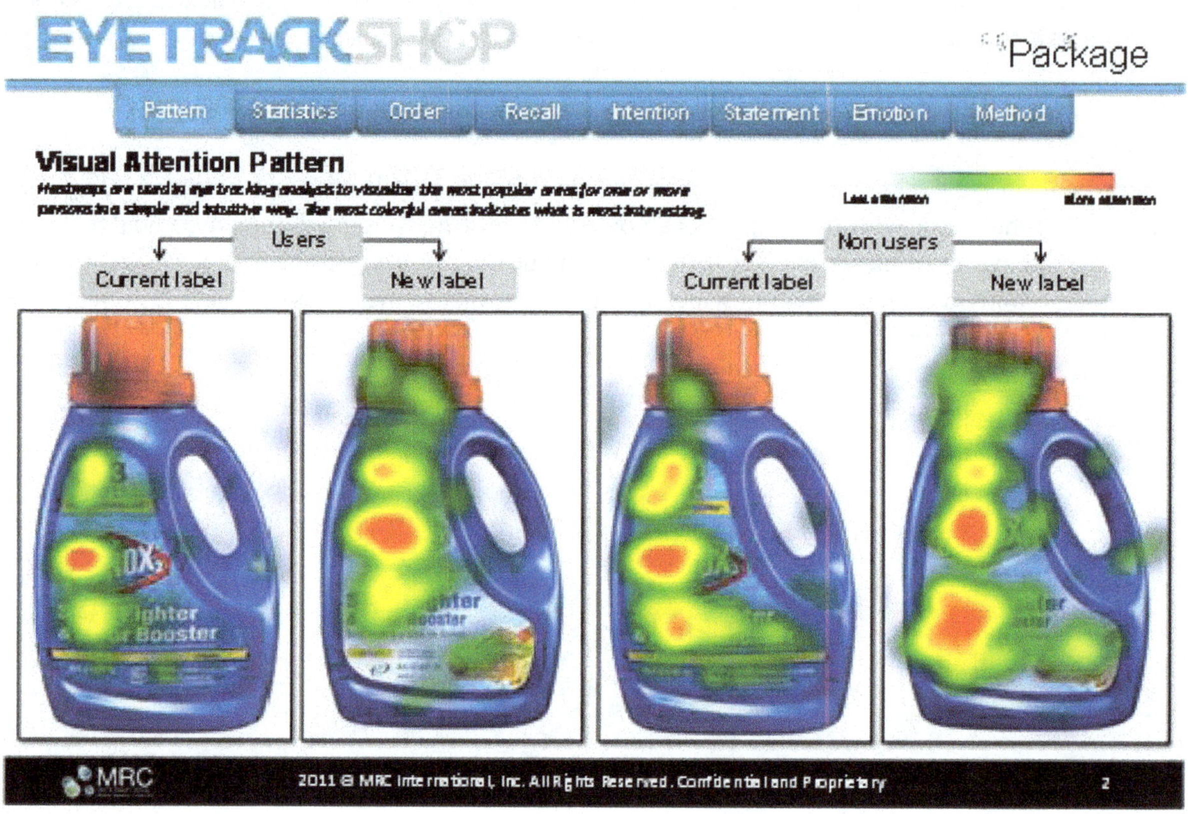

Figure 19. Heat Map and Gaze Plot for website usability
(http://imgmembers.com)

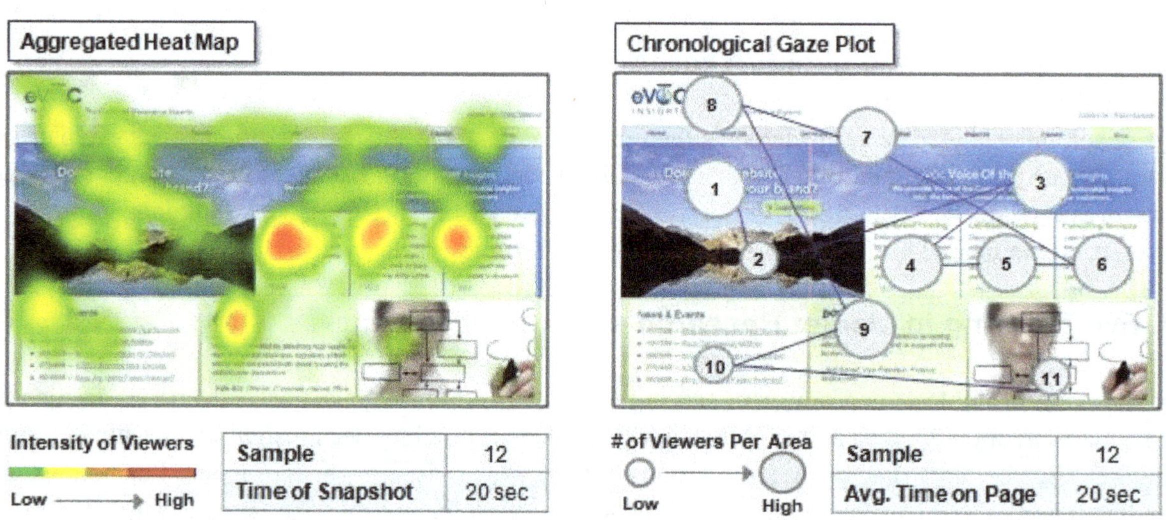

IV. Website Testing

Digital marketing utilizes eye tracking as a powerful tool for understanding usability and effectiveness of web pages. Gaze Patterns, fixations, blinks and saccades provide relevant information about user's interest on the website and areas of high attention.

V. Human Computer Interaction

Using eye control as interaction method for computers and devices is keen area of interest for researchers and tech geeks. Eye movements act as real time input for user-computer system. Utilization of eye movements in human – computer interaction remains an extremely encouraging methodology; its technical and market limitations are being diminished. However, computing through eye may result in Midas Touch problem in which an eye-gaze inspection could be wrongly interpreted as activation input.

VI. Driving Simulation

Eye tracking combined with human behavior analysis is used for simulation of automatic control systems and automobiles. This technology may help in hazardous situations involved due to human error like while using phone, high speed driving, state of sleepiness/drowsiness or sudden unconsciousness etc. Advancements in the field may result in enhanced safety measures in automobiles.

VII. Gaming

Gaming industry see eye tracking technology as a game changer improving the overall experience. Eye movement is also included as one of the input modes in the gaming setup instead of mouse, keyboard or gamepad. The technology is incorporated for PC games, Augmented or Virtual reality and Window devices. Assassin's Creed Origins, Hitman, Agents of Mayhem, Megaton Rainfall are some games that integrate gaze and eye tracking.

VIII. Educational Research

Eye movement is a tool utilized as a part of instructive research keeping in mind the end goal to comprehend the learning procedure, psychological load on students, and educating techniques. The outcomes help outline and enhance the learning environment. Eye tracking can help us discover social interaction pattern among students, between students and teacher, attention of students towards educational material, response towards various learning strategies. The WISO-Research Lab at the University of Hamburg in Germany has outfitted their lab with thirty eye trackers to add a new neuro/physiological-measurement dimension to research projects and understand cognitive processes behind decision making when running their economic research (https://www.tobiipro.com). The Slovak University of Technology (FIIT STU) in Bratislava has equipped their classrooms and labs with eye trackers to achieve both research and educational objectives.

IX. Assisted Typing

Eye tracking has a latest application in assisted typing (https://eyegaze.com/5-fascinating-uses-for-eye-tracking-technology/, 2019). Professionals will be able to navigate through the document without concentrating on the keyboard.

X. Eye Tracking in Virtual Reality

In Virtual Reality eye tracking can help in calculating the gaze points in 3D space. The combined technique of eye tracking and VR with the advantages of more natural stimuli, more natural movement, controlled environment and controlled data collection makes it possible to answer many research questions in a radically innovative way (Clay, Konig, & Konig, 2019).

LIMITATIONS

The technology is expensive and do requires huge investment in equipping the setup for experimentation. Also, the setup will require trained people for operation and supervision. Not every subject can comfortably work with the device and the calibration may require time. Even eye lashes and contact lens can cause hinderance in accurate quantization of eye movements. Though the technology has come up a long way but still its' accuracy is a matter of concern and hence psychological or medical researches don't consider eye gaze patterns as a sufficient and appropriate parameter to conclude the cognitive and emotional state of the subjects (Kok & Jarodzka, 2017). Eye developments reflect intellectual procedures, yet intellectual processes cannot be specifically derived from eye-tracking data.

FUTURE SCOPE

Eye Tracking technology has wide ranging applications and scope in the coming future. Investment in the technology can result in high accuracy and better results. Recording gaze patterns accurately can be helpful in medical research, gaming and Virtual reality. This technology if explored deeply has high potential of advancement. Eye gaze tracking has a wide history of exploration and can even be explored further owing to its advantages and applications.

CONCLUSION

Eye – Gaze tracking technology has a history of 100 years of exploration. In this paper we generally depict some illustrative investigations in the field of eye tracking, covering a few angles about various sorts of gadgets, existing methods in eye tracking, image processing and gaze data processing algorithms likewise, some outstanding applications in assistive innovation, human computer interface, virtual reality, neuroscience or e-learning. The type of method or gadget involved in the experimentation is strictly application oriented. The temporal and spatial accuracy, non – invasiveness, cost, high resolution, easy deployment are matters of interest for researchers enhancing the future scope of eye tracking technology to wide ranging applications hence making it a reliable tool.

REFERENCES

Al-Khalifa, H. S., & George, R. P. (2010). Eye Tracking and e-Learning: Seeing Through Your Students' Eyes. *eLearn, 2010*(6).

BaHammam, A. S., Nashwan, S., Hammad, O., Sharif, M. M., & Pandi-Perumal, S. R. (2013). Objective assessment of drowsiness and reaction time during intermittent Ramadan fasting in young men: A case-crossover study. *Behavioral and Brain Functions*, *9*(1), 32. doi:10.1186/1744-9081-9-32 PMID:23937904

Balan, O., Moldoveanu, A., Moldoveanu, F., Morar, A., & Asavei, V. (2013). Assistive IT for Visually Imapired People. *Journal of Information Systems & Operations Management*, *7*(2), 391–404.

Barea, R., Boquete, L., Mazo, M., & López, E. (2002). System for assisted mobility using eye movements based on electrooculography. *IEEE Transactions on Neural Systems and Rehabilitation Engineering*, *10*(4), 209–218. doi:10.1109/TNSRE.2002.806829 PMID:12611358

Bates, R., Istance, H., Oosthuizen, L., & Majaranta, P. (2005). Survey of de-facto standards in eye tracking. COGAIN conf. on comm. by gaze inter.

Beymer, D., & Flickner, M. (2003, June). Eye gaze tracking using an active stereo head. In *2003 IEEE Computer Society Conference on Computer Vision and Pattern Recognition Proceedings*, *2*, II-451.

Bhuiyan, N. (2017). *Survey on prescription pattern of eye diseases & eye related drugs*. Academic Press.

Brolly, X. L., & Mulligan, J. B. (2004, June). Implicit calibration of a remote gaze tracker. In *2004 Conference on Computer Vision and Pattern Recognition Workshop* (pp. 134-134). IEEE. 10.1109/CVPR.2004.366

Clay, V., König, P., & König, S. U. (2019). *Eye tracking in virtual reality*. Academic Press.

DC, D. (1999). *Military Standard: Human Engineering Design Criteria for Military Systems, Equipment and facilities*. Lockheed Human Factors Engineering Group.

Dhillon, H. S., Singla, R., Rekhi, N. S., & Jha, R. (2009, August). EOG and EMG based virtual keyboard: A brain-computer interface. In *2009 2nd IEEE International Conference on Computer Science and Information Technology* (pp. 259-262). IEEE. 10.1109/ICCSIT.2009.5234951

Drewes, H. (2010). *Eye Gaze Tracking for Human Computer Interaction* (PhD dissertation). www.ndltd.org

Duchowski, A. T. (2007). Eye tracking methodology. *Theory into Practice*, *328*(614), 2–3.

Goldberg, J. H., & Kotval, X. P. (1999). Computer interface evaluation using eye movements: Methods and constructs. *International Journal of Industrial Ergonomics*, *24*(6), 631–645. doi:10.1016/S0169-8141(98)00068-7

Goldberg, J. H., Stimson, M. J., Lewenstein, M., Scott, N., & Wichansky, A. M. (2002, March). Eye tracking in web search tasks: design implications. In *Proceedings of the 2002 symposium on Eye tracking research & applications* (pp. 51-58). 10.1145/507072.507082

Greene, H. H., & Rayner, K. (2001). Eye movements and familiarity effects in visual search. *Vision Research, 41*(27), 3763–3773. doi:10.1016/S0042-6989(01)00154-7 PMID:11712988

Grillon, H., Riquier, F., Herbelin, B., & Thalmann, D. (2006). Use of Virtual Reality as Therapeutic Tool for Behavioural Exposure in the Ambit of Social. *International Conference Series on Disability, Virtual Reality and Associated Technologies (ICDVRAT).*

Heide, W., Koenig, E., Trillenberg, P., Kömpf, D., & Zee, D. S. (1999). Electrooculography: Technical standards and applications. *Electroencephalography and Clinical Neurophysiology. Supplement, 52*, 223–240. PMID:10590990

Jacob, R. J. (1990, March). What you look at is what you get: eye movement-based interaction techniques. In *Proceedings of the SIGCHI conference on Human factors in computing systems* (pp. 11-18). 10.1145/97243.97246

Judd, D. B. (1975). Wys zeckiG. Color in Business, Science and Industry. *Wiiey, 19*, 420–461.

Kok, E. M., & Jarodzka, H. (2017). Before your very eyes: The value and limitations of eye tracking in medical education. *Medical Education, 51*(1), 114–122. doi:10.1111/medu.13066 PMID:27580633

Koller, M., Salzberger, T., Brenner, G., & Walla, P. (2012). Broadening the range of applications of eye-tracking in business research. *Analise, Porto Alegre, 23*(1), 71–77.

Krauzlis, R. J., Goffart, L., & Hafed, Z. M. (2017). Neuronal control of fixation and fixational eye movements. *Philosophical Transactions of the Royal Society B: Biological Sciences, 372*(1718), 20160205.

Lee, M. C., & Tsai, T. R. (2010). What drives people to continue to play online games? An extension of technology model and theory of planned behavior. *Intl. Journal of Human–Computer Interaction, 26*(6), 601-620.

Lukander, K. (2003). *Mobile usability-Measuring gaze point on handheld devices.* Master's thesis.

Lupu, R. G., & Ungureanu, F. (2013). A survey of eye tracking methods and applications. *Buletinul Institutului Politehnic din Iasi. Automatic Control and Computer Science Section, 3*, 72–86.

Majaranta, P., & Räihä, K. J. (2002, March). Twenty years of eye typing: systems and design issues. In *Proceedings of the 2002 symposium on Eye tracking research & applications* (pp. 15-22). 10.1145/507072.507076

Malmivuo, P., Malmivuo, J., & Plonsey, R. (1995). *Bioelectromagnetism: principles and applications of bioelectric and biomagnetic fields.* Oxford University Press. doi:10.1093/acprof:oso/9780195058239.001.0001

Masson, G. S., Yang, D. S., & Miles, F. A. (2002). Version and vergence eye movements in humans: Open-loop dynamics determined by monocular rather than binocular image speed. *Vision Research, 42*(26), 2853–2867. doi:10.1016/S0042-6989(02)00334-6 PMID:12450510

Morimoto, C. H., & Mimica, M. R. (2005). Eye gaze tracking techniques for interactive applications. *Computer Vision and Image Understanding*, *98*(1), 4–24. doi:10.1016/j.cviu.2004.07.010

Ohno, T., & Mukawa, N. (2004, March). A free-head, simple calibration, gaze tracking system that enables gaze-based interaction. In *Proceedings of the 2004 symposium on Eye tracking research & applications* (pp. 115-122). 10.1145/968363.968387

Picot, A., Charbonnier, S., & Caplier, A. (2010, May). Drowsiness detection based on visual signs: blinking analysis based on high frame rate video. In *2010 IEEE Instrumentation & Measurement Technology Conference Proceedings* (pp. 801-804). IEEE. 10.1109/IMTC.2010.5488257

Purves, D., Augustine, G. J., Fitzpatrick, D., Katz, L. C., LaMantia, A. S., McNamara, J. O., & Williams, S. M. (2001). Circuits within the basal ganglia system. In Neuroscience (2nd ed.). Sinauer Associates.

Rayner, K. (1998). Eye movements in reading and information processing: 20 years of research. *Psychological Bulletin*, *124*(3), 372–422. doi:10.1037/0033-2909.124.3.372 PMID:9849112

Rayner, K., Rotello, C. M., Stewart, A. J., Keir, J., & Duffy, S. A. (2001). Integrating text and pictorial information: Eye movements when looking at print advertisements. *Journal of Experimental Psychology. Applied*, *7*(3), 219–226. doi:10.1037/1076-898X.7.3.219 PMID:11676100

Rikert, T. D., & Jones, M. J. (1998, April). Gaze estimation using morphable models. In *Proceedings Third IEEE International Conference on Automatic Face and Gesture Recognition* (pp. 436-441). IEEE. 10.1109/AFGR.1998.670987

Rolfs, M. (2009). Microsaccades: Small steps on a long way. *Vision Research*, *49*(20), 2415–2441. doi:10.1016/j.visres.2009.08.010 PMID:19683016

Ryan, Schachat, Wilkinson, Hinton, & Sadda. (2012). *Retina*. Elsevier Health Sciences.

Savino, P. J., & Danesh-Meyer, H. V. (Eds.). (2012). *Color Atlas and Synopsis of Clinical Ophthalmology--Wills Eye Institute--Neuro-Ophthalmology*. Lippincott Williams & Wilkins.

Shih, S. W., & Liu, J. (2004). A novel approach to 3-D gaze tracking using stereo cameras. *IEEE Transactions on Systems, Man, and Cybernetics. Part B, Cybernetics*, *34*(1), 234–245. doi:10.1109/TSMCB.2003.811128 PMID:15369066

Singh, H., & Singh, J. (2012). Human eye tracking and related issues: A review. *International Journal of Scientific and Research Publications*, *2*(9), 1–9.

Snodderly, D. M., Kagan, I., & Gur, M. (2001). Selective activation of visual cortex neurons by fixational eye movements: Implications for neural coding. *Visual Neuroscience*, *18*(2), 259–277. doi:10.1017/S0952523801182118 PMID:11417801

Trattler, W. B., Kaiser, P. K., & Friedman, N. J. (2012). *Review of Ophthalmology: Expert Consult – Online and Print*. Elsevier Health Sciences.

Venkataramanan, S., Prabhat, P., Choudhury, S. R., Nemade, H. B., & Sahambi, J. S. (2005, January). Biomedical instrumentation based on electrooculogram (EOG) signal processing and application to a hospital alarm system. In *Proceedings of 2005 International Conference on Intelligent Sensing and Information Processing* (pp. 535-540). IEEE. 10.1109/ICISIP.2005.1529512

Vidal, M., Turner, J., Bulling, A., & Gellersen, H. (2012). Wearable eye tracking for mental health monitoring. *Computer Communications*, *35*(11), 1306–1311. doi:10.1016/j.comcom.2011.11.002

Wade, N. J. (2010). Pioneers of eye movement research. *Perception*, *1*(2), 33–68. doi:10.1068/i0389 PMID:23396982

Xu, G., Zhang, Z., & Ma, Y. (2006, July). Improving the performance of iris recogniton system using eyelids and eyelashes detection and iris image enhancement. In *2006 5th IEEE International Conference on Cognitive Informatics* (Vol. 2, pp. 871-876). IEEE. 10.1109/COGINF.2006.365606

Yoo, D. H., & Chung, M. J. (2005). A novel non-intrusive eye gaze estimation using cross-ratio under large head motion. *Computer Vision and Image Understanding*, *98*(1), 25–51. doi:10.1016/j.cviu.2004.07.011

Zhang, K., Zhao, X., Ma, Z., & Man, Y. (2010, November). A simplified 3D gaze tracking technology with stereo vision. In *2010 International Conference on Optoelectronics and Image Processing* (Vol. 1, pp. 131-134). IEEE. 10.1109/ICOIP.2010.346

Zhu, Z., Ji, Q., & Bennett, K. P. (2006, August). Nonlinear eye gaze mapping function estimation via support vector regression. In *18th International Conference on Pattern Recognition (ICPR'06)* (Vol. 1, pp. 1132-1135). IEEE.

Zimmer, C. (2012). Our strange, important, subconscious light detectors. *Discover Magazine*.

Chapter 8

Support of Gamification, Virtual, and Assistive Technologies in Intervening in Social and Behavioral Impairment

Hiten Rajpurohit
Dr. B. R. Ambedkar National Institute of Technology, Jalandhar, India

Arun Khosla
Dr. B. R. Ambedkar National Institute of Technology, Jalandhar, India

ABSTRACT

Neurodevelopmental disorders (NDDs) compromise the development and attainment of full social and economic potential of an individual. Technological intervention can play a big role and is capable of reducing the cost of present medical intervention. Games based on daily life activities can play big roles in improving social skills. One can easily customize games as per requirement or as specific to particular social skills for children to improve their respective social skills. Children find it easy to associate with these games since these games involve scenes related to their daily routine and don't involve any complex set of rules to be followed. Even parents, family members, and teachers can also help in playing these games at an initial level without any need for specialization or special training.

INTRODUCTION

Neurodevelopment is inter-association between various developmental functions like cognitive, emotional, sensory, social, behavioral functions and further, it also includes functional activities related to brain and genetics across the lifespan of an individual. Intrusion to above inter-association through genetics problems or due to environmental consequence can lead to abnormalities in performing above function which is one of the main cause of neurodevelopmental disorders.

DOI: 10.4018/978-1-7998-3069-6.ch008

Neurodevelopmental disorders (NDDs) are classified as a class of untimely disorders related to neurology, which includes intellectual disability (ID), Asperger syndrome (AS), autism spectrum disorders (ASDs) and disorders related to sensory, social, language, behavioral, cognitive and emotional disorders, etc.

In the last decade, there has been a significant evolution of technologies, high increment in data computational and processing capacity, and new discoveries in genetics fields have helped us to understand mutations activities that are related to neurodevelopmental disorders, which can be helpful for developing a treatment for such disorders. But as much has been not done in early intervention technologies since it does not involve big corporate, industry or MNCs in this field hence lack of resources and funding.

Neurodevelopmental disorders (NDDs) lead to a lack of social, behavioral and economics potential development of an individual in which one is capable. Technological intervention can play a big role and is capable of reducing the cost of present medical intervention.

Games based on daily life activities can play big roles in improving social skills. One can easily customize games as per requirement or as specific to particular social skills for children to improve their respective social skills. Children find it easy to associate with these games since these games involve scenes related to their daily routine and don't involve any complex set of rules to be followed. Even parents, family members, and teachers can also help in playing these games at an initial level without any need for specialization or special training.

Kinect based games use body movement as input by using a line of motion sensing sensor hence making interaction with game comfortable and playing game enjoyable since it did not involve extra devices to be connected to the body making it effective for children with Neurodevelopmental Disorders (NDDs). Microsoft Kinect based game can be played by hand movement, thus reducing the need for any physical input tools, gadget or any medium like mouse, virtual reality system, smart glasses, eye gaze tracker, video recorder, laser rangefinder, image recorder, scanner, joysticks, trackball, etc to be attached on body. Hence it can be easily used by children with Neurodevelopmental Disorders.

Kinect based games can enhance not only motor and sensory skills but also Social, Cognitive and Behavioral skills, which can help children with Neurodevelopmental Disorders in performing their daily life routine efficiently. If one can provide proper training and intervention regularly to children with Neurodevelopmental Disorders using Microsoft Kinect games based on daily life routine, definitely we can see improvement in their confidence while performing such activities and enhancement in their Social, Cognitive and Behavioral skills.

BACKGROUND

The present studies provide good evidence of the children with NDDs and their parent's satisfaction with technological intervention. However, findings should be interpreted with caution, more studies are important for better understanding of the Microsoft Kinect based games effects on NDDs patients in general. Some of the research work and different technologies and their potential use in support of gamification, virtual and augmented reality and WebPages in intervening the social and behavioral impairment have been discussed below:

The exploration of benefits which can be achieved through video games in various fields like social, medical, education and rehabilitation have been fired up in last decades, and one of the main reason for that is the irresistible interest of children in video games. Playing video games leads to an increase in mental activities, enhancement in focus and attention capabilities, social activities like sharing and turn-taking in between colleagues, enhancing social interaction among its users, which can be very helpful for children with Neurodevelopmental Disorders. Serious games can result in enhancing communication, emotional, behavioral and social interconnection among children with Neurodevelopmental Disorders [Bringas *et al.* (2016)].

Image and sound technologies have been important tools in the development of educational applications. These educational applications help children with neuro disorders to enhance their day to day life skills.These educational applications also help parents and caregivers of children with neuro disorders and learning disabilities to understand the requirements of their children by reducing miscommunication. Children interact with images or pictures in the application and associated audio clip will be played after that, it helps them to express their emotion and helps the parent to understand the requirement of their children more efficiently [Aziz *et al.* (2014)].

Kinect based technologies are some of the fast-growing technologies nowadays. Kinect is a motion-sensing input device and can track up to 6 skeletons at once, it also can detect and track the movement of 25 joints of the body simultaneously. Kinect support a large number of programming platform which make it first choice for the development of video-based games. One can use Microsoft Kinect for the detection of facial expression and eye gazing application. Kinect based technologies are widely used for rehabilitation purposes due to the large number of applications it provides and eases of maintenance and development of related programs. Due to its low cost, ease to portability, low maintenance requirement, and small size make it first choice for rehabilitation based application [OZCAN *et al.* (2017)].

Nowadays robots and humanoids have found great space in Neurodevelopmental disorders therapy. Humanoid or robots are made to works in an imitative environment specifically developed for interaction with children having Neurodevelopmental disorders. Yes, Humanoid or robots technologies are still in a dormant state and it is no match to real human interaction but still can provide good social interaction and can be utilized for teaching children basic social and behavioral interaction skills related to daily life activities [Dautenhahn *et al.* (2002)].

Proper utilization of Computer Assisted Technology (CAT) can be helpful in intervening patient with NDDs. Since significant advances in mixed media PC innovation over the previous decades have made refined PC diversions promptly accessible to people in general and when consolidated with the perception that most youngsters, incorporating those with NDDs, demonstrate a proclivity to PCs, specialists perceived the capability of PC innovation as a viable and effective device in research and treatment. This paper avoided web-based methodologies, to upgrade social, informative, and dialect improvement in people with NDDs by isolating the tremendous writing into four fundamental regions: dialect, feeling acknowledgment, the hypothesis of the psyche, and social abilities [Ploog *et al.* (2013)].

Children with NDDs mostly enjoy dynamic interaction with touch devices like mobiles and tablets. People find it easier while working with robots or humanoids, mobiles, tablets in the foreseeable environment. A quantitative and qualitative analysis was done to observe various aspects of social skills, behavioral skills, communication skills, focus, and attention capabilities enhancement over course of time while interacting with robot or humanoid, mobiles, tablets in the foreseeable environment using video recorded during the training interaction period [Fong *et al.* (2018)].

There is a lot of evidence related to role social and electronic media in improvising social interaction (like sharing, turn-taking skills) in children with NDDs. This innovation has helped children and teenagers with NDDs, their parents and caretaker to feel more comfortable while interacting with the outside world and people. People can easily access recourses from the American Academy of Child and Adolescent Psychiatry, American Academy of Pediatrics and many similar institutes and can take benefit of such facilities [Gwynette *et al.* (2018)].

In one of the research, Microsoft Kinect has been used for rehabilitation by using three different computer-assisted video games. Microsoft Kinect used to track body skeleton and 25 different body joints simultaneously to observe different aspects of balance while performing different physical activities like exercise and playing video games. Players need to move the avatar in games by using their hand movements. The system was consists of database and processing tools for further analysis and observing of therapies. The result shows the great interest of children in playing and interacting with such games and data collected was further used for clinical routine [Estepa *et al.* (2016)].

It has been observed that there is a rise in the interest of utilizing assistive technology in interdisciplinary research for children with NDDs for their rehabilitation, learning purposes. A lot of research has been in place to develop various interactive applications for easing complexity related to teaching purposes for children with NDDs. Various application has been developed mainly focusing on basic numerical, recognizing number and alphabet to support teaching and learning to autistic children. In one of the works, the researcher has developed an application to improve the learning skills of children with autism. The application was focused to teach numbers and alphabet using animation. The application consist of two-part one dealing with recognizing number and other with identifying numbers [Kamaruzaman *et al.* (2016)].

In another research work, Microsoft Kinect based games were developed focusing especially on enhancing social interaction skills (sharing, role-playing, turn-taking) in children with autism. The author has discussed, need of including children with special need in research work and designing various technologies to enhance their quality of life by improving their social interaction skills [Boutsika *et al.* (2014)].

Some have presented an overview of some of the past and present technologies in rehabilitation, early intervention, screening, diagnosis, therapy and study in neurodevelopmental disorders and related impairment providing direction for future research work. There is a lot of evidence and proof that how different technologies have been helpful in rehabilitation, early intervention, screening, diagnosis, therapy and study in neurodevelopmental disorders. Authors discuss different technological inventions used for NDDs kids like Robotics, Eye Tracking, Virtual Reality, Multimedia Toys, Mind Reading Devices, and Assistive Technology [Michel *et al.* (2004)].

The first very positive findings from an empirical study about the effectiveness of the use of a Kinect learning game for children with gross motor skills problems and motor impairments are very useful in further research work. This game follows the principles of a newly presented approach, called Kinems, which advocates that special educators and therapists should use learning games via embodied touchless interaction. children with dyspraxia and other related disorders such as autism, Asperger's Syndrome (AS), and Attention Deficit Disorder, can improve related skills. These games are innovative and are played with hand and body gestures [Altanis *et al.* (2013)].

Computer technologies such as affective computing, virtual reality, robotics, and Multitouch interfaces have been developed to support people with ASD. These innovative technologies, alone or in conjunction, can be used beneficially in a number of critical areas affecting individuals with autism, their families, and professionals who support them. Innovative technologies such as Eye Toy, Diamond Table, and Kinect have potential in training different skills (e.g. balancing, communication, motor skills) for individuals with ASD. The computer is popular and preferable among people with ASD because it is predictable, consistent, free from social demands and specific in focus of attention [Chen *et al.* (2012)].

A 3D computer vision system for cognitive assessment and rehabilitation based on the Kinect device has been developed. A system was developed focusing mainly on impairment like body balance-related impairment, left-right confusion impairment in children with neurodevelopment disorders using Microsoft Kinect. Data was accumulated by continuous monitoring and recording of body skeleton, movement of different 25 body joints and facial features using Microsoft Kinect. The Microsoft Kinect device was proved to be an affordable product which will be very useful in developing various applications in many fields such as rehabilitation, early intervention, screening, diagnosis, therapy and study in neurodevelopmental disorders and related impairment [González-Ortega *et al.* (2014)].

TECHNOLOGICAL INTERVENTION

Technology is changing human lives in such a rapid way which no one has ever imagined and the domain of autism has not remained exceptional. The use of technological intervention to teach children with NDDs is not a new concept. In fact, computer-assisted technology has been in use to teach students with NDDs from the last 4 decades.

Technological interventions are very helpful for training children with NDDs because these interventions can be easily customized, take less time to design and reduce the cost of a therapist and stress for taking early appointments. These special children have special needs and hence require a different kind of learning mechanisms as well as access to technological interventions that offer extra means of building links for an individual. This heightened focus includes services and interventions combined with technological advances that redefine how support and instruction can be provided.

There are various types of emerging technology tools such as Virtual Environment (VE), Collaborative Virtual Environment (CVE), Assistive Technology (AT), therapeutic robots, language tools, multimedia handheld devices, mobile apps, Computer Assistive Technology (CAT), Electronic Screen Media (ESM), floor/tabletop projectors that have been used to enhance different social and various other skills in children with ASD.

Robots and humanoid have found great space in Neurodevelopmental disorders therapy. Humanoid or robots are made to works in imitative environment specifically developed for interaction with children having Neurodevelopmental disorders. Yes, Humanoid or robots technologies are still in dormant state and it is no match to real human interaction but still can provide good social interaction and can be utilized for teaching children basic social and behavioral interaction skills related to daily life activities. Robots and humanoid can also be specifically customized as per some social condition in customized environment where it can interact with children and help them to enhance their communication skill which is one of major problem associated with children having NDDs, Enhancement in their communication capabilities will help to be more confident and self dependent and will further give sense of bulginess to society and surrounding.

Language remediation based applications can be used in speech-related impairment cases instead of using speech therapists hence reducing cost and time. These application and tools are easily available in the market, have low cost, required low maintenance, easy to customize as per application, are easily portable due to small size and low weight and hence are convenient for use in the house, educational institute, and learning centers.

Mobile and tablet technologies have been of great use in early intervention of children with NDDs. Their small size, low weight, easy to interact functionalities are some of the major reasons for their application in NDDs intervention. These can be used for video modeling, picture prompt, speech application development or all together in a single device which can help to enhance not only social and motor skills but also the imaginative capabilities of an individual. The application developed for mobile and tablets are giving promising result in enhancing communication skills, social skills, behavioral skills and increase in imagination, focus and attention capabilities.

Floor projections are more interactive and can be easily customized as per requirement and space available. In Floor projections, games can be planned as per requirement like solo, dual, multi or group playing. The other advantages of these technologies are that they are safe to use, easily customizable, take less time to prepare the required environment as compare to real games, less effective due surrounding such as public and other environmental factors like air, light, Etc. Floor projections give a sense of real-world and help in a great way for children with NDDs since they can perform outdoor activities inside the home in a controlled environment. Floor projections have been great technology which has resulted in improving social and motor skill of children with NDDs and also reducing the stress of parent which they used to feel while sending their children outside for playing outdoors games.

Virtual Reality (VR) can create an interactive virtual environment that can be easily customized as per need. It can help in teaching different social and environmental situations and records their behavior for further analysis of children with NDDs. VR has been one of the promising technology for providing social skill training to children with NDDs. VE has been used widely nowadays in a large number of educational institute, learning centers, and rehabilitation centers.

Kinect based games related to daily life routines, work and schedule can play big roles in improving behavioral impairments. People can easily modify and define games as per their needs and requirement or specific behavioral skill for individuals to improve their respective behavioral skills. People find it easy to associate with these games because they involve different levels and scenes related to daily life routines, work and schedule and don't involve any further complex set of rules to be followed or pre-training. Even parents, family members, caretakers, and teachers also can help in playing these games at the beginning without any requirement of pre-specialization and pre-training. Microsoft Kinect based games uses body movement as input signals by using special set of line of motion sensing sensors hence making interaction completely touchless which further enhance game comfortable and it makes playing game enjoyable since it did not involve peripheral devices to be connected to body for getting input signals making it effective in both hyper and hypo sensitive cases.

RELATED WORK

In the last two decades, researchers have grown interested in developing innovative technologies of interaction with children having NDDs [Bringas *et al.* (2016)]. They use the movement of different parts and joints of the body, facial changes or changes in expression, etc to interact with children having Autism. Electronic devices like computers, smartphones, tablets, gaming devices, and smart television have a major role in enhancing various skills including social skills. The aim of such interventions is to enhance focusing capabilities and body movement, which are parts of primary skills required for good social interaction [Chen *et al.* (2012)].

Video modeling which includes video games and storytelling using video play also have a big part in enhancing confidence and teaching the social skill in children with NDDs [Bringas *et al.* (2016)]. Serious games are also used extensively in various scenarios, such as medical and education and have made a significant mark in enhancing various skills if practiced regularly [Bringas *et al.* (2016)]. Nowadays multi-touch tabletop interfaces have played a major role in improving skills like turn-taking and improving coordination skills by allowing multi-user to play the game or use touch screens simultaneously [Chen *et al.* (2012)]. Likewise, interacting technologies like Eye tracker, Kinect, Virtual Reality (VR) system can also be used to enhance various skill in children with NDDs from social to motor and cognitive skill [Lahiri *et al.* (2013)].

Kinect is auxiliary equipment provided by Microsoft to use with gaming console Xbox 360 that allow one to have control gaming object, sound, songs, music, videos and movies with voice commands or by body parts movement without any need of additional input devices such as a keyboard, track Ball, microphone, joystick, light pen or mouse [Zhang *et al.* (2012)]. Games based on Kinect have a greater role in improving motor, problem-solving and social skill, these games use various body joint movements and voice commands to control and play the game [Altanis *et al.* (2013)]. To summaries, the previous research has solved some problem and have achieved some success, but there are many problems still exist to be resolved such as model for earlier intervention usually involve set of complex rules to be followed, but how can one expect children with NDDs to understand rule easily so it is most unfair to use such intervention for analysis and evaluating child performance.

We have developed game based on daily life routines like waking up, walking to restroom, walking till dining table, roaming in corridor, crossing road, walking till bus, exploring surrounding, walking in garden, public places like bus stand, railway station counter or standing in queue for foods in mess to provide real-life scenario so that one can find it easy to relate themselves to game. We have used Kinect to capture hand movement of the subject as input to the system. Movement of gaming object will be ass according to the movement of the hand, one needs to reach destination crossing various hurdles on reaching destination there will music to encourage subject. People can try a different level based on their problems and complexity requirement. Following two-approach have been used:

1. After deep discussion with parents and therapists, we have observed that each child is more attractive to some of the specific color. We have changed path and wall around the correct path from initial point till destination with those colors and observed performance of peoples with and without specific color on path and wall to measure improvement in their efficiency.
2. In this approach we have used daily life hurdles like water, traffic on roads, traffic signal, quality of road and zebra line on the road to teach peoples which path to be chosen and when and how to crossroad.

From approach 1 We have tried to understand whether a strip of specific color and signal in the home can be brought in use for helping one to reach their home independently after getting down from the bus. The same approach can be used in public places like banks, bus stand, railway station or airport for the individual with NDDs to reach particular counter for public services such as ticket counter. Figure 1 describes the scene 1 without any specific color on the outer wall of the path till destination while figure 2 describes the scene 2 without any specific color (Sky Blue) on the outer wall of the path till destination. It was observed that the outcome of scene 2 was better than scene 1 while playing the game.

Approach 2 is generalized to teach some basic behavioral skill which needs to be followed while crossing the road.

A good, easy and affordable way of helping peoples with NDDs is to provide them with computer assistive technology aimed at easing the impact of the NDDs effect. For example, peoples who are at the mild stage of the NDDs may have mental power related issues like remembering the different activities to carry out during their daily life routine as well as the procedure involved in the routines. A technology-aided program can help counter these issues may involve the use of a computer-assisted technologies such tablet, wristband or Smartphone, which is programmed to alert the peoples related to individual about the activities that is at the appropriate place and at given time and to provide them sensory signals based on sound or light regarding the steps to carry out further [Kerkhof *et al.* (2016); Lancioni *et al.* (2014); Lancioni *et al.* (2017); Lancioni *et al.* (2018); Wang *et al.* (2017)].

Figure 1. Scene 1 from Game

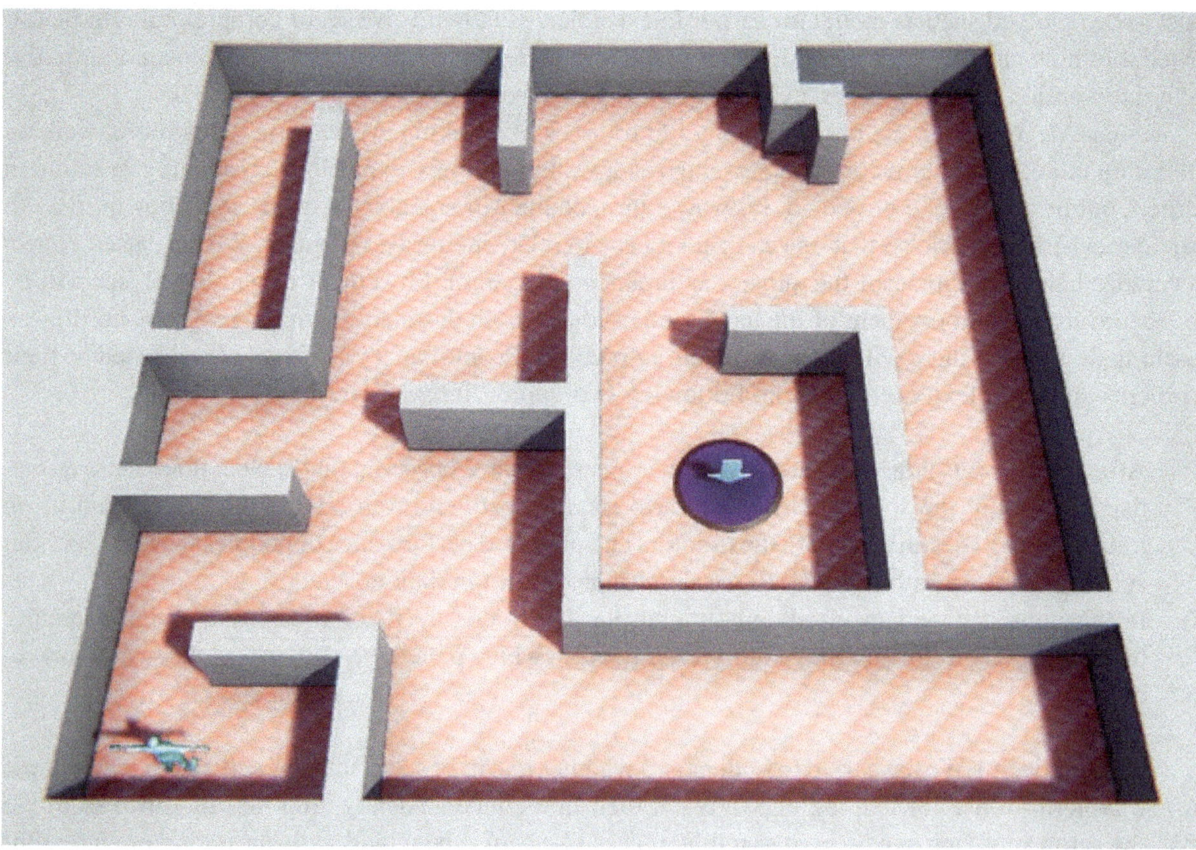

Figure 2. Scene 2 from Game

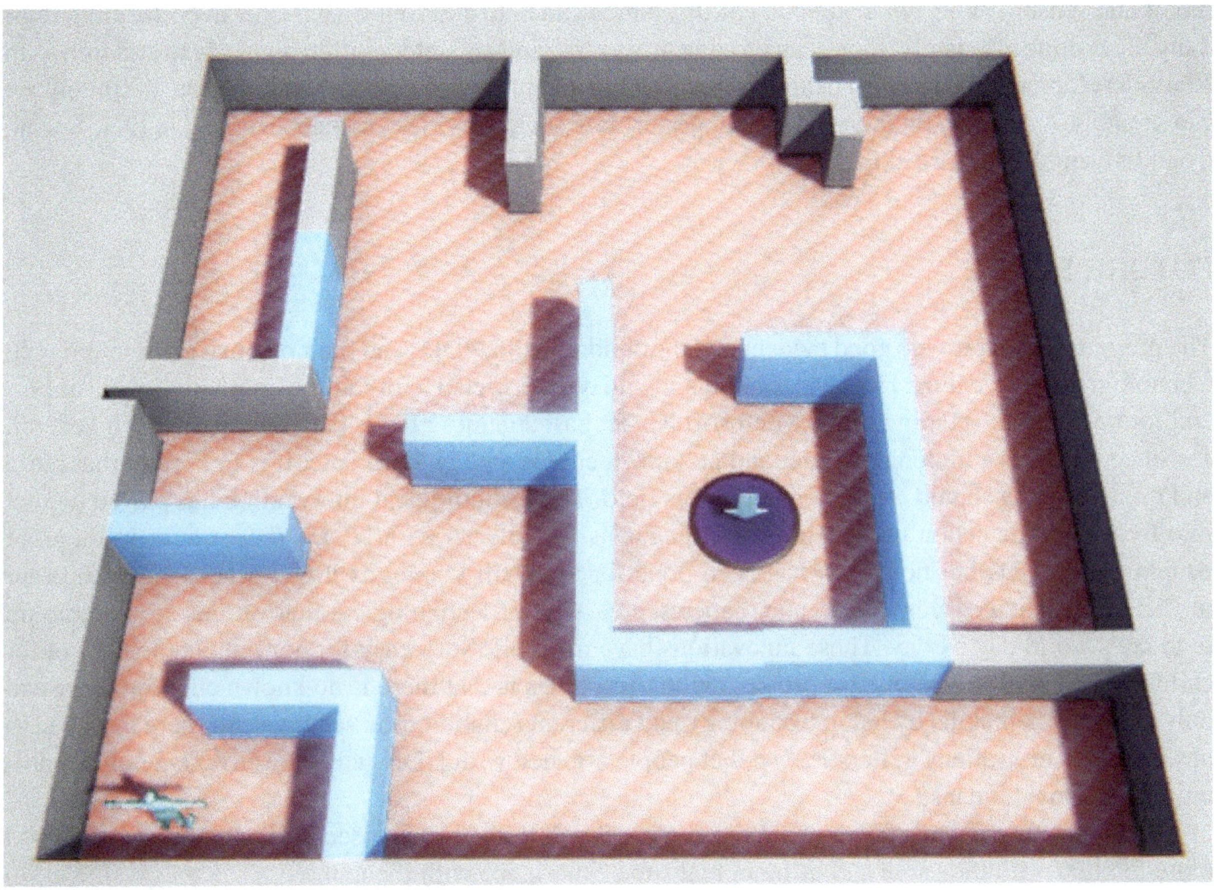

CONCLUSION

Games based on daily life activities can play big roles in improving social skills. One can easily customize games as per requirement or as specific to particular social skills for children to improve their respective social skills. Children find it easy to associate with these games since these games involve scenes related to their daily routine and don't involve any complex set of rules to be followed. Even parents, family members, and teachers can also help in playing these games at an initial level without any need for specialization or special training.

Kinect based games use body movement as input by using the line of motion sensing sensor hence making interaction with game comfortable and playing game enjoyable since it did not involve extra device to be connected to the body making it effective in both hyper and hypo sensitive cases of NDDs.

Microsoft Kinect based game can be played by hand movement. Thus reducing the need for physical input tools, gadgets or any medium like the mouse, virtual reality system, smart glasses, eye gaze tracker, video recorder, laser rangefinder, image recorder, scanner, joysticks, trackball, etc to be attached on body. Hence it can be easily used by children with NDDs.

In addition to social skill Kinect based games will also help in improving motor skills as well as sensory skills. Kinect based games have been developed earlier also for the children with NDDs but they were primarily focused to improve motor skills only. New developed games can enhance not only motor and sensory skills but also Social Skills, which can help children with NDDs in performing their daily life routine efficiently. If one can provide proper training and intervention regularly to children with Neurodevelopmental Disorders using Microsoft Kinect games based on daily life routine, definitely we can see improvement in their confidence in performing such activities and enhancement in their Social, Cognitive and Behavioral skills.

FUTURE SCOPE

The present studies provide good evidence of the children with NDDs and their parent's satisfaction with technological intervention. However, findings should be interpreted with caution, more studies are important for better understanding of the Microsoft Kinect based games effects on NDDs patients in general.

Since NDDs is a lifelong disorder and no known cure is available till date. It is important that more and more research should be carried out in this field. The technological intervention has played a great role from early detection to screening and diagnosis of children with NDDs. There exist millions of people with NDDs but not much has been done for them till known as it has been done with other medical issues like cancer, AIDS, and diabetes, etc. A lot of technological innovations are coming up in today's world day by day. These innovations have made life very easy for normal people but not for children with NDDs. The biggest problem with this NDDs is that there is no known cure for it, we can only enhance their skills by using technology and different rehabilitation schemes. So there is a need to develop new innovations in this field so that people affected with NDDs can take advantage of technology like normal humans

Further, as future work, 3D view of the street, school, home can be used in-game to make the child more familiar with the game and bring in real-time experience with the game.

REFERENCES

Altanis, G., Boloudakis, M., Retalis, S., & Nikou, N. (2013). Children with motor impairments play a kinect learning game: First findings from a pilot case in an authentic classroom environment. *J Interact Design Architect*, *19*, 91–104.

Aziz, M. Z., Abdullah, S. A., Adnan, S. F., & Mazalan, L. (2014). Educational App for Children with Autism Spectrum Disorders (ASDs). *Procedia Computer Science*, *42*, 70–77. doi:10.1016/j.procs.2014.11.035

Boutsika, E. (2014). Kinect in education: A proposal for children with autism. *Procedia Computer Science*, *27*, 123–129. doi:10.1016/j.procs.2014.02.015

Bringas, J. A. S., León, M. A. C., Cota, I. E., & Carrillo, A. L. (2016, October). Development of a videogame to improve communication in children with autism. In *Learning Objects and Technology (LACLO), Latin American Conference on* (pp. 1-6). 10.1109/LACLO.2016.7751751

Chen, W. (2012). Multitouch tabletop technology for people with autism spectrum disorder: A review of the literature. *Procedia Computer Science*, *14*, 198–207. doi:10.1016/j.procs.2012.10.023

Dautenhahn, K., & Billard, A. (2002). Games children with autism can play with Robota, a humanoid robotic doll. In Universal access and assistive technology (pp. 179-190). doi:10.1007/978-1-4471-3719-1_18

Estepa, A., Piriz, S. S., Albornoz, E., & Martínez, C. (2016, April). Development of a Kinect-based exergaming system for motor rehabilitation in neurological disorders. *Journal of Physics: Conference Series*, *705*(1), 012060. doi:10.1088/1742-6596/705/1/012060

Fong, T., Nourbakhsh, I., & Dautenhahn, K. (2003). A survey of socially interactive robots. *Robotics and Autonomous Systems*, *42*(3-4), 143–166. doi:10.1016/S0921-8890(02)00372-X

González-Ortega, D., Díaz-Pernas, F. J., Martínez-Zarzuela, M., & Antón-Rodríguez, M. (2014). A Kinect-based system for cognitive rehabilitation exercises monitoring. *Computer Methods and Programs in Biomedicine*, *113*(2), 620–631. doi:10.1016/j.cmpb.2013.10.014 PMID:24263055

Gwynette, M. F., Sidhu, S. S., & Ceranoglu, T. A. (2018). Electronic Screen Media Use in Youth With Autism Spectrum Disorder. *Child and Adolescent Psychiatric Clinics of North America*, *27*(2), 203–219. doi:10.1016/j.chc.2017.11.013 PMID:29502747

Kakkar, D. (2018, January). A Study on Machine Learning Based Generalized Automated Seizure Detection System. In 2018 8th International Conference on Cloud Computing, Data Science & Engineering (Confluence) (pp. 769-774). IEEE.

Kakkar, D. (2018, February). Accounting For Order-Frame Length Tradeoff of Savitzky-Golay Smoothing Filters. In 2018 5th International Conference on Signal Processing and Integrated Networks (SPIN) (pp. 805-810). IEEE.

Kakkar, D. (2019). Influence of Emotional Imagery on Risk Perception and Decision Making in Autism Spectrum Disorder. *Neurophysiology*, *51*(4), 281–292.

Kamaruzaman, M. F., Rani, N. M., Nor, H. M., & Azahari, M. H. H. (2016). Developing user interface design application for children with autism. *Procedia: Social and Behavioral Sciences*, *217*, 887–894. doi:10.1016/j.sbspro.2016.02.022

Kerkhof, Y. J., Graff, M. J., Bergsma, A., de Vocht, H. H., & Dröes, R. M. (2016). Better self-management and meaningful activities thanks to tablets? Development of a person-centered program to support people with mild dementia and their carers through use of hand-held touch screen devices. *International Psychogeriatrics*, *28*(11), 1917–1929. doi:10.1017/S1041610216001071 PMID:27425002

Lahiri, U., Bekele, E., Dohrmann, E., Warren, Z., & Sarkar, N. (2013). Design of a virtual reality based adaptive response technology for children with autism. *IEEE Transactions on Neural Systems and Rehabilitation Engineering*, *21*(1), 55–64. doi:10.1109/TNSRE.2012.2218618 PMID:23033333

Lancioni, G., Singh, N., O'Reilly, M., Sigafoos, J., Alberti, G., Chiariello, V., ... Campodonico, F. (2018c). A smartphone-based technology package to support independent activity in people with intellectual disability and blindness. *Internet Technology Letters*, *2018*(5), e34. doi:10.1002/itl2.34

Lancioni, G., Singh, N., O'Reilly, M., Sigafoos, J., D'Amico, F., Pinto, K., ... Caffò, A. (2017). A technology-aided program for helping persons with Alzheimer's disease perform daily activities. *Journal of Enabling Technologies*, *11*(3), 85–91. doi:10.1108/JET-03-2017-0011

Lancioni, G. E., Bosco, A., Olivetti Belardinelli, M., Singh, N. N., O'Reilly, M. F., Sigafoos, J., & Oliva, D. (2014). Technology-based intervention programs to promote stimulation control and communication in post-coma persons with different levels of disability. *Frontiers in Human Neuroscience*, *8*, 48. doi:10.3389/fnhum.2014.00048 PMID:24574992

Lancioni, G. E., O'Reilly, M. F., Sigafoos, J., Campodonico, F., Perilli, V., Alberti, G., ... Miglino, O. (2018a). A modified smartphone-based program to support leisure and communication activities in people with multiple disabilities. *Advances in Neurodevelopmental Disabilities*, *2*. doi:10.100741252-017-0047-z

Lancioni, G. E., O'Reilly, M. F., Sigafoos, J., D'Amico, F., Buonocunto, F., Devalle, G., ... Lanzilotti, C. (2018b). A further evaluation of microswitch-aided intervention for fostering responding and stimulation control in persons in a minimally conscious state. *Advances in Neurodevelopmental Disorders*, *2*(3), 322–331. doi:10.100741252-018-0064-6

Lancioni, G. E., & Singh, N. N. (Eds.). (2014). *Assistive technologies for people with diverse abilities*. New York: Springer. doi:10.1007/978-1-4899-8029-8

Lancioni, G. E., Singh, N. N., O'Reilly, M. F., Sigafoos, J., D'Amico, F., Pinto, K., ... Caffò, A. O. (2018d). Promoting supported ambulation in persons with advanced Alzheimer's disease: A pilot study. *Disability and Rehabilitation. Assistive Technology*, *13*(1), 101–106. doi:10.1080/17483107.2017.1297856 PMID:28287045

Michel, P. (2004). *The use of technology in the study, diagnosis and treatment of autism*. Final term Paper for CSC350: Autism and Associated Developmental Disorders.

Ozcan, M.O., Doyuran, T., & Beynek, B. (2017). *A Survey on the Use of Microsoft Kinect for Physical Rehabilitation*. Academic Press.

Ploog, B. O., Scharf, A., Nelson, D. S., & Brooks, P. J. (2013). Use of Computer-Assisted Technologies (CAT) to Enhance Social, Communicative, and Language. Development in Children with Autism Spectrum Disorders. *Journal of Autism and Developmental Disorders*, *43*(2), 301–322. doi:10.100710803-012-1571-3 PMID:22706582

Tanu, T., & Kakkar, D. (2018). *Strengthening risk prediction using statistical learning in children with autism spectrum disorder*. Advances in Autism.

Wadhera, T., & Kakkar, D. (2019). Eye Tracker: An Assistive Tool in Diagnosis of Autism Spectrum Disorder. In Emerging Trends in the Diagnosis and Intervention of Neurodevelopmental Disorders (pp. 125-152). IGI Global.

Wadhera, T., Kakkar, D., Kaur, G., & Menia, V. (2019). Pre-Clinical ASD Screening Using Multi-Biometrics-Based Systems. In Design and Implementation of Healthcare Biometric Systems (pp. 185-211). IGI Global.

Wang, R. H., Sudhama, A., Begum, M., Huq, R., & Mihailidis, A. (2017). Robots to assist daily activities: Views of older adults with Alzheimer's disease and their caregivers. *International Psychogeriatrics*, *29*(1), 67–79. doi:10.1017/S1041610216001435 PMID:27660047

Zhang, Z. (2012). Microsoft kinect sensor and its effect. *IEEE MultiMedia*, *19*(2), 4–10. doi:10.1109/MMUL.2012.24

Chapter 9
Yoga Therapy on Cognitive Function in Neurodevelopmental Disorders

Artchoudane Soccalingam
https://orcid.org/0000-0002-7826-0430
Center for Yogic Sciences, Aarupadai Veedu Medical College and Hospital, India & Vinayaka Mission's Research Foundation, India

Meena Ramanathan
Centre for Yoga Therapy Education and Research, Sri Balaji Vidyapeeth, India

Ananda Balayogi Bhavanani
Centre for Yoga Therapy Education and Research, Sri Balaji Vidyapeeth, India

ABSTRACT

Neurodevelopmental disorders (NDDs) are birth imperfections that cause dysfunction in cognitive and sensory processes and impairment in motor function, communication, and behavior. The major factors responsible for increasing incidence of NDDs are genetic, psychosocial, and excessive use of drugs. Yoga alleviates neurological problems and NDDs. Asana is a physical movement with breath awareness that facilitates the development of body awareness, concentration, and memory and provides vital energy for children with neurodevelopmental disability. Yoga therapy improves sensory coordination and motor imitations that enable persons with cognitive disabilities to make meaningful response by the integration of senses and functions of central nervous system.

INTRODUCTION

The global estimate for disability is raised due to increasing stress, chronic illness or chronic psychological distress in parents. World Health Organization estimates that 15% of the world's population live with some form of disability, of whom 2-4% experience significant difficulties in cognitive function (Suresh,

DOI: 10.4018/978-1-7998-3069-6.ch009

2019). Cognitive impairments is a major part of neurodevelopmental disorders (NDDs) which include disabilities in the functioning of the brain that affect a child's behaviour, memory or ability to learn. The characteristics of neurodevelopmental disorders are dysfunction in cognitive and sensory processes and impairment in motor function, communication and behavior. Presently, there is no biomarker to diagnose, assess or differentiate between NDDs, rather it is categorized into discrete disorder entities based on clinical presentation e.g. intellectual disabilities, attention deficit hyperactivity disorders (ADHD), autism spectrum disorder (ASD), dyslexia, learning disabilities and motor disorders. There is no intervention that completely treats NDDs since the causes are unknown.

SIGNIFICANT KNOWN CAUSES FOR NDDs

Attention-deficit hyperactivity disorder is a neurological disorder disruptive behavior characterized by symptoms of inattention, hyperactivity, impulsivity occurring more severely than typical for other individuals in the same stage of development (American Psychiatric Association, 2000). Pastor and Reuben (2008) have reported that children with ADHD frequently have other states of neurological disorders, half of the children with ADHD have a learning disability and one fourth have a conduct disorder. Other disorders, including anxiety disorders, depression and cognitive impairments can be expressed with signs and symptoms that resemble those of ADHD.

Origin of Neurodevelopmental Disorder in Various Phases (Stromland, 1994)

1. Preconception (from genetic)
    a. period of dividing zygote, implantation and bilaminar embryo (up to 2 weeks);
    b. common sites of action (also highly sensitive to teratogens; 3 to 7 weeks)
        i. central nervous system and heart
        ii. eye, heart, arm and leg
        iii. ear and teeth
        iv. palate
2. Gestation (emotional health of mother and also less sensitive to teratogens from environment like thalidomide, diethylstilbestrol, ionizing radiation, methylmercury, lead; 8 to 38 wk)
    i. Central nervous system
    ii. Eyes
    iii. External genitalia
    iv. Ear, teeth and palate
    v. Heart
    vi. Arms and legs
3. Postnatal (from second-hand tobacco smoke and lead)

Cognitive dysfunction (CD) is a generalized NDD characterized by significantly impaired intellectual and adaptive functioning. Mullin et al. (2013) suggested that an individual with NDD has genetically defective proteomes and defined NDD mechanisms at levels of complexity higher than the traditional single genes or proteins. However genetic defects are associated with one or multiple genotypes and the problems intrinsic to categorical NDD. Yasin et al. (2018) found that reduced effect of complex protein

CHD8 (chromodomain helicase DNA-binding protein), haplo insufficiency, or loss-of function mutations of CHD8 produce a distinct NDD, with a cognitive and behavioral profile beginning with developmental delay, progressing to CD and/or ASD, and with other neurofunctional features, such as anxiety. In NDDs, the genomic defects range from large chromosomal deletions 1q21.1, 16p11.2 and 22q11.2 to single-nucleotide polymorphisms (SNPs). Thus the large number of genes affected by these deletions of one or all that cause disorders with overlapping phenotypes like smaller genetic modifications, specifically SNPs in non-coding regions and this deletion syndrome closely associates with NDDs.

Intake of Steroids and Other Drugs May Cause NDDS

a. Corticosteroids: Administration of corticosteroids in patients with Preterm premature rupture of membranes is associated with endometritis and chorioamnionitis which may affect fetus that might lead to a 4% reduction of fetal head circumference, 11% in cranial volume, infant's poor developmental, intellectual and behavioral outcomes that are associated with small head circumference (French et al., 1999). There is no evidence that negative effect of repeated corticosteroids cause major neurodevelopmental disorders. Hence it is recommended to avoid repeated corticosteroid courses in women with Preterm premature rupture of membranes (PPROM) (Vermillion, Soper and Chasedunn-Roark, 1999). Every single dose of corticosteroid induces an increase in the count of maternal white blood cells that affects metabolism which may lead to gestational diabetes, influence the augmentation of amino acid concentration and increases glucose levels in maternal plasma (Mariotti, Marconi and Pardi, 2004).
b. Tocolytics: Slotkin and Seidler (2013) found that autonomic dysfunction in individuals exposed prenatally to terbutaline; in light of the connection between terbutaline and autism, these results could also contribute to autonomic dysregulation seen in children with this disorder. Both Nifedipine and Ritodrine cause increased pulse rate and fetal heart rate and decreases maternal systolic and diastolic blood pressure (van Geijn et al., 2005). Van Geijn et al. (2005) found myocardial infarction in about 4% of women and congestive cardiac failure or pulmonary edema in 2% of women on extended administration of nifedipine that may lead to asymptomatic mitral valve prolapse or ventricular septal defect.
c. Magnesium sulfate: This may lead to hypocalcemia and an increased risk of osteopenia and bone fractures in newborns (Asli et al., 2012). It may be used as long term treatment for neuroprotection, preeclampsia and as the short term treatment for acute preterm labor; in such cases lowest possible dose of magnesium sulfate should be used.
d. Stromland (1994) have found the affect of thalidomide in fetus during gestational days between 20th and 24th day may increase the risk of NDDs such as autism and more than one system are susceptible and different pathology may occur depending upon the dose and amount of exposure. However cesarean sections were more frequently performed in thalidomide embryonic mothers because of pelvic and uterine malformations.

However, neurodevelopmental disorders have a complex combination of genetic, biological, psychosocial and environmental risk factors which results from parents rather than any one clear cause. Such a wide range of environmental risk factors may affect neurodevelopment, including maternal use of alcohol, tobacco, or illicit drugs during pregnancy; direct correlation of socio-economic position to occupation, education, income, wealth, and place of residence; and low birth weight or premature delivery.

Other research findings also suggested that children, who are prenatally exposed to elevated levels of polychlorinated biphenyls (PCBs) through diet, have neurodevelopmental defects, including lowered intelligence and behavioural deficits such as attention and impulsive behavior (Sagiv et al., 2010). Thus the analysis of environmental chemicals, lead, mercury, PCBs, phthalates and organophosphate pesticides are disease causing factors for ADHD or other developmental disorders.

SIGNIFICANT UNKNOWN CAUSES FOR NDDs

The physical, mental, and psychic conditions of parents are known to be the cause for NDDs as explained by sage Thirumoolar in Thirumandiram, a classical treatise on yoga in Tamil. Process of pregnancy is affected by the physical, psychological and emotional health condition of the father and mother at the time of union and conceptison leading to many disabilities including ADHD, ASD, learning disabilities, intellectual disability, conduct disorders, cerebral palsy, impairments in vision and hearing, and down's syndrome (Natarajan, 2002).

When the father has any disease related to respiration that affect the movement of prana or vital energy during intercourse or after intercourse. Sage Thirumoolar described about birth imperfections in the second chapter of Thirumandiram, a classical text on yoga. *Paigindra vayukkuraiyir kuralaagum; paigindra vayu villaikkin mudamaagum; paigindra vayu naduppadir koonaagum; paigindra vayu mathark killaip paarkkile* (Thirumandiram, 464) which means if the man (biological father) is short of breath during the mid-act of intercourse then the infant will be born a dwarf; if he blows feeble breath during mid-act of intercourse then the infant will be born with defective limbs; if he halts breath during the mid-act of intercourse then the infant will be born with a hunchback (Natarajan, 2002). This can be attributed to chromosomal deletion of progeny, birth imperfection and NDDs.

When mother has any disease related to bowel and bladder that affect the movement of prana (imbalance in samana vayu and apana vayu) at the time of union. Sage Thirumoolar described about the infant born with dumb, deaf and blind in the same chapter of Thirumandiram. *Maadha udharam malamigil mandanaam; maadha udharam jalamigil moongaiyaam; maadha udharam irandokkil kannillai; maadha udharatthil vanda kuzhavikke* (Thirumandiram, 465), which means if the bowels of woman (biological mother) are heavy exceedingly then the infant will be born dullard; if her bladder is full then the infant will be born dumb; and if her bowel and bladder is full and heavy exceedingly then the infant will be born blind (Natarajan, 2002). This can be attributed to gut-brain dysfunction, autonomous dysfunction and NDDs in progeny.

According to Yogic scriptures, sage Thiruvalluvar described about disability in Thriukkural, a classical text on yoga. *Poriinmai yaarkkum pazhiandru arivuarindu aalvinai inmai pazhi* (Thirukkural, 618) means the physical or mental disability is no disgrace to anyone. But to be without knowing what should be known, and to be effortless, is indeed disgraceful (Effort, 2019). The aim of yoga practice is to overcome all types of sufferings and provides perfect platform to build holistic health, harmony and happiness.

Yoga is a spiritual science for the integrated development of physical, mental, emotional and spiritual aspects. It normalizes physiological and psychological functioning of human being where one able to control the disturbances and mental fluctuations. WHO defines health as "The state of complete physical, mental and social wellbeing and not merely absence of disease or infirmity" and Yoga is the unique tool that helps attain that state.

TRADITIONAL PRACTICES OF YOGA FOR NDDs

Yogi Svatmarama described the potential and effectiveness of yoga in Hatha Yoga Pradipika (HYP), *Yuva vrddhotivrddho va vyadito durbalo'pi va abhyasat siddhim apnoti sarvayogesh va tandritah* (HYP, I: 64), which means that any individual who is young, old or even very old, diseased or weak but not lethargic in the pursuit of different forms of yoga attains improvement and perfection through practice (Ramanathan and Bhavanani, 2017).

Yoga may be one of the best tools that could help eliminate NDDs from the society. Sage Gheranda codified the importance of yoga in Gheranda Samhita (GS) and says, *Ghatastha yogam yogash tattvajnanasya kaaranam* (GS. 2), meaning that the human body is like an unbaked clay pot that needs to be baked and made fit, through the fire of yoga sadhana (Gheranda, 1895). Further this process enables one to develop physical, mental and psychological wellbeing to attain happiness. Swami Gitananda (1976) says *Yoga is a way of life*, by which one can rediscover best in life. According to Ayurveda health is defined as, *Sama dosha sama agnischa sama dhatu mala kriyaaha prasanna atma indriya manaha swastha iti abhidheeyate* (Sushruta Samhita, 15:41), which means health is perfect only when the three doshas (vata means movement having ether and air elements, pitta means transformation having fire and water elements and kapha means solidarity having water and earth elements) are balanced, balanced agni (digestive fire: digestion, assimilation and metabolism), balanced dhatus (plasma, blood, muscle, fat, bone, marrow, and reproductive tissue), efficacy of all the excretory functions (physiological functions of urination and defecation) are in perfect order with a pleasantly disposed and contented mind, senses and spirit (Bhavanani, 2013).

Yoga is basically different from other conventional medical practices and removes the root cause of disease. Ill health occurs when the mind is not contented that may lead to sensual afflictions and disturbed excretion causing imbalanced dhatus and intoxicated digestion which results in imbalanced dosha and perverted guna or behavior. Yoga consists of various elements that address problems of children with autism spectrum disorder. Yogasana practice allows one to relax, tone the muscles, massage the internal organs, slow down breathing, regulate the flow of prana, relaxation and meditation which calm down the mind and balancing the emotions.

Yogic techniques allow internal cleansing, *Dhautir vastistathaa netih laulikeee traatakam tathaa Kapalabhaatish cha itaani shatkarmaani samaacharet* (GS. 12), which means various internal cleansing practices including dhauti, basti, neti, lauliki, trataka and kapalabhati are essential for purification in order to free the body and mind from disease and disorders (Gheranda, 1895). Yoga improves prana or vital energy and others consider it to mean mental force. Yoga practice makes the body strong and steady that is important for a person to copulate successfully for healthy progeny.

ENHANCING OVERALL HEALTH AND WELLNESS IN INDIVIDUAL WITH NDDs

a. Yoga for Lifestyle Disorders

Yoga recognizes human being as a combination of three bodies and five layers. An individual pertains to the following i) gross body refers to physical layer, ii) subtle body refers to energy layer, mental layer and wisdom layer and iii) causal body refers to bliss layer (Binorkar, 2014). The kind of lifestyle followed by a person is integrally related to good health in its true sense. Ill health arises when the three bodies are not in harmony with one another and are not properly aligned. Such state results in low vital force, poor health and susceptibility to various diseases.

Yoga has different techniques used for enhancing physical fitness, mental strength and spiritual elevation. Yoga practice helps to connect with one's innermost self through mindfulness exercise involving asana, controlled breathing i.e. pranayama and meditation. Asana helps strengthen the body, meditation sharpens one's focus, and breath calms the mind and heals the body (Bhavanani, 2017). When these three, mind, body and breath are in harmony, ultimately the result is improvement in stress, relaxation, mental clarity, flexibility, fitness and overall well-being.

b. Yoga for Gastro Intestinal Disorders

The symptoms of gastro intestinal disorders (GID) are always associated with inflammation in intestinal tract, irritable bowel syndrome, bloating, chronic constipation and other digestion related problems. GID is very common in children with ASD because most of the children don't chew or mix the food properly with saliva (Gorrindo, 2013; Buie et al., 2010). Children with ASD are usually averse to fruits, vegetables or essential supplement food for daily balanced diet that changes intestinal bacteria associated with gut microbiota which in turn affects vagal stimulation resulting into altered basal ganglia function (Williams et al., 2012). Gastro-intestinal disorder in children with ASD results in vomiting, flatulence, bloating, constipation, abdominal pain and also urine and fecal incontinence problems (Hanney et al., 2012).

Increased incidences of inflammatory bowel disease (IBD) in women are twice as much as in men and the most prevalent functional gastro intestinal disorder (Grundmann and Yoon, 2010). IBD may cause hormonal changes during menstrual cycle and pregnancy which may affect the health of mother and progeny (Mulak, Tache and Larauche, 2014). It is a disorder of motor and sensory functions of gastro intestinal tract and are found to have a strong association with psychiatric disorders (Fauci, Braunwald and Isselbacher, 1998; Whitehead, Palsson and Jones, 2002).

According to Ayurveda, Agni regulates all metabolic processes and maintains the overall health and zeal. The main causative factor ascribed for IBD is the malfunctioning of various agnis, that is, jathara agni (digestive fire) which effects both bhuta agni and dhatva agni which lead to stress in mind and consequentially impairs the function of bowel and bladder, menstrual cycle and pregnancy (Sushruta Samhita, 2010; Vagbhata, 2011,p.411). It also affects prana (life force), ojas shakti (conserved vital energy), tejas (inner radiance) such that the changes are visible in color, strength, health, enthusiasm, plumpness and complexion (Sushruta Samhita, 2010, p.512). According to the scriptures of Ayurveda and Yoga, health at the physical level can only be accomplished by i) integration of breath coordinated with body movement; ii) when body is stilled and mind becomes calm; iii) when breath is steady then emotions are balanced; and iv) balance among all aspects of psychophysiological function of an individual. Asana, breathing practices and meditation helps in digestion related problems as well as psychological problems like concentration, increasing attention span and memory power (Narasingharao, Pradhan and Navaneetham, 2016). Dynamic exercises and loosening exercises helps to channelize excessive energy which reduces hyperactiveness of children with ASD. Hence, Yoga is a form of alternative therapy for autistic children to cope with the overload of stimuli in their day to day life.

c. Yoga for Respiratory Illness

Stress appears to be particularly related to the occurrence and severity of several conditions such as bronchitis, obstructive pulmonary disorders, or psychiatric disorders. Increased respiratory rate have been linked to the presence of emotional upset through several pathways including direct physiological effects of emotion or stress on the airways, the effect of emotion on self-care, and the effect of having a chronic physical disease on emotional state. The acute effect of stress in fight-flight action and physical mobilization causes sympathetic arousal, bronchodilation and hyperventilation. Psychosocial functions and environmental factors affect respiration. A wide range of air pollutants which have been detected that influence feeble breath, shortness of breath, wheezing, nasal allergy, sore throat, chronic bronchitis, asthma, emphysema and lung cancer (Charyulu, 1999).

Breathing supplies vital energy and sustains life as it connects body, mind and emotions. Yoga can prevent and cure respiratory infections such as pneumonia and tuberculosis, lung cancer and chronic obstructive pulmonary disease (COPD) which in turn increases vital capacity and vital energy or prana (Artchoudane et al., 2018; Doijad and Surdi, 2012). Several studies reported that yoga has a profound effect on lung functions of the individuals (Agnihotri et al., 2018). However respiratory changes with yoga in which it improves maximum oxygen uptake and decreased perceived exertion unlike exercise. Hence yoga improves vital energy or ojas shakti in individual which results in healthy progeny. Yoga improves physiological and psychological process through different breathing techniques along with coordinated smooth body movements in children with autism (Radhakrishna, Nagarathna and Nagendra, 2010).

d. Yoga for Sleep Disorders

Sleep disorders of children with ASD include insomnia, sleep apnea, refusing to go to bed, sleepiness during day time, etc., and sleeping patterns are irregular which affect the routine of the entire family that causes stress particularly to parents who are the primary caretakers and constant support. Initiating and maintaining sleep for longer period among children with ASD is very difficult. Several studies have suggested that there are significant sleep problems with autistic children (Cohen et al., 2014). The sleep disorders exacerbate symptoms of autistic children who behave aggressively during daytime which makes disturbed sleep among family members (Schreck, Mulick and Smith, 2004). Children with ASD have higher co-morbidity burden than the general pediatric population, with higher rate of psychiatric illness, seizures and GI disorder (Klukowski, Wasilewska and Lebensztejn, 2015).

Yoga improved digestion related problems and enhanced sleep during night without any interruption for longer period compared to pre-intervention (Narasingharao, Pradhan and Navaneetham, 2017).

MANAGEMENT OF NDDs

In NDDs, the major perception of ASD is sensory process dysfunction, impairment in social communication and increased stereotype behavior which can be correlated with a combined disintegration of cognitive function, musculoskeletal function and cardiovascular function (Artchoudane et al., 2019).

1.a. Sensory Process Dysfunction

Artchoudane et al., (2019) have showed that sensory process dysfunction is common in children with ASD that cause impaired behavior such as over reactivity, repetitive stereotyped behavior, lack of responsiveness and social interaction, self-injurious, aggression and attention. Watling et al. (1999); Hughes, 2007; Wallace et al. (2010); Bauman and Kemper (2005); Baron-Cohen et al. (2000); Markram and Markram (2010) have found the limitations of functional behavior due to dysfunction in sensory process, growth of brain gets arrested and decelerated, that is, thinning of the cortex area which involves auditory, visual and cognitive performance, and formation of emotional memory. Sensory process abnormalities or sensory stimuli overload cause self-stimulatory behavior such as self-injury, self-aggression and hetero-aggressive behaviors that are found in children with high function ASD and low function ASD (Rojahn et al., 2001). However poor integration of sensory input or sensory defensiveness can be correlated with difficulty in attention and regulation, no playful activities, excessive nervousness and difficulty to calm after physical activity (Kenny, 2002).

1.b. Role of Yoga as Sensory Integrating Process

Yoga acts as a complementary therapy for children with ASD which improved sensory processes, focus, concentration and enhanced physical balance and flexibility. Koenig et al. (2012) have studied that yoga improves sensory process and resulted in significant positive changes. Gulati et al. (2018) have suggested that longer period of yoga therapy results in positive changes including health, sensory, communication and sociability and found even two weeks of yoga therapy improved behavior, aggression and calmness in children with ASD. Thus several studies have proved that yoga improves neurological problems and NDDs (Khalsa et al., 1999; Segal et al., 2010; Orme-Johnson D, 2006; Orme-Johnson DW, 2006; Zeidan et al., 2011; Newberg et al., 2010). Yogasana practice is a physical movement with breath awareness which facilitates the development of body awareness, concentration and memory, provides vital energy for children with neurodevelopmental disability (Ramanathan and Bhavanani, 2017).

2.a. Impaired Cardiovascular Function

The presence of single ventricle (SV) in fetus suggests that this causes alterations in cerebrovascular resistance and blood flow distribution between brain and placenta (Donofrio et al., 2003; Kaltman et al., 2005; Williams et al., 2013). Verrall et al. (2019) have found that NNDs are common in neonates undergoing complex surgery for congenital heart disease (CHD). Goff et al. (2012) have found that premature birth with CHD has greater risk for neurodevelopmental impairments.

2.b. Role of Yoga in Cardiovascular Function

Streeter et al. (2012) have found that yoga improves parasympathetic nervous system and gamma amino butyric acid (GABA) activities which improved cardiac function and reduces allostatic load among children with ASD. Thus it elicits improvement in cognitive function, elevates brain activity and self-regulatory mechanisms targeted behavior including self-stimulatory and repetitive behaviors, attention and emotion regulation such as anxiety, aggression, depression. Yoga practices are mind-body medicine which may be a beneficial adjunct therapy for patients with Cardiovascular diseases and Cardiovascular risk factor (Yeh et al., 2009).

3.a. Impaired Musculoskeletal Function

In children with ASD, physical impairments include dysfunctional posture and muscle tone (Jong et al., 2011), hypotonia (Ming, Brimacombe and Wagner, 2007), balance problems (Minshew et al., 2004), movement or motor skill deficits (Green et al., 2009), gait pattern differences (Calhoun, Longworth and Chester, 2011) and fine and gross motor problems (Provost, Heimerl and Lopez, 2007) which reflect the general issues of musculoskeletal function. Extensive research and anecdotal reports suggest functional effects of muscle weakness are widespread and common in children with ASD (Bhat, Landa and Galloway, 2011).

3.b. Role of Yoga in Musculoskeletal Function

Madanmohan et al. (2003) and Bhavanani et al. (2011) have studied that yoga therapy improves lung function, strength of inspiratory and expiratory muscles as well as skeletal muscle strength and endurance. Hence it is suggested that yoga can also improve muscle strength and overall health in children with ASD.

SOME YOGIC TOOLS FOR SPECIAL CHILDREN

Each practice to an individual child or group must be under the guidance of yoga therapist/professionals so that the child will be able to follow .

a) Enhancement of Cognitive function: Hakarakriya, Bhujangini kriya, Kukurukriya and Simhakriya. The movement with sound practice improves cognitive function actively against painful emotions and thereby one looses destructive impact.
b) Improvement in Behavior: Tadasana, Vrkshasana, Trikonasana, Sarvangasana, Matsyasana, Halasana, Dhanurasana, Pavanamuktasana and Vakrasana. These practices help balancing, controlling and managing a stressful situation.
c) Improvement in self-dejection (avoiding): Vamana Dhauti, Dugdhaneti and Trataka. These are the unique techniques allow one for refusal to face a problematic or stressful situation and act accordingly.
d) Improvement in hetero-aggressiveness: Kayakriya and Shavasana. These are the best practice to improve one's neuromuscular coordination and the state of depersonalization and derealization.
e) Empowerment: Nasarga Mukhabhastrika, Bhramari pranayama and Pranava pranayama. These practices allow living with one's own nature.

IMPACT OF YOGA PRACTICES ON CHILDREN WITH NDDs

Yoga therapy has impact on various aspects of musculoskeletal, cardiovascular and cognitive function in children with special needs. It has been observed that both internal processing and external processing of children with NDDs are significantly improved through breath-movement coordination, awareness and resonating brain waves. Chanting for children with NDDs have shown that significant improvement in synchronized cardiovascular rhythms, respiratory signals and cerebral blood flow, and thus it entrains a particular brain activity or body rhythm which creates one-pointedness in the mind. Pranayama with chanting (Pranava pranayama) improved the pattern of breathing thereby reducing hostile behavior, anxiety and facilitating relaxation (Ajmera et al., 2018).

DISCUSSION

The aim of this chapter was to investigate the effects of yoga therapy on cognitive function in children with NDDs and to present the basis of yoga therapy applied to children's rehabilitation. It empowers the application of yoga therapy to children with NDDs in clinical settings and promotes the therapeutic potential of yoga. Present modern science bloomed with the shadow of knowledge which deals with only one layer of the human being and is insufficient for unresolved issues and termed those as *unknown causes*. Recognizing complete knowledge from yogic texts like *Bhagavad Gita, Thirumandiram, Hatha Yoga Pradipika, Gheranda Samhita, Patanjali Yoga Sutra, Ananda Sutra and Brahma Sutra* for research may resolve various health issues for the present generation facing unresolved diseases and disorders. Bitter health situations of present generation suffering over a life time from NDDs and various stress related disorders can be improved by efficient application of yoga therapy. Children with NDDs are not yet able to sit still with proper attention direction. Yoga programs for autistic children that include chanting *AUM* has been shown to harmonize respiratory signals, cardiovascular rhythms and cerebral blood flow, and entrains a particular brain activity or body rhythm and creates one-pointedness in the mind (Sequeira and Ahmed, 2012; Shannahoff-Khalsa DS, 2010; Bernardi, et al., 2001; Khalsa DS et al., 2009; Schmidt, Trainor and Santesso, 2003). Streeter et al. (2012) and Ajmera et al. (2018) have studied that pranayama improved deep breathing patterns thereby reducing anxiety and facilitating relaxation. Yoga therapy promotes the ability to exchange information to and fro through all the senses that enables persons with cognitive disabilities to make meaningful responses through the integration of senses and functions of central nervous system. Improvement in functions such as attention, emotion, cognition, coordination, arousal levels, and activities of autonomous system are seen and perceived in children with ASD. Effect of yoga therapy on various areas are alleviating NDDs and behavioral characteristics sensory processing dysfunction, motor impairments, communication disorders, cognition and social interaction.

Yoga therapy acts as evidence-based holistic solution for clinical studies with the aid of which neuroscience research is able to reach desired destination with outcomes including relief of clinical symptoms of the disease, facilitated expression of feelings and skills, greater relaxation, as well as improved family and social QoL. Regular and continued long term practice of yoga may slow down motor, facial, vocal, and auditory cues that impact cognitive performance and motor imitation skills of children with ASD. Yoga therapy is seen to enhance brain functioning and help restore self-regulatory mechanisms like self-stimulatory and repetitive behaviors as well as attention and emotion regulation in children with ASD.

Menon (2015) spent many a troubled days trying to train yoga to kids whose intellectual disabilities were severe and they were trained for five days per week for one hour daily, after 2 to 5 months yoga practice became an important means for their self-development and rehabilitation, they showed marked improvement in span of attention, sensory-motor coordination, gross and fine motor skills, overall stability of posture and ability to follow instructions correctly without much time-lapse. Ramanathan and

Ramanathan and Bhavanani (2017) have found that yoga improves loco-motor skills, psycho-motor co-ordination, eye-hand coordination, attention span, immunity, appetite, sleep and promotes overall health in children with ASD. Hence yoga therapists and teachers must have patience, confidence, gradually develop mutual trust, friendship and establish a strong bond with humane and yogic ethical approach in children with ASD.

Children with NDDs are expressed as heterogeneous condition and certain behaviours may change with development. Yoga has been found extremely effective in improving basic skills. Regular practice of Yoga by the children with NDDs helps sustain attention span, improve cognitive function ability to comprehend and follow instructions, aids sensory-motor co-ordination as well as brings stability to gesture and postures. Repeated and regularity of yoga practice stimulates the firing of various types of sensory and motor neurons in brain, that in turn re-wiring new neural pathways. Yoga helps significant rehabilitation of physically and mentally handicapped as well visually impaired children. Yogic breathing techniques improve neuromuscular function and alteration in the primary thalamo-cortical level (Telles and Naveen, 1997; Telles et al., 1993). Yoga improved cognitive functions in breast cancer patients and in menopausal women (Vadiraja et al., 2009; Chattha et al., 2008). Several studies have reported that yoga improves cognitive function (Alexander et al., 2013; Soderstrom et al., 2012). Hence yoga has more significant improvement in relationships and enhancement of a variety of social, emotional, behavioural, and cognitive functions that can be attributed to improve cognitive function in children with NDDs (Grensman et al., 2018; Diamond and Lee, 2011).

CONCLUSION

Yoga improved brain functioning, elevated brain activity and also helped restore self-regulatory mechanisms including self-stimulatory and repetitive behaviors as well as attention and emotion regulation. Yoga is being identified as a treatment method that can optimize health outcomes for children with NDDs. Yoga enhances children's emotional balance, cognitive power and attention and decreases negative thought patterns, negative behavior, emotional and physical arousal, anxiety and reactivity. Yoga therapy also helps as protective and curative factor for children with NDDs. More longitudinal studies with strong methodological strategies are required to understand the cognitive function and overall health benefits of yoga therapy delivered for the same.

REFERENCES

Agnihotri, S., Gaur, P., Bhattacharya, S., Kant, S., & Pandey, S. (2018). Benefits of Yoga in Respiratory Diseases. *Indian J. Pharm. Biol. Res, 6*(4), 10-13.

Ajmera, S., Sundar, S., Amirtha, G. B., Bhavanani, A. B., Dayanidy, G., & Ezhumalai, G. (2018). A comparative study on the effect of music therapy alone and a combination of music and yoga therapies on the psycho-physiological parameters of cardiac patients posted for angiography. *J Basic ClinAppl Health Sci, 2*(1), 163–171. doi:10.5005/jp-journals-10082-01145

Alexander, G. K., Innes, K. E., Selfe, T. K., & Brown, C. J. (2013). "more than I expected": Perceived benefits of yoga practice among older adults at risk for cardiovascular disease. *Complementary Therapies in Medicine*, *21*(1), 14–28. doi:10.1016/j.ctim.2012.11.001 PMID:23374201

Allen, S., & Anita, M. (2014). Yoga: Therapy for Children on the Autism Spectrum. *Academic Exchange Quarterly Summer, 18*(2).

American Psychiatric Association. (2000). *Diagnostic and Statistical Manual of Mental Disorders* (Fourth Edition Text Revision). Washington, DC: American Psychiatric Association.

Artchoudane, S., Bhavanani, A. B., Ramanathan, M., & Mariangela, A. (2019). Yoga as a therapeutic tool in autism: A detailed review. *Yoga Mimamsa, 51,* 3-16. Doi:10.4103/ym.ym_3_19

Artchoudane, S., Ranganadin, P., Bhavanani, A. B., Ramanathan, M., & Madanmohan, T. (2018). Effect of adjuvant Yoga therapy on pulmonary function and Quality of life among patients with Chronic Obstructive Pulmonary Disease: A randomized control trial. *J Basic ClinAppl Health Sci, 2*(3), 117-122.

Asli, G., Melek, C., Ozgur, B., & Kuscu, N.K. (2012). Sudden Death of a Pregnant Woman in Third Trimester with No Risk Factor. *Case Reports in Obstetrics and Gynecology*. . doi:10.1155/2012/951480

Baron-Cohen, S., Ring, H. A., Bullmore, E. T., Wheelwright, S., Ashwin, C., & Williams, S. C. R. (2000). The amygdala theory of autism. *Neuroscience and Biobehavioral Reviews*, *24*(3), 355–364. doi:10.1016/S0149-7634(00)00011-7 PMID:10781695

Bauman, M. L., & Kemper, T. L. (2005). Neuroanatomic observations of the brain in autism: A review and future directions. *International Journal of Developmental Neuroscience*, *23*(2-3), 183–187. doi:10.1016/j.ijdevneu.2004.09.006 PMID:15749244

Bernardi, L., Sleight, P., Bandinelli, G., Cencetti, S., Fattorini, L., Wdowczyc-Szulc, J., & Lagi, A. (2001). Effect of rosary prayer and yoga mantras on autonomic cardiovascular rhythms: Comparative study. *BMJ (Clinical Research Ed.)*, *323*(7327), 1446–1449. doi:10.1136/bmj.323.7327.1446 PMID:11751348

Betts, D. E., & Betts, S. W. (2006). *Yoga for children with autism spectrum disorders*. Jessica Kingley Publishers.

Bhat, A. N., Landa, R. J., & Galloway, J. C. (2011). Current perspectives on motor functioning in infants, children, and adults with autism spectrum disorders. *Physical Therapy*, *91*(7), 1116–1129. doi:10.2522/ptj.20100294 PMID:21546566

Bhavanani, A. B. (2013). A closing word. In *Yoga Chikitsa: Application of yoga as a therapy* (1st ed.). Pondicherry, India: Dhivyananda Creations.

Bhavanani, A. B. (2017). Role of yoga in prevention and management of lifestyle disorders. *Yoga Mimamsa*, *49*(2), 42–47. doi:10.4103/ym.ym_14_17

Bhavanani, A. B., & Udupa, K. (2011). A comparative study of slow and fast suryanamaskar on physiological function. *International Journal of Yoga*, *4*(2), 71–77. doi:10.4103/0973-6131.85489 PMID:22022125

Binorkar, S. V. (2014). Yoga – The Non-Pharmaceutical Approach for Lifestyle Disorders. *Journal of Yoga & Physical Therapy*, *4*(04), e116. doi:10.4172/2157-7595.1000e116

Buie, A. T., Campbell, D. B., Hyman, S. L., & Jirapinyo, P. (2010). Evaluation, Diagnosis, and Treatment of Gastrointestinal disorders in Individuals with ASDs: A consensus report. *Pediatrics*, *125*(Supplement 1), S1–S18. doi:10.1542/peds.2009-1878C PMID:20048083

Calhoun, M., Longworth, M., & Chester, V. L. (2011). Gait patterns in children with autism. *Clinical Biomechanics (Bristol, Avon)*, *26*(2), 200–206. doi:10.1016/j.clinbiomech.2010.09.013 PMID:20934239

Charyulu, K. V. (1999). *Environment Education*. New Delhi, India: Neelkamal Publishers.

Chattha, R., Raghuram, N., Venkatram, P., & Hongasandra, N. R. (2008). Treating the climacteric symptoms in Indian women with an integrated approach to yoga therapy: A randomized control study. *Menopause (New York, N.Y.)*, *15*(5), 862–870. doi:10.1097/gme.0b013e318167b902 PMID:18463543

Cohen, S., Conduit, R., Lockley, S. W., Rajaratnam, S. M., & Cornish, K. M. (2014). The relationship between sleep and behavior in autism spectrum disorder (ASD): A review. *Journal of Neurodevelopmental Disorders*, *6*(1), 44. doi:10.1186/1866-1955-6-44 PMID:25530819

Diamond, A., & Lee, K. (2011). Interventions shown to aid executive function development in children 4-12 years Old. *Science*, *19*(6045), 959–964. doi:10.1126cience.1204529 PMID:21852486

Doijad, V. P., & Surdi, A. D. (2012). Effect of short term yoga practice on pulmonary function tests. *Indian Journal of Basic and Applied Medical Research*, *3*(1), 226–230.

Donofrio, M. T., Bremer, Y. A., Schieken, R. M., Gennings, C., Morton, L. D., Eidem, B. W., ... Kleinman, C. S. (2003). Autoregulation of cerebral blood flow in fetuses with congenital heart disease: The brain sparing effect. *Pediatric Cardiology*, *24*(5), 436–443. doi:10.100700246-002-0404-0 PMID:14627309

Effort, M. (2019). 618 - பொறியின்மை யார்க்கும் பழியன்று அறிவறிந்து ஆள்வினை இன்மை பழி. *Manly Effort - Wealth - Thirukkural*. Available at: https://www.thirukkural.net/en/kural/kural-0618.html

Fauci, A. S., Braunwald, E., & Isselbacher, K. J. (1998). *Harrison's Principles of Internal Medicine*. New York: McGraw Hill.

French, N. P., Hagan, R., Evans, S. F., Godfrey, M., & Newnham, J. P. (1999). Repeated antenatal corticosteroids: Size at birth and subsequent development. *American Journal of Obstetrics and Gynecology*, *180*(1), 114–121. doi:10.1016/S0002-9378(99)70160-2 PMID:9914589

Gitananda Giri Swami. (1976). *Yoga: Step-by-Step*. Pondicherry, India: Satya Press.

Goff, D. A., Luan, X., Gerdes, M., Bernbaum, J., D'Agostino, J. A., Rychik, J., ... Gaynor, J. W. (2012). Younger gestational age is associated with worse neurodevelopmental outcomes after cardiac surgery in infancy. *The Journal of Thoracic and Cardiovascular Surgery*, *143*(3), 535–542. doi:10.1016/j.jtcvs.2011.11.029 PMID:22340027

Gorrindo P. (2013). *Gastrointestinal dysfunction in Autism*. Academic Press.

Green, D., Charman, T., Pickles, A., Chandler, S., Loucas, T., Simonoff, E., & Baird, G. (2009). Impairment in movement skills of children with autistic spectrum disorders. *Developmental Medicine and Child Neurology*, *51*(4), 311–316. doi:10.1111/j.1469-8749.2008.03242.x PMID:19207298

Grensman, A., Acharya, B. D., Wändell, P., Nilsson, G. H., Falkenberg, T., Sundin, O., & Werner, S. (2018). Effect of traditional yoga, mindfulness–based cognitive therapy, and cognitive behavioral therapy, on health related quality of life: A randomized controlled trial on patients on sick leave because of burnout. *BMC Complementary and Alternative Medicine*, *18*(1), 80. doi:10.118612906-018-2141-9 PMID:29510704

Grundmann, O., & Yoon, S. L. (2010). Irritable bowel syndrome: epidemiology, diagnosis and treatment: an update for healthcare practitioners. *Journal of Gastroenterology and Hepatology*, *25*(4), 691–699. doi:10.1111/j.1440-1746.2009.06120.x PMID:20074154

Gulati, K., Loganathan, N., Mooventhan, A., Lahiri, A., & Telles, S. (2018). Effect of yoga therapy on the symptoms of sensory processing disorder in autistic individuals. *Yoga Mimamsa*, *50*(2), 60–61. doi:10.4103/ym.ym_9_18

Hanney, N. M., Jostad, C. M., LeBlanc, L. A., Carr, J. E., & Castile, A. J. (2012). Intensive behavioral treatment of urinary incontinence of Children with Autism Spectrum Disorders: An archival analysis of procedures and outcomes from an outpatient clinic. *Focus on Autism and Other Developmental Disabilities*, *28*(1), 26–31. doi:10.1177/1088357612457987

Hughes, J. R. (2007). Autism: The first firm finding = under connectivity? *Epilepsy & Behavior*, *11*(1), 20–24. doi:10.1016/j.yebeh.2007.03.010 PMID:17531541

Jong, D. M., Punt, M., Groot, D. E., Minderaa, R. B., & Hadders, A. M. (2011). Minor neurological dysfunction in children with autism spectrum disorder. *Developmental Medicine and Child Neurology*, *53*(7), 641–646. doi:10.1111/j.1469-8749.2011.03971.x PMID:21569013

Kaltman, J. R., Di, H., Tian, Z., & Rychik, J. (2005). Impact of congenital heart disease on cerebrovascular blood flow dynamics in the fetus. *Ultrasound in Obstetrics & Gynecology*, *25*(1), 32–36. doi:10.1002/uog.1785 PMID:15593334

Kenny, M. S. (2002). Integrated Movement Therapy™: Yoga-Based Therapy as a Viable and Effective Intervention for Autism Spectrum and Related Disorders. *International Journal of Yoga Therapy*, *12*, 71.

Khalsa, D. S., Amen, D., Hanks, C., Money, N., & Newberg, A. (2009). Cerebral blood flow changes during chanting meditation. *Nuclear Medicine Communications*, *30*(12), 956–961. doi:10.1097/MNM.0b013e32832fa26c PMID:19773673

Khalsa, D. S., Ray, L. E., Levine, S., Gallen, C. C., Schwartz, B. J., & Sidorowich, J. J. (1999). Randomized controlled trial of yogic meditation techniques for patients with obsessive-compulsive disorder. *CNS Spectrums*, *4*(12), 34–47. doi:10.1017/S1092852900006805 PMID:18311106

Klukowski, M., Wasilewska, J., & Lebensztejn, D. (2015). Sleep and gastrointestinal disturbances. *Dev Period Med*, *19*(2), 157–161. PMID:26384115

Koenig, K. P., Buckley-Reen, A., & Garg, S. (2012). Efficacy of the Get Ready to learn yoga program among children with autism spectrum disorders: A pretest–posttest control group design. *The American Journal of Occupational Therapy*, *66*(5), 538–546. doi:10.5014/ajot.2012.004390 PMID:22917120

Madanmohan, T., Lakshmi, J., Udupa, K., & Bhavanani, A. B. (2003). Effect of yoga training on hand-grip, respiratory Pressures and pulmonary function. *Indian Journal of Physiology and Pharmacology*, *47*(4), 387–392. PMID:15266949

Mariotti, V., Marconi, A., & Pardi, G. (2004). Undesired effects of steroids during pregnancy. *The Journal of Maternal-Fetal & Neonatal Medicine*, *16*(2), 5–7. doi:10.1080/jmf.16.2.5.7 PMID:15590425

Markram, K., & Markram, H. (2010). The intense world theory—A unifying theory of the neurobiology of autism. *Frontiers in Human Neuroscience*, *4*, 224. doi:10.3389/fnhum.2010.00224 PMID:21191475

Menon, P. (2015). *How Yoga Could Help 'Rewire' The Brains Of Mentally Disabled Children*. Retrieved from http://www.huffingtonpost.in/dr-praseeda-menon/how-yoga-could-helprewir_b_8336520.html#

Ming, X., Brimacombe, M., & Wagner, G. C. (2007). Prevalence of motor impairment in autism spectrum disorders. *Brain & Development*, *29*, 565–570.

Minshew, N. J., Sung, K., Jones, B. L., & Furman, J. M. (2004). Underdevelopment of the postural control system in autism. *Neurology*, *63*(11), 2056–2061. doi:10.1212/01.WNL.0000145771.98657.62 PMID:15596750

Mulak, A., Tache, Y., & Larauche, M. (2014). Sex hormones in the modulation of irritable bowel syndrome. *World Journal of Gastroenterology*, *20*(10), 2433–2448. doi:10.3748/wjg.v20.i10.2433 PMID:24627581

Mullin, A. P., Gokhale, A., Moreno-De-Luca, A., Sanyal, S., Waddington, J. L. V., & Faundez, V. (2013). Neurodevelopmental disorders: Mechanisms and boundary definitions from genomes, interactomes and proteomes. *Translational Psychiatry*, *3*(12), e329. doi:10.1038/tp.2013.108 PMID:24301647

Narasingharao, K., Pradhan, B., & Navaneetham, J. (2016). Sleep Disorder, Gastrointestinal Problems and Behaviour Problems Seen in Autism Spectrum Disorder Children and Yoga as Therapy: A Descriptive Review. *Journal of Clinical and Diagnostic Research : JCDR*, *10*(11), VE01–VE03. doi:10.7860/JCDR/2016/24175.8922 PMID:28050484

Narasingharao, K., Pradhan, B., & Navaneetham, J. (2017). Efficacy of Structured Yoga Intervention for Sleep, Gastrointestinal and Behaviour Problems of ASD Children: An Exploratory Study. *Journal of Clinical and Diagnostic Research : JCDR*, *11*(3), VC01–VC06. doi:10.7860/JCDR/2017/25894.9502 PMID:28511484

Natarajan, B. (2002). *Thirumandiram - A Tamil Scriptural Classic of Thirumoolar* [English Translation]. Chennai, India: Sri Ramakrishna Math Publications.

Newberg, A. B., Wintering, N., Khalsa, D. S., Roggenkamp, H., & Waldman, M. R. (2010). Meditation effects on cognitive function and cerebral blood flow in subjects with memory loss: A preliminary study. *Journal of Alzheimer's Disease*, *20*(2), 517–526. doi:10.3233/JAD-2010-1391 PMID:20164557

Orme-Johnson, D. (2006). Evidence that the transcendental meditation program prevents or decreases diseases of the nervous system and is specifically beneficial for epilepsy. *Medical Hypotheses*, *67*(2), 240–246. doi:10.1016/j.mehy.2006.03.034 PMID:16723189

Orme-Johnson, D. W., Schneider, R. H., Son, Y. D., Nidich, S., & Cho, Z. H. (2006). Neuroimaging of meditation's effect on brain reactivity to pain. *Neuroreport*, *17*(12), 1359–1363. doi:10.1097/01.wnr.0000233094.67289.a8 PMID:16951585

Pastor, P. N., & Reuben, C. A. (2008). Diagnosed attention deficit hyperactivity disorder and learning disability: United States, 2004-2006. *Vital and Health Statistics*, *10*, 237. PMID:18998276

Provost, B., Heimerl, S., & Lopez, B. R. (2007). Levels of gross and fine motor development in young children with autism spectrum disorder. *Physical & Occupational Therapy in Pediatrics*, *27*(3), 21–36. doi:10.1080/J006v27n03_03 PMID:17613454

Radhakrishna, S., Nagarathna, R., & Nagendra, H. R. (2010). Integrated approach to yoga therapy and autism spectrum disorders. *Journal of Ayurveda and Integrative Medicine*, *1*(2), 120–124. doi:10.4103/0975-9476.65089 PMID:21836799

Ramanathan, M., & Bhavanani, A. B. (2017). *Yoga for Children with Special Needs*. Ministry of Ayush. Available from: https://moayush.wordpress.com/2017/05/09/yoga-for-children-with-specialneeds/

Ramanathan, M., & Bhavanani, A. B. (2018). Addressing Autism Spectrum Disorder through Yoga as a Complementary Therapy. *J Basic ClinAppl Health Sci*, *2*(2), 3–7. doi:10.5005/jp-journals-10082-01123

Rojahn, J., Matson, J. L., Lott, D., Esbensen, A. J., & Smalls, Y. (2001). The Behavior Problems Inventory: An instrument for the assessment of self-injury, stereotyped behavior, and aggression/destruction in individuals with developmental disabilities. *Journal of Autism and Developmental Disorders*, *31*(6), 577–588. doi:10.1023/A:1013299028321 PMID:11814269

Sage, G. (1895). *The Gheranda Samhita: A Treatise on Hatha Yoga* (S. C. Vasu, Trans. & Ed.). Bombay, India: Theosophical.

Sagiv, S. K., Thurston, S. W., Bellinger, D. C., Tolbert, P. E., Altshul, L. M., & Korrick, S. A. (2010). Prenatal organochlorine exposure and behaviors associated with attention deficit hyperactivity disorder in school-aged children. *American Journal of Epidemiology*, *171*(5), 593–601. doi:10.1093/aje/kwp427 PMID:20106937

Samhita, S. (2010a). Nibandha Samgraha commentary chikitsa, 15/3, ed: 2010. Chaukhambha Sanskrit sansthan. Varanasi.

Samhita, S. (2010b). Nibandha Samgraha commentary sutra, 35/27, ed:2010. Chaukhambha Sanskrit sansthan. Varanasi.

Schmidt, L. A., Trainor, L. J., & Santesso, D. L. (2003). Development of frontal electroencephalogram (EEG) and heart rate (ECG) responses to affective musical stimuli during the first 12 months of post-natal life. *Brain and Cognition*, *52*(1), 27–32. doi:10.1016/S0278-2626(03)00006-X PMID:12812802

Schreck, K. A., Mulick, J. A., & Smith, A. F. (2004). Sleep problems as possible predictors of intensified symptoms of autism. *Research in Developmental Disabilities*, *25*(1), 57–66. doi:10.1016/j.ridd.2003.04.007 PMID:14733976

Segal, Z. V., Bieling, P., Young, T., MacQueen, G., Cooke, R., Martin, L., ... Levitan, R. D. (2010). Antidepressant monotherapy vs sequential pharmacotherapy and mindfulness based cognitive therapy, or placebo, for relapse prophylaxis in recurrent depression. *Archives of General Psychiatry*, *67*(12), 1256–1264. doi:10.1001/archgenpsychiatry.2010.168 PMID:21135325

Sequeira, S., & Ahmed, M. (2012). Meditation as a Potential Therapy for Autism: A Review. Autism Research and Treatment. doi:10.1155/2012/835847

Shannahoff-Khalsa, D. S. (2010). *Kundalini Yoga Meditation for Complex Psychiatric Disorders: Techniques Specific for Treating the Psychoses, Personality, and Pervasive Developmental Disorders*. New York: WW Norton & Company.

Slotkin, T. A., & Seidler, F. J. (2013). Terbutaline impairs the development of peripheral noradrenergic projections: Potential implications for autism spectrum disorders and pharmacotherapy of preterm labor. *Neurotoxicology and Teratology*, *36*, 91–96. doi:10.1016/j.ntt.2012.07.003 PMID:22813780

Soderstrom, M., Jeding, K., Ekstedt, M., Perski, A., & Akerstedt, T. (2012). Insufficient sleep predicts clinical burnout. *Journal of Occupational Health Psychology*, *17*(2), 175–183. doi:10.1037/a0027518 PMID:22449013

Streeter, C. C., Gerbarg, P. L., Saper, R. B., Ciraulo, D. A., & Brown, R. P. (2012). Effects of yoga on the autonomic nervous system, gamma-aminobutyric-acid, and allostasis in epilepsy, depression, and post-traumatic stress disorder. *Medical Hypotheses*, *78*(5), 571–579. doi:10.1016/j.mehy.2012.01.021 PMID:22365651

Stromland. (1994). Autism in thalidomide embryopathy: a population study. *Developmental Medicine & Child Neurology, 36,* 351.

Suresh, P. A. (2018). Global prevalence of autism: A mini-review. *SciFed Journal of Autism*, *2*, 1.

Telles, S., Joseph, C., Venkatesh, S., & Desiraju, T. (1993). Alterations of auditory middle latency evoked potentials during yogic consciously regulated breathing and alternative states of the mind. *International Journal of Psychophysiology*, *14*(3), 189–198. doi:10.1016/0167-8760(93)90033-L PMID:8340237

Telles, S., & Naveen, K. V. (1997). Yoga for rehabilitation: An overview. *Indian Journal of Medical Sciences*, *51*, 123–127. PMID:9355699

Vadiraja, H. S., Raghavendra, R. M., Nagarathna, R., Nagendra, H. R., Rekha, M., Vanitha, N., & ... . (2009). Effects of a yoga program on cortisol rhythm and mood states in early breast cancer patients undergoing adjuvant radiotherapy: A randomized controlled trial. *Integrative Cancer Therapies*, *8*(1), 37–46. doi:10.1177/1534735409331456 PMID:19190034

van Geijn, H. P., Lenglet, J. E., & Botte, A. C. (2005). Nifedipine trials: Effectiveness and safety aspects. *BJOG*, *112*(1), 79–83. doi:10.1111/j.1471-0528.2005.00591.x PMID:15715601

Vermillion, S. T., Soper, D. E., & Chasedunn-Roark, J. (1999). Neonatal sepsis after betamethasone administration to patients with preterm premature rupture of membranes. *American Journal of Obstetrics and Gynecology*, *181*(2), 320–322. doi:10.1016/S0002-9378(99)70555-7 PMID:10454676

Verrall, C. E., Blue, G. M., Loughran-Fowlds, A., Kasparian, N., Gecz, J., Walker, K., ... Winlaw, D. (2019). 'Big issues' in neurodevelopment for children and adults with congenital heart disease. *Open Heart, 6*(2), e000998. doi:10.1136/openhrt-2018-000998 PMID:31354955

Wallace, G. L., Dankner, L., Kenworthy, L., Giedd, J. N., & Martin, A. (2010). Age-related temporal and parietal cortical thinning in autism spectrum disorders. *Brain, 133*(12), 3745–3754. doi:10.1093/brain/awq279 PMID:20926367

Watling, R., Deitz, J., Kanny, E. M., & McLaughlin, J. F. (1999). Current practice of occupational therapy for children with autism. *The American Journal of Occupational Therapy, 53*(5), 498–505. doi:10.5014/ajot.53.5.498 PMID:10500858

Whitehead, W. E., Palsson, O., & Jones, K. R. (2002). Systematic review of the comorbidity of irritable bowel syndrome with other disorders: What are the causes and implications? *Gastroenterology, 122*(4), 1140–1156. doi:10.1053/gast.2002.32392 PMID:11910364

Williams, B. L., Hornig, M., Parekh, T., & Lipkin, W. I. (2012). Application of novel PCR-based methods for detection, quantitation, and phylogenetic characterization of Sutterella Species in intestinal biopsy samples from Children with Autism and gastrointestinal disturbances. *mBio, 3*(1), 1–11. doi:10.1128/mBio.00261-11 PMID:22233678

Williams, I.A., Fifer, C., Jaeggi, E., Levine, J.C., Michelfelder, E.C., & Szwast, A.L. (2013). The association of fetal cerebrovascular resistance with early neurodevelopment in single ventricle congenital heart disease. *Am Heart J, 165,* 544. doi:10.1016/j.ahj.2012.11.013

Yasin, H., Gibson, W. T., Langlois, S., Stowe, R. M., Tsang, E. S., & Lee, L. (2018). A distinct neurodevelopmental syndrome with intellectual disability, autism spectrum disorder, characteristic facies, and macrocephaly is caused by defects in CHD8. *Journal of Human Genetics*. doi:10.103810038-019-0561-0 PMID:30670789

Yeh, G., Wang, C., Wayne, P., & Phillips, R. (2009). Tai chi exercise for patients with cardiovascular conditions and risk factors: A systematic review. *Journal of Cardiopulmonary Rehabilitation and Prevention, 29*(3), 152–160. doi:10.1097/HCR.0b013e3181a33379 PMID:19471133

Zeidan, F., Martucci, K. T., Kraft, R. A., Gordon, N. S., Mchaffie, J. G., & Coghill, R. C. (2011). Brain mechanisms supporting the modulation of pain by mindfulness meditation. *The Journal of Neuroscience : The Official Journal of the Society for Neuroscience, 31*(14), 5540–5548. doi:10.1523/JNEUROSCI.5791-10.2011 PMID:21471390

Chapter 10
21st Century Education for Special Needs Students:
A Teacher's View and an Instructional Approach

Harpreet Kaur Dhir
https://orcid.org/0000-0002-6347-5586
Hacienda La Puente Unified School District, USA

ABSTRACT

Education is a human right—including students who have conditions requiring special education services. The purpose of this chapter is to promote inclusive education for students with learning disabilities due to diagnoses such as attention deficit hyperactivity disorder, autism, and more. A literature review includes a discussion pertaining to the elements of appropriate teaching methods compatible with developing 21st-century competencies for general education and special education students within the same classroom setting. Relative to employing strategies of differentiation and scaffolding while increasing cognition through experience-based lessons, this chapter provides examples from the author's classroom instructional plans. The content through action (CTA) method is presented as an ideal approach conducive to integrating 21st-century competencies through experiential lessons to teach the required content to students of various abilities. The chapter ends with recommendations on creating systemic change through building a support system at an organizational level.

INTRODUCTION

According to the Millennium Developmental Goals (MDG), educational rights equate to human rights leading to practicing cultural, social, political, and civil rights (Crosco, 2013). One of the eight goals of MDG is the goal of promoting primary education for all students at various levels of ability. The focus on advocating for education is included in six Education for All (EFA) goals which were established by

DOI: 10.4018/978-1-7998-3069-6.ch010

1500 participants from across the international borders. The EFA goals contain the emphasis on improving the quality of education ranging from early childhood to adulthood (Hinzen, 2013).

The global south did not meet the EFA goals which were due to be achieved by 2015. Educating the marginalized communities, including the students with learning disabilities, is a global issue (Mukherjee, 2017). The intergovernmental agencies as well as the non-profit groups have taken a lead to eliminate discriminatory practices around the globe, but exclusion continues to persist. According to Sider (2014), international collaboration to create educational equity required authenticity and trust, the recognition of diversity in creating educational programs, and economic development. Current technological advances might bridge the gaps in education by creating cross-cultural communication among the students and help understand the diversity existing in each community and organization such as a school.

BACKGROUND: LITERATURE REVIEW

India is one of the countries situated in the global south which did not meet the EFA goals. Due to religious, ethnic, and linguistic diversity, fully including special needs students in a general education setting has faced challenges. Mukherjee (2017) illustrated the background concerning the issues of exclusion and inclusion in a context such as India. According to the author, exclusionary practices were caused by the creation of nation-states in the colonial era on the ethnic and cultural lines creating an issue of majority culture imposing its values on the minority groups. Children from certain castes, tribes, gender, religion, and socio-economic class were excluded from their right to educational equity. The idea of inclusion as a global construct, influenced by the countries with developed economies such as the United States of America, has been associated with social justice, equity, and human rights. Inclusion is a complex issue in a country like India where a vast variety of subgroups could make educational equity difficult to monitor.

In the context of Indian diversity, Tagore's philosophy of education provided direction and inspiration to promote education for all. Tagore built an experiment school at Shantiniketen where progressive vision included the practice of democratic ideals, environmental sustainability, and inclusive learning for all (Pridmore, 2009). Implementing a model of human-centered teaching, embedded with diverse learning methods, Tagore encouraged students to experience education rather than to acquire information.

At Shantiniketen, arts played a role of making curriculum come to life through experiential learning. Tagore believed education led an individual to self-determination and freedom; freedom of mind, heart, and will (Lesar, 2015). The core beliefs of Tagore, concerning experiential learning, related to the theory of Constructivism. The theory of Constructivism is relevant to teaching the learning-disabled students in the inclusive setting of mainstream classrooms where experiential learning can lead to cognitive development (Dewey & Jackson, 1990).

The Theory of Constructivism

To understand the relevance of the theory of Constructivism in promoting inclusivity, learning about the foundations of the theory is important. The Social Development Theory of Lev Vygotsky formed the basis of constructivist thinking (Clark, 2018). Vygotsky, in Clark (2018), described the process of learning initiating with social interactions followed by cognitive development. Dewey and Jackson (1990) believed the development of mind was possible through social experiences and considered the human-mind to be a social entity by nature. The contextual experience preceding the cognitive development drives the instruction for all students. Clark (2018) clarified the concept of the Zone of Proximal Development (ZPD) which was designed by Vygotsky to differentiate the levels of understanding through assessing what students were able to accomplish without assistance, what students could do with guidance, and what student were not able to accomplish despite the guidance (Clark, 2018). ZPD level helped to identify an appropriate point of instruction for each student which facilitated the progress of individual students in the classroom.

Through testing, observation, portfolio evidence, or oral discussions, ZPD determination provides information on the appropriate strategies to be implemented for increasing student achievement. This method of approaching instruction is inclusive as teaching begins from the learning level of students, and learning is supported using strategies such as scaffolding. Scaffolding or supplemental support is provided to students during discussions and to assist in completing other assignments (Clark, 2018). Providing support based on the diverse needs is a hallmark of Constructivism as founded by Dewey and Jackson (1990) who advocated for an inclusive classroom to mirror the qualities of a democratic society where people of various backgrounds cooperated for the system to function (Cohen & Howlett, 2017).

The tenets of Constructivism include viewing all knowledge as a construct of the human mind and was subject to revision as a practical matter (McWilliam, 2016). The subjective nature of the constructivist perspective could be viewed as an action-based change and progress (McWilliam, 2016). Constructivism entails using knowledge in a variety of ways as a method of developing higher level thinking skills (Waddington & Weeth, 2016). Dewey believed in embedding multiple subjects, such as math and science, in human life beyond the textbooks (Waddington & Weeth, 2016) making the concepts of each subject comprehensible and relevant through experience.

Ensuring Educational Equity

Constructivism, derived from the social learning theory of Vygotsky, presented the idea of giving support to students at appropriate times and levels of understanding (Clark, 2018). This, arguably, could be a component of defining educational equity. Examining the program plan of a K-12 public-school district in the Los Angeles County facilitated the understanding of educational equity. The vision of the district was to provide all students with rigorous and culturally responsive learning for academic achievement and successful civic life. As a part of the vision to meet the needs of all students, the district had developed five objectives of which Objective One was dedicated to equity and access.

Objective One consisted of strategic initiatives by:

- Connecting students to the necessary supports within and outside the school along with progress monitoring.
- Providing professional training for all educators.
- Recruiting and retaining the staff reflecting the diversity of the schools.
- Identifying priority standards by content and grade level.
- Providing a challenging curriculum and access to technology to all students.

Creating an equity and access plan to promote educational equity is critical in any educational institute. Implementation of standards-based reforms continues to be insufficient to establish equitable learning for all students. The standards-based reforms have been criticized for marginalizing the minority students of color, the English Language Learners (ELL), and students in special education programs (Bartlett, Otis-Wilborn, & Sim, 2015). Providing access to alternative ways to differentiate teaching and learning might be necessary for some students in meeting the educational needs.

Providing Alternatives

Differentiation is a part of the equitable learning process to meet the needs of various students. Instructional approaches will need to combine different strategies such as direct instruction, modeling, guided practice, discussions, cooperative learning, small group or one on one instruction, and on-going feedback (Pappas, 2009). The purpose of instruction is to develop learning at three levels: surface, deep, and transfer (Fisher & Frey, 2016) with transfer of learning being the goal. Providing alternatives needed to include reflections on matching specific routines with the appropriate level of learning. A variety of strategies to deliver instruction would provide alternative methods to reach each student in the classroom while maintaining high expectations for all regardless of the ability levels.

Developing Systematic Support Systems

Indicators of high-quality programs are worth the examination in creating equitable access to education. Academic language is developed using language frames and discussions to increase the level of conversational quality. How language is used by teachers and students indicated the meeting of the goals (Frey & Fisher, 2010). Implementing strategies to check for understanding, scaffolding instruction, and providing corrective feedback contributes to the supportive learning for the diverse population present in the classrooms.

At a systems level, developing a vision would be necessary to build systems of support for improving the instructional practices and establishing mutual understanding of the indicators of success (Frey & Fisher, 2010). Response to Intervention (RTI), a scientific and research-based program, assists in identifying the needs of the students by collecting data through screening, offering appropriate interventions, and progress-monitoring to inform further modifications. Progress monitoring is an essential component of RTI. Rinaldi, Averill, and Stuart (2011) reported the structure of the RTI model as built on the layers or tiers ascending with the objective of bringing majority of students to proficiency in Tier One. Tier Two consists of providing supplemental teaching or interventions as needed in case of a student's inadequate response to learning the core curriculum. Tier Three includes intensive individualized instruction either within the general education mainstream classrooms or in the designated programs for the special needs students. Each tier entail systems of progress-monitoring to support the students.

Developing Concrete Targets

Additionally, to promote inclusive education, equity includes having access to education based on concrete targets for academic and social-emotional progress. Methods for curricular planning need to be examined conducive to building equity in the instruction. Backwards design begins by identifying the standards and objectives including assessment tools or strategies (Pappas, 2009) to develop concrete targets. Developing skeletal structures of the curriculum assisted in developing the targets (Guskey, 2009). The skeletal structure consisted of essential core of the standards at each grade level. To avoid mechanistic teaching, the recommendation was to write the essential learning goals in broad terms to be agreed on by the subject-area educators. These curricular skeletons lead to developing the specific target areas.

An important part of establishing the targets is to consider the evidence of learning to measure the achievement of learning goals. Students need to demonstrate the understanding with participation in activities, artifacts, and the recall of facts in order to continue progressing on the continuum of standards (Marcoux, 2011). Portfolios were reported to be the ideal repository of evidence to demonstrate on-going development toward meeting the essential standards (Marcoux, 2011). Agreements on the development of a curricular skeleton and instruments of gathering evidence will lead to developing short-term and long-term targets at the organizational level.

Educational equity can be achieved by supporting the learning of diverse students through methods such as scaffolding, progress monitoring, establishing clear targets, and methods of demonstrating understanding at the higher cognitive levels. Clark (2018) emphasized the importance of the "knowledgeable other" or the teacher in learning to occur. Establishing equity needed to consider professional development for teachers to strengthen and enhance the programs.

21st-Century Teaching and Learning

The definition of 21st-century education, driving the educational initiatives in the United States, was established by the Partnership for 21st-Century Skills (P21) framework. The P21 framework advocated for all students to be prepared in competencies necessary for transitioning from school to college and career (Donovan, Green, & Mason, 2014; Hunt, 2013). Support systems established at the organizational level and identifying student outcomes were essential to implementing the competencies in teaching. Additionally other existing frameworks informing the 21st-century competencies are from EnGauge 21st-Century Skills, Organization for Economic Cooperation and Development (OECD), and United Nations Educational, Scientific, and Cultural Organization (UNESCO) (Chalkiadaki, 2018). Some of the common skills present in these multiple frameworks, as compiled by (Chalkiadaki, 2018), are creativity, critical and divergent thinking, collaboration, civil competence in becoming a global citizen understanding diversity, digital competence, leadership and entrepreneurship, communication in multiple languages, physical and emotional well-being, and more. The four Cs entailing communication, creativity, critical thinking, and collaboration are the focus of this chapter as presented in the framework of Partnership for 21st-Century Skills (P21) (Donovan et al., 2014).

The Essential Components

Additional necessary structured systems of support to develop the four Cs of 21st-century competencies include the alignment of standards and assessment, curriculum and instruction, providing professional development for teachers, and developing a learning environment compatible with the recommendations of the framework (Hunt, 2013). Achievement outcomes need to be based on the required areas of learning and innovation skills including the four Cs of communication, collaboration, critical thinking, and creativity, along with information media and technology skills (Hunt, 2013). The components of the 21st-century education posed a challenge for educators to reform instructional practices in order to develop the competencies for all students regardless of the ability level to meet the EFA goals at the local and national levels.

The Four Cs

From the areas listed under 21st-century competencies in P21, the components of four Cs (Donovan et al., 2014) had a direct impact on the classroom instruction leading to developing life and career skills while embedding technology within the learning environment. Creativity, one of the four Cs, is defined as innovation conducted through the process of designing and revising the prototypes while critical thinking is a necessary component connected to problem-solving (Dhir, 2019). Collaboration and communication or collaborative communication, other components of the four Cs, are based on social interactions considered essential to learning according to the tenets of Constructivism (Dewey & Jackson, 1990) and multimedia resources can enable collaboration and communication (Dhir, 2019).

While integration of technology is unavoidable in the context of the modern world, the initial phase of learning needs to begin with social interactions situated in the realm of the four Cs. The technology enters the world of learning as a tool for developing the innovations further, recording the ideas, communicating and presenting the findings, and reflecting on the learning. During a Visual and Performing Arts (VAPA) training with the Disney Imagineers, I asked the legendary Marty Sklar (contemporary of Walt Disney) of his views on the use of technology versus hands-on experience in the innovative creations at Disneyland. My concern was based on the prevalent views of educators associating the time spent on computer to 21st-century education. Marty Sklar's response was consistent with constructivist views. He considered technology essential to Disney films, live shows, and theme park innovations, but the role of technology was to be used as a supportive tool. Human experiences were important to innovation prior to selecting appropriate technical tools to enhance the functions of the designs. The importance of sharing this anecdote is to reinforce the idea of experience as a basis for developing cognition and enriching the learning through technology in the context of a classroom. The four Cs of the P21 framework engage the students in learning through experiential process in a way which leads to the use of technology as a tool (Donovan, Green, & Mason, 2014; Henriksen, Mishra, & Fisser, 2016) to improve creation and presentation. Technology, by itself, is insufficient to fulfill the development of 21st-century competencies associated with the four Cs.

Teacher Perceptions and Role in Inclusive Education

Teachers have been playing an important role in driving school programs related to the students with learning disabilities. The attitudes and perceptions held by the educators could influence the instructional choices which impact the students. Defining the role of an instructor in teaching a student with special needs was important in guiding the discussion. A general education teacher in a full inclusion classroom was considered to hold a primary role in educating all the students regardless of the classifications. A special education teacher held a supportive role of leading the educational teams to provide individualized guidance to students with severe disabilities (Ruppar, Roberts, & Olson, 2017). The collaboration between the general education and the special education teacher has been an effective strategy where the perspectives of both teachers led to the positive results with an outcome of increased achievement for the students (Xin, Hunt, Thouless, & Tzur, 2018).

Teachers have been facing challenges such as difficulty implementing the non-negotiable aspects of special education including teaching a student with special needs using the individualized plan (Bartlett, Otis-William, & Sim, 2015) while addressing the needs of the students in the general education program simultaneously. Learning about the characteristics of students with disabilities, understanding the influence of culture and traditions on all individuals adding to the layers of inclusion and diversity, and modifying the classroom environment to accommodate students with special needs are associated with what teachers need to know for an effective instructional program (Scott & Temple, 2017). The challenging task of teaching special education students within the general education setting can be achieved by implementing appropriate teaching methods conducive to inclusivity.

The characteristics of expert teachers, who instruct students struggling with academic or social areas, are described as innovative problem-solvers. Context-specific expertise of an educator can lead to students to develop deep knowledge of the required content (Ruppar, Roberts, & Olson, 2017). An individualized instruction could occur by developing positive relations with the students and becoming familiar with their attitudes and abilities. According to Ruppar, Roberts, and Olson (2019), developing an awareness of students' strengths and struggles can be beneficial in forming relations. Curriculum organization and instructional methods need to reform to build an inclusive environment welcoming diversity in schools.

Diversity Embedded in the Curriculum

The New Generation Science Standards (NGSS) and the Common Core State Standards (CCSS), implemented in the American public-school system, inherently value teaching across disciplines. Integration centered around literature could facilitate the connections between the NGSS and CCSS and the building of diverse mindset. The idea of diversity is not limited to a day celebrating the food and festivals of various cultures but is, instead, a curricular design enabling the students to build skills necessary for global citizenship (Meyer & Rhoades, 2006) inclusive of the special-needs students representing a slice of diversity in the world. Embedding respect for diversity in curriculum by using literature in the integrated units of study as a reference can provide students with a vantage point when learning the required content.

Reflections on Diverse Education

Respect for differences and awareness of similarities needs to become the norm to be taught through the curriculum-based lessons which raise the issues of diversity in an authentic manner to strengthen learning. Ford (2014) emphasized two main goals of education focused on diversity and inclusion. One goal was for the students to learn about others around them, and the second goal was to learn about themselves (personal biases and views). In increasingly diverse nations around the globe, educational institutions need to use curriculum to combat stereotypes and skewed cultural representations.

Literature used in the units of study could have images, plots, languages, morals and values, conflicts, and characters leading to an unintentional biased view toward students of diverse populations. When I immigrated to the United States at 14 years of age, I was enrolled in an English class where students were assigned the reading of A Christmas Carol. I interpreted the novel's storyline as representative of the society's views advocating the mainstream rejection of diverse beliefs. This interpretation led to pretending my family celebrating Christmas to avoid the risk of being identified as Scrooge among peers. Rudyard Kipling's Jungle Book was another offensive representation of the people of the Indian subcontinent as wild and uncivilized representative of the stereotypes existing in the colonial mindset. Students with special needs struggle with perceptions and stereotypes prevalent in the society. Mass shootings in the United States often lead to the discussions on mental health issues assuming the attacker to have such issues.

Molly's Pilgrims is a book on cultural diversity and would be an appropriate addition to the units of study where the issues of American identity are explored. Island of the Blue Dolphins provides a historical fiction examining the effects of the European colonialism on the North American tribes leading to the extinction of some of the cultures. Promoting literature in the curriculum which served to explore the issues of diversity rather than imposing majority values is needed in curriculum designs. More literature on diversity in society is needed for the elementary school students which includes characters with physical or emotional challenges as well. Theodore Taylor's chapter book for young readers entitled The Cay is about survival of two individuals (young white blind boy and an elderly black West Indian man) learning about each other as they are stranded on an island. Integrating books with themes of diversity allows students to experience the struggles of others and form personal interpretations. Fraise and Brooks (2015) asserted the educational institutions had traditionally imposed the dominant value systems. This needed to change to include the personal life experiences and views through literary reflections influencing inclusive education.

Diversity in a Unit of Study

A unit of study I had developed during my study of design-based learning at California Polytechnic University, Pomona provides an example of diversity in curriculum. Prior to teaching the first learning experience, the unit began with a background-building design challenge where students had to construct a creature with physical parts which helped it to move, get energy, and protect itself. Upon completion of the designs, each student's unique creature met the three criteria items. The designs had similarities and differences, and students respected each other's designs recognizing different ways each qualified as a creature. The culturally relevant pedagogy promoted the inclusion of students' diverse views embedded in the learning experiences (Chenowith, 2014) as represented by various designs qualifying as a creature. The conversation was extended to relate to the diversity of American citizens in terms of race, ethnicity, religion, language, and disabilities. To evaluate the diversity embedded in curriculum, the framework shown in Figure 1 can facilitate assessment.

The framework in Figure 1, designed to evaluate inclusivity domains, is inspired by the article of Meyer and Rhoades (2006) with a purpose of strengthening the integration of diverse education in the curriculum. According to the authors, diversity needs to be an integral part of the curriculum design and not to be ignored as an optional topic. The characteristics of including diverse learning styles and self-advocacy were consistently evident in the design lessons. Students created creatures based on individual prior knowledge, skills, subject knowledge, and life's experiences following a universally set criteria for each design challenge. Diversity was in action during the design activities as the students modified the models based on observing others, listening to peers justify how the individual creatures met the design criteria based on the unique physical external parts, and appreciating the different solutions for the same criteria. Meyer and Rhoades (2006) provided a definition of diversity in education to include developing members of society who can think critically and are socially active. Tasks where students innovate solutions, such as designing of a creature, are conducive to engaging all ability levels since the completion process is based on the individual potential of a learner rather than an external directive of right and wrong choices.

Figure 1. Curriculum diversity evaluation framework

Curriculum Diversity Evaluation Framework

Evaluation Framework Rubric	Scoring			NGSS Report Evaluation
1=Barely 2=Inconsistently	3= Consistently			
Includes diverse learning styles	1	2	3	All learning experiences included engineering design challenges where students created prototypes based on the individual skills, techniques, materials, and knowledge.
Promotes self-advocacy	1	2	3	Consistently, the tasks prompts the student to revise and justify the design modifications with the student assuming the role of an expert of the design.
Teaches citizenship	1	2	3	Some tasks implicitly taught a sense of community building through respecting other's designs and the places of the origins, but needs to be more explicit.
Develops an understanding of diversity of views and values in one community.	1	2	3	The tasks referred only to the engineered creatures. The unit needs more literature choices including the diversity of views on how cultures perceive the role of animals in their lives.

Bias in Curriculum

Some implicit components of bias were unintentionally included in a life-science unit I had developed to teach about animals. The biased areas were not explicit enough to be noticed at first. Learning experience on the classification of the animals included a sorting activity where students had to create groups based on physical traits. One of the items provided for sorting was a picture of a human family along with the pictures of animals. Some students struggled with the idea of perceiving humans as animals, whereas the others were comfortable with the idea of classifying humans as animals. My response to the students' concern was of affirming humans as animals based on scientific knowledge. This was an example of imbalanced approach where one biased view dominated the learning of the students (Meyer & Rhoades, 2006).

Realizing that for some students, viewing humans as animals could pose a conflict between the personal beliefs and the ideas established in the curriculum. The complexity of this issue is caused by religious beliefs beyond the cultural aspects representing diversity of values present in student populations. Being sensitive to the multiplicity of beliefs and ways of life through the spoken words, images presented in literature and other media, and the inclusion of the authenticity of students in performance tasks can develop inclusive learning environment. To curb the non-inclusive nature of my response, I allotted time to allow the students to present their views in a discussion format and write a persuasive essay on their position whether humans can or should not be classified as animals advancing the writing and language skills.

MAIN FOCUS OF THE CHAPTER

Inclusive Teaching

Teaching in a full-inclusion classroom could necessitate the employment of a variety of methods to meet the goals of the individualized plans as written for special needs students. According to Ledford et al. (2016), some students may learn best with direct instruction to acquire the necessary skills, and others might consider learning using a variety of methods with on-going reinforcement. Regardless of the instructional methods, providing a relevant context for the learning to occur was essential (Ledford et al., 2016). Selecting teaching methods is based on the specific needs of the students where instruction centers on the appropriate levels: surface, deep, or transfer (Fisher & Frey, 2016). The initial surface teaching would progress over time to deep learning and finally to the level of transfer where skills learned in one context can be generalized to other situations. For this progression to occur, the learning needed to consist of authentic problem-solving (Smith, 2016) giving students an opportunity to experience the concepts as relevant to personal lives.

An essential component of instructional setting was to arrange the class into groups for the purpose of collaboration or for instructional efficiency. Groupings could be in forms of a large whole class group, small group with four to five students, or in an individual one on one setting. Ledford et al., (2016) recommended the students to experience a variety of group settings along with the one on one setting. Learning in a variety of settings was considered ideal to support students with disabilities such as autism. "Efficiency of instruction" could be achieved by students interacting with peers and academically and socially benefitting from the interaction (Ledford et al., 2016) beyond the dependence on the direct instruction from the teacher as the only source of learning. In employing the collaborative and individual learning settings, monitoring the progress of the special-needs students would be based on the considerations related to the individual students.

Universal Design for Learning (UDL) method is based on neuroscience research involving neutral networks: recognition network, strategic network, affective network. The recognition network is concerned with fact gathering and categorizing. Organizing and expressing ideas is a part of the strategic network and connecting learning to emotional experiences is associated with the affective network (Scott & Temple, 2017). Implementing the three networks to deliver effective instruction at the conceptual level involved providing students with multiple means of representation of the same concept, multiple means of actions related to the concept, and multiple means of engagement with the concept. The freedom of accessing various representations of the concept created multiple opportunities for the struggling students to comprehend the complexities of a new concept.

Integrating reading and writing across the curricular areas was associated with developing literacy across disciplines. Artistic expression found in poetry and music facilitated the exploration of language in a creative manner (DeHart, 2019). Students with disabilities learned by relating to the concept and to the instructor on a personal level. The importance of teachers getting familiar with the students' likes and dislikes was important in developing relations with students (Ruppar, Roberts, & Olson, 2017). Allowing students to express their thinking artistically, as included in writing tasks, engaged students in learning through personally connecting to the assignments (DeHart, 2019). Halcrow (2018) established the connection between art and language as employing common cognitive processes. Tasks involving drama, role play, music, and other forms of art could bring relevance to oral language leading to the development of writing. Artistic expression developed skills of experimentation, experiencing language, and demonstrating learning through authentic tasks (Halcrow, 2018).

21st-Century Education and Inclusivity

21st-century learning needs must be examined through the shifts in the employee evaluations of the competencies required for today's work environment. Students with special needs are a part of this century's workforce along with their peers and need the skill development compatible with the demands of the society. According to Aslan (2015), employee observations and evaluations include the employee's ability to adapt, self-direct, be accountable and responsible, the degree of work quality and entrepreneurship, and social and intercultural skills. The focus of these evaluations is on individual characteristics and on the skills necessary for the job. Aslan (2015) stressed the schools, in addition to the skill-building, must integrate the recommendations of the Partnership for 21st Century Learning (P21) consisting of the four Cs of communication, collaboration, critical thinking, and creativity. The recommendations are applicable to all students including students with learning challenges.

The 21st century competencies of knowledge, skills, and expertise include the emphasis on academics along with the focus on life-long learning. The four C's of critical thinking, communication, creativity and innovation, and collaboration were the key ideas of the 21st-Century teaching and learning (Aslan, 2015). According to the author, developing independence, attitude of teamwork, empathy, punctuality, reliability, patience, digital skills, and presentation and discussion skills can strengthen the preparation for the jobs which might be in the market in the future. Organizing curriculum, instructional methods, and assessment as an aligned system will benefit the students with special needs.

Curriculum Development

Keeping the student needs in the forefront, experiences included in the curriculum must follow and be followed by other experiences. According to Soto (2015), the curriculum development process begins by establishing the rationale before setting the goals and objectives of the curriculum. Followed by the goals, the instructional strategies need to be compatible with teaching thinking skills and social attitudes before assessing the student performance.

Curriculum development is based on the needs of the students along with the needs of the society. According to Archambault and Masunaga (2015), Curriculum mapping tools could facilitate the development by including components allowing content analysis of the study. Visual representation of the program structure could be presented in sequential phases of laying the foundation, initiating the process of structuring the program, and integration of the system with skills and assessments. Organizing curriculum is the responsibility of the general education and special education teachers to identify short-term and long-term goals. Achieving the goals in the context of 21st-century education is dependent upon teaching methods which allow the integration of the four Cs.

Instructional Practices

Adaptation of appropriate instructional strategies need to consider the needs of each student. Familiarity with diverse student population with regards to race, ethnicity, language, and ability can lead to developing background knowledge necessary for designing instruction (Fisher & Frey, 2012). Along with building the background knowledge, the importance of teaching content area literacy is instrumental to develop 21st-century competencies. Ming (2012) considered instruction which consists of integrated curriculum across disciplines with having the potential to foster higher cognitive dimensions of critical thinking and problem-solving skills. The other strategies for developing content area strategies were authentic writing, collaborative tasks, discussions, graphic organizers, visual representations, and relevant textual sources. Rigorous instruction is not only reserved for students in the general education but is equally important for students in the special education programs.

I have taught students in mainstream general education classroom who were diagnosed with Attention Deficit Hyperactivity Disorder (ADHD) or autism of various degrees on the spectrum. Some students were successful with supportive interventions provided in the classroom such as proximity of seating, frequent monitoring, contract with rewards and consequences, sensory cushions, chewing gum to reduce anxiety, and more. Students with more intense needs were assigned an instructional paraprofessional personnel to support the academic and social needs of the learner in the classroom and on the playground. Rigorous instruction was implemented through modification of assignments by granting extended time, adjusting the length of the task, breaking the task in smaller chunks, and providing small group or individualized instruction. Identification of a student as a learning disabled or being diagnosed with other conditions does not translate to exclusion from being educated and being challenged in relation to the individual abilities.

Assessment

With the changing world, the assessment practices must change to evaluate the competencies as suited for the modern workplace. With reduced focus on testing rote learning and increased focus on experiential learning, assessments have been developed through two state consortia including Partnership for Reading for College and Career (PARCC) and Smarter Balanced Assessment Consortium (SBAC) (Pellegrino, 2014) as summative, annual standardized testing in California. The assessments are designed to reflect the expectations of the modern world as mentioned by the Gordon Commission of 2013. The standardized assessments are administered not only to assess the performance of individual students but to measure the educational organization's overall program as well. Pellegrino (2014) reported the formative assessments to measure individual achievement in the form of unit or end of the grading period. As a teacher who has worked with special needs students, the formative assessment is not only at the end of unit or grading period, but throughout the term. Traditional selected response assessments with multiple choice test items may inform the educators of the student's ability of recalling facts, but balanced assessments are needed to include multiple representations of student knowledge including performance-based tasks.

Traditional or alternative assessments can coexist depending on the purpose of evaluation. The three types of processes (networks) involved in learning such as recognition network, strategic network, and affective network (Scott & Temple, 2017) may require variations in the forms of assessment. To assess recognition network, a traditional assessment with selection of a response might suffice to assess learning of facts. But the assessment of strategic network will demand a demonstration of organizing and expressing ideas in form of an essay. Affective network associated with emotions will follow a problem-based experience where performance-based assessment will be appropriate.

Another reason for balancing assessment practice with a mixture of traditional and alternative assessments is to provide students with an opportunity to represent understanding using multiple means of engagement, action, and expression (Scott & Temple, 2017). In some cases, peer interaction in a small group could provide information on an individual student in the context of a group (Ledford et al., 2016). Accurate assessment of learning is essential to fulfill a component of systematic instruction (Ledford et al., 2016). No universal assessment method exists as the most effective system to evaluate the performance of special needs learners. The commonality between traditional or alternative assessment is to evaluate cognitive processes involved in the fact gathering phase of learning or at the stage of making connections requiring higher level thinking.

In addition to assessing student performance, program-level evaluation will benefit the educational organizations. Soto (2015) described the assessment of the instructional practices to be implemented for the purpose of evaluating the meeting of the established objectives. The author suggested assessing the instructional process at the beginning and at the end through documents and interviews. Documents of tests, questionnaires, artifacts, samples of work, and records along with observations and interviews provide evidence for evaluating the instructional program. From the scholarly literature, the assessment practices included program evaluations along with individual achievements.

The changing world has shifted the curriculum, instruction, and assessment practices. The challenges continue to be present in meeting the necessary shifts through the employment of appropriate teaching methods. Pellegrino (2014) lamented the financial resources used in producing large scale tests and in conducting research and development studies to produce the tests along with the loss of instructional time in administering the tests. The changing educational environment will need to confront the challenges obstructing progress requiring the examination of teaching practices including methods advocating standards-based curriculum integration.

Unpacking Standards

21st century educational shifts are embedded in the Common Core standards. Klock (2010) described the standards movement including the Common Core standards as developed by the subject specialists from national organizations of math and English teachers. The developers of the standards have claimed a non-prescriptive nature of the standards and did not provide any methodological information to facilitate the instructional practices. Through the process of unpacking or analyzing, teachers will be able to understand the content and skill-based details of the standard. The depth of understanding could lead to integration of common themes across the subject-specific content.

Curriculum Integration

Klock (2010) pointed at a disadvantage of Common Core standards to have emphasized math and English leaving other content areas behind. For that reason, planning the curriculum needed integration with social science, science, and other disciplines. The integration of math and science was implemented in a first-grade full-inclusion classroom where the students (general and special education) learned about the plant structure and the idea of biomimicry through the combination of three-dimensional solids.

Standards: CCSS and NGSS

Math: 1.G.2 (CCSS) Compose two-dimensional shapes (rectangles, squares, trapezoids, triangles, half-circles, and quarter-circles) or three-dimensional shapes (cubes, right rectangular prisms, right circular cones, and right circular cylinders) to create a composite shape, and compose new shapes from the composite shape. (Students do not need to learn formal names such as right rectangular prism.)

Science: 1-LS1-1. (NGSS) Use materials to design a solution to a human problem by mimicking how plants and/or animals use their external parts to help them survive, grow, and meet their needs. Examples of human problems that can be solved by mimicking plant or animal adaptations could include designing clothing or equipment for protection such as mimicking the shape of a tree to design an umbrella.

Integrated Lesson

The most essential component of an integrated instructional plan is the combination of prescriptive and descriptive designs of the curriculum. Stewart and Varner (2012) defined prescriptive curriculum centered around the idea of what should be learned, and the descriptive curriculum was concerned with the actual experiences in the classroom. Common Core standards have moved beyond the experiences focusing on application of knowledge (Stewart & Varner, 2012). Creating a narrative of problems, students learned about plants and shapes through the conceptual connections between the two standards.

Lesson Procedures: Classroom Example

Step 1: Students reviewed the names of two-dimensional and three-dimensional shapes connecting to their learning from kindergarten standards. Using picture cards and the shape blocks, the shapes were discussed using descriptive properties such as flat and curved surfaces and the number of faces and edges.

Step 2: Students were provided three-dimensional shapes to design shelters for their simulated nation named STEM Land with states such as coast, valley, desert, mountains, rainforest, and islands. The students belonged to the various states as citizens. The solution was necessary for constructing a shelter for the scientists who worked outdoors to study plants. Students designed the shelters by combining three-dimensional figures to protect the scientists from the weather conditions and other dangers.

Step 3: Students drew the shelter designs in the Plant Journal and described each shape solving a specific problem and assigning a justification for using the shapes for specific purposes. As an example, a cylinder might function as a water storage, a cube might make a food storage system, and a triangular pyramid could provide protection based on the pointy vertices on each end.

Step 4: A new problem was noticed by the scientists of STEM Land concerning the cutting of the forests causing harm to the environment. To work on the solution, students needed to design shape forests. Using the net patterns of the three-dimensional figures, students cut and formed the shapes.

Step 5: In the Plant Journal, students drew an illustration of a plant and labeled all external parts: roots, stem, leaves, flower, fruit, and thorns. They also included the description of the function of each part to help the plant survive and grow.

Step 6: Students worked in groups of four to analyze which three-dimensional solid figure could function as a root to absorb water, as a stem to carry water, as a leaf to make food, as a flower to attract insects to pollinate, as a fruit to store seeds, and as thorns for protection. This information was organized in the Plant Journals in categories and provided justifications for choosing certain shapes for certain functions similar to the plants. For example, many students selected cylinder to function as a stem based on the straw like shape of a cylinder.

Step 7: After each group developed a consensus on the shapes mimicking the plant function, each individual student built a shape plant following the model decided as a group. They illustrated the shape plant in the Plant Journal labeling each shape responsible for a certain function.

Step 8: Each group created a shape forest by placing all the shape plants on a tag board.

Opportunities for Extension

Students drew the shapes with all curved surfaces, all flat surfaces, and shapes with both curved and flat surfaces existing in the shape forest. Writing opinion paragraphs was taught to build skills of argument having students pursuade one shape forest better than the others by providing reasons for the claim. 21st-century teaching required a change in the curriculum planning and teaching practices (Stewart & Varner, 2012) where students must justify claims and confront counter-claims.

Unpacking the standards was essential in identifying connections between the two content areas. Integrating math and science, as discussed in the example, involved students by collaborating and communicating with each other to reach consensus. The critical thinking and creativity were involved throughout the instructional steps. The CCSS and NGSS standards were not designed to direct the teachers with an implementation method. Curriculum integration provided a path to include creativity, critical thinking, collaboration, and communication known as the four Cs.

SOLUTIONS AND RECOMMENDATIONS

Content through Action (CTA): A Teaching Method

CTA method is an ideal method for creating a learning environment which could engage the general education and special education students. The method encompasses the research supporting the role of the teacher as a guide, on assigning tasks embedded with authenticity and social interaction prior to teaching the content, and the integration of the multiple disciplines under a unifying theme. The three-dimensional process of the CTA method began with an experience addressing a problem and proceeded to teach content through the action-based experience.

Teaching using the CTA method engages the students through a social experience of problem-solving. Students prefer learning in an environment where an interactive experience leads the learning rather than a lecturing method (Sedden & Clark, 2016) where an instructor delivers information without allowing the students to experience the concept. The experiential learning consists of having direct experiences with the real-world problems to consider the personal views and the perspectives of others (Dhir, 2019). To accomplish the conceptual development, Content through Action (CTA) method (Dhir, 2019) was implemented embedding multiple strategies into a systematic approach.

Figure 2 includes an overview of an experience from a unit of study on being a socially responsible citizen which was implemented in the primary grades. Students assumed the role of community citizens as shown in Figure 2. The example consisting of the integration across disciplines to teach content-based lessons is included. The applicability of the CTA method is adaptable to any age or ability level of learning and can be adjusted to remove or add subject areas appropriate to the unit.

CTA method allowed the students to learn through the narrative style sequence of experience enabling the content to be presented in a comprehensible manner. The narrative-based sequence assisted in connecting the emotions to the abstract concepts from the required content as an interaction of the self with the society (Dhir, 2019). The transformation of the abstract ideas in the curriculum into the concrete experience will be beneficial to the special-needs students. Allowing multiple representations of a concept (Scott & Temple, 2017) is present in the CTA method. The multiplicity of the prototype designs and revisions was an integral component engaging the students on an authentic level which is necessary for the learning to occur. According to Dhir (2019), all students had the ability to learn based on the teaching methods combined with the efforts of the student.

The CTA method emphasized the role of teachers as a strategic step prior to launching instruction. Sifting through various curricular areas to plan a six to eight week-long unit, the challenge for the teacher is to connect the important concepts under one experience (Dhir, 2019). Role of a teacher in creating a narrative approach for the purpose of unifying the separate subjects is supported by seminal authors. Bruner (1986) considered teaching math or science without the humanistic stance as impossible since human mind employs language to express understanding. Gardner (2000) emphasized the need to integrate arts and sciences for the learning to be enhanced and transformation to occur. The special needs students can benefit from the integrated units embedded with a narrative involving problem solving. The process allows individual teacher to be able to design units considering the needs of the students in the classroom and integrate the required curriculum within the unit.

CTA method emphasizes the experience of a concept or a problem to occur prior to learning facts. Bruner (1986) promoted the idea of organizing human experiences using a narrative format as an interactive connection between the views of the self and the social world. Figure 3 includes the CTA process model using matryoshka dolls to represent the flow of the learning process where the largest doll contains the universal idea descending toward the smallest doll including the revision stage of the thinking process. The sequential flow consists of multiple stages of the experiential phase: principle container, problem and research container, action container, evaluate and research container, and revised action container (Dhir, 2019).

The students can experience the math concepts through the stages of the experience. Following the process, as shown in Figure 3, the students experience the broad unifying idea of preservation for the purpose of integrating social studies and science content of nature, artifacts, and ideas. Building a prototype of a preservation structure and researching other systems of preservation, students can develop an understanding of the design and function of the structures. The direct math instruction occurred in the next phase (See Figure 2). The idea of preservations serves as an example and can be replaced with other universal ideas as core concepts to integrate the segmented subjects based on the instructional needs.

A learner's role was emphasized in the CTA-based learning process. Having to reexamine the understanding from different perspectives through prototype building and conducting research, a learner is placed in a setting where experience is combined with research. Students learning through experience and research accomplish gaining the conceptual and procedural information simultaneously (Lynch, Chin, & Blazer, 2017). This unique journey of experiencing a concept and building a prototype through research allows the learner to shape an action and refine it through the process and increase the understanding along the way (Gopaul, 2011).

Figure 2 shows the overview of the learning process including the dimension of content learning after experiencing the concept. This dimension embedded two strategies: The integration of the four Cs (Donovan et al., 2014) and the content integration including the math strands of measurement and data. When designing the content-related lessons following the experience, the four Cs are employed to build the lesson structure involving the students to collaborate and communicate along with finding solutions to the problems through innovative creative methods.

The example in Figure 2 shows one math lesson in addition to the lessons related to the other subjects. A teacher utilizing the CTA method could expand the math lessons by extending the lesson with other math strands based on the needs of the students. Although the CTA method is more than an intervention program, the teacher may use the method as an intervention model to address the needs of those students lacking conceptual understanding of the subject-specific concepts. The procedural understanding of solving math problems in a traditional drill practice strategy did not help the students increase the mathematical understanding in my classroom. Beginning the unit by embedding the experience first, the conceptual knowledge grew resulting in an increased academic achievement. Employing the CTA method is beneficial in developing a systematic approach to building the conceptual knowledge.

Integrating Technology as a Tool

The competencies necessary for the 21st-century need to be examined to integrate the educational shifts in the instructional practices. Mishra (2013) viewed the 21st-century skills as being compatible to what technological education was equipped to offer to the students including skills such as creativity, flexibility, and independence in learning. My second-grade students in a low achieving and low socio-economic school with at least 95% of the students on free and reduced lunch program were introduced to the Google Classroom. The following year I implemented the use of Google Classroom while teaching first grade students in a school located in an affluent neighborhood. Both classrooms were full inclusion classrooms with general education students and special needs students. The increased participation and motivation to learn from online sources was evident in both schools. The students learned how to navigate through the virtual classroom in a pace that defied my preconceived notions of primary students (general and special needs) learning in an online setting.

Concerns involving the use of Google Classroom with primary-aged students emerged from the assumption of technology being difficult and requiring multiple lessons overtime for the students to begin using various features of the program. Contrary to my concern, students related to the online classroom without requiring reteaching as they explored the platform on their own and learned from peers when faced with a challenge. The state of being in a self-directed learning mode attracted the modern learners as they enjoyed the opportunity to learn in an authentic manner regardless of their designations as general or special needs student.

Frey, Schmitt, and Allen (2012) defined authenticity as having to do with the real world. The sense of control over their own learning authenticated the experience for them as realistic and taking them beyond the multiple-choice worksheets. They controlled the audio-visual resources as they paused the online presentations, replayed for clarity of information, and controlled the volume using the headphones. They were in-charge of participating in the online discussion without waiting to be called on. The self-directed, authentic learning increased the level of engagement.

Mishra (2013) asserted the self-directed learning can lead the students to practice innovation through problem solving and using the online resources to their advantage and is compatible with how the 21st-century students learn. The internal factors of a 21st-century learner include being the agents of their own learning with the supporting external factors of technological resources and problem-based classroom environment. The role of technology is limited to being an instructional strategy or a tool to enrich the CTA experience to benefit the overall learning process.

Figure 2. Content through Action overview reprinted with permission (Dhir, 2019)

Content through Action (CTA) **Overview: Experience Leading to Content Learning** The examples were provided from an integrated curriculum unit using the theme of social responsibility. The overview included the experience phase in the first and second dimensions and focused on the content in the third dimension.	
Dimensions of Study	**Experience and Content Instruction**
1st Dimension: The Experience First **Student's Role:** **Community Citizen**	Students designed a community prototype researching the elements of an existing community. In the context of the prototype community, the students found the potential problems and generated solutions while assuming the role of socially responsible citizens.
2nd Dimension: The Content Next Incorporate instructional structures to include the 4Cs: • Communication • Collaboration • Critical thinking • Creativity	Curriculum Integration Portfolio Examples: The teachers can integrate other subject areas to the list such as art. The special needs students can work individually or in groups with guidance: **Math reasoning and writing:** Measuring the linear dimensions of the community and recording in math journals. **Art:** Illustrate and label the parts of the community **Reading comprehension and writing:** -Writing a descriptive paragraph describing the community and the problems to be solved. -Reading the **science** text book and articles on the topics of how human innovations solved a problem impacting people's daily lives. -Read the **social science** textbook on the topics of community issues and how the issues were solved. Create a timeline of the life of a socially responsible leader. **Using technology:** -Research a present issue in the community and how citizens have been working to solve it. -publish and present the products using a platform such as the Google Classroom slides. -Watch videos and use other resources posted by the instructor for the learners to respond to.

Figure 3. Content through Action method reprinted with permission (Dhir, 2019)

Content through Action (CTA) Method

Part One: The Experience First

A. Content Connections: Teacher examines the content across disciplines to generate the unifying instructional themes

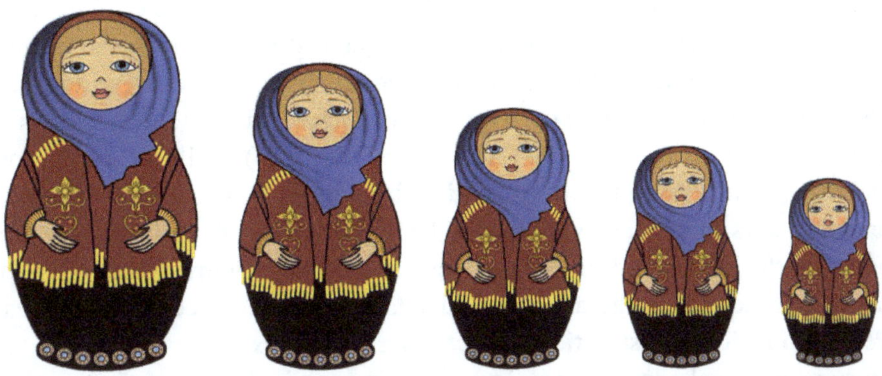

B. Principle container.	C. Problem and Research container	D. Action-Container	E. Evaluate and Research Container	F. Revised Action Container
Unifying multiple content areas	**Launching the Problem**	**Designing the first Prototype**	**Performance standards**	**Designing the revised Prototype**
Example:	Example:	Example:	Example:	Example:
Community Building	Problem: How do we develop a community of citizens who are socially responsible? Research: Examine existing solutions.	Forming a Prototype of a socially responsible community.	Evaluate the prototype against the standards Research the existing solutions again.	Multiple representations of the prototype and follow step E and F with each revision.

FUTURE RESEARCH DIRECTIONS

Changes in the programs for increasing student achievement can only be achieved if the processes are sustained through implementation fidelity. Management of the processes needs the financial as well as non-financial support of various organizations or community members. Continued research concerning teaching methods inclusive of special needs students in mainstream settings will establish the importance for the necessary changes in the instructional practices and may be instrumental in motivating other educators to engage in promoting inclusive education.

The implementation of the Common Core State Standards (CCSS) in the United States has contributed to a wide-spread change in the field of education for the past decade and serves as an example to the international educational community for the importance of building a supportive coalition for a systemic change. CCSS, despite the opposition from the politically conservative and liberal groups, succeeded in establishing its place via the financial support from Bill and Melinda Gates foundation, National Governor's Association, and from the Council of Chief State School Officers (Peterson, Barrows, & Gift, 2016). The support from the consortium has helped in sustaining the changes. Some of the incentive programs such as Race to the Top held contests between states to win rewards based on the level of CCSS implementation. Race to the Top initiative gave waivers to the states in fulfilling the No Child Left Behind requirements (Peterson, Barrows, & Gift, 2016). Building a coalition for policy-level decision making driving the shifts in instructional practices should engage teachers and other stakeholders. Personal views of teachers should also be accounted for in creating program fidelity as teachers are considered the most important component of the learning environment (Anagun, 2018). Further research is recommended in the areas of understanding the perspectives of educators and the stakeholders in regard to inclusive instructional practices.

The 21st-century educational concerns consist of aligning curriculum, instruction, assessment, and the learning environment. Writing a school plan can support accountability toward the desired systemic changes by listing the learning outcomes and the indicators of success. Evaluating the outcomes through local and regional benchmarks, curriculum planning, and appropriate teaching methods can contribute to the long and short-term changes. The school plan needs to be motivating, focused on developing the competencies, and including value-based rewards (Anagun, 2018). Accountability towards the school plan includes examining the role of teachers in the 21st-century classrooms. Using constructivist teaching to design the learning environment and implementing new approaches to learning should be a part of the accountability instead of solely focusing on evaluating the effectiveness of teachers in delivering lessons. Teachers and schools, both, need to be held accountable for integrating the four Cs of communication, collaboration, critical thinking, and creativity as a part of the school plan derived from the Partnership for 21st Century (Anagun, 2018).

CONCLUSION

The importance of inclusive methods of teaching where students with special needs and students from general population interact and learn together is essential for the progress of the society. Establishing an inclusive classroom may be challenging for some educators based on the views towards some intellectual disabilities influenced by the personal beliefs (Barrio, Miller, Ojeme, & Tamakloe, 2009). More information and training in the appropriate teaching methods might lead to including the special needs population within the mainstream classroom with appropriate supports in place, as modeled in the public schools across the United States. Training in effective communication to promote meaningful dialogue, providing accommodations, and collaborating with parents can enable instructors to create a positive learning environment inclusive of diverse students (Barrio, Miller, Ojeme, & Tamakloe, 2009).

Fidelity in sustaining the changes is important in progressing continuously. Community support along with appropriate teaching strategies will be necessary to implement and sustain the changes in integrating the teaching methods compatible with the development of 21st-century competencies. In the United States, CCSS has faced a sizable opposition, but the continuous implementation has established the place for the standards. Fidelity to removing barriers to implementation is necessary and can be achieved through training educators in appropriate teaching methods compatible with the demands of the modern world. Further research in identifying the barriers to implementing the 21st-century competencies is recommended.

ACKNOWLEDGMENT

This chapter is written in dedication to all the special needs students who have helped me to understand that their presence enriched the classroom experience for all their peers and instructors. This research received no specific grant from any funding agency in the public, commercial, or not-for-profit sectors.

REFERENCES

Anagün, Ş. (2018). Teachers' Perceptions about the Relationship between 21st Century Skills and Managing Constructivist Learning Environments. *International Journal of Instruction*, *11*(4), 825–840. doi:10.12973/iji.2018.11452a

Archambault, S. G., & Masunaga, J. (2015). Curriculum mapping as a strategic planning tool. *Journal of Library Administration*, *55*(6), 503–519. doi:10.1080/01930826.2015.1054770

Aslan, S. (2015). Is learning by teaching effective in gaining 21st Century Skills? The views of pre-service science teachers. *Educational Sciences: Theory and Practice*, *15*(6), 1441–1457. doi:10.12738/estp.2016.1.019

Barrio, B., Miller, D., Ojeme, C., & Tamakloe, D. (2019). Teachers' and parents' knowledge about disabilities and inclusion in Nigeria. *Journal of International Special Needs Education*, *22*(1), 14–24. doi:10.9782/17-00010

Bartlett, M., Otis-Wilborn, A., & Sim, N. J. (2015). CCSS: Rigor or righteousness in special education. *Journal of Reading Education*, (3), 23.

Bruner, J. (1986). *Actual minds, possible worlds*. Cambridge, MA: Harvard University Press.

Chalkiadaki, A. (2018). A systematic literature review of 21st century skills and competencies in primary education. *International Journal of Instruction*, *11*(3), 1–16. doi:10.12973/iji.2018.1131a

Chenowith, N. H. (2014). Culturally responsive pedagogy and cultural scaffolding in literacy education. *Ohio Reading Teacher*, *44*(1), 35–40.

Clark, K. R. (2018). Learning theories: Constructivism. *Radiologic Technology*, *90*(2), 180–182. Retrieved from http://www.radiologictechnology.org/content/90/2/180.full.pdf+html PMID:30420576

Cohan, A., & Howlett, C. F. (2017). Global conflicts shattered world peace: John Dewey's influence on peace educators and practitioners. *Education and Culture*, *33*(1), 59–88. doi:10.5703/educationculture.33.1.0059

Croso, C. (2013). Human rights are the key to the world we want. *Adult Education and Development*, *80*, 78–85. Retrieved from http://www.iiz-dvv.de/en/adult-education-and-development/editions/aed-802013-post-2015/articles/human-rights-are-the-key-to-the-world-we-want/

DeHart, J. D. (2019). Two Birds, One Stone: Exploring complex writing through poetry. *Knowledge Quest*, *47*(5), E1–E4.

Dewey, J., & Jackson, P. W. (1990). *The school and society and the child and the curriculum a centennial publication*. Chicago, IL: The University of Chicago Press.

Dhir, H. (2019). Planning curriculum for teaching thinking skills needed for 21st century education. In Handbook of research on critical thinking and teacher education pedagogy (pp. 107-133). doi:1 doi:0.4018/978-1-5225-7829-1.ch007

Donovan, L., Green, T. D., & Mason, C. (2014). Examining the 21st century classroom: Developing an innovation configuration map. *Journal of Educational Computing Research*, *50*(2), 161–178. doi:10.2190/EC.50.2.a

Fisher, D., & Frey, N. (2016). Making learning visible: Reflecting on John Hattie's ideology, new book, and upcoming conference session. International Literacy Association, 33(5).

Fisher, D., Frey, N., & Lapp, D. (2012). Building and activating students' background knowledge: It's what they already know that counts. *Middle School Journal*, *43*(3), 22–31. doi:10.1080/00940771.2012.11461808

Ford, D. Y. (2014). Why education must be multicultural. *Gifted Child Today*, *37*(1), 59–62. doi:10.1177/1076217513512304

Fraise, N., & Brooks, J. S. (2015). Toward a theory of culturally relevant leadership for school-community culture. *International Journal of Multicultural Education*, *17*(1), 6–21. doi:10.18251/ijme.v17i1.983

Frey, B. B., Schmitt, V. L., & Allen, J. P. (2012). Defining authentic classroom assessment. *Practical Assessment, Research & Evaluation*, *17*(2), 1–18. Retrieved from https://pareonline.net/genpare.asp?wh=0&abt=17

Frey, N., & Fisher, D. (2010). Getting to quality: A meeting of the minds. *Principal Leadership*, *11*(1), 68–70. Retrieved from https://www.fisherandfrey.com/journal-publications

Gardner, H. (2000). Project zero: Nelson Goodman's legacy in arts education. *The Journal of Aesthetics and Art Criticism*, *245*(3), 245. doi:10.2307/432107

Gopaul, B. (2011). Distinction in doctoral education: Using Bourdieu's tools to assess the socialization of doctoral students. *Equity & Excellence in Education*, *44*(1), 10–21. doi:10.1080/10665684.2011.539468

Guskey, T. R. (2009). Getting curriculum reform right. *School Administrator*, *66*(11), 38.

Halcrow, K. (2018). Imitation and innovation: Harnessing the principles of music pedagogy for the writing classroom. *Literacy Learning: The Middle Years*, *26*(3), 48–57.

Henriksen, D., Mishra, P., & Fisser, P. (2016). Infusing creativity and technology in 21st century education: A systemic view for change. *Journal of Educational Technology & Society*, *19*(3), 27–37. Retrieved from http://danah-henriksen.com/wp-content/uploads/2016/10/creativity-systemic-view.pdf

Hinzen, H. (2013). Lifelong learning for all – A potential global goal for the post 2015 education and development agendas! *Adult Education and Development*, *80*, 4–9. Retrieved from https://www.dvv-international.de/en/adult-education-and-development/editions/aed-802013-post-2015/articles/lifelong-learning-for-all-a-potential-global-goal-for-the-post-2015-education-and-development-agendas/

Hunt, M. W. (2013). [APP]ETITE for instruction: 21st-century learners in a video and audio production classroom. *Techniques*, *88*(8), 36-40. Retrieved from https://www.questia.com/magazine/1G1-349490089/app-etite-for-instruction-21st-century-learners

Klock, J. (2010). Building novel connections in an increasingly standardized world. *Teacher Librarian*, *38*(2), 15–18.

Ledford, J. R., Barton, E. E., Hardy, J. K., Elam, K., Seabolt, J., Shanks, M., ... Kaiser, A. (2016). What equivocal data from single case comparison studies reveal about evidence-based practices in early childhood special education. *Journal of Early Intervention*, *38*(2), 79–91. doi:10.1177/1053815116648000

Lesar, I. (2015). The role of the arts in Tagore's concept of schooling. *CEPS Journal*, *5*(3), 111-128. Retrieved from https://www.researchgate.net/publication/283659456_The_Role_of_the_Arts_in_Tagore's_Concept_of_Schooling

Lynch, K., Chin, M., & Blazar, D. (2017). Relationships between observations of elementary mathematics instruction and student achievement: Exploring variability across districts. *American Journal of Education*, *123*(4), 615–646. doi:10.1086/692662

Marcoux, E. (2011). Turning the standards toward the student – A metacognition aspect. *Teacher Librarian*, *38*(3), 67–68.

McWilliams, S. A. (2016). Cultivating constructivism: Inspiring intuition and promoting process and pragmatism. *Journal of Constructivist Psychology*, *29*(1), 1–29. doi:10.1080/10720537.2014.980871

Meyer, C. F., & Rhoades, E. K. (2006). Multiculturalism: Beyond food, festival, folklore, and fashion. *Kappa Delta Pi Record*, *42*(2), 82–87. doi:10.1080/00228958.2006.10516439

Ming, K. (2012). 10 Content-area literacy strategies for art, mathematics, music, and physical education. *The Clearing House: A Journal of Educational Strategies, Issues and Ideas*, *85*(6), 213–220. doi:10.1080/00098655.2012.691568

Mishra, P., Fahnoe, C., & Henriksen, D. (2013). Creativity, self-directed learning and the architecture of technology rich environments. *TechTrends*, *57*(1), 10–13. doi:10.100711528-012-0623-z

Mukherjee, M. m. (2017). Global design and local histories: Culturally embedded meaning-making for inclusive education. International Education Journal: *Comparative Perspectives, 16*(3), 32-48. Retrieved from https://www.academia.edu/37807740/Global_Design_and_Local_Histories_Culturally_embedded_meaning-making_for_Inclusive_Education?auto=download

Pellegrino, J. W. (2014). Assessment as a positive influence on 21st century teaching and learning. *Psicologia dell'Educazione*, *20*(2), 65–77. doi:10.1016/j.pse.2014.11.002

Peterson, P., Barrows, S., & Gift, T. (2016). After Common Core, states set rigorous standards. *Education Next*, *16*(3), 9–15.

Pridmore, J. (2009). The poet's school and the parrot's cage: The educational spirituality of Rabindranath Tagore. *International Journal of Children's Spirituality*, *14*(4), 355–367. doi:10.1080/13644360903293572

Rinaldi, C., Averill, O. H., & Stuart, S. (2011). Response to intervention: Educators' perceptions of a three-year RTI collaborative reform effort in an urban elementary school. *Journal of Education-Boston University School of Education,* (2), 43.

Ruppar, A., Roberts, C., & Olson, A. (2017). Perceptions about expert teaching for students with severe disabilities among teachers identified as experts. *Research and Practice for Persons with Severe Disabilities*, *42*(2), 121–135. doi:10.1177/1540796917697311

Scott, L., & Temple, P. (2017). A conceptual framework for building UDL in a special education distance education course. *Journal of Educators Online*, *14*(1), 48–59. Retrieved from https://eric.ed.gov/?id=EJ1133749

Sedden, M. L., & Clark, K. R. (2016). Motivating Students in the 21st Century. *Radiologic Technology*, *87*(6), 609–616. PMID:27390228

Smith, S. (2016). (Re)counting meaningful learning experiences: Using student-created reflective videos to make invisible learning visible during PjBL experiences. *Interdisciplinary Journal of Problem-based Learning*, *10*(1). doi:10.7771/1541-5015.1541

Soto, S. (2015). An analysis of curriculum development. *Theory and Practice in Language Studies*, *5*(6), 1129–1139. doi:10.17507/tpls.0506.02

Stewart, C., & Varner, L. (2012). Common Core and the rural student. *National Teacher Education Journal*, *5*(4), 67–73.

Waddington, D. I., & Weeth Feinstein, N. (2016). Beyond the search for truth: Dewey's humble and humanistic vision of science education. *Educational Theory*, *66*(1/2), 111–126. doi:10.1111/edth.12157

Xin, Y., Hunt, J., Thouless, H., & Tzur, R. (2018). Special Education and Mathematics Working Group. *Conference Papers -- Psychology of Mathematics & Education of North America*, 1515–1525.

KEY TERMS AND DEFINITIONS

Content Through Action (CTA): A constructivist-based teaching method where experiential learning develops the standards-based content knowledge across disciplines. CTA method engages students in learning the 21st-century competencies of critical thinking, creativity, collaboration, and communication.

Diversity: In the context of a classroom, the term diversity is used for a class of students who belong to various racial, ethnic, linguistic, economic, and religious backgrounds along with the differences in academic levels of achievement.

Experiential Learning: A unit of study where experiencing a universal idea through problem-solving drives learning.

General Education: An American public-school classroom instructional model where students are enrolled regardless of diverse backgrounds. Teachers deliver core curriculum to students without any individualized plans for learning.

Inclusive Classroom: A classroom model, where special education students are enrolled in the least restrictive environment of a mainstream general education classroom, is inclusive.

Special Education: An American public-school instructional model where special needs students with Individual Educational Plans (IEP) are supported by resource specialists, instructional aides, speech therapist, psychologist, occupational therapist, and adaptive physical education teacher.

Special Needs: Students with an Individual Educational Plans (IEP) based on the identified conditions or disabilities are classified as special needs students.

Chapter 11
Design Thinking for Technology Supporting Individuals With Neurodevelopmental Disorders in Developing Countries:
Participatory Design for Inclusivity

Adheesh Budree
https://orcid.org/0000-0002-7448-4453
University of Cape Town, South Africa

Harsha Kathard
University of Cape Town, South Africa

ABSTRACT

This research is concerned with analysing the value of using participatory design, and in particular the design thinking methodology, as a basis for the participative development of interfacing technology for use by individuals with neuro-developmental disorders, with a particular focus on developing economies with restrictions in budget and know-how. It becomes crucial as our knowledge expands to ensure that tools developed to assist individuals with neurological disorders to live a full and independent life are designed in conjunction with the users concerned. Inclusive design, however, is not limited to the technology itself, but rather taking into account the individual as well as the wider community in the design. Design needs to also be based in social accessibility to counter stigmas and ableism views. This study found that design thinking has proven to be an effective framework for involving individuals with neuro-developmental disorders to come up with solutions that address their needs and should be used in future implementations in order to assess the results.

DOI: 10.4018/978-1-7998-3069-6.ch011

INTRODUCTION

As medical insight progresses and strengthens, so too does our understanding of neuro-developmental disorders. It becomes crucial as our knowledge expands to ensure that tools developed to assist individuals with neurological disorders to live a full and independent life are designed in conjunction with the users concerned. However, the development cannot be limited to the individual, but caregivers and the wider community as well. This becomes increasingly difficult in developing economies such as South Africa and India, where socioeconomic inequality has led to unequal access to healthcare facilities and services. In these countries it becomes imperative to engage in creative methods in context-responsive practices to ensure equitable healthcare service delivery (Cloete, Wilson, Petersen & Kathard, 2015).

Based on this reality, it is necessary to investigate other methods of design for technology used by individuals with neuro-developmental disorder that are participative and inclusive in nature. According to Newell and Gregor (2000), an inclusive design perspective must include a larger variety of user characteristics and functionality, include representative users, manage accessibility for people with different types of disability, balance accessibility and ease of use for a variety of abilities, clearly specify characteristics and functionality of the overall user group, and provide any additional components for accessibility. Design Thinking is one such methodology and has been successfully used to address technology development for neurodevelopmental disorder users, as is extends User Centred Design to become User Sensitive Inclusive Design, which includes both experimental techniques and effective results communication methods for mainstream researchers and product developers (Newell and Gregor, 2000).

This chapter is concerned with assessing the value of using participatory design, and in particular the Design Thinking methodology as a basis for the participative development of interfacing technology for use by individuals with neuro-developmental disorders, with a particular focus on developing economies with restrictions in budget and know-how. The chapter presents multi-disciplinary literature across both the information technology and medical sciences bodies of knowledge in order to arrive at an assessment and recommendations for implementation of inclusive technology projects for people with intellectual disabilities such as neuro-developmental disorders across the developing world.

BACKGROUND AND RELATED WORK

Intellectual Disabilities and Neuro-developmental Disorders

According to 'International Classification of Functioning, Disability and Health' (ICF) published by the World Health Organization, the term disability is an all-encompassing term that includes activity limitations, physical and mental impairments, and participation restrictions, all which fall into a subset of a larger classification grouping which covers three main areas including environmental factors, body functioning and structure and activities and participation (WHO, n.d.). Mullin, Gokhale, Moreno-De-Luca, Sanyal, Waddington and Faundez (2013) specify neuro-developmental disorder (NDD) conditions as intellectual disabilities that are multifaceted in nature and are normally characterised by impairments in a large number of possible fields. These include cognition, communication, behaviour and/or motor skills. These typically are a result of abnormal brain development. Also falling within the NDD spectrum include communication disorders, intellectual disability, attention deficit/hyperactivity disorder (ADHD), autism spectrum disorder (ASD), and schizophrenia (Mullin et. al., 2013).

Disability in Developing Countries

Mitra (2005) posits a two-way interaction between disability and poverty, namely that disability intensifies the risk of poverty, while socio-economic conditions of poverty increase the risk of disability. In developing countries, disability has been found to be associated with multidimensional poverty and requires policy intervention and education as persons with disabilities account for a large portion of the working age population. However, simultaneously, people with disabilities have been found to have attained lower levels of education and as such experience lower employment rates than those without disabilities (Mitra, 2005; Mizunoya and Mitra, 2013; Mitra, Posarac, and Vick, 2013).

Safety nets play a large part in reaching individuals with disabilities to enable them to participate in opportunities to such as inclusive employment, growth and education. These safety nets include programs such as social insurance, public funding and livelihood programs. Such programs can be instrumental in enhancing the welfare of individuals living with disabilities as well as their caretakers through gaining their own sources of income and in turn giving them greater household bargaining power (Mitra, 2005; Mizunoya and Mitra, 2013; Mitra, Posarac, and Vick, 2013).

However, with a lack of necessary administrative capacity and knowledge in many developing countries, the implementation of such programs proves to be both difficult and costly. Community-based support and programs could be the solution, but in order for them to be successful exclusion and stigmatisation of people with disabilities has to be addressed (Mitra, 2005). Rohwerder (2018) highlighted the main drivers behind stigmatism of people with disabilities in developing countries, both personal and social, as:

- An absence of understanding and awareness of the causes behind disabilities and their related characteristics.
- Cultural or religiously rooted misunderstandings and fallacies around the cause of disabilities often derived from belief structures rooted in cultural or religious, resulting in people with disabilities classified as a source of indignity which has an impact on how they are treated.
- Misconceptions around the nature and abilities of individuals with disabilities, including financial contribution capability.
- The existence of prejudiced legislation and policies that merely reinforce discrimination.
- In many cases, the segregation of individuals with disabilities from mainstream society which entrenches those negative stereotypes.

Rohwerder (2018) further stated that perceptions towards disability differ both within developing countries, and also individual communities, and sometimes within families. Different levels of stigma are associated with differing types of impairments, with the severity of the impairment as well as how the impairment was acquired also playing a role in stigmatization. In sub-Saharan Africa, individuals with severe mental health conditions, albinism, intellectual disabilities and sensory disabilities were commonly found to experience a higher level of stigmatisation than those with physical disabilities. However, disabled individuals who are seen to participate in their communities are faced with less stigma than those with comparatively more severe disabilities. Stigma associated with a combination of gender as well as disability was found to be higher, with disabled female individuals experiencing double the disadvantage as compared to their male counterparts. Attitudes towards disability have also been found to be impacted by socio-economic status, with rural dwelling individuals with disabilities found to encounter more harmful practices than those in urban and metro areas (Rohwerder, 2018).

As such, assistive devices and inclusion awareness can be used to eliminate barriers to participation in communities and employability opportunities, and thus affording many with disabilities a path out of poverty. It has been found that is not necessarily the creation of disability-specific programs that allow for this inclusion, but rather ensuring that mainstream safety net programs are built to be disability inclusive (Mitra, 2005; Mizunoya and Mitra, 2013). Disability-only technology tends to perpetuate an ableist view, which is defined as an inclination to reflect abled individuals as superior to disabled individuals, with detrimental social effect (Shinohara, Kristen, Bennett, and Wobbrock, 2016).

Technology for Disabled People

Information Communications and Technologies (ICT) applications allow disabled individuals to better integrate economically and socially into the communities they belong to. The introduction of mobile phones and tablets have made a ground-breaking new medium for assistive technology widely available. A number of apps relating to disabilities and health are available. These apps, some free and others available for purchase, disseminate key information on subjects concerning disability as well as health issues. An example of such an app for intellectual disabilities is ezTasker, which can be used to notify Alzheimer's patients and individuals with other cognitive disabilities or neuro-developmental disorders to complete daily errands such as watering a plant (Khetarpal, 2014).

Technologies targeted at people with disabilities can be grouped into two categories, namely assistive technologies and accessible technologies. The World Health Organisation (WHO) defines Assistive Technology as technology that is adapted or specially designed to improve the functioning of individuals with disabilities (WHO, n.d.). Assistive technologies are normally proprietary devices built specifically for individulas with disabilities, while accessible technologies are devices or applications that are usable by individuals without disabilities but incorporate a degree of accessibility so that persons with disabilities can also make use of them. Though there are many proprietary assistive technologies on the market, there are fewer off-the-shelf mainstream technologies that incorporate usability for disabled users (Shinohara, Bennett, Pratt and Wobbrock, 2018).

According to Agree (2014), surveys conducted in the United States in the 1990s exposed a high incidence of technology usage among people, specifically adults, with disabilities, as well as finding that the use of multiple devices is commonplace. A study of clients conducted by the California Independent Living Centers (ILCs) found that disability from birth was a highly significant indicator of the acceptance of any technology as well as the number of devices used (Kaye, Yeager and Reed, 2008).

Use of technology by those with intellectual disabilities such as neuro-developmental disabilities have been shown to be less common. According to an American study of adults with intellectual disabilities, only 10% of individuals queried used technological devices, with the incidence lower for individuals with physical disabilities. In addition, the California ILC study found that individuals with intellectual disabilities were significantly less likely than their counterparts with physical disabilities to use technological devices, as well as make use of fewer devices, regulating for a significant number of covariates (Quinn, Behrmann, Mastropieri, Bausch, Ault and Chung, 2009; Wehmeyer, 1998).

The United Nation's Convention on the Rights of Persons with Disabilities (CRPD) has specified that individuals have the right to technology availability in order to ensure their equal and full entitlement of all essential freedoms and human rights. Though, access to relevant technology is currently limited in most countries, moreso in the developing world, with only between 5% and 15% of those requiring access having it freely available (Borg, Lindström and Larsson, 2011).

Participatory Design

User-Centred Design (UCD) allows for focus on the user and the user experience, which in turn allows the developer to focus on inclusion and the needs of the user. In theory, UCD welcomes users to contribute to the development procedure and focus on inclusivity issues associated with disability, providing opportunities for designers to engage with disabled users and gain familiarity with accessibility issues. However, in practice it has been found that few developments have successfully taken into account disabled users, and still focus primarily on able-bodied users (Sharp, Rogers and Preece, 2007).

Limited literature is currently available the use of Design Thinking in a neuro-developmental context. In a literature review conducted by Shinohara et. al. (2016), it has been theorised that disability cannot merely fall into the sphere of mainstream 'user experience', but rather requires a focus on accentuating accessibility and engaging with people with disabilities can assist developers to build more accessible technologies. Unlike mainstream UCD, disability-specific approaches that focus on accessibility design are better suited to cater for disabled users, and individuals with disabilities must be included in the design development itself as part of the overall community of people (Shinohara et. al., 2016).

User Centred Design allows developers to focus on the users as the centre of the design process. By involving people with disabilities as a normal part of such design, the process affords them the dignity of being treated in the same way as any other users of systems. There exists however, the possibility, of division between issues of "disabled rights" and goals and methodologies associated to research. There is a growing awareness of the rights of people with disabilities within the field which have been articulated in the ideas of Participatory Action Research (PAR), with individuals with disabilities involved in setting the research agenda, developing research questions, participating in the research as researchers, advisors, and consultants, testing research ideas, and evaluating the research results (Newell and Gregor, 2000).

User involvement has been found to be fundamental when dealing with individuals with neuro-developmental disorders in order to adequately represent the needs and requirements of these individuals where the condition is typified by communication impairments possibly to the level of being non-verbal learning difficulties, general learning difficulties or difficulties envisioning how they themselves or others might use the artefact (Coon and Watson, 2013).

Participatory design has therefore become key in accessible technology development, where in order to build a detailed view of task and user requirements drove a need for more human-centred design, in which the active participation of disabled users in the development process is required (Maguire, 2001). This involvement can take the form of interviews, focus groups and/or prototype testing which is then followed by repeated system evaluations. Moreover, the focus has shifted from merely the users to a much wider range of stakeholders either directly or indirectly involved in the system. In this way, the participants are not simply sources of information or system testers, but active contributors to the evolution of the system through idea generation and decision making. (Sanders and Stappers, 2008).

Sanders and Stappers (2008) highlight three main innovation strategies together with design methodologies as progressing from a focus on co-design and co-production towards a philosophy of co-creation. Co-design in healthcare propositions an incorporative design including medical professionals, patients and the community who work hand-in-hand throughout the design process, leading to a final solution that is then developed by professional developers. Co-production takes co-design a step further by including the core economy (which includes individual families, grouped neighbourhoods and the overall community), moving the balance of power, resources and responsibility from professionals to individuals. Co-creation occurs when users are fundamental to the planning, design, production and continuous development of accessible technology and services, allowing ordinary people to generate content and shape it to their requirements (Blomkvist and Holmlid, 2010). A key factor in ensuring inclusivity in the design process is practising empathic modelling or design, which was found to support inclusive design (Burçak and Halime, 2014).

Generating lasting and transformative technology for intellectually disabled individuals and their communities require participatory design that allows the questioning of the norms and expectations surrounding service practices and interactions. It requires proper engagement by all key stakeholders when required, allowing users to drive the design process and co-create flexible media or infrastructures that people can inhabit, possess and transform (Blomkvist and Holmlid, 2010).

Design Thinking for Inclusive Design

Design Thinking is a participatory design methodology centred in human participation, problem solving and co-design, and has come to the fore as one of the best human-centred design methodologies for technology development (Brown and Wyatt, 2010). Design thinking is normally used in situations where problems presented are complex and multidimensional making it difficult deal with using run of the mill requirements investigations and solutions. These are often referred to in Design Thinking literature as 'wicked problems' (Rittel and Webber, 1973).

Challenges faced by individuals with intellectual disabilities such as neuro-developmental disorders fall into the 'wicked problem' category in that they are characterised by a large number of intertwined complex issues across a heterogenous group that requires combining not only analytics and creativity but also empathy and understanding to come up with truly innovative (Withell and Heigh, 2013).

The iterative steps to approach a Design Thinking project are depicted in Figure 1 below.

Figure 1. Design Thinking Steps
(Source: https://joeyaquino.wordpress.com/2012/05/23/want-a-crash-course-in-stanfords-design-thinking-here-it-is-for-free-pt-1-empathy/)

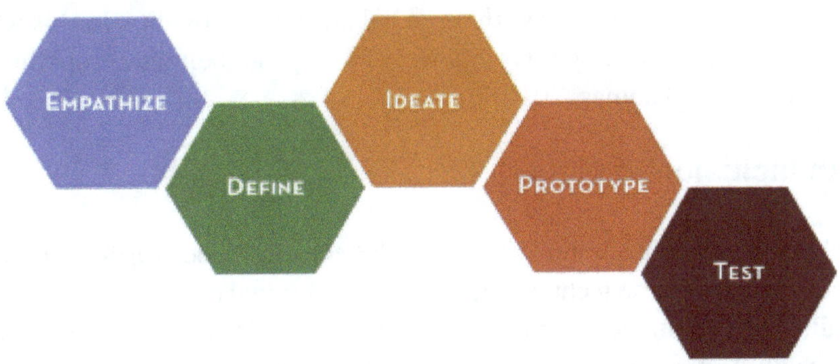

Each step in the process can be explained as follows (Dam and Siang, 2019):

Step 1: Empathise

- The first step is to understand the problem from an empathic perspective. This involves participation from users and experts in the field. Empathy allows for more human-centred design by allowing the user to put aside their own world beliefs to gain better insight into the user and their needs.

Step 2: Define

- The second step allows the designers to collate and understand the information that was gathered during the empathise step in order to define the core issues identified from a human-centred perspective.

Step 3: Ideate

- The Ideate step allows for the generation of ideas from all participants to address the issue. The focus of this step is to think out of the box and be creative in the problem-solving process.

Steps 4: Prototype

- Inexpensive, scaled down versions of possible solution are mocked up and iteratively assessed and refined within the team itself.

Step 5: Test

- Designers/developers and participant evaluators now test the product in an iterative manner to fine tune the final product. Results are often used to not necessarily just find a solution, but to redefine the problems and better understand the user, conditions of use, thought processes, behaviour, and feelings, and in order to empathise.

Empathic design strategies allow for a shift away from designing for the persona of an ideal user to revealing and discovering technological product opportunities for real people. As developers immerse themselves, design ideas come to the fore which provide for relevant design information and support for process ideation. Empathy has been shown to deepen a developer's understanding of people with disabilities, taking into account not only daily activities but social backgrounds, education, and cultural norms that in many cases may differ greatly from their own. By acquiring insight into the disabled people's aspirations, emotions and fears, the developer can draw on critical cues and inspiration which in turn leads to the creation of technology with more balanced functionality. In this way, by employing an empathic design strategy, the developer is empowered to expand their own empathic horizon together with the user (McDonagh and Thomas, 2010).

Designing With Inclusion in Mind

While assistive technologies have been shown to bridge the technical needs gap for people with disabilities, it is increasingly common that these technologies have conventional equals with similar capabilities. As an example, a Braille note taking device that is refreshable has similar functionality to a conventional laptop. By using disability-specific design and development approaches, developers are able to produce technologies that can assist individuals with disabilities, however in most cases due to the specificity of the approach only disabled individuals can use them. This is also the case of mainstream technology. This becomes counterproductive as the technology needs to be inclusive and break down the stigmas associated with ableism (Shinohara et. al, 2016). It becomes clear from literature that inclusion must consider a range of issues, such as disability, race, gender and class which need to be taking into consideration when designing for such a diverse range of people, of which people with disabilities are seldom included.

Research has found that contemporary conventional personal technologies are often still inaccessible, as developers behind these mainstream technologies neglect as a rule of thumb incorporation of accessible design unless specifically to satisfy legal requirements (Crutchfield, 2016). It has thus become fundamental in accessible technology development for individuals with intellectual disabilities to integrate accessibility within the design process and idea generation not as a separate topic, heuristic afterthought or legal obligation, but rather as part of the mainstream development process (Shinohara et. al., 2016). In order to do so, developers need to be exposed to disabled users, their caregivers and support structures and their requirements throughout the development process as it shifts the development thought process though awareness and empathy from exposure (Ludi, 2007; Shinohara et. al, 2016; Waller, Hanson, and Sloan, 2009).

The inclusion of individuals with disabilities in the design process has demonstrated a means to assist developers build accessible technologies. However, by only focusing on just disability outputs can result in creating separation of technologies between abled and disabled users, perpetuating ableism and othering of people with disabilities. This occurs regardless of whether the ability to create a holistic solution that is accessible to all exists or not. Raising awareness of benefits behind inclusive design must be focused on by putting the spotlight on understanding the specific characteristics of inclusion that shape design thinking when creating solutions for both disabled and non-disabled users (Shinohara et. al., 2016; Withell and Heigh, 2013). The key factors identified by Shinohara et. al. (2016) for successful combined usability are adapted to a development environment as follows:

- Perceptions of Accessibility
    - Challenges emerging from designing inclusive solutions including abled and disabled were unlike those faced when designing for a homogenous group, which can influence developer perception of difficulty or feasibility. This can be countered by learning expert disabled users experiences which can encourage developers to re-assess accessible design, without excluding abled user important non-functional needs.
- Functional and Non-Functional Factors
    - Bridging non-functional and functional requirements of both abled and disabled users can become challenging as entrenched ableist perceptions need to be overcome where the developer considers the disability before the person, and education around use of technology by disabled users has to be taken into account. The focus should not myopically be on the disability but take into account the user enjoyment of the interaction as well.
- Tensions and Opportunities
    - Rather than looking at the challenges of inclusive design as obstacles, developers should be encouraged to use these as tools to be creative and strategize out of the box.
- Changing Attitudes Toward Inclusive Design
    - Empathy is the key to building understanding, and reflection and open dialogue is recommended on an ongoing basis for developers to track issues, challenges with in-hand subject matter, or overcome issues within groups.

Shinohara et. al. (2016) found that most new developers do not naturally approach technology design with an understanding or appreciation of the requirements of disabled users. According to current social psychology literature, developer understanding around disability requirements are shaped by previous personal experience. Developers tend to approach inclusivity projects from a social and cultural stereotype of disability and preconceived, usually deficit, ideas around ability. This can lead developers to be uncomfortable with working with people with disabilities and the perpetuating of ableism perspectives, particularly in disability-specific approaches (Christiansen, 1999; Mead, 1962; Shinohara et. al., 2016).

It therefore becomes key for developers to engage with users with disabilities on an ongoing basis rather that treat the addition of functionality for disabled users as a theoretically based afterthought. By doing so, the developer is able to transcend merely an understanding of functional requirements, but also able to get a grasp of the non-functional requirements which are normally overshadowed. In addition, side-lining the disabled experience, can lead developers to feel self-conscious about and afraid to offend expert users due to society socializing disability-sympathetic, if not patronizing and ableist, behaviours. By allowing the working together of developers and users on design leads to an equal opportunity to influence overall design (Shinohara et. al., 2016)

However, including people with disabilities transcends merely face time with users, but rather melding disabled and non-disabled perspectives and functional/non-functional requirements throughout the design process. A method to create equal contribution is the creation of a socio-technical space for interaction within the project group. Frequently, it has been found that unique challenges arise from the intersection of both user groups. In this way, disabled users are considered a component of the entire user group and not merely as a smaller sub-set thereof (Ludi, 2007; Waller et. al., 2009; Shinohara, 2016).

However, significant changes to general user centred design philosophy is required to address the following issues (Newell and Gregor, 2000):

- Difficulty getting informed consent from some users,
- The users may not be able to communicate their thoughts, or even may be "incompetent" in a legal sense,
- The user may not be the purchaser of the final product,
- Payments may conflict with benefit rules,
- Users with disabilities may have very specialised and little known requirements,
- Different user groups may provide very conflicting requirements for a product,
- There can be ethical issues when involving users with disabilities in the design process, and may require clinician intervention.

In their follow-up study, Sinohara et. al. (2018) highlighted three key tenets out of their research for the humanising of disability in design. They based the perspective of design for social accessibility emphasizing incorporation of users with and without disabilities in designing for disability, the addressing of both social and functional factors simultaneously in design and development, and the inclusion of tools to encourage deliberation of social factors in accessible design.

Examples of Successful Design Thinking Inclusive Project: Autism&Uni Project

The Autism&Uni project is an example of a project that uses participation to inclusively design online tools for individuals with neuro-developmental disorders. Autism&Uni is a research initiative assisting youth on the autism spectrum to help them manage the transition from school into Higher Education (HE). The project, which began in 2013, was originally funded by the European Union's Lifelong Learning Programme till 2016, and thereafter has been taken over by Leeds Beckett University.

The project is centred around autistic users who are actively involved at every stage using the Design Thinking methodology, ensuring that they directly influence the project outcomes (Autism&Uni, 2019). Fabri, Andrews and Pukki (2016) reflected on the participatory design process that was used to develop the online Autism&Uni toolkit which provides autistic students with strategies and information to assist with managing challenges that could be encountered when transitioning to tertiary education. In particular, the process followed the principles of Design Thinking which hinges on participatory design. Feedback from the project on inclusive design with people with disabilities has been very promising. Some of the key findings according to Fabri, Andrews and Pukki (2016) were:

- The Design Thinking process proved to be an good framework for incorporating intellectually disabled users in the development of solutions that speaks to their requirements. The Autism&Uni project followed the five steps of the Design Thinking process in a systematic manner, with user involvement specifically in Step 1, 4 and 5, however there was no reason to suggest that the inclusive workshops could not be extended to these as well. This would create an ongoing process of user involvement throughout the entire design process.
- Another key finding was that the 'Empathise' stage could be further augmented by taking on methods such as focus group interviews and co-research activities, which would have broken the anxiety and inertia seen in the filling out of questionnaires in contrast to the success of spontaneous and informal discussions. This highlighted that the approach to data collection needs to be carefully considered in similar inclusive design projects.
- Running workshops combining the 'Prototype' and 'Test' stages seemed to work well with a small number of workshop participants (approximately 10) and simplified the process so that rigorous structuring was not required while still developing good feedback that in line with content to the structured workshops. The varying of structure can be used to find the optimal combination that can work specifically for the users on the project concerned.
- Common assumptions about individuals with intellectual disabilities were also thrown into question. One of these was the oversimplification that people with disabilities are predominantly visual thinkers and prefer images over text to impart information. The research results suggested the opposite is true for the Autism&Uni project participants who preferred text over visual distractions. Another assumption from literature was that people on the autism spectrum had little desire to share ideas and observations and lacked creativity presented in conventional methods. Observations from the Autism&Uni workshops found that participants showed their aptitude to add creatively and imaginatively to the design process uniquely in situations where they felt safe and comfortable. This highlighted that users' requirements need to be taken into account while preconceived ideas around disability need to be broken down.
- Some of the challenges faced were managing stressful situations for the participants in group work, as well as the limited number of respondents in terms of representativity.

In the Autism&Uni project, participants with intellectual disabilities were involved from the beginning of the project, which ensured the continuous connection with representatives from the overall community as team members were able to shape the research and deliberate on the findings. Effort has to now be put in place to ensure that ongoing participation through to and post the end of the Autism&Uni project is in place to ensure that the project results, publications and the toolkit developed are distributed openly with the wider community.

CONCLUSION

The objective of this research was to analyse the role of the Design Thinking process in promoting inclusivity in design of technologies for disabled individuals, in particular individuals with neuro-developmental disorders.

Inclusive design, however, is not limited to the technology itself, but rather taking into account the individual as well as the wider community in the design. Design needs to be based in social accessibility to counter stigmas and ableism views, in particular in areas where religious and cultural biases against people with disabilities exist. The focus therefore isn't on medical interventions, but rather on interventions that drive inclusion and real-world participation, which then drives true change (Inclusive Practices Africa, 2019).

This can be done by emphasizing incorporation of users with and without disabilities in designing for disability, the addressing of both social and functional factors simultaneously in design and development, and the inclusion of tools to encourage consideration of social factors in accessible design.

The research found that Design Thinking has proven to be an effective framework for involving individuals with neuro-developmental disorders to come up with solutions that address their needs, as has demonstrated in the Autism&Uni project.

It therefore warrants further investigation into the usage of Design Thinking in the development of technology for individuals with neuro-developmental disorders, and in particular being able to do so in an economically viable and sustainable manner that addresses these issues within a developing country context.

FUTURE RESEARCH RECOMMENDATIONS

This research has demonstrated that Design Thinking as an inclusive design methodology can be successful in providing for both non-disabled and disabled users functional and non-functional requirements. Further projects like Autism&Uni are required to assess on a wider scale the success of the methodology on inclusive design projects. These projects are key in strengthening interdisciplinary work to address the complex issue of disability inclusion and address contextual needs through the process as well as allow the process to highlight the appropriateness of creation with the user consistently involved in the process. This then extends the learnings around implementing the methodology to other forms, making it accessible to a wide variety of interdisciplinary areas that it can be used in.

REFERENCES

Agree, E. M. (2014). The potential for technology to enhance independence for those aging with a disability. *Disability and Health Journal, 7*(1), S33–S39.

Altay, B., & Demirkan, H. (2014). Inclusive design: Developing students' knowledge and attitude through empathic modelling. *International Journal of Inclusive Education, 18*(2), 196–217. doi:10.1080/13603116.2013.764933

Autism & Uni. (2019). Accessed at http://www.autism-uni.org/

Bigelow, K. E. (2012). Designing for Success. *Developing Engineers Who Consider Universal Design Principles., 25*(3), 211–225.

Blomkvist, J., & Holmlid, S. (2010). Service prototyping according to practitioners. In *Proceedings of 2nd Service Design and Service Innovation conference, ServDes.2010. Linköping Electronic Conference Proceedings, 60*. Linköping, Sweden: Linköping University Electronic Press.

Borg, J., Lindström, A., & Larsson, S. (2011). Assistive technology in developing countries: A review from the perspective of the Convention on the Rights of Persons with Disabilities. *Prosthetics and Orthotics International, 35*(1), 20–29. doi:10.1177/0309364610389351 PMID:21515886

Brown, T., & Wyatt, J. (2010). Design thinking for social innovation. *Development Outreach, 12*(1), 29–43. doi:10.1596/1020-797X_12_1_29

Christiansen, C. H. (1999, November). Defining Lives: Occupation as Identity: An Essay on Competence, Coherence, and the Creation of Meaning. *The American Journal of Occupational Therapy, 53*(6), 547–558. doi:10.5014/ajot.53.6.547 PMID:10578432

Cloete, T. L., Wilson, W. J., Petersen, L., & Kathard, H. (2015). Identifying a context-effective school hearing screening test: An emic/etic framework. *International Journal of Audiology, 54*(9), 605–612. doi:10.3109/14992027.2015.1014575 PMID:25766492

Coons, K., & Watson, S. (2013). Conducting Research with Individuals Who Have Intellectual Disabilities: Ethical and Practical Implications for Qualitative Research. *Journal on Developmental Disabilities, 19*(2), 14–24.

Crutchfield, B. (2016). *ADA and the Internet: ADA Settlements-Fitting Accessibility Compliance into Your Product Lifecycle*. SSB Bart Group.

Dam, R., & Siang, T. (2019). *5 Stages in the Design Thinking Process*. Access at https://www.interaction-design.org/literature/article/5-stages-in-the-design-thinking-process on 12/07/2019

Fabri, M., Andrews, P. C. S., & Pukki, H. (2016). Using Design Thinking to engage autistic students in participatory design of an online toolkit to help with transition into higher education. *Journal of Assistive Technologies, 10*(2).

Inclusive Practices Africa. (2019). *Disability Inclusion Drives Change*. Access at Inclusivepractices.co.za

Kaye, H.S., Yeager, P., & Reed, M. (2008). Disparities in usage of assistive technology among people with disabilities. *Assist Technol., 20*, 194-203.

Khetarpal, A. (2014). Information and communication technology (ICT) and disability. *Review of Market Integration, 6*(1), 96-113.

Ludi, S. (2007). Introducing Accessibility Requirements through External Stakeholder Utilization in an Undergraduate Requirements Engineering Course. *Proc. Soft. Eng., 07*, 736–743. doi:10.1109/ICSE.2007.46

Maguire, M. (2001). Methods to support human-centred design. *International Journal of Human-Computer Studies, 55*(4), 587–634. doi:10.1006/ijhc.2001.0503

McDonagh, D. and Thomas, J. (2010) Rethinking Design Thinking: Empathy Supporting Innovation. *Australasian Medical Journal - Health and Design 1, 3*(8), 458-464.

Mead, G. H. (1962). *Mind, self, and society from the standpoint of a social behaviorist.* Univ. of Chicago Press.

Mitra, S. (2005). *Disability and Social Safety Nets in Developing Countries.* Social Protection Discussion Paper No. 0509. World Bank.

Mitra, S., Posarac, A., & Vick, B. (2013). Disability and poverty in developing countries: A multidimensional study. *World Development, 41*, 1–18. doi:10.1016/j.worlddev.2012.05.024

Mizunoya, S., & Mitra, S. (2013). Is there a disability gap in employment rates in developing countries? *World Development, 42*, 28–43. doi:10.1016/j.worlddev.2012.05.037

Mullin, A. P., Gokhale, A., Moreno-De-Luca, A., Sanyal, S., Waddington, J. L., & Faundez, V. (2013). Neurodevelopmental disorders: Mechanisms and boundary definitions from genomes, interactomes and proteomes. *Translational Psychiatry, 3*(12), e329. doi:10.1038/tp.2013.108 PMID:24301647

Newell, A. F., & Gregor, P. (2000). User sensitive inclusive design—in search of a new paradigm. In *Proceedings on the 2000 conference on Universal Usability* (pp. 39-44). ACM. 10.1145/355460.355470

Quinn, B.S., Behrmann, M., Mastropieri, M., Bausch, M.E., Ault, M.J., & Chung, Y. (2009). Who is using assistive technology in school? *J Spec Educ Technol., 24*, 1-13.

Rittel, H., & Webber, M. (1973). Dilemmas in a General Theory of Planning. *Policy Sciences, 4*(2), 155–179. doi:10.1007/BF01405730

Rohwerder, B. (2018). *Disability stigma in developing countries.* Academic Press.

Sanders, E., & Stappers, P. J. (2008). Co-Creation and the New Landscapes of Design. *CoDesign, 4*(1), 5–18. doi:10.1080/15710880701875068

Sharp, H., Rogers, Y., & Preece, J. (2007). *Interaction design: beyond human-computer interaction.* Wiley.

Shinohara, K., Bennett, C. L., Pratt, W., & Wobbrock, J. O. (2018). Tenets for Social Accessibility: Towards Humanizing Disabled People in Design. *ACM Transactions on Accessible Computing, 11*(1), 6. doi:10.1145/3178855

Shinohara, K., Bennett, C. L., & Wobbrock, J. O. (2016). How designing for people with and without disabilities shapes student design thinking. In *Proceedings of the 18th International ACM SIGACCESS Conference on Computers and Accessibility*, (pp. 229-237). ACM. 10.1145/2982142.2982158

Waller, A., Hanson, V. L., & Sloan, D. (2009). Including accessibility within and beyond undergraduate computing courses. *Proc. ASSETS '09*, 155–162. 10.1145/1639642.1639670

Wehmeyer, M.L. (1998). National survey of use of assistive technology by adults with mental retardation. *Ment Retard., 36*(1), 44-51.

Withell, A., & Heigh, N. (2013). Developing Design Thinking Expertise in Higher Education. *2nd International Conference for Design Education Researchers*, Oslo, Norway.

World Health Organisation. (n.d.). *International Classification of Functioning, Disability and Health (ICF).* Accessed at https://www.who.int/classifications/icf/en/

Chapter 12
Brain-Computer Interface and Neurofeedback for Brain Training

Sheetal Bhatia
National Institute of Technology, Jalandhar, India

ABSTRACT

AT liberty and open correspondence is central to present day life. Human cerebrum PC interfaces (BCIs), which interpret estimations of the client's mind movement into PC directions, present developing types of without hands correspondence. BCI correspondence frameworks have since quite a while ago been utilized in clinical settings for patients with loss of motion and other engine issue and have not been executed with the expectation of complimentary correspondence between solid, BCI-gullible clients. Brain PC interface innovation speaks to an exceptionally developing field of research with application frameworks. Its commitments in therapeutic fields extend from avoidance to neuronal restoration for genuine wounds. Human intellect perusing and remote correspondence have their exceptional unique mark in various fields, for example, instructive, self-guideline, creation, advertising, security, just as games and excitement. It makes a shared comprehension among clients and the encompassing frameworks.

INTRODUCTION

The communication path among people and PCs has enormously advanced since the presence from time the ðrst business PC, the UNIVAC, in 1951. The best way to benchmark that convoluted bit of apparatus was an altered IBM electric and criticism to clients was given via a Tektronix oscilloscope. Present day PCs are totally portable and despite the fact that they are for the most part constrained by a mouse and a console, a few elective human-machine interfaces have been created during the most recent two tennar utilizing haptics, speech and deem

Human brain PC interfaces (BCI), which interpret estimations of the client's cerebrum movement into PC directions to control outside gadgets, present developing types of sans hands correspondence. BCI spellers are virtual consoles that translate cerebrum movement designs enabling clients to choose characters

DOI: 10.4018/978-1-7998-3069-6.ch012

in arrangement to spell words and, eventually, uninhibitedly convey (Shuhaida, Azuan & Osman, 2007). BCI consoles copy manual consoles, which broaden the client by enabling them to physically show their constant contemplations, interface with the web and convey remotely. BCI correspondence frameworks, including spellers, have since a long time ago been utilized in clinical settings to encourage correspondence in instances of quadriplegia, anarthria and amyotrophic sidelong sclerosis. These frameworks are frequently created utilizing electroencephalography (EEG) (Yahud & Osman, 2007), which takes into consideration versatile, adaptable and moderate gadgets BCI can possibly reform correspondence, but then its potential for making free correspondence in solid clients is generally unexplored Here we present another and proficient non-obtrusive framework, utilizing meager terminal electroencephalography (EEG), that permits free correspondence between people dependent on constant mind action interpreting.

Obscuring Paths Between Mind and Machine

As science grows our comprehension of the world it can lead to the development of new innovations. These can bring enormous benefits, yet in addition challenges, as they change society's relationship with the world. Researchers, designers and more extensive society must guarantee that we augment the advantages from new advances while limiting these difficulties. The Royal Society has set up an Emerging Technologies Working Party to analyze such improvements and make points of view.Truth be told, we as of now have the main outward neural interface framework to be tried in people (AAPB, 2003). It is called BrainGate and comprises of a variety of miniaturized scale terminals, embedded into the piece of the mind worried about controlling arm developments. Sign from the small scale anodes are decoded and used to control the development of a cursor on a screen, or the movement of a mechanical arm.

A significant element of these frameworks is the requirement for some sort of criticism. A patient must have the option to see the impact of their willed examples of thought on the development of the cursor. What's surprising is the capacity of the cerebrum to adjust to these fake frameworks, figuring out how to control them better.Innovation is starting to guarantee methods for revamping these associations, however is it our resourcefulness or the brain, that is getting it going? Neural interface innovations have the potential to bring significant advantages to society.These incorporate extraordinary treatments for individuals with conditions, for example, stroke, epilepsy, loss of motion or despondency (Bennett et al., 1990). They offerpotential outcomes for upgraded fixation, basic leadership and coordinated effort. They could likewise add to enhancements in singular wellness and prosperity, as well as empowering more secure homes, streets and work environments, for instance by checking for weakness.Numerous individuals overall as of now advantage from restorative neural interface advancements. Much of the time, their conditions have demonstrated sedate safe and 'electroceuticals' have accomplished what pharmaceuticals could not. Cochlear inserts that substitute harmed portions of the ear give hearing for around 400,000 individuals (Sreeja et al., 2017). A great many individuals with conditions, for example, Parkinson's ailment, dystonia and basic tremor have been treated with profound mind stimulation Outside, wearable interfaces incorporate a scope of gadgets that help individuals who have had a stroke in their recovery. Individuals generally incapable to impart have had the option to explain words utilizing mind flag alone, giving them an precious methods for connection.

Neurofeedback and Basic Learning Thoery

Following the chronicled strings of neurofeedback no drugs or careful intercessions by any means! Since this worldview runs counter to continuation restorative as well as scientific convention as educated in the greater part of our therapeutic and scholarly organizations of higher adapting, such another worldview is viewed as utter horror and has the right to be disregarded if not really hated by most Human services control specialists in these foundations (Demos, 2005). Thomas Kuhn, the researcher thinker, is said to have noticed that before another worldview is acknowledged, the vast majority of the disciples of the more established worldview must have kicked the bucket (Thompson et al., 2009) Neurofeedback, in spite of being 40 years old, is still in the phase of improvement as another worldview and the wellbeing care foundation is to some degree concentrated on keeping it in that technique (Shaw, Zaichkowsky, & Wilson, 2012). It would be full-grown to recollect that in the mid 70s we built up biofeedbackers and felt that the PCs could never supplant the tough, dependable remain solitary biofeedback units (Khambhati et al., 2013) .Who could know how inconceivably quick the science and improvement of PC innovation would advance.Not very numerous years back the electrical sign created by the mind and showing up on the scalp were viewed as excessively little, excessively arbitrary, and too unimportant to possibly be considered earnestly as an analytic pointer of cerebrum movement. Be that as it may, with the appearance of such achievements as scaled down electronic circuits and those of Fast Fourier Transform chip, complex filtering, huge impedance preamps, lownoise organic amplifiers, and exact simple to advanced converters, PCs would now be able to be programed to operate the EEG information in manners constrained distinctly by the inventiveness of the programmers and equipment creators.

This part of the book will tends to the subject of how to arrange the neuromodulation impacts coming about because of broadly contrasting neurofeedback approaches created over the most recent four decades Along with This part will endeavor to assess the condition of the field as of now. The goal is to perceive the shared characteristics among the different methodologies on the first hand and in those of the clinical discoveries on the next one. This will give rise to acodification of an insignificant arrangement of cases that deliver to cover the shared characteristics in the middle of the procedures, and it leads to a basic order plot for the different clinical discoveries (Beutler & Davidson, 1995). The proof for such a negligible arrangement of cases will be showed to a great extent by reference.Neurofeedback innovation is a PC data the board framework, which empowers to change mind biopotentials with a functioning interest of a patient himself. To achieve this, a present adequacy of a certain EEG-cadence utilizing different PC implies is reflected in parameters of light and additionally sound criticism signals appearing to a patient so as to show him a cognizant mind control of the force of possess musical EEG parts to accomplish attractive healing impacts. In the event that a human progressively can hear or see a sufficient impression of his own biopotentials, at that point he has an chance to figure out how to alter them in a course required. From the start the accomplished impacts are present moment, in any case, over the span of preparing in the vast majority this aptitude is fortified. Consequently, NFB offers assistant offices for nondrug recovery of different mind pathologies (Fedotchev et al., 2017). As a rule, NFB framework comprises of five components or on the other hand handling steps: a cerebrum signal gathering, signal starter handling, recognizing key highlights, input signal age, and a versatile preparing. After EEG recording, the information are to begin with handled (e.g., ancient rarity identification, evacuation, and remedy), with age and determination of highlights, what's more, criticism signal calculation and documentation. The last step shuts the criticism circuit, where a member endeavors to figure out how to utilize a criticism sign to change the mind action as indicated by guidelines. All the vital steps are taken on an ongoing premise. The recognized highlights, when in doubt, reflect quantitatively the movement level of a specific cerebrum territory or arrange, and an input sign transmits the data on the relating changes in the cerebrum condition. Members are prepared to discover and adjust the systems so as to change deliberately the condition of their minds as per the starter directions . An underlying phase of building up NFB innovation was a arrangement of inquires about completed by Kamiya in the 60-ies of the only remaining century (Dinov & Leech, 2017), which showed the human ability to change deliberately the force of ghostly parts of his own EEG . Hence, this reality filled in as the reason for advancement various clinical NFB applications to treat numerous infections through direct revision of electric procedures in cerebrum (Budzynski et al., 2009). The instruments of restorative activity of NFB are still unclarified, however numerous investigations are committed to their comprehension . As indicated by one idea, potential components of NFB are improvements of neural systems remembering the expansion for their worldwide interconnection and neuroplasticity. Other specialists consider NFB to play out the alteration of cerebrum electric action vibrations set up for such a homeostatic level, which gives an ideal balance between neural system adaptability and soundness. By present time there has been increased positive clinical experience of NFB application for a wide range of sicknesses. Among them there are consideration deficithyperactivity issue, learning handicap, stroke, awful mind damage, uncontrolled epilepsy, substance misuse, gloom, chemical imbalance, headache, dietary issues, torment disorders and other pathologic conditions. It ought to be noticed that in any case the starting point of manifestations (Hinds et al., 2014). NFB preparing hold out assistant offices for recovery through direct re-training of electric forms in the mind.

A Categorization of Neuromodulation Advancements

Rewording Robert Bly, formost may contend that "brain is here to seek its own joy" and that it leads to way off in to whatever connects with that could be its interests it, or what it plays with it, or mirrors it. Provided that fairly unobjectionable supposition, one may contend that clear guidelines to "succeed" might be discretionary even in the input worldview. Criticism might be adequately compensating inherently to assemble the process even in the undermined cerebrum. One may moreover discuss on the job of volition in Sterman's feline research (Sterman et al., 1969). Positively the felines were strategizing to obtain nourishment. At the point when one of them took place to trigger nourishment remunerate while occupied with an intricate stretch development, she along these lines rehashed a similar development time and with expectations of rehashing her prosperity. The methodology may well have been counter-profitable at last. Be that as it may, no matter. It was compensating enough to be supported. Past encountering nourishment as a compensate, for which no extraordinary arrangement should be made, zero more appears to be required. It appears that we cannot choose over a basic or even a magnified job in EEG criticism. Then again, maybe very little is lost, as the accompanying story delineates. An individual experiencing preparing with NeuroCarePro programming (reference as www.zengar.com) communicated its fulfillment with the involvement at ending of the session, however couldn't resist vocalizing the disturbance with the way that the CD meant to be Siegfried Othmer, Ph.D. 7 tuning in to continued interfering with progression of music, I feel vastly improved, resting all things considered, however would you be able to request that her utilization another CD that doesn't have skips (Birbaumer, 2007). He had unmistakably not known that the skips were the carriers of data pertinent to mind in truth the main one's his brain was accepting but then the procedure plainly impacted. In addition to the fact that he was irritated with the breakage in the music, yet his brain as well was. Furthermore, the brain got onto more data to work than that he would have been. It didn't get that flawless relationship motor long to make sense of point that it was a piece of an intelligent framework and was being assumed as a functioning job. Also, similarly the way brain will fuse a tennis racket like an expansion of arm when it is grabbed, brain will quickly proper input circle just as a feature of its circle of impact. Plainly we should comprehend neurofeedback till attainable ptiches in brain. Formerly that undertaking is cultivated, we can get the job of volition to the talk, as it emphatically enhances the input procedure in most genuine circumstances. So now at this pont in time an alternate question along these lines should be asked, which is the reason is there to such an extent speciation happening in EEG input by any stretch of the imagination? What are the developmental specialties that enable the entirety of the strategies to endure till the current time? Maybe we simple live in an early multiplication stage with solidification to pursue laterby. This will ideally be explained in what pursues. At any frequency, our present assignment of essentially arranging those different structures are tested by the entirety of the assorted variety which is as of now surviving. Hence the simple classicfication can be done as following.

NEUROMODIFICATION TECHNIQUES

Research at Wadsworth Centre: Noninvasive BCI- Brain-Computer Inteface

The essential objective of wadsworth focus BCI program is to develope EEG bci frameworks that can give severly crippled inviduals an elective methods for correspondence as well as control. We have indicated the individuals with or without engine disabilites can figure out how to control sensriomotor rythms recorded from the scalp to move a PC cursor in one or 2D and we have additionally utilized the P300 occasion related potential as a control sign to make descrete determinations. In general, our reseraches demonstrates that there are a few methodologies that may furnish options for people with serious engine incapacities. We are currently assessing the common sense and viability of a BCI correspondence framework for day by day use by such people in their homes (Renard et al., 2010). The EEG is composed to a degree of detail and exactness that is hard to observe with our traditional estimation instruments (Barkley, 1992). Despite what components of the signal we decide to concentrate on, yet others must stay out of center or off-screen totally. In the event that one decides to see the EEG with high-recurrence goals, for model, the isolation into unmistakable, thin, thoroughly delineated frequencies bands is very striking. As of the reason this cannot be minor to mastermind, it has to be imperative to brain work. The division line in-between two recurrence systems is a stage limit, that is, a district where stage can experience an irregularity. Inside a specific recurrence run that characterizes an axle, the stage differs easily and ceaselessly all through. Correspondingly, the spatial appropriation of a neuronal get together should be described by a cover stage variety up the get together. On the off chance that a stage limit subsists at the edges of such a neuron gathering, as anyone may presume it is probably going to be darkened by and by bioelectromagnetism. At long last, correspondence between neuronal congregations at some expel from each other is dependent upon stage arrangement (Renton et al., 2018). It pursues, at that point, that the CNS must oversee stage in perfect detail all together to manage the domain that a nerve troupe directions in recurrence space, to portray the dimensional impression which involves on cortex, also to set up, keep up distal correspondence with neuronal congregations somewhere else on cortexInconspicuous obstruction with this procedure will at that point incite the mind's pertinent reaction. The impedance is regarded to be unobtrusive on the off chance that it basically tweaks rather than upsets the progressing action. Neurofeedback completely meets this rule, and incitement methods are equipped for meeting it whenever led at adequately low drive levels. Both input and incitement systems are most grounded in the event that they encroach upon the part of brain work that is with the quick the board of the mind, and that is the connected stage or, identically, that of the prompt recurrence of parcel. This representation for neuromodulation represents intensity of the lens and for the intensity of upgraded reward recurrence preparing in criticism. It additionally represents the perception in QEEG-based work that intelligence preparing seems more grounded than sufficiency based preparing. In LENS, the upgrade gives the stage reference. On account of the ROSHI, the boost stage contrasts between the two sides of the equator. In the recurrence enhanced criticism, which is ordinarily directed with a solitary divert in bipolar montage, the one site is provided reference for another. Similar remains constant in lucidness preparing with two-channel montage: the first site leads to the stage reference for the other. In EEG proceduring with a bipolar montage, the net resultant signal is a solid capacity of relative stage. This is a fundamental statepoint, and it's anything but a conspicuous one. The peruser is alluded to a point by point conduct towards of this subject in Putman and Othmer. By excellence of normal mode dismissal in the differential intensifier, movement that is Parallel-sided between the two locales isn't seen at its yield, and in this manner can't ever be remunerated. What's more, in the event that it can't be remunerated, at that point concerning everything else it is adequately being repressed. The final impact is to compensate separation of movement in-between two locales, which is the genuine remove state. The methodology was formerly examined with between hemispheric situations at similar locales, which we utilized Or maybe only for certain years (Othmer & Othmer, 2007). Clinical results in terms of consistent execution tests would have been distributed for this technique, exhibiting improved results regarding before information (Putman et al., 2005). Taken a gander at in the above manner, even this explicitly focused on remuneration based preparing can be viewed as having a proscriptive as opposed to a prescriptive angle: the condition of synchrony, of stage congruity, is banished. On the other hand, the system rewards everything except for the state of synchrony. And since the main thing blocked from progress is the synchrony condition, concerning the expansive remaining stage area the method can even be viewed as having a non-recommended view point too: the stage relationship isn't as a rule firmly obliged (APA, 1993). The preparation itself adds up to an unobtrusive, nonstop challenge that falsehoods to a great extent in the stage space. It must be recognized now that the strength of stage is not evident from the science. Undoubtedly, plentifulness contrasts among those of the two destinations involved as a similarly as unequivocally into the outcome. Since the overall job of adequacy and stage, all things considered, circumstances isn't self-evident, their particular jobs can be explained with a Monte Carlo computation in which trial circumstance is reproduced in all of its normal changeability. This has been finished with presumption of arbitrariness in relative stage and in the plentifulness at the two destinations (Putman & Othmer, 2006). An almost complete avoidance of remunerations is found for relative stage under 40 degrees in this reenactment. In genuine EEGs there will be some limited connection in amplitudes, along with the ones which just serves to fortify the placed stage reliance. On the off chance that the difference in the plentifulness proportion is stuck, at that point the genuine fluctuation must be represented in the stage.

Monitoring Brain Using EEG Techniques

A few systems have been utilized to screen brain activites, for example,

(1) Electroencephalography (EEG),
(2) Magnetoencephalography (MEG),
(3) Functional Attractive Resonance Imaging (fMRI),
(4) Functional Near-Infrared Spectroscopy (fNIRS),
(5) Single Photon Emission Tomography (SPECT), and
(6) Proton Outflow Tomography (PET).

Every technique has its individual qualities just as advantages and disadvantages. Be that as it may, for a few reasons potential contrasts which can be estimated in-between different scalps are altogether different in those could be estimated when cathodes were embedded legitimately in brain. For example, the movement of potential generators can be estimated legitimately by:

1. A superposition of possibilities produced in various regions of cortex is estimated utilizing scalp anodes conserding brain tissue and alcohol are conductive.
2. The adequacy of initially created potential contrasts is lessened as a result of the resistive characteristics of tissue in that of the potential generators what's more, terminal (for example alcohol, skin, bone of the skull).
3. Limits brought about by cell layers and different inhomogeneities (for example liquorskull, skull-skin) in-between potential generators and terminals impact the adequacy of EEG flag as a component of their recurrence.

Along these lines, the situations for EEG anodes ought to be picked as it were, which all cortex areas are secured. For moreover applications, this is generally entire cortex.

A globally acknowledged standard for anode arrangements is the 10–20 framework (cathodes are set at separations of 10 or 20% of the length of a few associations between few reference focuses) presented in 1957 by International EEG Organization. Cathodes were put by the 10–20 framework. Three of the anatomical reference focuses necessarily be resolved before 10–20 framework anode positions which are:

1. Nasion: The one onset of the nose on the skull, below the forehead.
2. Inion: The bony protuberance which marks the transition between skull and neck.
3. Pre-auricular reference point: located before the cartilaginous protrusion of the acoustic meatus (the auditory canal)

The name for a specific cathode position mirrors the anatomical district of the cortex above which it is found. Fp represents frontopolar, F represents frontal, T represents worldly, C represents focal, P represents parietal, O stands for occipital and A represents auricular while G means the ground terminal. Indeed numbers mean the correct piece of the head, odd numbers allude the left part. For the most part, there are two classifications of relics can be recognized in EEG estimations which are natural and specialized. The natural ancient rarities are brought about by the recorded subject and specialized ancient rarities are brought about by the EEG recording gadget (APA, 1994; Hughes et al., 1994). The wellsprings of numerous natural curios are dipoles beginning for instance from solid exercises which are a lot more grounded than the EEG related dipoles. A superposition of the two kinds of dipoles causes relics in the sign which are frequently portrayed by huge pinnacles or vacillations of a specific morphology. Once in a while, in any case, they can scarcely be recognized from the genuine EEG (Gimeno & Lin, 2017).

Other natural antiquities impact the contact among skin as well as terminal or the electrical riches of the path between potential generators and anodes.

BCI Challenges and Provided Solutions

Building up the correspondence interface utilising human brain signals has confronted a great deal of difficulties (Abdulkader & Mostafa, 2015).They can be ordered as specialised and ease of use. Specialised difficulties are worried about the framework obstructions uniquely those in regards to EEG highlights attributes. Ease of use difficulties portray the restrictions influencing the degree of human acknowledgement

Technical Issues

A few issues related to the recorded electrophysiological possessions of the brain signals which consolidate non-linearity, non-stationarity and uproar, small getting ready sets and the companying dimensionality censure.There are as yet numerous difficulties in the reconciliation of BCIs into powerful prosthetic gadgets (Murphy et al., 2016). These difficulties remember satisfactory spatiotemporal goals for translating data recorded from the cerebrum for naturalistic control, unraveling an adequate number of degrees of opportunity to keep up normal developments, reconciliation of input systems, facilitating the innovative help required for joining of the BCI and diminishing the intrusiveness of parts while keeping up the life span of sign procurement. Also, various ongoing examinations have concentrated on gadgets contained completely inside the CNS that make counterfeit connections between related territories. Here, we center around the favorable circumstances and weaknesses of different ways to deal with interfacing BCI gadgets with the sensory system, in light of results from both pre-clinical and clinical examinations. We feature the difficulties related with the usage of high devotion BCI gadgets to a clinical setting, potential strategies for beating these difficulties, and the differentiation between gadgets that control outward tasks and those that control activities natural for the CNS.

Figure 1. Flow chart to describe the technical challenges in BCI

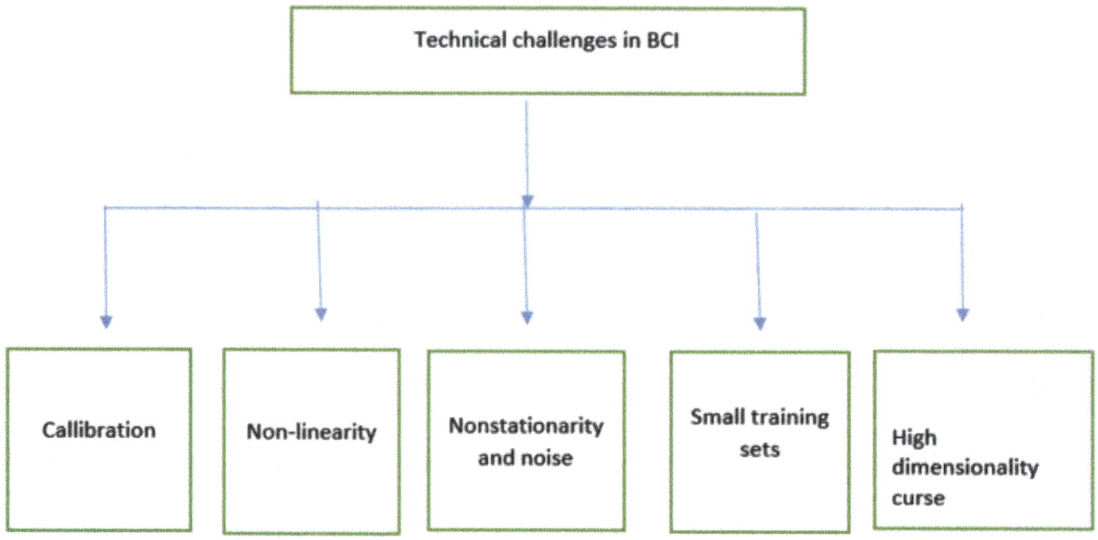

Non-Linearity

Human brain is a profoundly unpredictable nonlinear framework in which clamorous conduct of neural gatherings can be identified. Accordingly EEG sign can be better described by nonlinear powerful techniques than direct strategies.

Nonstationarity and noise: Nonstationarity property of electrophysiological brain signals speaks to a significant issue in building up a BCI framework . It begins a persistent difference in the utilized flag after some time either between or inside the account sessions. The psychological and passionate state foundation through various sessions can contribute in EEG signals fluctuation. Additionally weariness and fixation levels are viewed as a feature of interior nonstationarity factors. Clamor is additionally a major donor in the difficulties confronting the BCI innovation and causing the nonstationarity issue. It incorporates undesirable sign brought about by changes in terminal position, and ecological clamor . A blend of development antiques, for example, electrical action delivered by skeletal muscles electromyogram (EMG) and sign made by eye developments and squinting Electrooculogram (EOG), is likewise reflected in the procured sign bringing about challenges in recognizing the fundamental example.

Small-Scale training sets: The preparation sets are generally little, since the preparation procedure is affected by convenience issues. Albeit vigorously instructional courses are viewed as tedious and requesting for the subjects, they give the client important experience to manage the framework and figure out how to control his / her neurophysiological sign (Rogala et al., 2016).Therefore a huge test in planning a BCI is to adjust the exchange off between the mechanical multifaceted nature of deciphering the client's mind signals and the measure of preparing required for fruitful activity of the interface .

High dimensioality curse: In BCI frameworks, the signs are recorded from numerous channels to protect high spatial precision. As the measure of information expected to appropriately portray various signs increments exponentially with the dimensionality of the vectors, different component extraction strategies have been proposed. They assume a significant job in recognizing qualities. Along these lines the classifier execution will be influenced uniquely by the modest number of particular characteristics rather than the entire recorded signs that may contain repetition. By and large, it is prescribed to use, in any event, five to ten fold the number of preparing tests per class as the quantity of measurements (Cochrane, 2010). Be that as it may, this arrangement can't be supported in a profoundly dimensional condition as the BCI framework, causing the extending of the dimensionality revileProposed solutions:

A few arrangements have been explored to stand up to and limitthe inñuence of the recently referenced specialized issues.They are spread over different BCI framework parts. The fol-lowing areas clarify some utilized techniques for improvingthe execution of BCI based frameworks

Noise Benefits in Array of BCI

Noise can improve the exactness of cerebrum PC interface (BCI) frameworks. Added substance Gaussian clamor can profit varieties of troupe bolster vector machines (ESVMs) that characterize P300 or engine symbolism (MI) exercises in electroencephalogram (EEG) signals. It leads to procced towards, that these clamor benefits in 64-channel EEG signals from the BCI Competitions II dataset IIb and BCI Competitions III dataset II for the P300 speller worldview and in 3-channel EEG signals from the BCI Competitions II dataset III and BCI Competitions III dataset IIIa for MI grouping frameworks. It likewise show that clamor can improve the precision of EEG arrangements dependent on confined direct positions in business recording frameworks, for example, the 14-channel Emotiv Epoc headset. The test results show that clamor can furnish classifiers with higher precision and can diminish the information assortment time for P300 grouping. The outcomes additionally show that preparation ESVMs with a connected unique dataset and commotion included datasets can improve MI characterization. Clamor can improve the exactness of P300 grouping for both intra-subject and between subject arrangement frameworks for different clients. Expansion of commotion can essentially influence the parameters of polynomial portion capacities and the quantity of help vectors of the SVM. This prompts a development of the edge between two parallel hyperplanes that in the end improve the grouping exactness. Molecule swarm advancement (PSO) can be utilized to look for the ideal commotion power.

Seperability of Multiple Classes

AI systems are utilized to make an interpretation of client's aim into a substantial decision. They segregate and recognize the chose class. They have been utilized, for instance, to defeat a few constraints related with little preparing sets, single preliminary, and furthermore the changeability among sessions and inside individual sessions. They likewise intend to accomplish better and appropriately, higher ITR results. Next we show three diverse AI calculations, for example, straight discriminant investigation (LDA), bolster vector machine (SVM), and k closest neighbors (KNN).

CONCLUSION

Neurointerface innovations are coming into use in medication to substitute or recuperate helpful capacities in individuals unequipped for playing out these capacities due to neuromuscular issue or wounds, just as to treat a wide scope of ailments and disarranges without meds. Brain PC interface innovation empowers to help repay engine and tangible capacities, contribute to the recuperation of affectability of harmed body territories, makes it conceivable to play out an out-understanding checking to identify and avert possibly perilous conditions (e.g., epileptic seizures). It will give the recuperation of some lost capacities in deadened patients. Due to mind PC interface innovation deadened patients can, by demonstrations of will, type on a screen and press virtual on-off catches accessible for their self-administration of gadgets. Eventually, by a multi-type participation of nervous system specialists, analysts, doctors, engineers and mathematicians the referenced abilities of cerebrum PC interface innovation will be finished by quickened instruction programs and focused on memory recovery that will empower to broaden altogether the circle of its clinical application for both diagnostics of sicknesses and screening of hazard gatherings, and furthermore for successful amendment of different obsessive conditions(Sylvan & Christodoulou, 2010). Neurofeedback innovation was at first arranged on clinical applications, and at this point it has been effectively tried in treatment and remedy of countless sicknesses and disarranges going from consideration deficithyperactivity issue and chemical imbalance to chronic drug use also, immunodeficiency. Regardless of various unsolved issues, at this point a neurofeedback innovation shows up to be, in any event, an extremely helpful enhancement for the existing treatment offices. Looking forward, due to the advancement of progressively flawless research conventions, the utilization of current innovations of human mind imaging what's more, ideal association of input signals (e.g., in the type of music), interface advancements can induce key positions in clinical practice. Brain signals reflect the dealt with practices and controlling behavior of the cerebrum or the effect of the got information from other body parts either identifying or inside organs (Rockstroh, Elbert, Birbaumer, & Lutzenberger, 1990). Cerebrum Computer Interfacing gives a coordinating office among mind and outside equipment. BCI applications have pulled in the assessment arrange. A couple of assessments have been displayed in this paper with respect to the creating excitement for BCI application fields, for instance, helpful, definitive, transportation, games and incitement, and security and check fields. It in like manner shows the various contraptions used for getting cerebrum signals. These record contraptions are isolated into two principal groupings: nosy and non-prominent. Prominent class, which requires installing restorative technique, is commonly required for essential stifled conditions because of their higher accuracy rates achieved either spatially or briefly. Of course, the non-meddlesome class, as referenced as of now, has been commonly spread in other application fields on account of its central focuses over the prominent one. Various troubles and issues acted like a result of utilizing cerebrum signals have furthermore been discussed nearby certain plans offered by different computations at various BCI planning sections.

REFERENCES

Abdulkader, S. N., Atia, A., & Mostafa, M. S. M. (2015). Brain computer interfacing: Applications and challenges. *Egyptian Informatics Journal, 16*(2), 213–230. doi:10.1016/j.eij.2015.06.002

Afshar, P., Khambhati, A., Stanslaski, S., Carlson, D., Jensen, R., Dani, S., ... Denison, T. (2013). A translational platform for prototyping closed-loop neuromodulation systems. *Frontiers in Neural Circuits, 6*, 117. doi:10.3389/fncir.2012.00117 PMID:23346048

American Psychiatric Association. (1994). *Diagnostic and Statistical Manual of Mental Disorders: DSM-IV*. Washington, DC: American Psychiatric Association.

American Psychological Association. (1993). *Promotion and dissemination of psychological procedures.* An unpublished task force report for Division 12. Washington, DC: American Psychological Association.

APB (Association of Applied Psychophysiology and Biofeedback). (2003). *Ethical principles of applied psychophysiology and biofeedback*. Wheat Ridge, CO: Association for Applied Psychophysiology and Biofeedback.

Barkley, R. A.(1992). *Is EEG biofeedback treatment effective for ADHD children?* ChaADDer Box.

Bennett, B. E., Bryant, B. K., VandenBos, G. R., & Greenwood, A. (1990). *Professional liability and risk management*. Washington, DC: American Psychological Association. doi:10.1037/11102-000

Beutler, L. E., & Davidson, E. H. (1995). What standards should we use? In S. C. Hayes & V. M. Follette (Eds.), *Scientifi c standards of psychological practice: Issues and recommendations*. Academic Press.

Birbaumer, N. (2007). *A brain computer interface for restoration of movement following stroke*. Neuro Connections.

Budzynski, T. H., Budzynski, H. K., Evans, J. R., & Abarbanel, A. (Eds.). (2009). *Introduction to quantitative EEG and neurofeedback: Advanced theory and applications*. Academic Press.

Cochrane, K. (2010). *Comprehensive neurofeedback training in the context of psychotherapy for transformational change* (Doctoral dissertation). International University for Graduate Studies.

Demos, J. N. (2005). *Getting started with neurofeedback*. New York: W. W. Norton & Company.

Dinov, M., & Leech, R. (2017). Tracking and optimizing human performance using deep reinforcement learning in closed-loop behavioral-and neurofeedback: A proof of concept. *bioRxiv*, 225995.

Duffy, F. H., Hughes, J. R., Miranda, F., Bernard, P., & Cook, P. (1994). Status of quantitative EEG (QEEG) in clinical practice: 1994. *Clinical Electroencephalography*.

Fedotchev, A. I., Parin, S. B., Polevaya, S. A., & Velikova, S. D. (2017). Brain–computer interface and neurofeedback technologies: current state, problems and clinical prospects. *Современные технологии в медицине, 9*(1).

Fedotchev, A. I., Parin, S. B., Polevaya, S. A., & Velikova, S. D. (2017). Brain-computer interface and neurofeedback technologies: current state, problems and clinical prospects (review). *Sovremennye tehnologii v medicine, 9*(1), 175-184.

Gimeno, H., & Lin, J. P. (2017). The International Classification of Functioning (ICF) to evaluate deep brain stimulation neuromodulation in childhood dystonia-hyperkinesia informs future clinical & research priorities in a multidisciplinary model of care. *European Journal of Paediatric Neurology, 21*(1), 147-167.

Hinds, O., Wighton, P., Dylan Tisdall, M., Hess, A., Breiter, H., & Van Der Kouwe, A. (2014). Neurofeedback using functional spectroscopy. *International Journal of Imaging Systems and Technology, 24*(2), 138–148. doi:10.1002/ima.22088 PMID:24999293

Murphy, M. D., Guggenmos, D. J., Bundy, D. T., & Nudo, R. J. (2016). Current challenges facing the translation of brain computer interfaces from preclinical trials to use in human patients. *Frontiers in Cellular Neuroscience, 9*, 497. doi:10.3389/fncel.2015.00497 PMID:26778962

Putman, J. A., & Othmer, S. (2006). Phase sensitivity of bipolar EEG training protocols. *Journal of Neurotherapy, 10*(1), 73–79. doi:10.1300/J184v10n01_06

Renard, Y., Lotte, F., Gibert, G., Congedo, M., Maby, E., Delannoy, V., ... Lécuyer, A. (2010). Openvibe: An open-source software platform to design, test, and use brain–computer interfaces in real and virtual environments. *Presence (Cambridge, Mass.)*, *19*(1), 35–53. doi:10.1162/pres.19.1.35

Renton, A. I., Mattingley, J. B., & Painter, D. R. (2018). An open interface system for non-invasive brain-to-brain free communication between naive human participants. *bioRxiv*, 488825.

Rockstroh, B., Elbert, T., Birbaumer, N., & Lutzenberger, W. (1990). Biofeedback-produced hemispheric asymmetry of slow cortical potentials and its behavioural effects. *International Journal of Psychophysiology*, *9*(2), 151–165. doi:10.1016/0167-8760(90)90069-P PMID:2228749

Rogala, J., Jurewicz, K., Paluch, K., Kublik, E., Cetnarski, R., & Wróbel, A. (2016). The do's and don'ts of neurofeedback training: A review of the controlled studies using healthy adults. *Frontiers in Human Neuroscience*, *10*, 301. doi:10.3389/fnhum.2016.00301 PMID:27378892

Royal Society. (2019). iHuman: blurring lines between mind and machine. Royal Society.

Shaw, L., Zaichkowsky, L., & Wilson, V. (2012). Setting the balance: Using biofeedback and neurofeedback with gymnasts. *Journal of Clinical Sport Psychology*, *6*(1), 47–66. doi:10.1123/jcsp.6.1.47

Shuhaida, Y., Azuan, N., & Osman, A. (2007). *Prosthetic hand for the brain-computer interface system*. Academic Press.

Sreeja, S. R., Rabha, J., Samanta, D., Mitra, P., & Sarma, M. (2017, December). Classification of moator imagery based EEG signals using sparsity approach. In *International Conference on Intelligent Human Computer Interaction* (pp. 47-59). Springer.

Sterman, M. B., & Egner, T. (2006). Foundation and practice of neurofeedback for the treatment of epilepsy. *Applied Psychophysiology and Biofeedback*, *31*(1), 21–35. doi:10.100710484-006-9002-x PMID:16614940

Sylvan, L. J., & Christodoulou, J. A. (2010). Understanding the role of neuroscience in brain based products: A guide for educators and consumers. *Mind, Brain and Education : the Official Journal of the International Mind, Brain, and Education Society*, *4*(1), 1–7. doi:10.1111/j.1751-228X.2009.01077.x

Thompson, T. W., Hinds, O., Ghosh, S., Lala, N., Triantafyllou, C., Gabrieli, S., & Gabrieli, J. (2009). Training selective auditory attention with real-time fmri feedback. *NeuroImage*, *47*, 22. doi:10.1016/S1053-8119(09)70339-8

Yahud, S., & Osman, N. A. (2007). Prosthetic hand for the brain-computer interface system. In *3rd Kuala Lumpur International Conference on Biomedical Engineering 2006* (pp. 643-646). Springer. 10.1007/978-3-540-68017-8_162

Chapter 13
Role of Artificial Intelligence in Modeling Psychometrics to Detect Neurodevelopmental Disorders:
Use of AI to Understand Human Behavioral Aspects

Navjot Singh
Alert Enterprise, India

Amarjot Kaur
Alert Enterprise, India

ABSTRACT

The objective of the present chapter is to highlight applications of machine learning and artificial intelligence (AI) in clinical diagnosis of neurodevelopmental disorders. The proposed approach aims at recognizing behavioral traits and other cognitive aspects. The availability of numerous data and high processing power, such as graphic processing units (GPUs) or cloud computing, enabled the study of micro-patterns hundreds of times faster compared to manual analysis. AI, being a new technological breakthrough, enables study of human behavior patterns, which are hidden in millions of micro-patterns originating from human actions, reactions, and gestures. The chapter will also focus on the challenges in existing machine learning techniques and the best possible solution addressing those problems. In the future, more AI-based expert systems can enhance the accuracy of the diagnosis and prognosis process.

DOI: 10.4018/978-1-7998-3069-6.ch013

INTRODUCTION

The use of Machine Learning (ML) for clinical diagnosis of different diseases such as cancer or cardiovascular diseases in modern day is rapidly increasing. Various other health domains utilizes ML and Artificial Intelligence (AI) techniques for rapid and accurate clinical diagnosis (Brinker et al., 2018). AI-based systems seems very promising, but poses numerous challenges in the clinical diagnosis of neurodevelopmental disorders (Faghri et al., 2017; Mannini & Sabatini, 2010). The core of modern-day ML applications is the ability of machines to classify and recognize the input data with the correct label at scale. The ML based systems learn from patterns and predict the correct class to assist clinicians for early and efficient detection of Neurodevelopmental disorders.

If we have to differentiate one person from another, in general terms their behavior is one of the most important aspects to look into. There are numerous studies available on this topic that are conducted in the last few decades analyzing the psychological and emotional state of human beings to identify their behavioral traits and the behavioral shift. The detection of the disorder on the basis of behavioral traits sounds very promising, but at the same time it is very challenging. The major roadblock is the mapping of the statistical approaches to real-life scenarios such as scalability requirement. Some of the other challenges are:

- Identifying contextually suitable implementation of algorithms is not explicitly explored and defined (Nathalia et al., 2018).
- Very few examples of successfully scalable machine learning implementations and generalization of models (Wadhera & Kakkar, 2019).
- Consuming nontraditional sources of structured and unstructured data for robust machine learning solutions.
- Digitizing information without human bias is messy.
- Building real-time ML solutions using scalable data pipelines need a multi-domain understanding which makes it a difficult process (Li et al., 2016).

Through this chapter, we will learn and explore the most advanced ways i.e., data-driven and ML based approaches to solve the above-mentioned challenges. Additionally, we will also focus on the introduction to relevant ML algorithms and their methodology for disorder detection. Afterward, the impact of different channels of collecting and processing information on the accuracy is detailed to improve the bottom-line performance extraordinarily. Finally, towards the end of this chapter, we will propose a solution on how to weigh different aspects of processed information and use them temporarily for practical scenarios to address the existing challenges in a better way.

Background of Artificial Intelligence and Machine Learning

As the name suggests, AI is a means of incorporating human intelligence into machines. The act of machines performing tasks without being explicitly coded for that particular task only, but trained on general-purpose scenarios using labeled data on those scenarios is called artificial intelligence (Tanu & Kakkar, 2018). Inside AI, ML is a field of study, which gives computers an extraordinary ability to learn micro-patterns through algorithms which otherwise cannot be processed manually. This ability to understand micro-patterns enables machines to perform certain tasks without being explicitly instructed to do so. The primary objective is to let machines learn without human assistance and adjust their actions according to the situation. The major area where machine learning had the biggest breakthroughs in recent years is classification. The classification algorithms need labeled data on which we train them to predict the class for unseen data. For example, a model is first trained on 100 images of cats and 100 images of dog. And, on exposing it to an image of either cat or dog, it explicitly predicts the correct class, even when that image was not part of the original images data corpus.

Types of Machine Learning

The core use cases of ML always rely on data and find the pattern from that data to exhibit intelligent behavior. This process can differ in many ways, for example: what type of data we are using, what is the level of information available about the datasets, what is the granularity of the metadata available, what channels are feeding the data into the algorithms at what frequency and a lot of other factors. We can pick one most important question from these and dive further deep into it, i.e., what is the level of information available about the data or we can simply call it labels.

Supervised Machine Learning

Supervised machine learning is a technique that uses a data set to teach a pattern to a system so that it can predict similar outcomes on unseen data. For example: X1-Y1 is the training data and while detecting it will find Y2 only if X2 is provided as testing data. The process of learning from labeled data gives machines enormous power to predict unseen classes of data with highest precision rates, which are too close to humans in current data ML algorithms and at the largest scales, which humans cannot achieve. The steps involved in solving a given problem using supervised machine learning are as follows:

- The very first step is to decide what type of data we need, for example, in case of handwriting recognition we need to decide whether we need the full text or one word or just a character as labeled data. This demand - a complete understanding of the problem and availability of different data sets to train the system and find a solution in terms of a supervised machine learning model.
- The second important step is to gather the data. We need to know what is the real-world use of the proposed algorithm. In referenece to this, we have to gather input values as well as their corresponding output values in the form of a labeled dataset. This can be done with the help of human experts and automated rule-driven softwares or any other way of crowdsourcing the labels for a data set.
- Identify the input for the learned algorithm. The accuracy is highly dependent on how we represent the input object. The input object is transformed into a feature vector, which involves descriptors of a given object. There should not be too many features to avoid the disadvantages due to the dimensionality issues. However, there should be enough features to correctly predict the output.
- Once the function is identified, we need to choose the right learning algorithm for it. The examples of a few algorithms are Support Vector Machines, Neural Networks, and Decision Trees, etc.
- Once the design is complete, we need to run the learning algorithm on the training data after defining the control parameters if required by the selected algorithm. We also need to maintain a subset of the labeled data as testing or validation set. Afterwards, adjust the parameters to optimize the accuracy while validating against the testing data set.

- The last step is cross-validation and optimization of the validation data set by adjusting the parameters, if required. It is important to know that in this step the accuracy would be measured on a validation set selected from the training dataset to avoid the problem of model overfitting. This step ensures that the algorithm performs accurately in versatile environments.

Few other factors important to consider while using supervised machine learning are:

One of the major factors to be considered while training a machine learning algorithm is the heterogeneity of the data. It means we need to consider the discrete classes and choose algorithm accordingly. If there are too many heterogeneous values in the data, we need to choose algorithms like decision trees while other algorithms like SVMs, neural networks and logistic regression in the same class need the data to be scaled for better performance. Other factors to consider are:

- Data redundancy: If the training data contains a lot of redundant information, the algorithm performs poorly because of numerical instabilities. We need to use regularization methods to solve issues of data redundancy.
- Monitoring parameter interaction: The interaction of different parameters will help in deciding the type of algorithm. If there is a direct interaction between the parameters, then the linear algorithms are preferred. In case of complex interactions, sophisticated algorithms like decision trees and neural networks are considered. Hence, it becomes important to study the interaction between parameters through measures like correlation coefficient and others
- Understanding labeled data: The label is simply a representation of a row of data or an entity in the dataset. If we take an example of a corpus of 500 photos of dogs and cats, we will need 500 labels to explicitly describe each one of these images. Worldwide, the amount of data available is growing enormously. International Data Corporation says by 2025 worldwide data will grow 61% per annum to 175Zettabyte from current 33 Zettabyte, with as much of the data residing in the cloud as in data centers. Just for reference, a Zettabyte is a trillion gigabytes. Now multiply that 175 times. The scale is no doubt huge and as we know the AI in machines is supported by data, this generates a lot of questions. Some of which are: would it will be able to have the ML-driven AI which will grow exponentially as the data grows; would machines become incredibly intelligent that they start to manipulate human beings and finally be able to harm us. There is another factor amidst all these facts that out of the total available data, a very small fraction is a labeled data. Thus, it becomes a bottleneck in the growth of AI, but having said that we are right now at a stage where we can create absolute intelligent systems which can learn from the experiences ingesting labeled data. And, when asked about an unlabeled scenario, one can tag it with the right predicted result. The dependency of ML on labeled data will be best studied when we know the types of learning in ML algorithms.

Unsupervised Machine Learning

While it might sound interesting how ML techniques enable computers to learn the patterns by experiencing them from the data and then able to decide in any scenario how to act. It is also very interesting that we do not need to explicitly define any rule (Marlin, Kale, Khemani, & Wetzel, 2012). Today the data available in the world is abundant, so we can create any intelligent system in any domain up to the intensity we want. Innovation in solutions dependent upon ML algorithms is however capped because of strong dependency upon providing the context to machines through data labeling before they can learn from that data. This dependency kept many innovations away from the machine learning world for the longest time. This area of ML which work without the need of labeled data, is called unsupervised machine learning.

Unsupervised ML is a set of self-organizing algorithms that finds unknown patterns in the data without the need for previously labeled data sets. It is the most important area of ML after supervised machine learning algorithms. There are few hybrid algorithms combining supervised and unsupervised MLs, which scientists have used in the recent past are called semi-supervised ML algorithms.

The majority of algorithms in unsupervised machine learning use cluster analysis while others use principal component analysis. The beauty of cluster analysis algorithms is that they help segment the data sets based on patterns such as density, frequency, occurrence for the analysis, without need of any prior information. One of the main applications of unsupervised machine learning is density estimation in statistics that further solves many bottleneck problems. The other important area where unsupervised machine learning is used includes data summarization or explaining data features. Other contrast between two areas of ML is that supervised ML uses conditional probability distribution methods, while unsupervised ML intends to infer from a priori probability distributions (Wadhera et al., 2019).

Some of the most common algorithms used in unsupervised learning include:

- Clustering which involves hierarchical clustering, k-means, mixture models, density-based clustering, OPTICS algorithm.
- Anomaly detection such as Local Outlier Factor.
- Neural Networks include autoencoders, deep belief nets, Hebbian Learning and various others.
- Approaches for learning latent variable models such as
  - Expectation–maximization algorithm (EM)
  - Method of moments
  - Blind signal separation techniques
    - Principal component analysis
    - Independent component analysis
    - Non-negative matrix factorization
    - Singular value decomposition

Deep Learning

Modern-day ML has an important subset called deep learning. It is AI-based that imitates the working of the human brain to process data and create patterns for deeper understanding and decision making. Like a human brain, it involves neurons, here considered as statistical models, are responsible for information exchange to meet an objective of learning a pattern from the given data sets. The deep learning technique can be used for both supervised and unsupervised machine learning (Kakkar, 2019). It can consume structured as well as unstructured data sets. The core functionality of deep learning algorithms depends upon neural networks, hence it is sometimes also called as deep neural networks. With the easier and greater availability of the faster processing system like GPUs over the cloud as well as offline, the deep learning field has really taken off in recent years.

Supervised machine learning algorithms, despite their dependency on labeled data, are most widely used because of high accuracy and recall performance. If tuned on a fine quality data, the performance can be very optimal. In the few cases, the accuracy of these algorithms can be more than 90% of precision and recall. Hence, we will evaluate different applications of supervised machine learning which are useful in understanding the behavioral traits.

The case we are studying through this chapter is a very generic and practical life problem. Hence, it may need multiple algorithms to address a robust solution. We can study how those use cases are useful from the following sections:

USE CASES OF SUPERVISED MACHINE LEARNING FOR BEHAVIORAL ANALYSIS AND HUMAN DECISION-MAKING ASSESSMENT

Handwriting Recognition

The process of handwriting recognition is useful to identify what is written by hand and in some cases, who has written it or simply whose handwriting it is (Champa & AnandaKumar, 2010). The input data for handwriting recognition can be ingested from sources such as paper documents, photographs, touch screen mobile phones, and touch screen kiosks, etc. It can be digitally converted from hard copy to soft copy through techniques like optical character recognition or intelligent word recognition. One can even use this technique to recognize the pen-tip movements on a computer screen or a kiosk or a magnetic plate. A good handwriting recognition algorithm can handle formatting and perform segmentation of characters with good accuracy.

One of the recent breakthroughs in handwriting recognition is the ability to identify people from their handwriting. There is a difference in how biometric systems look at your handwriting, it is not only observe writing but also analyze the way of writing. They study the writing speed and rhythm as well as how much pressure you apply while writing. It is because of granularity with which the system analyzes the writing patterns and shape of words. The accuracy of identifying the person from handwriting or any other general classification task using the handwriting is at par with the human's accuracy. The handwriting recognition is one such application of AI which can help you identify a person's handwriting, we can also do other classification tasks taking analogy from this problem on how it is being solved using handwriting data as the source. Let us see how it helps us uncover the behavior of an individual.

The human psychology can also be adjudged by analyzing their handwriting through the written text with the help of modern-day AI algorithms, which can represent written text as an individual signatory feature. The handwriting of a person can vary from time to time-based upon the emotional aspects such as emotional state, any kind of disorder or behavioral patterns.

There is more than one example of how handwriting is used to exhibit human emotions and psychology. For example, many famous artists such as William Shakespeare, William Wordsworth and Samuel Taylor Coleridge (to name a few) all have written in their very specific style of writing. There is a particular area study called graphology, which employs projective techniques to study the details and description of the strokes of handwriting. Traditionally, there are many applications of graphology i.e. understanding handwriting ranging from employment profile to psychological analysis, marital compatibility, medical diagnosis, and graphotherapy.

The different factors, which are considered while analyzing handwriting, are as follows:

- Slant: The inclination of letters from the vertical edge. If we consider the psychological point of view, it represents the dependency of an individual on others.
- Baseline: The horizontal direction of written lines is studied and represents the level of optimism of an individual, for example, the ascending lines are associated with more optimistic people while the defending ones represent more pessimistic people
- Speed: The speed of writing represents intellectual assimilation, mental processing and the ability of the individual to comprehend something. This aspect allows us to measure intellectual levels, the ability to adjust to new scenarios as well as activity and temper of the person. one can also measure the professional performance of a person through the analysis of the speed of handwriting.
- Flow Continuity: This aspect through the collection of words represents the ability to cohesion one's personality.
- Pressure: The pressure with which mark is printed on sheet represents the intensity of the energy. It is also a measure of emotional security while the individual performs some actions. Other aspect which pressure can measure is how much conviction a person day-to-day things in himself or herself.
- Layout: It represents how much clarity the writer has in his ideas, we can also infer how good they are with their time management, adapting to the social norms and other similar aspects of the personality.
- Dimension: The width of characters is the most easily quantifiable aspect. One can simply measure the difference between the size of characters written under different circumstances. It can measure the self-esteem levels along with other aspects like the self-concept and degree of introversion and extroversion or self-confidence.
- Connection shape: The way connections between words is made represents the alignment with different types of cultures and situations.

With all the above-shared examples and features, we can conclude that recognizing handwriting can easily classify an individual on multiple aspects. We can classify different individuals using the features of handwriting in different behavioral classe. With this, one can easily identify the behavioral and the decision-making model for an individual. This concept is promising enough to conclude that the behavior can be analyzed using handwriting and sophisticated AI algorithms if used in the right way which is quantifiable and scalable.

Speech Processing

Speech is one of the most intuitive channels through which humans transfer information and hence communicate. The information that speech signals carry is multidimensional. It is also evident that speech signals are free-flowing waves of sound so digitizing these signals comes with its challenges as well as opportunities. In this section, we will touch upon the points which involve digitization of speech signals, processing the unstructured form of the data using machine learning and how it relates to the behavioral analytics.

The speech processing lies at the intersection of digital signal and natural language processing. Let us briefly look at these definitions.

The use of computers or sophisticated digital signal processors for processing digital signals to perform signal processing tasks is attributed to Digital Signal Processing. The signals processing represents the samples of continuous variables in the form of numbers. These variables lie in the domain of space, time and frequency. Natural Language Processing (NLP) is an area of study and manipulation of natural language through text and speech using ML or statistical algorithms primarily. This field of study is at least five decades old, but in recent years, it has seen a boom with the advent of modern-day AI domains like deep learning and fast processing power of modern-day computers.

The information contained in the speech signals is very granular in nature and contains many structured as well as unstructured data points. There are multiple use cases where speech processing is pivotal in providing the unique solutions, let us study one of the use cases to identify common challenges and solution to achieve the objective of speech processing. Through this use case, we will also get an insight into where else we can use a speech signal processing technique through analogy to solve known as well as unknown problems in the domain of behavioral analytics. There are multiple use cases of speech processing like virtual assistants, voice identification apps, call center automation, neurocomputational speech processing and speech coding.

Voice Recognition

Voice recognition is identifying the words a person is speaking using the features of the voice signal. The primary question answered here is what the person is speaking. This use case can simplify the task of identifying a person from an unknown speech signal by passing it to a model that is trained on the pre-labeled speech signals. Facilitating business use cases like speech to text or voice biometrics i.e. identifying the same person through voice command for security purposes. The solution to voice identification problem holds a lot of potentials. Speaker recognition is at least 4 decades old area of study to identify the speaker from the voice. These acoustic patterns reflect both anatomies and learned behavioral patterns.

Generally, one second of sound is read 16000 times, hence we have an array representing a sound signal with 16000 different readings, which are amplitudes of sound at these many points. Once the sampling is done correctly, the data is fed into a neural network algorithm. however, its direct processing would be difficult because of the natural noise in the data. Thus, there is a need to do some preprocessing on the audio data before consuming it. One way to preprocess the audio is to group the sample data into chunks of 20 milliseconds so that there is an array of numbers for 20 second period representing the audio data at finer granularity with less noise. To understand the patterns of these 20-millisecond chunks of data, spectrogram is a common technique in audio preprocessing. Now that we have completed the preprocessing and have the audio data in a easy format, we can feed this data into a deep neural network. Once we train the neural network on this data, split it into 20-millisecond chunks. The algorithm tries to identify the correct word spoken at each data point level. Once we consume the entire audio data through the neural network, we know the most probable spoken word at a chunk level. The next step is to stitch the words together and identify what a person is saying and even who is saying that if the analysis is done at more granularity and unique pattern for a person identified through it.

This all might sound like a very useful proposition, but at the same time, there are challenges as well in this field as all other areas. Some of those challenges are like bad quality data, background noise, reverb and echo, accent variations and other similar issues. However, if all of these respective challenges are addressed to some level, we have a world-class human-like system which identifies what someone is saying and who is saying and even the other aspect which we are interested in is the behavioral analytics so let's look into in the following text.

Speech Processing and Behavioral Analytics

While we are studying how behavioral traits in human beings affect decision making and play an important role in the assessment and intervention of multiple aspects. It is worth paying attention to one of the strongest channels of exhibiting human behavior and exploring it with the use of AI. In this section, we will focus on how speech processing unlocks human behavior analysis through the granular study of the micro patterns occurring in the speech waves.

The human behavior is complex in nature as well as heterogeneous as it gets varyingly characterized by individuals who themselves can have multimodal nature. Speech cues offer an important method to measure and model human behavior. We have studied in earlier sections that one second of speech contains 16000 unique data points or even more, which means it becomes signature every time we speak something with the specific feeling. It can represent one second of speech or emotion or we speak something in varied conditions. This very fact is extremely useful to imagine how we can look into the behavior of someone and profile it by fingerprinting on the parameters we want to measure. If in nonprofessional terms we take an example of a kid who feels excited in a certain environment (playground) and replies in a tone that is more vibrant which is only observed when the kid is in that particular environment. We can very easily identify what is the nature of the emotions of that kid by training a machine learning model on varying environments. This gives a great insight into analyzing the behavior using the speech signal through applications of supervised machine learning.

While it is clear that there is a strong connection between speech signal processing and behavioral analytics, it has its challenges. Some of them are listed as follows:

- It is a bit hard to define the notion of emotions because of their subjective nature and people interpret them differently.
- The annotation of an audio signal is another subjective task which makes it complex such as how many emotions need label and at what level i.e. a word, or character for sentence.
- The speech data is the most free-flowing and publicly available data, but at the same time collecting the neutral and bias-free data is a difficult task. Also, it becomes ambiguous to decide that training data.
- Labeling the speech data is more difficult than labeling the image or text data because of its subjective nature and difficult annotation measures. The labeled data has to go through multiple stages of validation from different individuals before we start using it.

Through this section, we can conclude that speech is the real reflection of the emotional state and behavioral aspect of an individual, it can show the patterns, which affect the decision making, and help in assessment and intervention of different parameters. While this is a research area from a few decades, the recent advancement looks very promising and the future of speech analytics for behavioral insights looks rewarding.

Emotion Recognition Through Facial Expressions

We studied speech as one of the most important channels of information in humans. While exchanging information through speaking into a natural language has some conscious and some subconscious element to it, we are going to study about another very important channel of information to look into behavioral traits of human beings, which has relatively subconscious element into it as compared to speech as we studied previously.

With the latest advancement in the computer vision space, we can study the images more extensively as well as intensively (Wadhera & Kakkar, 2019). We can go up to better granularity while classifying images or exploring their content. Nowadays it is the fact that we have started to study one of the most valuable sources of information about humans, i.e. human faces, with better accuracy and scalability. The face biometric has become more popular as it increased accuracy of face identification. Even smartphone manufacturers started providing the inbuilt feature of recognizing face features for biometric purpose and dozens of other innovative applications have started to emerge (Tanu & Kakkar, 2018). While recognizing faces have become easy, scalable and accurate, it is worth mentioning that the next wave of innovation has started to emerge with recognizing micro-patterns on the face to identify the human emotion and process behavioral analysis. Let us look into the methodology of studying faces with the use of deep learning techniques and how the facial emotion and behavior recognition helps to study behavior of individuals.

Whether it is human or machine, the process of facial recognition follows a generic process which is defined through three steps as follows:

1. The first step is to identify where exactly in the image the face exists and how many faces are there. This process is also called face detection. It is relatively easy as compared to identifying the micro-patterns and doing the low-level analysis of the facial expression which is the overall objective of this entire larger exercise
2. Once the face is detected, the next step is to identify the facial features. These features are the representation of the face in the picture. The examples of facial features are the shape of the facial components describing the skin texture in the overall area.
3. The third step is to analyze the motion of the facial features. This can be the movement of the facial muscles to identify whether the face in the picture is laughing or is it happy, angry, surprised or joyful.

In all the above-mentioned steps, one common thing is we are analyzing the image. Let us look into how the image is analyzed and how we represent the imagery data as numbers to be consumed by the deep learning algorithms such as the Convolutional Neural Network (CNN).

One of the most efficient algorithms to be used for image-based analyses is CNN. Using CNNs we do not consume the entire pixel set of an image, but use a convolved feature map that is smaller than the original input image. It represents the actual image and can discriminate that image from others. It is obvious that we lose some information using this methodology, but still, we can meet the end goal that is detecting the features.

These days we have the processors available, which can compute at very high speeds. This fact has become the core reason for the success of image-based Analytics solutions. CNN based facial emotion recognition is one of the most successful use cases which has reportedly achieved accuracy comparable to humans. The faster processing power means the ability to process more pixels at a larger scale and the granularity of the analysis while analyzing images. As we can analyze images at better granularity, we can infer more information from them such as the micro pattern showing the changing emotions at the micro-level. One can also analyze the change in emotions concerning two different changing scenarios such as external conditions for certain situations which an individual is exposed to. One fine example of this can be asking a set of questions to an individual at the workplace versus asking the same set of questions to a similar individual at home. This will show the change in behavior of a person when they are at work as compared to when they are at a relatively easy comfort zone such as home.

Since the last few decades, there have been many types of research that show the facial expressions convey the behavioral intentions of the expresser in a scene. While emotion is a mental situation, which is exclusively unique for every individual and at the same time it is a private aspect. There can be legal aspects of measuring emotions, behavior or personality of someone if the right consent was not taken so the scientific approach that we discussed in the section also has that challenge like any other disruptive technology or scientific innovation out there. Other observations worth mentioning here are that these days the cameras in public places are becoming a common practice, hence government needs to regulate this technology to avoid the misuse, especially when the video stream from these cameras is not protected using extra precautionary measures (Champa & AnandaKumar, 2010).

While we talked about the technology and its challenges now let us look at the positive aspect. The ability to measure one's emotion or behavior from an image can prove as a revolutionary technique to areas like medical diagnosis. The live video that has an average of 15 to 35 frames per second can be very easily processed by using regular GPU. This is not the end as the cloud-based infrastructure can be very easily leveraged with a personal computer and an internet connection and probably above the average camera to start measuring emotion and start logging them in real-time into a database. Once we have the real-time stream of data coming into the database, we can build an application on top of that with web or mobile interface and have patients, as well as medical practitioners, use that application for monitoring of emotional and behavioral parameters. The advantage of using search methods for measuring behavior is that these methods are fully automated, hence there is no scope of error, unlike the other manual methods. We can also process dozens, hundreds or even thousands of patients' data in parallel by finding the computational availability.

Use of AI Techniques in Understanding Human Behavioral Traits

While AI is a subject of research for the last few decades, but there have been few revolutionary breakthroughs in this domain because of the high availability of data and computation power in the cloud as well as on-premise. These new technologies can automate a few tasks which human beings perform repeatedly so that humans can focus on more intelligent tasks. It is extremely overwhelming to see new inventions and breakthroughs in the world of AI to a level that it is now able to not only mimic the intelligence, but also understand what humans want. The new wave in AI is about understanding human behavior and emotions pertaining to changing situations and environmental factors (Tanu & Kakkar, 2018). This ability of the AI algorithm helps them stand out especially in areas like medical diagnosis.

Let us take an example of a psychology practitioner to understand human behavior while medical counseling. If we go to the very fundamental level of a psychology counseling session, we can easily infer that, the psychologist would ask a few questions to the patient and in return patient will reply. The good psychologist will know that the words which the patient is speaking do not carry 100% of his/her emotions. The core channels of information in this kind of scenario are tone of the patient while he or she is speaking, their body language, there facial expressions for any other parameter which can be seen or heard by a human being. This means that the majority of information about anyone's behavior is carried either in speech signals or in the form of imagery data or we can say images or videos.

While we have observed many interesting applications in the previous sections, where either speech signals for the video data is processed to understand the behavioral intent of an individual, let us look at one more example retinal images being a basis to predict factors responsible for neuro-developmental disorders as follows:

It has been observed that ML can do classifications tasks very efficiently as compared to humans doing the same thing. In the case of retinal images, the AI algorithm produces results by decoding the personality of a person through the appearance of the retina and understanding the changes in the pattern of an image at the micro-level to identify how the behavioral and emotional aspects vary with respect to the changing external scenarios. The analogous scenarios like detecting & classifying retinal images have been researched upon so far. This shows the promising future of using retinal images as the basis to detect behavioral changes.

Neurodevelopmental Disorders Identification and Behavioral Traits

While neurodevelopmental disorders are a group of heterogeneous conditions that are shown by any kind in the skill acquisition for any disturbance in the same. It can be into social, language, and cognition for motor domains. The single most important aspect of preventing neurodevelopmental disorders is its diagnosis at a very early stage. It is very interesting to observe that if we improve the single key parameter indicator i.e. the turnaround time for the detection of abnormal behavior due to neurodevelopmental disorder, we can not only improve the prognosis but also avoid any kind of further loss due to this disorder. While studying the applications of AI for decoding human behavior throughout the chapter, we have observed that all the natural channels of information can be leveraged to the undefined limits. The quality of results will only depend upon the quality of data and the computer power.

Whether it is handwriting or speech or facial expressions all of these sources of information are implicit and they best reflect the subconscious behavior and emotional journey of the patient. These information streams can be consumed and classified in real-time using ML and we can guide these insights with explicit information such as clinical records or EHRs of a patient to obtain more informed insights. The solution is discussed in the next section as follows.

PROPOSED SOLUTION

While we discussed a few sophisticated techniques to study micro patterns, let us look into the image shown which connects the dots and shows how all of these techniques can be useful in the present and future researches.

Figure 1. Block diagram reflecting the behavioral traits modeling using Supervised Machine Learning for disorder identification

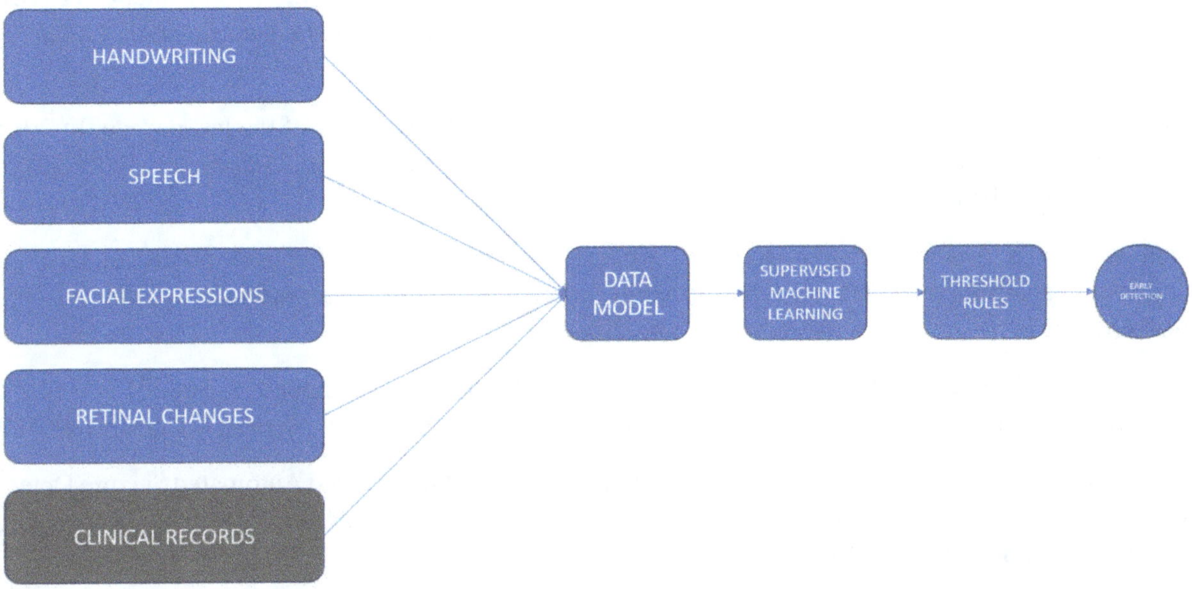

The figure shows the comprehensive approach of ingesting data from multiple sources instead of just relying on traditional clinical records data. There are multiple stages of the proposed solution which leverage the topics we discussed in detail throughout the chapter. One may follow below-listed steps to build a solution using the proposed methodology:

- Ingest data from multiple sources in a data lake using Big Data architecture
- Normalize the data at a common level so that disparate data types can be correlated
- Process the speech, image, text and transactional data to extract features and model the data
- Use classification algorithms to classify into desired classes.
- Once the classification results are obtained, we may use them differently depending upon what is the precision of a particular model and what is the significance which it holds in the overall objective, we may use thresholds and rules at this stage
- The last step is to identify the diagnosis results using pre-defined rules and consuming the incoming streams of processed data in the form of the knowledge base.

CONCLUSION

We can conclude that AI can play a pivotal role in the early detection and mitigation of any level of neurodevelopmental disorders and hence, acting as an important tool to diagnose and cure the disorders. The expert system based on behavioral traits and human decision-making process can make the system more robust and accurate. The proposed solution discussed in the last section is specific to the problem domain and one can add on more traits to generalize the system. In the future, more generic and standardized frameworks are yet to be explored both scientifically and technologically.

REFERENCES

Brinker, T. J., Hekler, A., Utikal, J. S., Grabe, N., Schadendorf, D., Klode, J., ... von Kalle, C. (2018). Skin cancer classification using convolutional neural networks: Systematic review. *Journal of Medical Internet Research, 20*(10), e11936. doi:10.2196/11936 PMID:30333097

Căleanu, C. D. (2013, May). Face expression recognition: A brief overview of the last decade. In *2013 IEEE 8th International Symposium on Applied Computational Intelligence and Informatics (SACI)* (pp. 157-161). IEEE. 10.1109/SACI.2013.6608958

Champa, H. N. & AnandaKumar, K. R. (2010, August). Automated human behavior prediction through handwriting analysis. In *2010 First International Conference on Integrated Intelligent Computing* (pp. 160-165). IEEE.

Faghri, F., Hashemi, S. H., Babaeizadeh, M., Nalls, M. A., Sinha, S., & Campbell, R. H. (2017). *Toward Scalable Machine Learning and Data Mining: the Bioinformatics Case*. arXiv preprint arXiv:1710.00112

Kakkar, D. (2018, January). A Study on Machine Learning Based Generalized Automated Seizure Detection System. In *2018 8th International Conference on Cloud Computing, Data Science & Engineering (Confluence)* (pp. 769-774). IEEE.

Kakkar, D. (2018, February). Accounting For Order-Frame Length Tradeoff of Savitzky-Golay Smoothing Filters. In *2018 5th International Conference on Signal Processing and Integrated Networks (SPIN)* (pp. 805-810). IEEE.

Kakkar, D. (2019). Influence of Emotional Imagery on Risk Perception and Decision Making in Autism Spectrum Disorder. *Neurophysiology, 51*(4), 281–292. doi:10.100711062-019-09822-8

Kakkar, D. (2019, March). Automatic Detection of Autism Spectrum Disorder by Tracing the Disorder Co-morbidities. In *2019 9th Annual Information Technology, Electromechanical Engineering and Microelectronics Conference (IEMECON)* (pp. 132-136). IEEE.

Kakkar, D. (2020). Drift-Diffusion Model Parameters Underlying Cognitive Mechanism and Perceptual Learning in Autism Spectrum Disorder. In *Soft Computing: Theories and Applications* (pp. 847–857). Singapore: Springer.

L'Heureux, Grolinger, Elyamany, & Capretz. (2017). *Machine Learning With Big Data: Challenges and Approaches*. Academic Press.

Li, L. E., Chen, E., Hermann, J., Zhang, P., & Wang, L. (2017, July). Scaling machine learning as a service. In *International Conference on Predictive Applications and APIs* (pp. 14-29). Academic Press.

Mannini, A., & Sabatini, A. M. (2010). Machine learning methods for classifying human physical activity from on-body accelerometers. *Sensors (Basel), 10*(2), 1154–1175. doi:10.3390100201154 PMID:22205862

Marlin, B. M., Kale, D. C., Khemani, R. G., & Wetzel, R. C. (2012, January). Unsupervised pattern discovery in electronic health care data using probabilistic clustering models. In *Proceedings of the 2nd ACM SIGHIT international health informatics symposium* (pp. 389-398) 10.1145/2110363.2110408

Nascimento, N., Alencar, P., Lucena, C., & Cowan, D. (2018, October). A context-aware machine learning-based approach. In *Proceedings of the 28th Annual International Conference on Computer Science and Software Engineering* (pp. 40-47). IBM Corp.

Tanu, D. K. (2019). Analysis of Weighted Visibility Graphs in Evaluation of Austim Spectrum Disorder and Epilepsy Relationship. *ICTESM-2019: 1st International Conference: with theme International Conference on Current Trends in Engineering, Sciences and Management*, 37-43.

Tanu, T., & Kakkar, D. (2018). *Strengthening risk prediction using statistical learning in children with autism spectrum disorder*. Advances in Autism.

Wadhera, T., & Kakkar, D. (2019). Eye Tracker: An Assistive Tool in Diagnosis of Autism Spectrum Disorder. In Emerging Trends in the Diagnosis and Intervention of Neurodevelopmental Disorders (pp. 125-152). IGI Global.

Wadhera, T., Kakkar, D., Kaur, G., & Menia, V. (2019). Pre-Clinical ASD Screening Using Multi-Biometrics-Based Systems. In *Design and Implementation of Healthcare Biometric Systems* (pp. 185–211). IGI Global. doi:10.4018/978-1-5225-7525-2.ch008

Wadhera, T., Kakkar, D., Wadhwa, G., & Raj, B. (2019). Recent Advances and Progress in Development of the Field Effect Transistor Biosensor: A Review. *Journal of Electronic Materials*, *48*(12), 7635–7646. doi:10.100711664-019-07705-6

Chapter 14
Activity Recognition System Through Deep Learning Analysis as an Early Biomarker of ASD Characteristics

Abirami S. P.
Coimbatore Institute of Technology, India

Kousalya G.
Coimbatore Institute of Technology, India

Balakrishnan P.
VIT University, India

ABSTRACT

Autism spectrum disorder (ASD) is a very high-flying area of research in the current era owing to its limited and on-going exploration. This chapter aims to bridge the gap of such late realization of autistic feature through machine intervention commonly known as computer vision. In this chapter, basic summarization of important characteristic features of autism and how those features could be measured and altered before a human could recognize are proposed. The chapter proposes a model for activity identification of the autistic child through video recordings. The approach is modelled in a way that consists of two phases: 1) Optical flow method detects the unusual frames based on motion pattern. 2) Each of these detected frames are fed to convolution neural network, which is trained to extract features and exactly classify if the particular frame under consideration belongs to usual or unusual class. This examines the various activities, time delay, and factors influencing the motion of the autistic child under constrained scenarios proving maximum accuracy and performance.

DOI: 10.4018/978-1-7998-3069-6.ch014

INTRODUCTION

Autism spectrum disorder is found to be one of the major concerns of parents in the recent years owing to the wide exposure of its presence. The darkened part is that most of the people are unaware of the basic characteristics of autism to identify them. ASDs are neurodevelopmental disorders with high prioritized features like impaired social communication, atypical repetitive behaviors, restrictions in range of interests, anxiety disorders and even includes language impairment that emerge during the age of 6 months to 3 years on average. This target of proper guidance could be achieved at a higher rate only with the help of early identification and early diagnosis of autistic feature in the child. Many studies and survey suggests that the parents were able to map the characteristics of their child shown at their earlier stage of development with the autistic character only after a long period of identification. This is due to the lack of granular analysis of their children characteristics and insufficient knowledge about autism and its various observation characteristics.

The autism spectrum disorder is mainly due to the impairments made in their five sensory organs that either makes the children to under react or over react and in certain case leading to neutral and repetitive behaviours respectively which is found to be purely a neurodevelopmental disorder. These differences in the behaviour should be monitored, analysed and differentiated. To perform this series of task every parent should be aware of such neurodevelopmental disability and their impacts. Also, such developmental activities could be mapped against the autism symptom before approaching the clinical trials. This is made with the help of computer vision where the analysis could be turned out as an application through handheld devices.

Early identification and early diagnosis of such autism could help the parents to bring the child to their specific field of interest. The very early diagnosis of autism is at the age of 3 months, is the point where the child tends to recognize the mother. As there are varied reasons behind this activity such as lower vision, poor eye contact, etc., the abnormality could only be identified and not concluded. Hence the autistic feature could never be solely being authorized unless the symptoms are examined further. This model helps the parents to identify the difference in the behaviour pattern and can be made prior to clinical evaluation and analysis. This minimizes the effort of clinical traits supporting the clinical advisor and the parents.

Earlier diagnosis of autism spectrum disorder is limited by various factors. Some of the commonly well known and discussed pitfalls are as follows: i) knowledge on developmental stages of the infant and toddler with and without autistic characteristics. ii) use of traditional and convolution methods such as questionnaire formats of diagnosis, iii) improper classification of unusual behaviour along with the non typically developing communicational and social behaviours, iv) delay in the acceptance state of the parents to acknowledge their child to be autistic and v) lack of awareness and proper guidance in bring up the children at the right age which is to be specific in months. Understanding and eliminating the difficulties influenced by the society could comfort, improve and support the autism child, family and the autistic society.

The proposed activity recognition system is built so as to find if the action of the autistic child is relevant to the object and also to find the time delay in performing the action. At the initial stage the system is modelled to find the activity recognition using Optical Flow algorithm. The optical glow algorithm figures out the presence of subject and then analyzes the activity made by the subject with respect to the object. Along with activity analysis, this model focuses in analysing the time delay in action of the subject (autistic child) with respect to an object.

Use of cameras to record such activities has resulted in large video data which are hard to maintain and process. Such surveillance videos are characterized by multiple entities performing concurrent activities. Though the actions are monitored through video record, those are Non-intelligent video surveillance that requires continuous monitoring by human, These surveillance videos are very costly, problematic and also very difficult and challenging to watch over all the videos continuously by an individual to monitor and alert the abnormal activity of the autistic children. Therefore an intelligent video surveillance is necessary to be built that monitors the human activities in real-time. This intelligent system could then categorize the usual and unusual activities in the video before a human could recognize.

Since video is a sequence of frames, it is necessary to capture the interactions between the frames and identify motion pattern. The task lies in generating motion influence map for frames using optical flow value. Optical flow is the pattern of motion of blocks of image objects between two consecutive frames. Such motion influence map can effectively depict,

1) Movement speed.
2) Movement direction.
3) Size of the objects with their interactions within a frame sequence.

The model for activity recognition is then extended as a model involving Convolution Neural Network which categorizes the activity using feature extraction and classification. The paper aims in developing both the models as optical flow algorithm is not semantic in some scenarios whereas Convolution Neural Network provides better results in terms of accuracy and performance. The system as a whole at the final stage proposes a model that makes use of Optical flow based motion influence map generation and Convolution Neural Network to effectively monitor and detect unusual activities.

State of Art

The state of art deals with the nature of autism, characteristics of autism, early diagnosis of autism, defects and delay in detection through regular methods, computer intervention in diagnosis, influence of video based detection, abnormality detection through video analysis and various techniques employed respectively thus finally heading towards the importance and need for the proposed work in the paper.

From the perspective of neurodevelopmental sciences, autism is found to be one of the important exploring disorders among children and adults. Though the reasons behind this neurodevelopmental disorder vary in a wide range such as genetics alteration, societal impacts, etc., the Autism Spectrum Disorder (ASD) is found to impact the behaviours and communication deficits in children. These deficits do not hinder the development of the child unless they are not identified and treated.

Many researchers belonging to the field of medical, occupational therapy, computer fields join hands in solving the problem of early identification and diagnosis of ASD. This in turn will support parents and clinical diagnosis process to shape the children in a better way with respect to their interest. Support for diagnosis of autism makes people realize the capability, deficiency, difficulties, and most importantly their neutral to aggression parameters. The indicators of autism predominantly appear by the age of 2 years that stands as a point of start for the diagnosis. Henceforth the regular observation and proper clinical trials could be carried out. Though the age of 2 years seems to be an early identification source comparing the life time, it is observed that the identification could still be untimely identified with proper supporting mechanisms.

Many findings confirmed the behaviours of autism such as

- being very aggressive
- being neutral on most of the time
- being non responsive in nature
- having repetitive behaviour
- troublesome in gathering words
- showing anxiety, engaged in hand flapping
- Posing and exposing body posture
- Facial expression
- walking on the toe tip
- inappropriate responses in subject with respect to the object
- Processing unique word / activity or signs for n iterations
- no proper gaze on humans
- Likelihood in loneliness and self exclusion

Shyam Sundar et al. (2013) suggested that the expressions possessed by the children could provide an informative biomarker about the autism influenced person characteristics. As the facial expression could be identified, the way similar approach is that the body expressions are useful in analyzing and identifying behavioral aspects of the children under autistic consideration.

Rehg et al. (2011) suggested that the vision based techniques are employed for various analyses such as head posture variations, fractal structure of face, expressions of the face. Apart from this the author suggests strong insights on the activity recognition system as an early biomarker of autism that explains the social and communicative behavior of the children in a dyadic interaction or on par with any object. This activity recognition through computer vision based technique gives the basic level of engagement in the child during the interaction or activity.

Dworzynski et al. (2012) suggested that as the emotional behavior, communication plunge and other behaviors face the higher level and cognitive functioning dropping to lower level would result in the higher increase of the probability in autism diagnosis. The author also suggests the frequency of change in the child behavior over time is a resultant effect of quicker change in then sensory profile and functioning of neurons.

John et al. (2017) briefed that the early diagnosis of autism will enrich health care units that deals with neurodevelopmental disorder to support the parents, care takers and the entire surrounding of the autistic child as they confront the difficulties and challenges in raising the autistic child in a better way. The author also pointed that educating such parents and their families about the features, challenging behaviors, support factor, ways to involve the children in situations, easy and smooth handling of the children and also some treatment measures to keep the children in state will definitely support the family which in turn will prop up the autistic child. Through this the family would never experience the feel of self centric rather the sense of family centric or autism society centric.

Many researchers suggest that it is the duty of the physicians to alert the caregivers on their own well being towards the child. Maintaining such collaborative relationships with the child, family and caretakers, any clinical assistants would ease the diagnosis process. This could also enhance the feasibility of proving appropriate training in communication skills, behavioral skills, and comprehensive development and even identify the facts that hinder the children ability to act stable in their likeliness. This widens the intervention window of the autistic child.

Apart from these support to the autistic child that is provided after ages of diagnosis, Michail et al. (2015) suggested that their sensory, vestibular and visual processing is much important to maintain the body in a stable state. The author also concludes that the children with high functioning of autism will find it more difficult in balancing their body and even head in a steady state. The work also suggests that this imbalance of body could be an early biomarker to intervene autism within 36 months. This is because it is observed that any children under normal development would balance themselves and starts stepping within 36 months of age. When the former specified case fails in any children, it is the immediate next step to have a keen understanding behind the lag of steps in the children.

Anna et al. insights that there was only minimal number of study conducted in relation with neural correlates. This neural correlates involves the time perception in autism spectrum disorder that correlates the change of functions over time period expressing as any communication and behavioral deficits. This in analyzed in the way of knowledge that the subtle impairments of low level functioning neurons would have an adversary affect that cascades over time to results in the high functioning of disability. To identify and analyze autism the model needs to be build on a time dependent learning methods for more accurate results.

Abirami et al. suggested that the autism spectrum could be diagnosed at an early state through facial expression analysis .Through the results, the authors suggests that the children with specific facial expression over a time period could likely to fall under the category of autistic feature in the near further. The proposed method using computer intervention makes the autistic feature analysis possible at an early stage. The authors were able to identify the predominantly expressed expression in ASD that could be combined with the motion analysis to analyse the likeliness and behavioural response of the child.

Manoranjan et al. suggested that the video surveillance is a key to detect and identify objects excluding the man power. The author discussed various applications that accommodated the video analysis and surveillance such as crowd analysis, healthcare, elderly support, abnormality detection, any type of suspecting etc.

Motion detection for various applications has been done based on Optical flow algorithm. In the proposed work of Rensso Victor et al, anomalous events in crowd places are detected using spatiotemporal feature descriptor specifying histograms of optical flow orientation, magnitude and entropy based on optical flow information. The two principal morphological operations used are dilation and erosion. Threshold based segmentation is done to discriminate foreground from background. Assumptions are made for threshold values and for detecting congestion.

Mariem Gnouma et al, approached a new foreground detection architecture based on information extracted from the Gaussian mixture model (GMM) incorporating with the uniform motion of Magnitude of Optical Flow (MOF) for human action recognition. Fast dynamic frame skipping technique is used to avoid frames that contain irrelevant motion. Human action classification is done using sparse stacked auto encoder combined with Soft Max classifier.

Recently, Mohammad et al. specified that deep learning approaches have paved an efficient way for image processing. Particularly Convolution Neural Networks (CNN) has been used for feature extraction and image classification. The author presents Fully Convolution Neural Network (FCN) based architecture for time-efficient anomaly detection and localization. The system adapts a pre-trained classification CNN to FCN for generating video regions to describe motion and shape concurrently. This concerns two main tasks, feature representation and cascaded outlier detection.

Another solution proposed by Wenqing Chu et al. provides method for abnormal event detection based on jointly optimizing the sparse coding and the unsupervised feature learning for video data. To exploit the spatiotemporal information of the inputs, the deep 3-dimensional convolution network (C3D) is used. The research work performed dictionary learning for generating spatiotemporal features and then obtained the sparse coding results followed by constructing multiple level similarity trees.

For video analytics, analysis should be based on time series and in that case recurrent neural networks can be used. In Bharat Singh et al. proposed work; a multi-stream bi-directional recurrent neural network is used for fine-grained action detection. It uses a bidirectional Long Short Term Memory for action detection task. LSTM layer is trained on complete videos containing multiple actions. Instead of representing motion information using a sequence of flow fields, the author suggests to use a sequence of corresponding pixel displacements called pixel trajectories. Output from multi-stream network is fed to LSTM which provided nominal accuracy.

Another method using motion of the objects is given by Shifeng Li et al. In the proposed work, anomaly detection based on two global grid motion templates which are able to capture the motion distribution, space and scale information was modelled. It contains maximum and minimum threshold to capture the upper and lower bound motion patterns of trained samples and compute the similarity between templates and testing samples.

With the key advantage of the current technological solutions to detect anomalies the proposed paper suggest in integrating the optical flow motion detector inculcated with the CNN. This proposed system suggests an intelligent video monitoring system for autistic child that analysis the time delay taken by the autistic child to perform an action. The system could also detect any abnormal activity done by an autistic child when he / she undergoes any stress, aggression or temperament as the system is modelled for the positive well behaviour possessed by the children. Such unusual activity detection is defined in this paper through identification of motion patterns that do not conform to the expected behaviour. This could be achieved by specifying and distinguishing the activities as 'usual' and 'unusual' that could occur and that should not occur respectively. This ensures better results in terms of accuracy, sufficiency and specificity to autistic features. On detecting such abnormal behaviours and anomalies, every parent of the children who could fall under the category of autism could be benefited at an early stage before appearing to clinical analysis.

The proposed system could further be improved by employing this early intervention parameter into a handheld application which in turn could be integrated with the facial expression and emotional analysis along with the Chat questions finalized and approved by the autism society to detect autism and level of autism at an initial stage.

Dataset Description and Pre Processing

The data for the analysis of the proposed system in collected from countable children with and without autistic feature within the age of two years and later the sample analysis was also made in analysing videos of autistic children presented over the internet. The videos analysed from he internet source had a varied age groups within 6 years approximately. As the video is generally the sequence of frames, they are processed sequentially. In order to satisfy the processing requirements and the capacity of computation, the dimensions of the input video is chosen to be 320 x 240. Further, the RGB frames are converted to gray scale where a gray scale image consists of only the intensity information of the image rather than the apparent colors. RGB vector with three dimensional spaces is converted into gray scaled vector of one dimensional space with the inculcation of predefined function in OpenCV.

Proposed Methodology

The basic system architecture of the proposed methodology in depicted in the Fig.1. There are three main stages of the proposed methodology namely i) input processing stage in which the video frames are captured and pre processed, ii) optical method of identifying abnormal/unusual activity that produces intermediate results for analysis and iii) computation of unusual activity based on computational neural network.

Figure 1. System Architecture of the proposed system

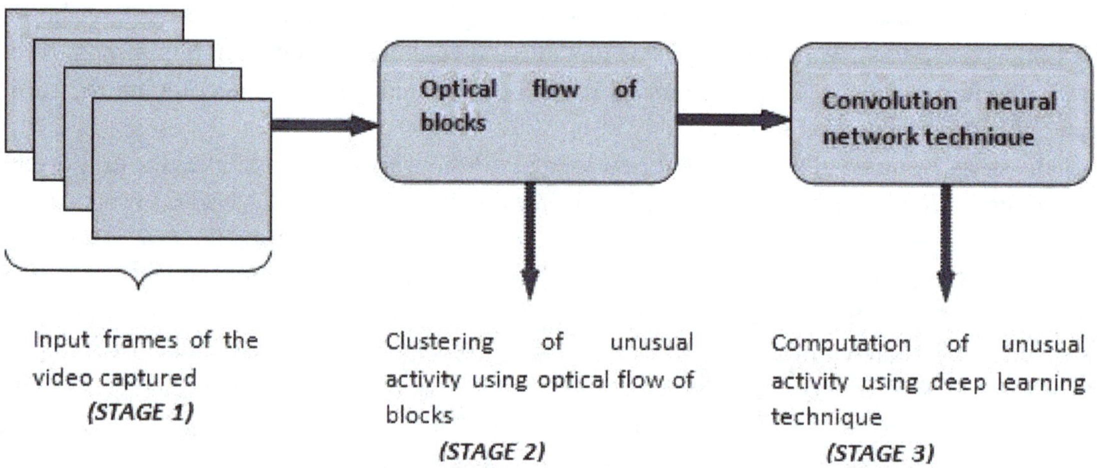

The detailed working flow graph of the proposed methodology is shown in Fig.2. The diagram is sub divided into two parallel towers contributing to stage 2 and stage 3 of the system architecture. The stage 2 explains the separation of optical flow of blocks and the process of how the individual blocks are integrated to form the mega blocks out of which the unusual activity and the time delay to detect the unusual activity could be measured. The application of neural network based analysis of unusual activity is specified in stage 3 of the flow diagram. The figure distinctively explains about how the proposed model integrates the two stages through the flow of frames identified under motion influence blocks towards the input frame to the neurons of the convolution input layer. The figure also explains the pre processing step on the input frames collected through the video capture.

Figure 2. Flow diagram of the proposed system

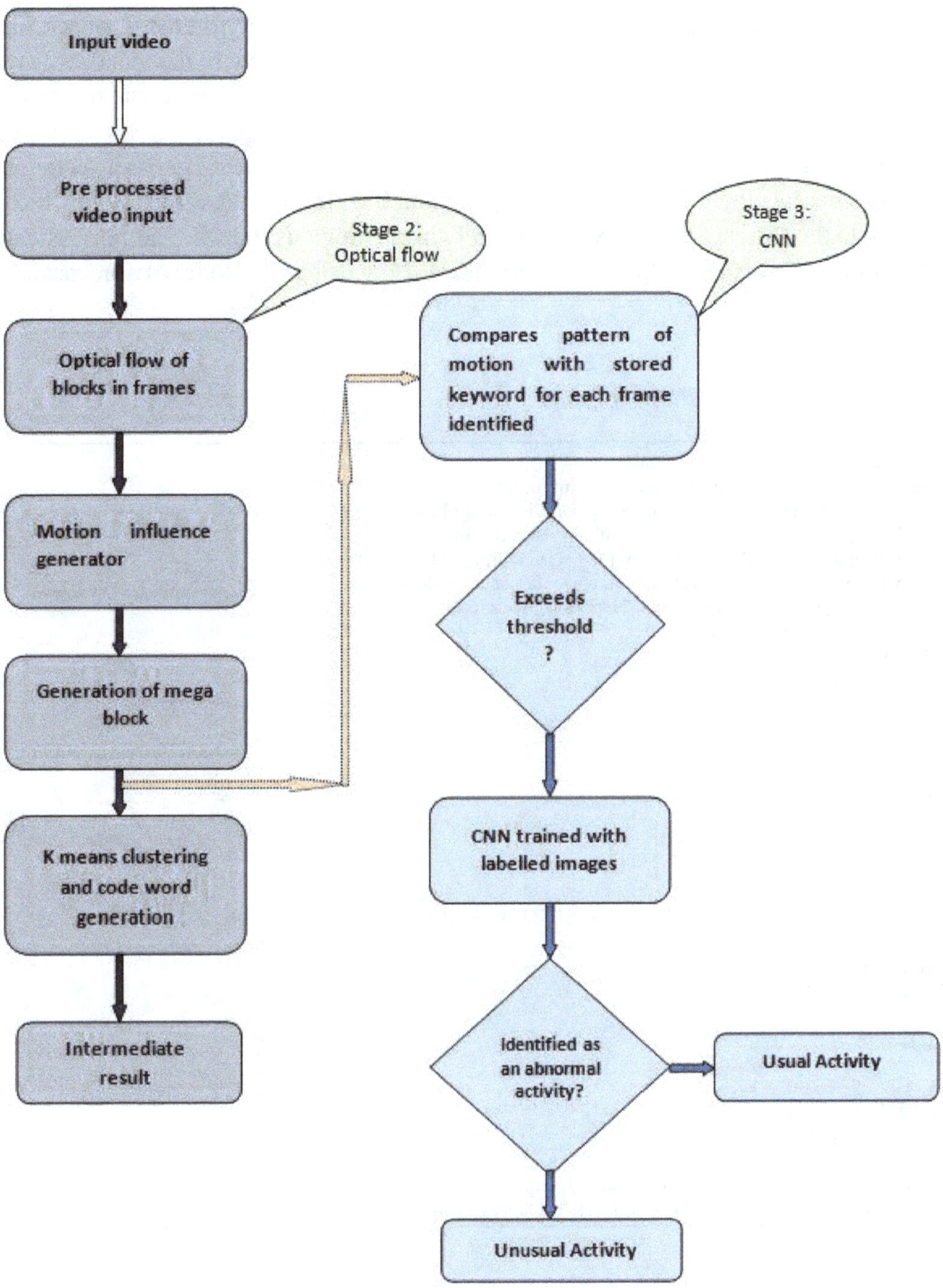

Optical Flow of Frames and Blocks

Before the optical flow of frames is identified, the input video undergoes pre- processing. The pre-processing involves in segregation of frames over the captured video in a rate of 60 frames per second. The 60 frames are then dropped in random intervals and are reduced to its half quantity. This random drop of frames ensures that no new action in a frame is missed out in the filtered /dropped frames.

After the pre-processing step, optical flow is computed for each frame in the video, which in turn is an input where optical-flow is computed for each pixel in a frame using FarneBack algorithm. Optical flow is defined as a pattern of motion of objects, surfaces, and edges apparently visualized in a visual scene due to the relative motion between an observer and the scene. Optical-flow is a vector of the form (r, θ), where, r represents the magnitude of each pixel and θ represents the direction in which the each pixel has moved to the corresponding pixel moderately in the previous frames. The calcOpticalFlowFarneback () function in OpenCV computes a dense optical flow using the Gunnar Farneback's algorithm as shown in Table 1.

Table 1. Algorithm for Optical Flow of Frames

```
Input: Flow image from the video and flow matrix
Step 1: Initialize the number of rows and columns in the frame block
Step 2: For every index, i in the value matrix, compute optical flow of blocks
 opFlowOfBlocks[i[0]/block_row][i[1]//Block_col][0] += magnitude[i[0]][i[1]]
 opFlowOfBlocks[i[0]//block_row][i[1]//block_col][1] += angle[i[0]][i[1]]
Step 3: for every index value I in the optical flow, compute the center of blocks
 opFlowOfBlocks[i[0]][i[1]][i[2]] = float(value)/(block_row*block_col)
 value = opFlowOfBlocks[i[0]][i[1]][i[2]]
Step 4: if(i[2] == 1):
 angle = math.degrees(val)
 if(angle > 337.5):
 k = 0
 else:
 q = angle//22.5
 a1 = q*22.5
 q1 = angle - a1
 a2 = (q+2)*22.5
 q2 = a2 - angle
 if(q1 < q2):
 k = int(round(a1/45))
 else:
 k = int(round(a2/45))
opFlowOfBlocks[i[0]][i[1]][i[2]] = k
 theta = value
 Step 5: if(i[2] == 0):
 r = value
 x = ((i[0] + 1)*block_row)-(block_col/2)
 y = ((i[1] + 1)*block_row)-(block_col/2)
 blocks_centre[i[0]][i[1]][0] = x
 blocks_centre[i[0]][i[1]][1] = y
Step 6: return the computer optical flow of blocks with the centre block value
opFlowOfBlocks,block_row,block_col,block_row*block_col,blocks_centre
```

Motion Influence Generation

The key task lies in finding the motion patterns using optical flow. The motion influence value of the current block ('X') is calculated based on the fact that neighbouring blocks ('Y') are more influenced rather than the distant blocks. The threshold distance and angle for block 'x' is calculated using its optical flow value and these are compared with the Euclidean distance calculated between block 'x' with the surrounding blocks 'y' and also the angle between them. If the Euclidean distance is less than the threshold and if the angle between the blocks lies between the threshold angles, then the block 'y' is considered to be under the influence of the block 'x'.

Then a number of smaller blocks are grouped into a larger block. The Motion Influence value of such a block is the summation of motion influence values of all the smaller blocks constituting a larger block. Table.2 explains the algorithm for computing motion Influence Generator.

Table 2. Algorithm for Motion Influence Generator

Input: Optical flow of blocks **Step 1**: compute the threshold distance of the block **Step 2**: compute the threshold angle of the blocks **Step 3**: compute the centre of the blocks using x1 = block-centre[block1_i[0]][block1_i[1]][0] y1 = block-centre [block1_i [0]][block1_i [1]][1] x2 = block-centre [block2_i [0]][block2_i [1]][0] y2 = block-centre [block2_i [0]][block2_i [1]][1] slope(m) = float(y2-y1)/(x2-x1) **Step 4**: compute the Euclidean distance using Eu_dist = float(((x2-x1)**2 + (y2-y1)**2)**0.5) **Step 5**: compute the angle between blocks as if(block1_angle-block2_angle < 0): block1_angle = math.degrees(block1_angle) block2_angle = math.degrees(block2_angle) return math.radians(360 - (block1_angle - block2_angle)) return block1_angle - block2_angle **Step 6**: using the computed values fron step 1 to step 4, compte the motion influence block as MIV[i[0]][i[1]][int(opFlowOfBlocks[i[0]][i[1]][1])] += math.exp(-1*(float(eu_distanceDist)/opFlowOfBlocks[i[0]][i[1]][0]))

Create Mega Blocks

From the motion influence generator value, the mega blocks of frames are framed using the algorithm as specified in Table.3. These mega blocks are created that depicts the influencing circumference of the subject which makes it certain that these is no loss in the data field spread over the frames.

Table 3. Algorithm for Mega Block Creation

Input: motion influence frames, number of rows and number of columns **Step 1**: Compute motion influence value, MIV using number of frames, number of rows and number of columns **Step 2**: For every frame in the MIV For every index value i in the frame Compute the mega block motion onfluence vector as [MIV_mega[i[0]//n][i[1]//n][frame_count]),(frame[i[0]][i[1]])] MIV_mega[i[0]//n][i[1]//n][frame_ount] = np.array(list(map(sum, zip(*temp)))) **Step 3**: return the MIN_mega with its coordinates

Codewords Generation

Clustering is performed on these larger blocks to generate a concatenated feature extraction. It is done using openCV K-means clustering method with Spatio-temporal features using the mentioned syntax and centres returned are saved as codewords.

```
ret, labels, cw = cv2.kmeans(np.float32(MIV_mega[row][col]), cluster_n, None, criteria,10,flags)
```

These codewords model the pattern of usual activities that can occur in the respective area. Such codewords are saved in a Numpy file with .npy extension which has to be used in training phase.

Training and Testing

The training phase takes the input video which has normal activities that can take place in an autistic positive environment. The aforementioned steps are carried out on the input and the results of training phase are the codeword's.

The testing phase takes the input video which involves unusual activities of autistic children. The same steps carried out in training phase are done until the generation of motion influence value for larger blocks. Then the saved codeword's are loaded and they are compared with the motion influence value.

A minimum distance matrix over the larger blocks is constructed, in which the value of an element is defined by the minimum Euclidean distance between a feature vector of the current test frame and the codeword's in the corresponding larger block. We find the highest value in the minimum distance matrix as the frame representative feature value and is compared with the defined threshold value. If it exceeds the threshold, then it is more likely to occur as unusual activity in that frame. Then block level detection occurs to find out in which blocks unusual motion pattern occurs

Classification Using Convolutional Neural Network

Convolution neural network being one of the most predominantly notable deep leaning approch for image data process inspite of its complexity in developing the internal deep neural network architecture. The CNN takes the input and process through the following stages namely

- Convolution layer
- Max pooling layer
- Fully connected network

The proposed methodology aims in applying the CNN to the frames identified under the optical flow of blocks technique so as to attain maximum efficiency and accuracy. This is because, the optical flow method detects a frame as unusual based on motion pattern which may be inaccurate in certain scenarios. So these frames are subjected to feature extraction and classification using CNN at the end. Though the video is processed in alive stream under optical flow of blocks, the video is subdivided into number of frames and the frames are fed as input to the optical flow, processeed using megablock creation and the resultant local optimum abnormality detected frames and fed into the convolution layer of CNN.

The CNN architecture is designed in the way of involving two hidden layers acting with Relu activation function . These two hidden layers converge into the fully connected layer so as to ensure maximum true positive situation. This CNN method of analysing motion and finding the abromality in the system minimizes the fasle positive and true negative values. On each hidden layer the blocks of N frames are taken as input along the block_row, block_column and block_centre.

As this is a supervised learning, the model is trained using labelled images consisting both usual (labelled as 0) and unusual activities (labelled as 1). In this method the images are pre-processed to have 200 x 200 dimension and gray scaled. These images are passed in batches to the model and the neural network is trained. 20% of data is used for validating the proposed CNN model. The loss and accuracy metrics for training and validation are visualized with much improved accuracy.

Fig. 3 explains the working of convolution neural network with two hidden layer. The CNN model takes the input as frames computed from the optical flow of blocks. These frames will hold the motion influencing portion of the frames focus to be trained over the neural network. The process of CNN involving two hidden layer constituting convolution and max pool layer correspondingly is depicted. The number of hidden layers is restricted to two as the increase in the number of hidden layers could require improved computational facility through high processing hardware. The fully connected layer results in either normal or abnormal activity which is then be activated with ReLU activation function so as to produce the desired output of unusual activity. The ReLU linear activation function is specifies as

$f(x) = x$; for all values of x over (0,n)

which defines the fact that increase in the value of x will have a linear impact on $f(x)$, say $f(x)$ could be *maximum (0,x).*

The proposed system makes use of Jupyter notebook for implementing python code for CNN. Keras, which is an open-source neural network library, is used to implement the CNN which is using Tensorflow as backend proving better and easy implementation of video and image pressings and analysis. The proposed methodology makes use of sequence model to perform training and testing.

RESULTS AND INSIGHTS

The proposed method is implemented over a countable number of autistic subjects under constrained experimental setups. This is because of the privacy and concern of the children information. In spite of this difficultly the papers ensures to employ computer vision based early identification of autism. The video was captured from three children possessing with and without autism considered within three different situations. The results are compared with each category of children and then time delay in processing the activity was also performed. The unusual activity of both the category of children could be identified with change in the dimensionality of the frame classified under blocks. These results and insights made out of the proposed work suggests the parents and clinicians that the child behaves abnormal in normal situations pointing to the delay in their action thus proving the children may fall under autistic category in the near feature due to the developmental delay and abnormal behaviour.

Scenario 1: On the first modelling of video capture, the children were not subjected to any object under influence. That is in turn, the children were set to make movements of their own and through their natural sensory processing system in a contactless environment. During this video analysis it was found that the children with autism functionality showed varied movements in a limited period of time ranging a difference between 2 sec to 3 sec. The children were found to make repetitive movements which further indicate the presence of autistic feature. On the other hand on examination of a regular developing child, the movements of the children were also found to rapidly change within a minimum specified amount of time but the repetition in movements were not present. This is because the regular developing children do not perform the same task as they fall under boredom category.

Figure 3. Working of CNN with Optical Flow of Blocks

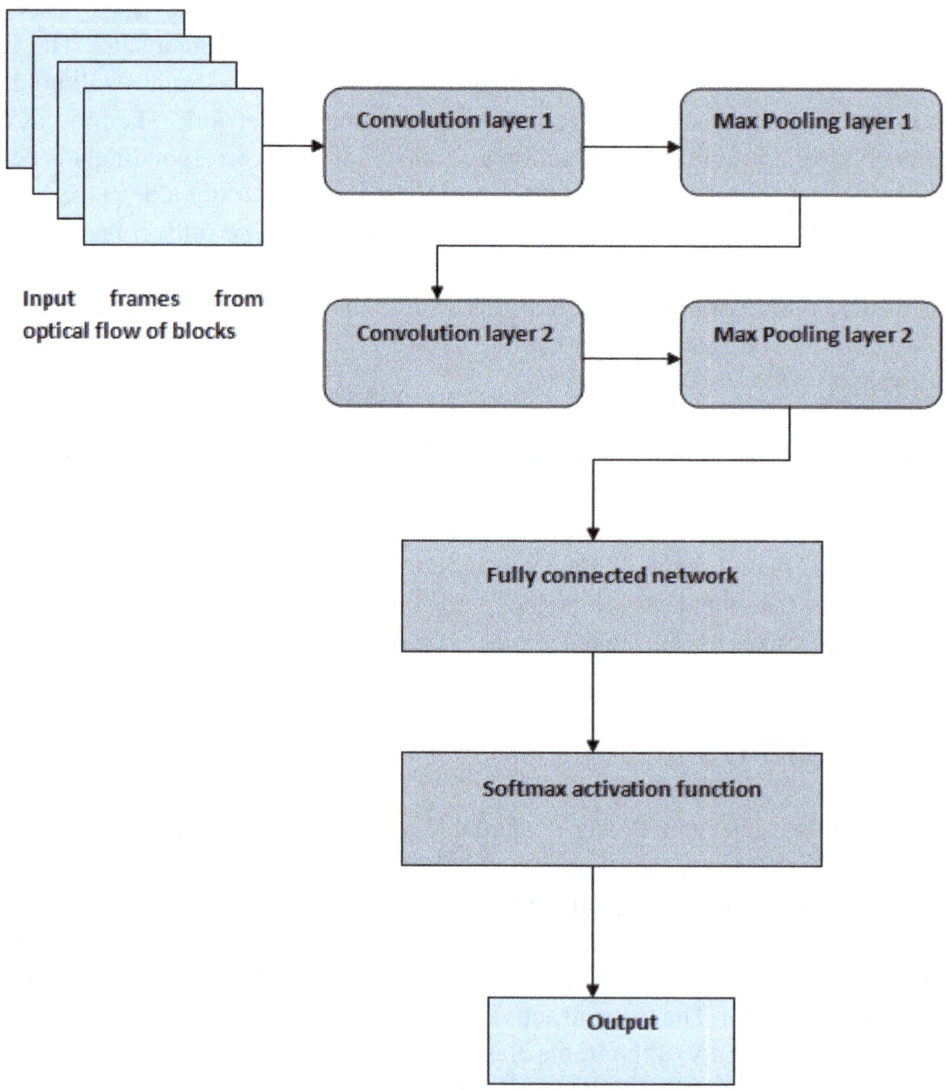

Figure 4. Variation in Blocks of autistic children under Scenario 1

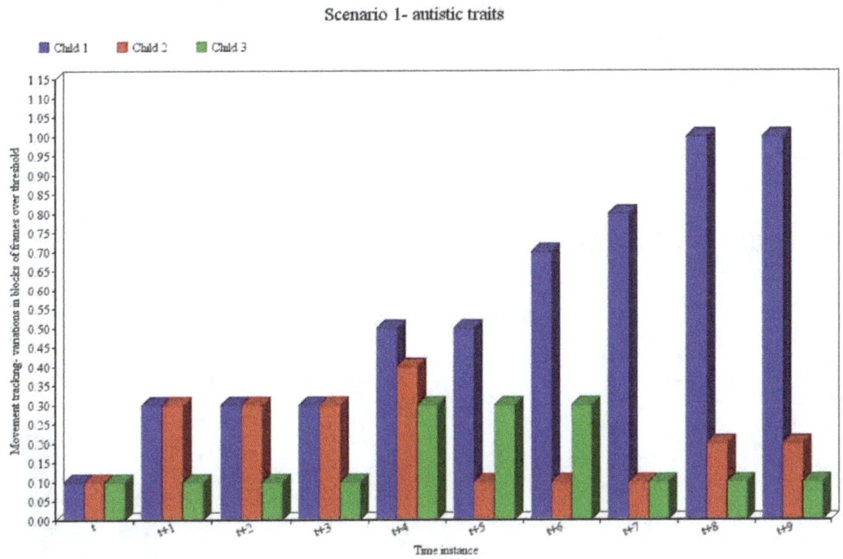

Figure 5. Variation in Blocks of non autistic children under Scenario 1

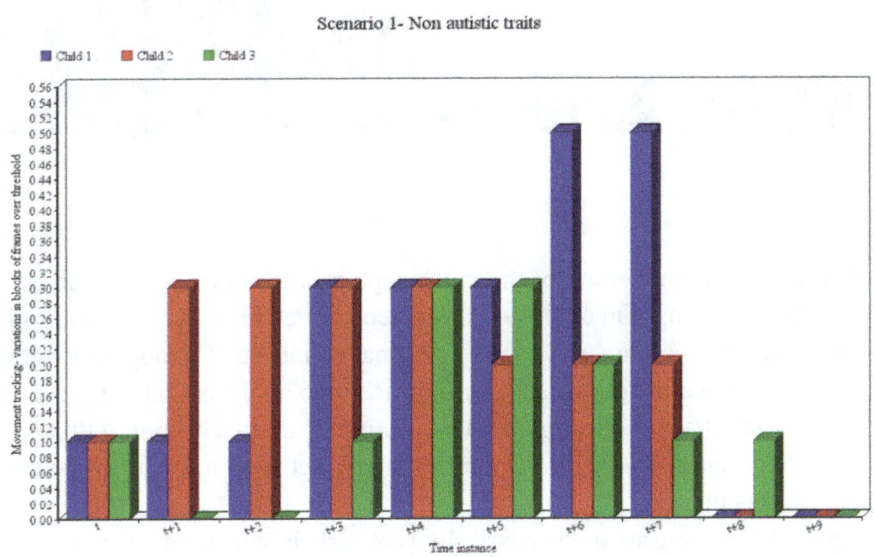

Fig.4 and Fig.5 explains the variations in blocks of frames for autistic and non autistic children respectively under the Scenario 1. The graph takes the time series along x- axis and the differentiated no of blocks long the y-axis. The variations could be used to analyse and diagnose the movement tracking abnormality when the variation in the blocks goes beyond the threshold. For example the child 1 in the Scenario 1 on monitoring for t to t+n time series, the child makes a varied movement along time. Though the graph specifies the gradual movement of activity of the child, the real time observations shows a drastic change in movement. This is to prove that the movement in frames could be granularly analysed that could neither be analysed nor visualised in our naked eyes. Since the dropping of frames could be made during analysis, care should be taken to ensure that dropping of frames in the video sequence must be carefully adjusted in the processing so as to avoid that there is no drastic unusual movement shown by the child.

Figure 6. Variation in Blocks of autistic children under Scenario 3

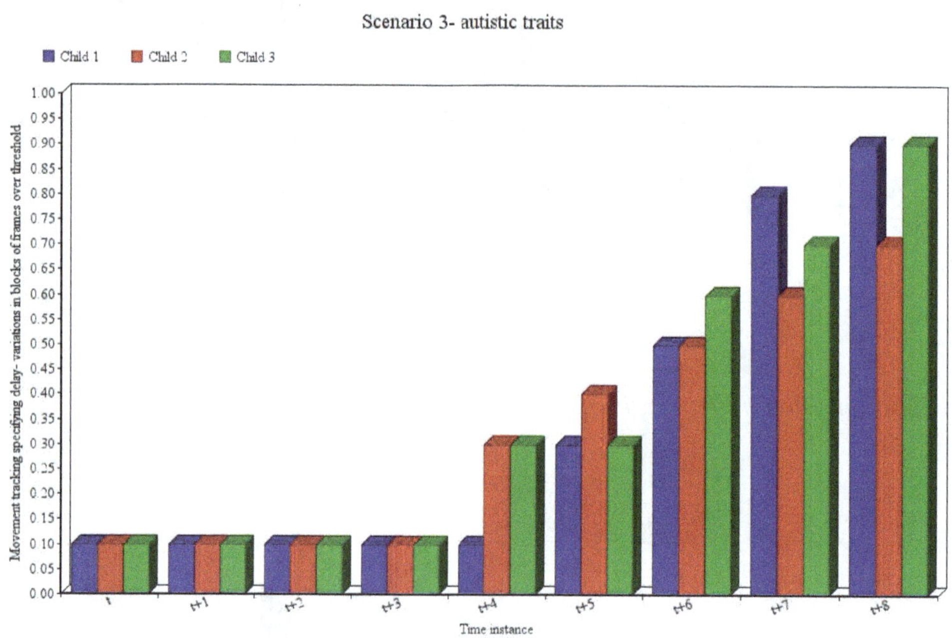

Scenario 2: On the second modelling of the video capture, the children were subjected to an object that is fixed to be a human being. On analysing the video of the children for about 2 minutes run, the children with high functioning autism were not able to make their head steady which made the head to bang in the air. There were two insights made during this video analysis that are i) the head movement control ability due to vestibular processing could be minimum in the children with autism; ii)the time taken by the autistic children to view and respond to the object took a longer period when compared over typically developing children.

Of the second modelling, there are many possibilities of early intervention of autism in children. Since the entire methodology is proposed in support with supervised learning, with high functioning autism as a class label, the following insights could be made in a most accurate manner.

i) Any children at the age of maximum 3 to 4 months must be capable to balance the head. Once this fails, there might be a possibility to fall autistic.
ii) Any children at the age of 4 months again in maximum must be able to sense the mother and make any facial reaction. In reference with the authors previous work of facial expression, if there in any

hindrance of making any facial expression with the mother at least during breast feeding, then the child should be carefully monitored. This suggests the parents as an early biomarker of autism.

Figure 7. Variation in Blocks of non autistic children under Scenario 3

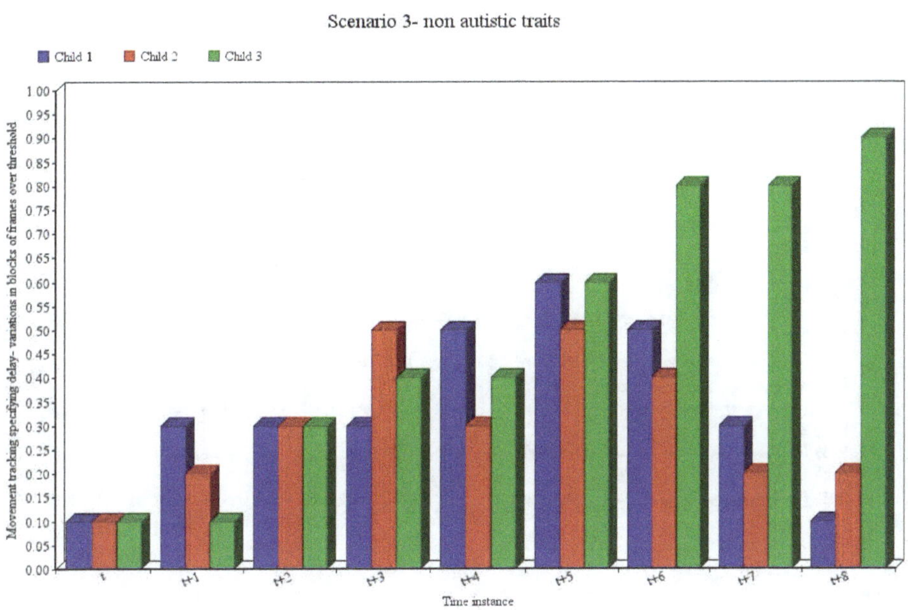

Scenario 3: The third modelling of video capture was made in an intention to make the children play around with an object so as to identify the rate of fall of interest over time. The following analysis were made out of this scenario; i) the children delayed in grabbing the object; ii) the children found to hold the object for a longer period with no movement; iii) the children made repetitive actions on the object and iv) the children with no sign of boredom excludes the object which was achieved by a analysis of direct change of movement.

Fig.5 and Fig.7 depicts the time delay exhibited in autistic child and non autistic child under the Scenario 3. It is observed that the movement of the children remains stable for a longer period of time in the autistic traits. Whereas, it was found that there was a reasonable change in the variation of blocks for non autistic traits. This stable movement in the variation analysis suggests that the children tend to focus on the object and there occurs a developmental delay in responding to the object. Such delays in responsiveness hold true for the autism characters that has to be further analyzed under varied circumstances.

After the analysis of the video captured, the parents' were confirmed about these insights made in the children, it was ended up hearing that the symptoms were seen in the children at an early stage but the darkest spot is that they were not able to map these characteristics until diagnosed by a clinician after years of maturity. Feeding this sole idea into the technology, the proposed method supports the early diagnosis of autism and stands as a key biomarker of autistic society under proper setup.

Figure 8. Accuracy and Loss validation over no of epochs

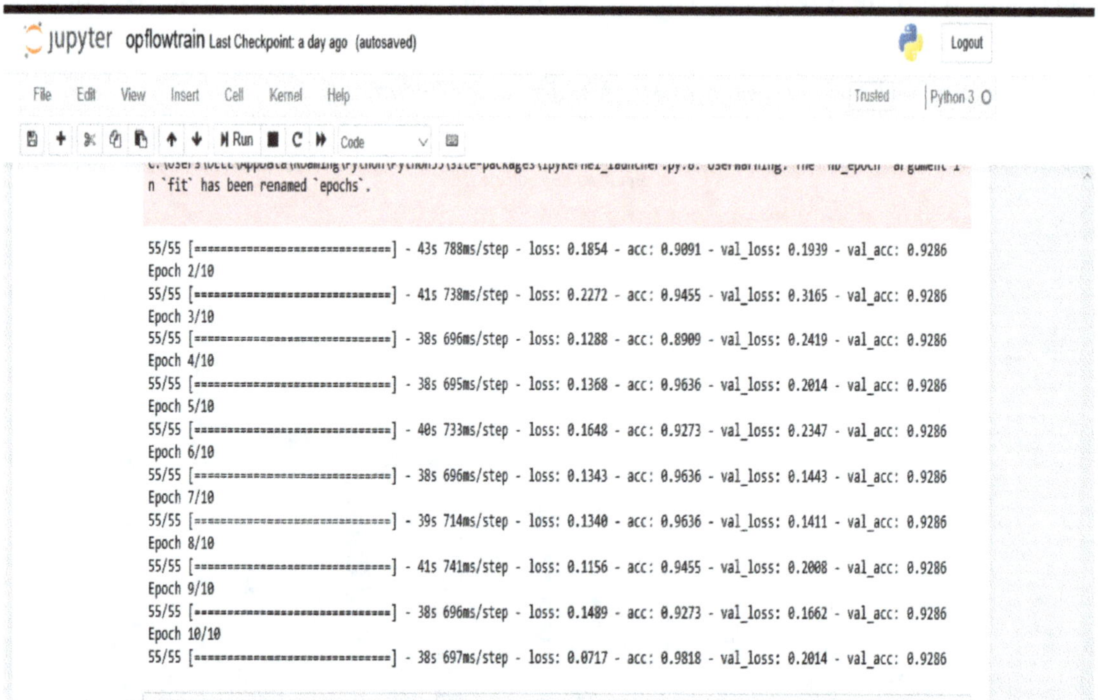

Figure 9. Comparison of Training Loss over Validation

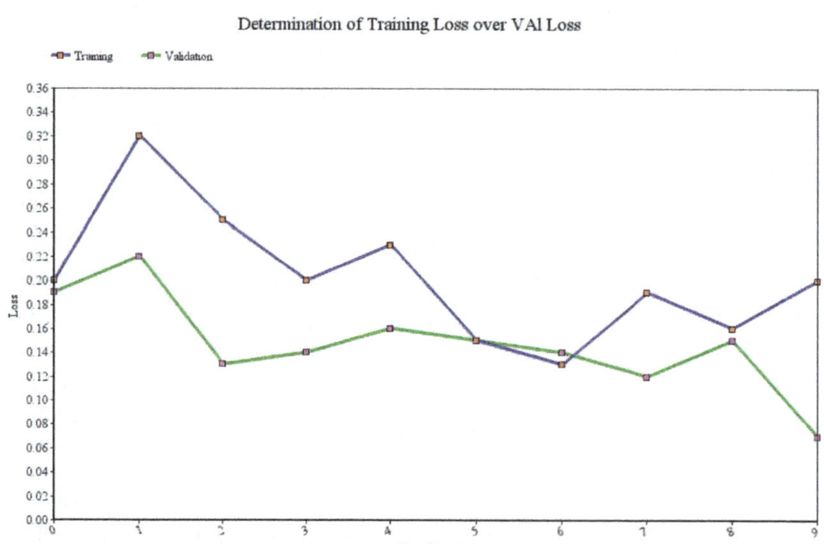

Figure 10. Comparison of Accuracy over the various proposed models

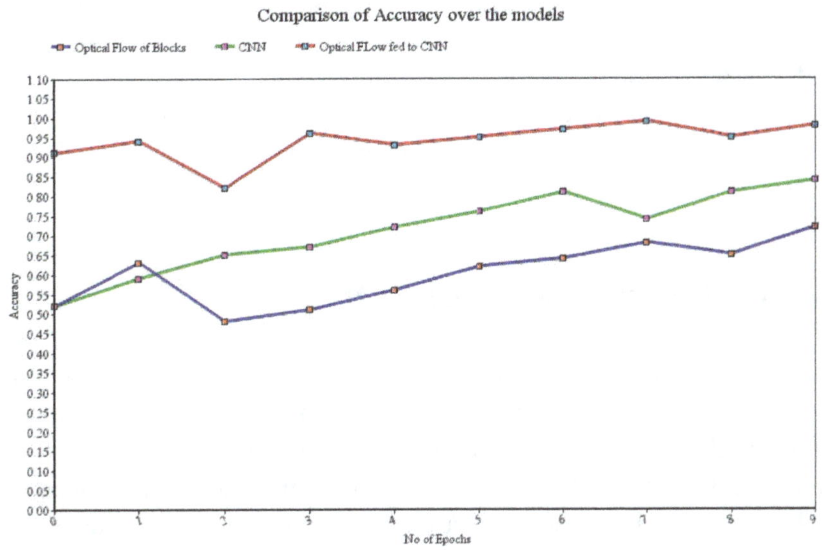

Fig.8 depicts the change in accuracy and loss function with the increase in number of epochs. On validation, the accuracy was found to be 92%on an average analysis with the integration of optical flow of blocks with convolution neural network compared over the techniques implemented individually.

Fig.9 specifies graphically the determined and comparative of the loss function between the testing and validation phases.

Similarly, Fig.10 specifies the comparison of accuracy obtained over the proposed models with respect to the number of epochs.

Finally, the major insights of the proposed models holds 1) the parents are guided at an earlier stage 2) the abnormal activities of the autistic child could be analysed 3) the object or any action that makes the autistic child to go aggressive, wild or even neutral could be identified, 4) on the other hand the object that influences the interest in the child could also be analysed, 5) the time taken by the child to respond to an action could be evaluated and most importantly 6) appropriate action for their activity could be taken in prior to their action as this could not be made through in-person communication and activity analysis. It takes time for every human to receive, analyse, predict and reciprocate a reaction. The system provides maximum accuracy and performance for the distributed video data collected for evaluation. The further improvement of the early biomarker is planned to integrate with the expression analysis modelled for autistic children in the authors' previous work. This could result in appropriate identification of the characteristic feature of the child prior to clinical trials and minimize the time and effort taken by questionnaire pattern of analysis such as Q-chat, M-chat, ISAA, etc.

This analysis over video capture could be used to find the interestingness of any child over any object say even human. Though the proposed system makes several real time insights the analysis was made in a scenario based execution which could be varied in a larger range in real time. In order to solve this and to bring maximum efficiency in the proposed system, the techniques could be modelled using a complete 360% video surveillance camera that monitors the every movement of the child and triggers an alarm using sensors. Though this seems to be very cost consuming, this could end with a better accuracy. But the similar could be made on a small scale to feed a small video clip of the children and make the system analysis the time delay and the rate of change of time in every action. This could further be improved in integrating the basic correlated questionnaire, facial expression and facial emotions into a single unit. The proposed model makes an attempt to suggest a technology based early intervention method for prior and easy diagnosis of autism. The paper does not conclude that the children with unstable movement or unusual activity will be an autistic child rather suggests that the child may fall under autism in the near future.

CONCLUSION AND FUTURE ENHANCEMENT

The proposed work focused on major autistic features to concern and the important factors that support for the early intervention of autism through computer vision. The proposed work confine that the use of facial expression and the activity recognition in every child could support for the autism diagnosis at a faster convergence rate compared to the complementary methods such as questionnaire formats in clinical analysis. The major insight made is that the balance of the child is made a true positive state with the working of sensory and vestibular impacts that touches the neurodevelopmental delay and hindrance. The proposed model examines the activity of the child using optical flow of motions technique and then extended in accompanying the convolution neural network based motion analysis. Apart from the simple execution of CNN for the input activity captured in frames, the proposed methodology takes the input from the output of the optical flow based activity recognition which proves better in accuracy compared to the execution of the corresponding techniques individually. The proposed system proves an early biomarker that clues the parents and clinical analysis that the child with abnormal motion and physical activity could fall under the category of autism in the near feature although no guarantee of high functioning autism is possible without the integration of other diagnosis methodology and further examination. The major challenge lies on the data collection that the activity of the children could not be captured using a 360 degree surveillance camera. The next prioritized challenge was the computing ability to process a minute video of high quality. Though the task lies easy in detecting human object in frames, the maximum difficulty was found to eliminate the false positive values in the frame. A simple change in the posture of the child was detected abnormal and the CNN improved in eliminating such false positive values.

The proposed system was designed as a sub task of developing a mobile based application that supports the parents to examine their children at home in prior to approaching the clinical specialists. The ultimate vision of the project is to incorporate the basic formatted and analysed feature based questionnaire along with facial expression and motion detection in handheld devices. This could ease the way of diagnosis and gives a better indication to the parents about autism.

REFERENCES

Abirami, S. P., Kousalya, G., & Karthick, R. (2018). Identification and exploration of facial expression in children with ASD in a contact less environment. *Journal of Intelligent & Fuzzy Systems*, *36*(3), 2025–2032.

Adrien, J. L., Lenoir, P., Martineau, J., Perrot, A., Hameury, L., Larmande, C., & Sauvage, D. (1993). Blind ratings of early symptoms of autism based upon family home movies. *J AM Acad of Child Adoles Psychiatry*, *32*(3), 617–626. doi:10.1097/00004583-199305000-00019 PMID:7684363

Bartak, L., Rutter, M., & Cox, A. (1975). A comparative study of infantile autism and specific development receptive language disorder. I. The children. *The British Journal of Psychiatry*, *126*(2), 149–159. doi:10.1192/bjp.126.2.127 PMID:1131465

Bone, D., Bishop, S. L., Black, M. P., Goodwin, M. S., Lord, C., & Narayanan, S. S. (2016). Use of machine learning to improve autism screening and diagnostic instruments: Effectiveness, efficiency, and multi-instrument fusion. *Journal of Child Psychology and Psychiatry, and Allied Disciplines*, *57*(8), 927–937. doi:10.1111/jcpp.12559 PMID:27090613

Bone, D., Goodwin, M. S., Black, M. P., Lee, C. C., Audhkhasi, K., & Narayanan, S. (2014). Applying machine learning to facilitate autism diagnostics: Pitfalls and promises. *Journal of Autism and Developmental Disorders*, 1121–1136. PMID:25294649

Bone, D., Lee, C. C., Black, M. P., Williams, M. E., Lee, S., Levitt, P., & Narayanan, S. (2015). The psychologist as an interlocutor in autism spectrum disorder assessment: Insights from a study of spontaneous prosody. *Journal of Speech, Language, and Hearing Research: JSLHR*, *57*(4), 1162–1177. doi:10.1044/2014_JSLHR-S-13-0062 PMID:24686340

Chu, W., Xue, H., Yao, C., & Cai, D. (2018). Sparse Coding Guided Spatiotemporal Feature Learning for Abnormal Event Detection in Large Videos. *IEEE Transactions on Multimedia*, *21*(1), 246–255. doi:10.1109/TMM.2018.2846411

Colque, Caetano, Lustosa de Andrade, & Schwartz. (2016). Histograms of Optical Flow Orientation and Magnitude and Entropy to Detect Anomalous Events in Videos. *IEEE Transactions on Circuits and Systems for Video Technology*, *27*, 673–682.

Doumas, M., McKenna, R., & Murphy, B. (2015). Postural Control Deficits in Autism Spectrum Disorder: The Role of Sensory Integration. *Journal of Autism and Developmental Disorders*, *46*(3), 853–861. doi:10.100710803-015-2621-4 PMID:26446773

Duvekot, van der Ende, Verhulst, Slappendel, van Daalen, Maras, & Greaves-Lord. (2016). Factors influencing the probability of a diagnosis of autism spectrum disorder in girls versus boys. *SAGE Journals, 21*(6), 646 – 658.

Dworzynski, K., Ronald, A., Bolton, P., & Happé, F. (2012). How different are girls and boys above and below the diagnostic threshold for autism spectrum disorders. *Journal of the American Academy of Child and Adolescent Psychiatry*, *51*(8), 788–797. doi:10.1016/j.jaac.2012.05.018 PMID:22840550

Filipek, P.A., Accardo, P.J., & Baranek, G.T. (1999). The screening and diagnosis of autistic spectrum disorders. *Journal of Autism Developmental Disorder, 29*(6), 439–84.

Gepner, B., Mestre, D., Masson, G., & De Schonen, S. (1995). Postural effects of motion vision in young autistic children. *Neuroreport, 6*(8), 1211–1214. doi:10.1097/00001756-199505300-00034 PMID:7662910

Gnouma, M., Ladjailia, A., Ejbali, R., & Zaied, M. (2019). Stacked sparse auto encoder and history of binary motion image for human activity recognition. *Multimedia Tools and Applications, 78*(2), 2157–2179. doi:10.100711042-018-6273-1

Gowen, E., & Hamilton, A. (2013). Motor abilities in autism: Are view using a computational context. *Journal of Autism and Developmental Disorders, 43*(2), 323–344. doi:10.100710803-012-1574-0 PMID:22723127

Grossman, R. B. (2015). Judgments of social awkwardness from brief exposure to children with and without high-functioning autism. *Autism, 19*(5), 580–587. doi:10.1177/1362361314536937 PMID:24923894

Hollocks, M. J., Ozsivadjian, A., Matthews, C. E., Howlin, P., & Simonoff, E. (2013). The relationship between attentional bias and anxiety in children and adolescents with autism spectrum disorders. *Autism Research, 6*(4), 237–247. doi:10.1002/aur.1285 PMID:23907924

John, N. (2017). The Early Origins of Autism. *Child and Adolescent Psychiatric Clinics of North America, 26*(3), 555–570. doi:10.1016/j.chc.2017.02.008 PMID:28577609

Joseph, R. M., Tager-Flusberg, H., & Lord, C. (2002). Cognitive profiles and social-communicative functioning in children with autism spectrum disorder. *Journal of Child Psychology and Psychiatry, and Allied Disciplines, 43*(6), 807–821. doi:10.1111/1469-7610.00092 PMID:12236615

Kroncke, Willard, & Huckabee. (2014). Assessment of Autism Spectrum Disorder: Critical Issues in Clinical, Forensic and School Settings. Springer Publications.

Li, S., Yang, Y., & Liu, C. (2018). Anomaly Detection based on two global grid motion templates. *Signal Processing Image Communication, 60*, 6–12. doi:10.1016/j.image.2017.09.002

Lord, C., Risi, S., Lambrecht, L., Cook, J., Edwin, H., Leventhal, B. L., ... Rutter, M. (2000). The autism diagnostic observation schedule generic: A standard measure of social and communication deficits associated with the spectrum of autism. *Journal of Autism and Developmental Disability, 24*, 659–685. doi:10.1007/BF02172145 PMID:11055457

Mubashir, M., Shao, L., & Seed, L. (2015). A survey on fall detection principles and approaches. *Neurocomputing, 100*, 144–152. doi:10.1016/j.neucom.2011.09.037

Rajagopalan, Dhall, & Goecke. (2013). *Self-Stimulatory Behaviours in the Wild for Autism Diagnosis*. IEEE Explore.

Rehg, J. M., Abowd, G. D., Rozga, A. A., Romero, M., Clements, M. A., & Sclaroff, S. (2013). Decoding children's social behavior. IEEE CVPR.

Sabokrou, M., Fayyaz, M., Fathy, M., Moayed, Z., & Klette, R. (2018). Deep-anomaly: Fully convolution neural network for fast anomaly detection in crowded scenes. *Computer Vision and Image Understanding, 172*, 88–97. doi:10.1016/j.cviu.2018.02.006

Singh, Marks, Jones, Tuzel, & Shao. (2016). A multistream bidirectional recurrent neural network for fine grained action detection. *The IEEE Conference on Computer Vision and Pattern Recognition (CVPR)*, 1961-1970.

Somogyia, E. (2016). Visual feedback increases postural stability in children with autism spectrum disorder. *Research in Autism Spectrum Disorders, 29*, 48–56. doi:10.1016/j.rasd.2016.06.001

Sorte, Patil, & Bhamare. (2016). Motion Detection Using Optical Flow And Standard Deviation. *IEEE International Conference on Automatic Control and Dynamic Optimization Techniques*, 295-300.

Stagg, S., Slavny, R., Hand, C., Cardoso, A., & Smith, P. (2013). Does facial expressivity count? How typically developing children respond initially to children with autism. *Autism*, 704–711. PMID:24121180

Tripathi, R. K., Jalal, A. S., & Agrawal, S. C. (2018). Suspicious human activity recognition: A review. *Artificial Intelligence Review, 50*(2), 283–339. doi:10.100710462-017-9545-7

Vostanis, P., Smith, B., Chung, M. C., & Corbett, J. (1994). Early detection of childhood autism: A review of screening instruments and rating scales. *Child: Care, Health and Development, 6*(3), 165–177. doi:10.1111/j.1365-2214.1994.tb00378.x PMID:8062410

Wu, Zaheer, Hu, Manmatha, Alexander, Smola, & Krahenbuhl. (2016). Compressed video action recognition. *The IEEE Conference on Computer Vision and Pattern Recognition (CVPR)*, 6026-6035.

Young, R. L., Brewer, N., & Pattison, C. (2003). Parental identification of early behavioural abnormalities in children with autistic disorder. *Autism, 7*(2), 125–143. doi:10.1177/1362361303007002002 PMID:12846383

Zwaigenbaum, L., Bauman, M. L., Choueiri, R., Kasari, C., Carter, A., Granpeesheh, D., ... Natowicz, M. R. (2015). Early intervention for children with autism spectrum disorder under 3 years of age: Recommendations for practice and research. *Pediatrics, 136*(Suppl 1), 60–81. doi:10.1542/peds.2014-3667E PMID:26430170

Chapter 15
Comparative Study on ASD Identification Using Machine and Deep Learning

Rajandeep Kaur
Dr. B. R. Ambedkar National Institute of Technology, Jalandhar, India

Rajneesh Rani
National Institute of Technology, Jalandhar, India

ABSTRACT

Autism spectrum disorder (ASD) is a neurodevelopment disorder that consists of a lack of social interaction and repetitive behavior of a person. It must be diagnosed at an early stage; otherwise it may adversely affect the life of that person. However, ASD consists of numerous overlapping neurodevelopment disorders such as autism and schizophrenia, which share some common brain structures. The medical image analysis is very popular to identify and segment different diseases in healthcare. In recent years, due to the tremendous changes in imaging devices, neuroimaging has recorded a great increase in identifying neuropsychiatric disorders. Moreover, MRI (magnetic resonance imaging) is a powerful non-invasive medical imaging to distinguish between these overlapping diseases by extracting brain connectivity. The researchers have applied numerous algorithms to understand common and distinctive brain connectivity features for these disorders. This chapter will focus on state-of-the-art techniques based on machine and deep learning with their comparative analysis and challenges of ASD.

INTRODUCTION

Autism spectrum disorder (ASD) is a lifelong neurodevelopment disorder with core symptoms of social impairment like repetitive behavior, interaction and communication problem in a person. Autism was firstly discovered by Kanner in 1943 (Pratap A., Kanimozhiselvi, 2014). He described it as unusual behavior present in children from birth to 30 months. The onset of ASD is usually at the time of birth or during the first three years of life. Studies show that some demographic attributes like gender and

DOI: 10.4018/978-1-7998-3069-6.ch015

race vary among ASD and healthy individuals such that males are four times more prone to ASD than women (Baio, J., Wiggins, L., Christensen, D. L., Maenner, M. J., Daniels, J., Warren, Z., … & Durkin, 2018). Some other factors such as environmental, socio-economic and risk related at the time of birth also affects the growth and general behavior of child which may further lead to ASD (Geetha, Sukumar, Dhivyadeepa, Reddy, & Balachandar, 2018).

Worldwide, there is one patient of ASD in 100 and in the United States; this prevalence is 1 in 68 (Mertz, 2017). In India, 1 in 500 children to 1 in 166 children are prevalent to have and this rate has increased from the last few decades. Currently, more than 2 million people in India affected from autism (Barua & Daley, n.d.). There are several reasons which may cause ASD, however, exposure to toxic metal-based pollutants play a significant role (Bhargavan, 2019). The other reasons include lack of care, stress, maternal illness, and lack of nutrition food for mothers and some other reasons related to birth of child.

To cope up with this problem, the different methods were proposed which mainly includes screening test, imaging of children and brain imaging based on machine learning (Thabtah, 2018) and deep learning (Razzak, Naz, & Zaib, 2018). The screening test is subjective and slow method while imaging is objective and more reliable testing method (Borràs-Ferrís, Pérez-Ramírez, & Moratal, 2019). Furthermore, in case of imaging of patients, the images of children taken and movement of eyes, hands, arms etc. observed to detect ASD. However, it is not so appropriate way for infants, also, behavioral observations may lead to misdiagnosis (Hyde et al., 2019).

The medical imaging such as MRI (Magnetic Imaging Resonance), CT (Computer Tomography), PET (Position Emission Tomography), US (Ultrasound), DSA (Digital Subtraction Angiography), and X-ray are popular imaging methods that are used to understand the different parts of the body and to detect different diseases. The brain imaging, which is part of medical imaging, is a reliable and quantitative approach to detect numerous brain diseases and connections. Brain imaging includes MRI (Magnetic Resonance Imaging), fMRI (functional Magnetic Resonance Imaging), rs-fMRI (resting-state functional Magnetic Resonance Imaging), sMRI (structural Magnetic Resonance Imaging), and dMRI (diffusion Magnetic Resonance Imaging) which are used by most of the state-of-art methods. The fMRI of brain slice, taken from ABIDE dataset, with axial view, coronal view, and sagittal view is represented in Figure 1 (Di Martino et al., 2014). Moreover, MRI is a powerful tool that helps to develop a method that is capable to find autism at an early stage. In addition, the identification of ASD can be done in less time and the treatment of a child can be started early which is required for the betterment of a child and his/her family (Borràs-Ferrís et al., 2019).

Figure 1. fMRI of brain slice representing Axial View, Coronal View and Sagittal View

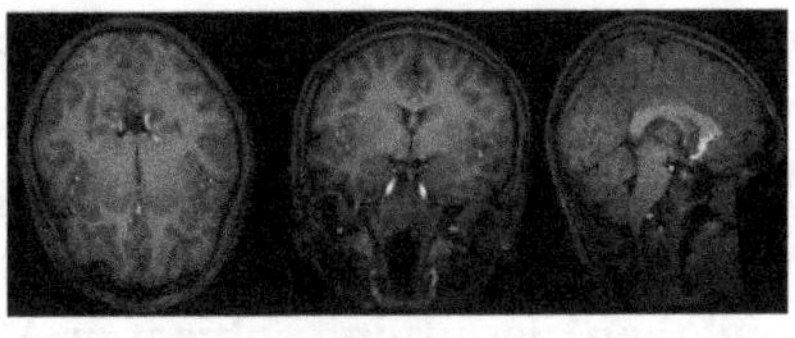

The neuroimaging such as structural MRI and functional MRI, is a powerful tool in diagnosing ASD by investigating the structure and function of the brain. Different structural and functional characteristics of brain assist researchers to distinguish between ASD and healthy subjects. The abnormalities in gray and white matters are one of the characteristic to discriminate between ASD and TD (Typical Development). In addition to this, the change in volume of brain and the cortical surfaces are other factors to distinguish the children with ASD (Ha, Sohn, Kim, Sim, & Cheon, 2015).

Nowadays, the tremendous advancement in learning algorithms gives a new direction to medical applications. Therefore, algorithms of machine learning surpass the human performance and performing better in various fields such as medical image analysis. Consequently, the machine learning algorithms have been used by numerous researchers to do more inventions in different fields. Many researchers used these techniques to do advancement in numerous medical applications like identification of children with ASD, Tumor detection, organ detection, segmentation of landmark etc. (Litjens et al., 2017). Further advancement in hardware like GPUs (Graphical Processing Units) gave birth to deep learning techniques. The GPUs help to speed up work using the parallel pipeline. In addition, many researchers used this technology to improve the performance of neural networks. Due to this, deep learning becomes the most attractive way to perform computation and do the analysis of large data. Majority of papers published by various researchers, in medical imaging filed, from 2015 are based on deep learning (Ker, Wang, Rao, & Lim, 2017).

From the above, it is clear that the autism has been increased from the last few decades and there is a need for a reliable method that can detect ASD so that the medication and other therapies can be started on time. Therefore, to develop a reliable ASD diagnosis method and to provide a better life for autistic children are the main motivation behind this research.

Objectives of Proposed Chapter

The statistics show that the problem of ASD is increasing by leaps and bounds which causes numerous problems for patients as well as for their family members. Thus, it becomes essential to develop a reliable method that can identify ASD at an early stage within a significant amount of time and accuracy. Various researchers have proposed numerous algorithms using machine and deep learning to diagnose patients with ASD and delineate standard biomarkers. The main objective of the chapter is to elaborate on various techniques based on neuroimaging such as fMRI and sMRI. The second objective is to elaborate on the basic architecture with basic steps that can be followed to propose a new and better algorithm to diagnose ASD. However, as this process consists of various challenges, thus, the last objective is to recognize the different challenges associated with this process.

Basic Architecture of Identifying ASD Using Neuroimaging

The neuroimaging, a kind of digital imaging, plays a significant role in diagnosing patients with ASD. The researchers have used different steps to achieve results. However, there are some steps which can be followed to classify patients with ASD as compared to healthy group. The important steps used in this process are data acquisition, feature extraction, feature selection, sampling, dividing data into training and test set and applying classifier and then classifying subject in ASD or Non-ASD classes (Thabtah, 2018). The basic architecture of diagnosing ASD using neuroimaging is depicted in Figure 2.

There are some steps that are optional and may be omitted like feature selection and noise removal. The feature selection is used when a large number of features are extracted from input data and may cause overfitting or have insignificant information. Similarly, the noise removal step can be used if the input image contains some noise due to some reasons like unwanted movement of patient. Thus, it makes the image unusable and can damage important information. However, noise removal is avoided in medical images.

Figure 2. Basic Architecture of Identifying ASD using Image Processing

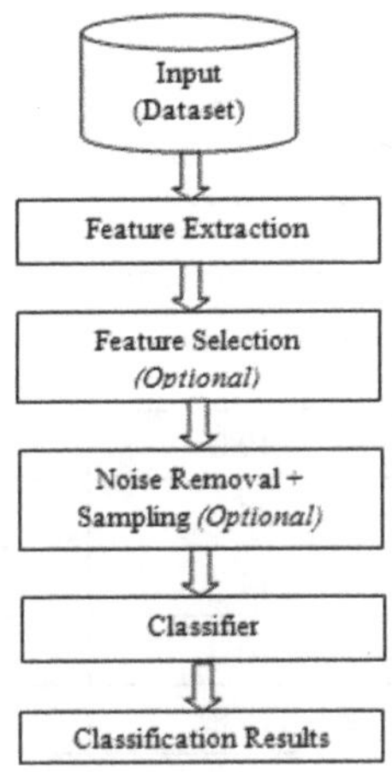

The architecture of identifying ASD may vary from one technique to others. However, this architecture includes basic steps to classify subjects into ASD and non-ASD groups. The description of these steps is given below:

Input from Dataset - Firstly, the required data is acquired from a dataset that will be in the form of MRI. The ABIDE (Autism Brain Imaging Data Exchange) is a consortium which provides previously collected data from 17 different site as described in Table 1. The ABIDE data is available at http://fcon_1000.projects.nitrc.org/indi/abide/ which consist of 1035 (ASD 505, HC 530) resting-state - fMRIs (Di Martino et al., 2014). It is freely available dataset and used by most of the researchers for performing their experiments (Borràs-Ferrís et al., 2019; Heinsfeld, Franco, Craddock, Buchweitz, & Meneguzzi, 2018)

The data available in ABIDE contains rs-fMRI images 878 male and 157 female subjects. Thus, most of the studies have been done on male subjects with ASD as compared to female subjects (Aghdam & Sharifi, 2018; Eslami, Mirjalili, Fong, Laird, & Saeed, 2019). Also, males are four time prominent to ASD as compared to females (Baio, J., Wiggins, L., Christensen, D. L., Maenner, M. J., Daniels, J., Warren, Z., … & Durkin, 2018).

Feature Extraction & Selection - The data is considered as features and the next task is to extract significant features from this given input. In the case of large numbers of features, many researchers applied feature selection (Chanel et al., 2016). The purpose of this step is to select the most significant features which affect the result most. The purpose of this step is to train the classifier only with the most informative features and to dodge the problem of over-fitting.

Table 1. Summary of ABIDE Dataset

Site	ASD			Healthy Control		
	Total Subjects	M/F Count	Average Age	Total Subjects	M/F Count	Average Age
Caltech	19	M 15, F 4	27.4	18	M 14, F 4	28.0
CMU	14	M 11, F 3	26.4	13	M 10, F 3	26.8
KKI	20	M 16, F 4	10.0	28	M 20, F 8	10.0
Leuven	29	M 26, F 3	17.8	34	M 29, F 5	18.2
MaxMun	24	M 21, F 3	26.1	28	M 27, F 1	24.6
NYU	75	M 65, F 10	14.7	100	M 74, F 26	15.7
OHSU	12	M 12, F 0	11.4	14	M 14, F 0	10.1
OLIN	19	M 16, F 3	16.5	15	M 13, F 2	16.7
PITT	29	M 25, F 4	19.0	27	M 23, F 4	18.9
SBL	15	M 15, F 0	35.0	15	M 15, F 0	33.7
SDSU	14	M 13, F 1	14.7	22	M 16, F 6	14.2
Stanford	19	M 15, F 4	10.0	20	M 16, F 4	10.0
Trinity	22	M 22, F 0	16.8	25	M 25, F 0	17.1
UCLA	54	M 48, F 6	13.0	44	M 38, F 6	13.0
UM	66	M 57, F 9	13.2	74	M 56, F 18	14.8
USM	46	M 46, F 0	23.5	25	M 25, F 0	21.3
Yale	28	M 20, F 8	12.7	28	M 20, F 8	12.7
Total	505	M 443, F 62		530	M 435, F 95	

M- Male, F-Female

Noise Removal - Further, the fMRI may be noisy due to some reasons like MRI scanner problem, head movement of patient etc. Thus, to convert the noisy data into meaning data, the image preprocessing packages are used. The most common packages are SPM, FSL, AFNI, and Brain and Voyagar (Yang, Sarraf, & Zhang, 2018).

Sampling of Data - In machine learning or deep learning, a large dataset is required to train the system properly to improve the accuracy of the algorithm. However, the dataset provided online like ABIDE contains a total of 1035 rs-fMRI images which may not be sufficient to train the algorithm, especially in the binary classification problem. Some researchers used oversampling to avoid this unbalanced data problem. When the instances of a class with fewer instances are enhanced to maintain the balance of both classes is referred to as oversampling while in under-sampling, the class with majority instances is reduced to balance the class instances. Thus, many researchers performed oversampling on data to balance it (Dennis P. Wall, Dally, Luyster, Jung, & DeLuca, 2012). However, under-sampling is avoided in medical data as it may lead to loss of data and may provide incorrect results (Thabtah, 2018).

Selection of Classifier - Lastly, the selection of classifiers is done to classify subjects in ASD and a healthy group. Some commonly used classifier with fMRI data are k-nearest neighbors, Logistic Regression, Support Vector Machines (SVM), Gaussian Naive Bayes (GNB), Fisher's Linear Discriminant Analysis (LDA). However, it is necessary to select appropriate classifier to achieve high performance (Pereira, Mitchell, & Botvinick, 2009). The data is decomposed into training and test set using some methods like cross-validation method. The classifier is firstly trained with the training set and the performance of the system is tested on the test set. Sometimes, the classifiers perform well with the training set but not with the test set. This phenomenon is known as overfitting. To avoid, this problem, it is important to divide data properly into two sets.

Classification Results - There are different parameters used to measure the performance of the classifier, however, the commonly used parameter are accuracy, sensitivity, specificity, F-measure, precision and area under curve (AUC) (Altay & Ulas, 2018; Dekhil et al., 2018).

The steps above mentioned are not key steps that have to follow strictly, however, these are just for guidance can others steps can be added or removed to develop an algorithm.

BACKGROUND

Several research studies have proposed new techniques to automate the process of identifying ASD instead of relying upon screening tools which may be biased as well as takes more time. The researchers used magnetic resonance imaging of the brain to understand the functional connectivity among various brain components and how children with autism have different brain connectivity as compared to neurotypical children (Bos et al., 2014; Du, Fu, & Calhoun, 2018). However, some studies showed contradictory results because of variation in dataset size, age or gender of subject, fMRI acquisition method or severity of ASD (Borràs-Ferrís et al., 2019). It can be observed that most of the researchers used machine learning and further moving to deep learning for providing fast and better results. The next section will explain the work done by various researchers with accuracy as a performance parameter.

LITERATURE REVIEW

Many researchers have proposed various techniques to identify autism in children by using subjective as well as objective methods. The aim of most of the researchers is to find some standard biomarkers for early and accurate detection of autism. Some state-of-art techniques proposed by various researchers to diagnose ASD are given in this section. These studies are mainly divided into three parts. The first and second part contains the research studies for detecting ASD based on deep and machine learning respectively. The third part contains the research studies for finding functional connectivity of brain which will be further helpful in finding ASD.

Research Studies for Detecting ASD Based on Deep Learning

(Eslami, Mirjalili, Fong, Laird, & Saeed, 2019) proposed a new framework, ASD-DiagNet, to identify patients who suffered from ASD using fMRI data. The proposed technique used autoencoder and single-layer perceptron (SLP) jointly and applied on 1035 subjects (505 ASD, 530 TC) taken from ABIDE open access dataset to evaluate its results. The proposed technique was used for feature selection and classification. In order to enhance the training set, the data augmentation technique has been proposed using linear interpolation. The method achieved a maximum of 80% and an average 70.1% classification accuracy and a huge improvement in execution time as compared to state-of-the-art techniques. An improvement of 2% has been observed in accuracy and the method proposed can perform well for small and large datasets.

(Aghdam, Sharifi, & Pedram, 2019) proposed a novel technique to diagnose ASD in young children using a convolutional neural network. In the proposed work, the dynamic classifier along with a static classifier has been used. The data of young children of age 5 to 10 have been collected to detect ASD at an early age. The data of 116 (54 ASD, 62 TC) individuals have taken from ABIDE-I and 343 (156 ASD, 187 TC) individuals have taken from ABIDE-II. After preprocessing the data, data reduction has been performed using the Fourier transform. The accuracy obtained was 0.7273, 0.7 and 0.7045 from ABIDE-I, ABIDE-II, and combination of ABIDE-I and ABIDE-II dataset respectively. The Adamax and Adam optimizers have also been employed, in which, the adamax optimizer tends to have fewer errors.

(Heinsfeld et al., 2018) developed a deep learning-based technique to detect ASD (Autism Spectrum Disorder) and identify brain patterns of patients. The author focused to find out different neural patterns of functional connectivity of the brain using rs-fMRI (resting-state functional Magnetic Resonance Imaging). The proposed method used two stacked denoising autoencoders and a multilayer perceptron (MLP) to extract knowledge in a better way. The output of the system was represented in two classes: ASD (Autism Spectrum Disorder) or TC (Typical Control). The correlation between fMRI data represented that some areas like anterior and posterior brain areas are negatively while some areas are positively correlated. This underconnectivity among different brain areas helped to distinguish between ASD and TC groups. The proposed technique has been applied on rs-fMRI images taken from ABIDE (Autism Brain Imaging Data Exchange) open-access dataset and achieved 70% of accuracy.

(Dvornek, Ventola, & Duncan, 2018) proposed a novel method by combining phenotypic (Age, Sex, Handedness, Full IQ, Eye Status) and rs-fMRI data for classifying subjects with autism. Both types of data have been combined and fed into a neural network to classify subjects with ASD from typical control (TC). The experiments have been performed on 1100 subjects (529 ASD and 571 TD) taken from the ABIDE dataset using several neural networks. The proposed method outperformed than some recent work and achieved 70.1% accuracy. In the future, the architecture of sMRI can be improved and more behavioral measures can be included for better accuracy.

(Kong et al., 2018) proposed a novel deep learning-based technique to identify autism. In this technique, a two-sparse autoencoder along with a softmax layer is used to form a deep neural network. The author constructed a network of ROIs (Region of Interest) which consists of brain features. Further, the F-score ranking method had been applied to select the most important 3000 features. The 182 subjects (78 ASD, 104 TC) for the experiment has taken from the ABIDE-I dataset with an average age of 15 years. The proposed method used to classify ASD from TC (Typical Control) group and achieved accuracy as 90.39% and area under curve (AUC) was 0.9738. In addition, the sensitivity and specificity are 84.37%, 95.88% respectively for the NYU dataset.

(Jain, 2018) proposed a method to extract features from rs-fMRI data and used graph Convolutional Neural Network to distinguish between subjects with autism and typical control. The fMRI data is converted into graphical representation to represent connectivity between different regions of the brain. The author did an experiment on the ABIDE dataset using Harvard Oxford (HO) for analysis. Later on, CC400 atlas has been used to perform voting. The combination of both atlases performed better and achieved 70.23% accuracy. The author also included some phenotypic features like age, gender, fiq, piq, and viq to evaluate the effect of these features on the model.

(Khosla, Jamison, Kuceyeski, & Mert, 2018) proposed a novel volumetric CNN based to classify subjects with ASD from typical control. The proposed method had applied on 774 ABIDE-I subjects (379 ASD, 395 TC) and 393 ABIDE-II subjects (163 ASD, 230 TC) which qualified manual quality assessments. For ROI extraction, seven types of atlases used which includes Harvard- Oxford (HO), Craddock 200 (CC200), Eickhoff-Zilles (EZ), Talaraich and Tournox (TT), Dosenbach 160 (DOS160), Automated Anatomical Labelling (AAL) and Craddock 400 (CC400). The proposed method achieved 73.30% accuracy with HO atlas which was better than state-of-the-art techniques. The author used the group-averaged saliency map for different atlases. However, the individual atlas can be visualized using saliency map and analyzed in the future.

(Aghdam & Sharifi, 2018) made use of deep belief network on sMRI (structural - MRI) and rs-fMRI (resting-state fMRI) data to identify autism in young children. The data of 185 subjects (116 ASD and 69 TC) of age group 5 to 10 years has been taken from ABIDE-I and ABIDE-II and the main emphasis was given on gray matter, white matter and rs-fMRI data. After the preprocessing of fMRI images, the images are segmented into 116 ROIs. Later on, after parcellation, the fusion of sMRI matters and rs-fMRI has been performed to improve the results. The proposed algorithm provided maximum accuracy as 65.56% with a depth 3 deep belief network. In addition to this, other performance parameters such as sensitivity, specificity, and F1 score are reported as 84%, 32.96%, and 74.76% respectively. The work can be further extended by considering the geographical area and a large dataset can be taken for better results.

(Yang et al., 2018) introduced a technique by using deep learning-based framework LeNet-5, to classify subjects with autism using fMRI images. The work has been performed on subjects whose data was taken from ABIDE-I of age ranging from 9 to 20. Initially, the data of 100 (50 ASD, 50 TC) subjects have taken from the database, however, after screening only 27 (11 ASD, 16 TC) subjects have been chosen for the analysis. The proposed technique was applied to the preprocessed images using slice-level image classification. The proposed method outperformed than state-of-the-art techniques in terms of sensitivity and specificity. In the future, work can be further extended by locating brain pathology and help to identify a standard biomarker for autism.

Research Studies for Detecting ASD Based on Machine Learning

(Andriamananjara, Muntari, & Crimi, 2019) used Support Vector Machine (SVM) and dynamic functional connectivity measures to show distinct and overlapping features of schizophrenia and autism spectrum disorder. The fMRI data for ASD was obtained from ABIDE-II comprising 54 subjects (31 ASD, 23 TC) of age between 7 to 50 years. The dataset for schizophrenia subjects was obtained from COBRE dataset with 146 subjects (70 SZ, 74 TC) of age between 18 to 65 years. The majority of subjects from both datasets were male. In the initial step, windowing and person correlation were used to process the data and later on scores are provided to brain regions to identify ASD or SZ by comparing with the control group. The author showed some common features for both ASD and SZ which need to be further carried out for research.

(Mastrovito, Hanson, & Hanson, 2018) presented that there are some differences as well as similarities between two neurological disorders; Autism Spectrum Disorder (ASD) and Schizophrenia (SZ). The author used the Support Vector Machine (SVM) classifier to classify both disorders. However, it was also mentioned that it has not been proved that whether machine learning algorithms are successful in distinguishing between ASD and Schizophrenia. The resting-state data of cohort subjects (27 ASD, 27 SZ) has been taken from the Center for Biomedical Research Excellence (COBRE) for SZ and from

ABIDE for ASD. The RFE method was used to distinguish between subjects with ASD from the control group and subjects with SZ from the control group by identifying connectivity features. However, there are more common features and few features to discriminate between these two types of population. Thus, the work can be further extended to identify more features to distinguish between two populations in a better way.

(Sartipi, Shayesteh, & Kalbkhani, 2018) proposed a new technique based on GARCH variance series on rs-fMRI data to detect autism. In the proposed method, double-density dual-tree discrete wavelet transform (D3TDWT) is used to segment the ROI of each subject into time-frequency sub-bands. In the next step, for feature extraction, Generalized AutoRegressive Conditional Heteroscedasticity (GARCH) model is used. After selecting the most significant features using a two-sample t-test algorithm, the support vector machine with five-fold cross-validation is applied to verify results. The fMRI data of 468 (ASD 222 and 246 TC) subjects have been taken from six different sites (YALE, PITT, UCLA, SDSU, NYU, and TRINITY). To provide clear results, gender was used as phenotypic data. The proposed method achieved 71.6%, 93.7% classification for male and female subjects respectively. In the future, more phenotypic information can be added and work can be performed on a large dataset.

(Xiao et al., 2017) proposed a new technique to diagnose ASD in toddler using MRI based brain features. The MRI data of 85 toddlers (46 ASD, 39 TD) has been taken to do study. The support vector machine, naïve bayes, and random forest machine learning classifiers have been applied on input data to test the performance of these classifiers. The feature like cortical thickness, volume, and the surface has been selected and evaluated by different classifiers. It has been observed that some brain regions, like left hemisphere, played an important role in discriminating ASD as compared to other regions. The random forest method showed the best result with an accuracy of about 80%, specificity, and sensitivity about 81% and area under curve (AUC) about 0.88. However, it has been as concluded that the random forest is an optimal approach for small datasets.

(Kassraian-Fard, Matthis, Balsters, Maathuis, & Wenderoth, 2016) compared different machine learning algorithms on rs-fMRI images of 154 subjects (77 ASD, 77 TD) taken from publically available ABIDE dataset. In addition, the author discussed basic guidelines for applying machine learning classifiers as well as its pitfalls. To balance the data under-sampling is used. The six classifiers Logistic Regression (LR), Lasso Regularized Logistic Regression (LassoLR), Support Vector Machine (SVM), Probabilistic Neural Network (PNN), Linear Discriminant Analysis (LDA) and Gaussian Naïve Bayes (GBN) are applied to fMRI data. The SVM outperformed with 63% accuracy while the accuracy of GNB is reported as 57% which was least among all classifiers. The author concluded that the reason behind less accuracy may be the variation between data collected from different sites. Moreover, the dataset is very small to do experiments and high-dimensional which may lead to overfitting problem. These pitfalls need to be improved in future research.

(Chanel et al., 2016) proposed a voxel based approach on two types of data (task-based and rs-fMRI based) to distinguish between ASD patients from the typical control group. In task-based data includes facial expression and body reactions of actors. The method used machine learning classifier Support Vector Machine (SVM) and Recursive Feature Elimination (RFE) method. The authors focused on social motivation as the main feature which was captured by the classifier. The experiments have been performed on 29 adults (15 ASD and 14 TD) RFE method performs significantly well and may be helpful in identifying biomarkers to detect patients with ASD. The accuracy of the proposed method lies between 69% and 92.3%. However, the dataset size was limited and needs to expand in the future.

(Zhang et al., 2016) used fiber clustering tractography segmentation for predicting connectivity alterations in white matter in patients with autism. The reason to use a clustering-based segmentation technique was that it provides better results than traditional methods. The diffusion weighted imaging data of 150 males (70 ASD and 80 TD) with similar age, distribution is taken for evaluation. After extracting fiber tracts, feature selection has been applied to select the most relevant fiber tracts. To check the viability of the proposed algorithm, the author used the support vector machine (SVM) classifier because of its high dimensionality feature and it is capable of capturing multivariate relationships among different regions. The maximum accuracy was achieved as 81.33% which was better than the parcellation-based approach.

(Plitt, Anne, & Martin, 2015) showed that rs-fMRI was useful in finding the functional connectivity of the brain and further identifying patients with ASD. The work has been done on in-house fMRI images, which were taken using a GE, Signa 3T whole-body MRI scanner, of same age and IQ cohort of 118 individual males (59 ASD; 59 TD). Also, the data of 178 individuals were obtained from the ADIBE dataset for replication. After preprocessing, the author extracted three sets of regions of interest (Power, Destrieux and DiMartino) and applied leave-one-out cross-validation (LOOCV) using nine popular machine learning classification algorithms to classify ASD vs. TD. Further, it has been observed that L2LR and L-SVM outperformed than other considered classification algorithms in terms of accuracy.

(Katuwal, Cahill, Baum, & Michael, 2015) did experiment on sMRI images of 734 male subjects (373 ASD, 361 TC) taken from the ABIDE dataset. The three types of machine learning classifiers (support vector machine, random forest, and gradient boosting machine) have been applied to input data on individual sites and across the sites. The accuracy of the system has been improved after augmenting age and IQ morphometric features. The highest accuracy is achieved as 97% on CAL site individually with five significant features. The least accuracy 64% was reported on the UCLA site with two features. The author concluded that a more promising technique can be developed if a large dataset is provided using a deep learning algorithm.

(Zhou, Yu, & Duong, 2014) proposed a graph theory and machine learning-based technique to predict different characteristics of ASD and identify subjects with autism. The data of 280 children (127 ASD and 153 TD) has been taken from the multi-center Functional Connectome Project. After selecting 22 features, the authors applied the mRMR algorithm to select the most significant features. The random tree method achieved 70% accuracy with 6 primary features and 98% accuracy with 4 primary features for classifying children with ASD from TD. The author concluded that caudate volume, caudate-cortical fcMRI, IFG pars opercularis and triangularis fcMRI as most significant features that helped to improve the accuracy of classification prediction.

(Nielsen et al., 2013) find out the connectivity between different brain regions using preprocessed rs-fMRI data taken from the ABIDE dataset. The ABIDE dataset contained rs-fMRI images data of 964 subjects (447 ASD, 517 TC) from 16 for sites. The connectivity matrix along with phenotypic features like age, gender, age-squared and handedness; given as input to leave-one-out classifier. The highest accuracy achieved by the proposed method was 60%. It has been also noticed that the accuracy obtained by state-of-art techniques that were using data from a single site was better; however, it becomes less for multisite.

Research Studies for Finding Functional Connectivity of Brain

(Du et al., 2018) showed that the functional connectivity of the brain was a promising method of predicting brain disorders such as Schizophrenia, ASD, attention deficit hyperactivity disorder (ADHD).

The functional connectivity can be static or dynamic which can be used to investigate such problems. Furthermore, the brain regions can be decomposed into regions of interest and the sliding window can be augmented in static functional connectivity for a better understanding of brain regions. There are various state-of-the-art studies which had used different features of brain data to diagnose neuro-disorders; however, this was one of the challenges to choose correct features for better results. Other challenges are validating results, accurate classification, and evaluation of the proposed model which needs considerable attention in the future.

(Bos et al., 2014) did experiment on rs-fMRI images of 56 male children (27 ASD, 29 TC) of age between 6 to 16 years to observe connectivity between and within brain network. The data is taken from a lab using MRI scanner and preprocessing has been done using SPM8. For data analysis, the group independent component analysis has been done to decompose the data into brain networks. Further, ten components selected which showed a high cross-correlation. It has been investigated by authors that there was no difference within network connections; however, reduced connectivity between two higher-order networks of ASD has been observed. Moreover, in the right insula, connectivity in DMN has increased in children with ASD and decreased in the case of typical control group. The dataset taken for research is small and may be extended in future research.

(Lynch et al., 2013) investigated the functional connectivity between DMN (default mode network) of 39 young children (20 ASD, 19 TC) who have the same age, gender, and IQ. DMN helps to understand the connectivity between brain regions while doing any activity. After acquiring fMRI images using a 3T GE Signa scanner, preprocessing is done. Later on, ROIs are extracted and connectivity between these ROIs has observed using multivariate regression. In the case of children with ASD, the hyperconnectivity has been observed in the posterior cingulate and retrosplenial cortices with the predominately medial and anterolateral temporal cortex. Further, connectivity between social impairment and ASD has also been observed.

(Barttfeld et al., 2012) performed a study on subjects with ASD to define different brain connectivity patterns in different states. The data has been acquired from 24 right-handed adult subjects (12 ASD, 12 TC). The data has been preprocessed using statistical parametric mapping software and six predefined functional networks (cingulo-opercular (OP), frontoparietal (FP), occipital (OC), sensorimotor (SE), default brain network (DEF) and cerebellum (CER) were used to define ROIs. Later on, an analysis was done on the ADOS score to obtain results. It has been concluded that the connectivity between brain networks is dependent on the state and provides more information about changes in brain networks as compared to a direct comparison of brain networks.

Summary of Existing Work

Numerous techniques have been proposed by various research studies for diagnosing ASD. The comparative analysis of these techniques is given in Table 2. From this Table, it can be observed that many researchers have performed their work on fMRI images using machine or deep learning. The last col-

Table 2. Summary of Existing Work

Reference	Dataset	Type of Data	Algorithm	Average Age	Sample Size	Accuracy (in %)
(Nielsen et al., 2013)	ABIDE	rs-fMRI	Leave-one-out Classifier		447 ASD,517 TC	60
(Zhou et al., 2014)	Functional Connectcome Project	MRI	Graph Theory and Machine Learning	13.5±6.0 ASD, 14.56±5.7 TD	127 ASD,153 TC	70
(Plitt et al., 2015)	ABIDE	rs-fMRI		17.66±2.72, 18.3±3.05)	59 ASD,59 TC	76.67
(Chanel et al., 2016)	Clinical Patients	rs-fMRI and task based	SVM and REF	28.6 ASD, 31.6 TD	15 ASD,14 TC	69 - 92.3
(Zhang et al., 2016)		diffusion weighted imaging		11.11±2.45	70 ASD,80 TC	81.33
(Heinsfeld et al., 2018)	ABIDE	fMRI	Deep Learning		505 ASD,530 TC	70
(Mastrovito et al., 2018)	COBRE- SZ ABIDE-ASD	MRI	SVM	> 18	27 ASD,27 SZ	
(Aghdam & Sharifi, 2018)	ABIDE	rs-fMRI, sMRI	Deep Belief Network	5 to 10	116 ASD,69 TC	65.56
(Kong et al., 2018)	ABIDE-I	MRI	DNN	15	78 ASD,104 TC	90.93
(Dvornek et al., 2018)	ABIDE	rs-fMRI	Deep Learning		529 ASD,571 TC	70.1
(Katuwal et al., 2018)	Clinical Routine Patients	MRI	RF	3 to 4	15 ASD,18 TC	
(Khosla et al., 2018)	ABIDE-I and II	rs-fMRI	3D CNN	5 to 64	379 ASD, 395 TC 163 ASD, 230 TC	73.30
(Jain, 2018)	ABIDE	Rs-fMRI	Graph CNN	5 to 64	539 ASD,573 TC	70.23
(Eslami et al., 2019)	ABIDE	fMRI	Deep Learning		505 ASD,530 TC	70.1

ASD- Autism Spectrum Disorder, TC- Typical Control, SZ- Schizophrenia

umn indicates the accuracy achieved by various algorithms. The highest accuracy is 90.93% which is achieved by (Kong et al., 2018). However, the author used a very small dataset with 182 subjects only. The accuracy achieved by other researchers is around 70%. It indicates that future research must be done to propose a new algorithm with enhanced accuracy.

Different Methods of Detecting ASD

Autism is a lifelong disorder that causes various problems for patients like communication, behavior and restricted activity, thus, it must be detected as early as possible. There are numerous methods used by clinical psychologists or clinical experts to diagnose it which are depicted in Figure 3.

The testing tools for autism are mainly categorized as screening or non-screening tools. The screening tools are subjective and may include a set of questions that need to answer a child or his/her parents (Guo et al., 2018). The psychiatric, psychologist or physician evaluate the result and identify whether child has autism or not. These types of methods need more time and only experts will be able to interpret the result and further diagnose autism.

Figure 3. Testing Tools of Autism

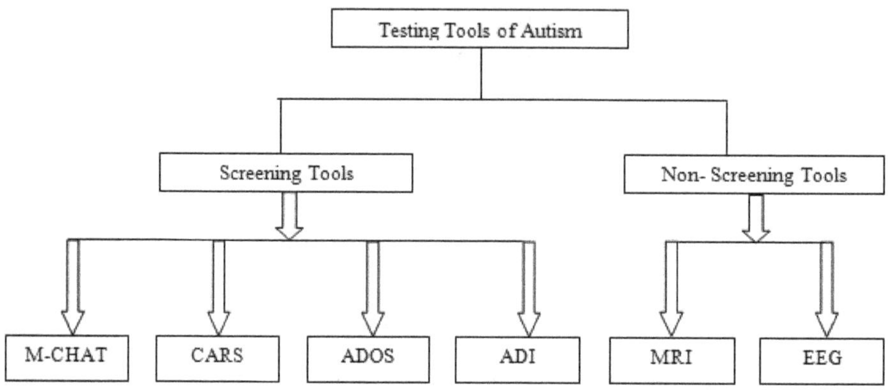

The non-screening tools are objective and mainly include MRI based or EEG signal based method. In the case of MRI method, the input is an image of brain connectivity while in EEG based methods, the input is brain signals. The non-screening tools are more powerful and reliable to detect patients with ASD. The description of various diagnostic tools is given below:

1. **M-CHAT (Modified-Checklist for Autism Toddlers)** - This is a screening tool that consists of some questions and used to diagnose autism in toddlers who are 16 to 30 months old. The methods have been improved from the last few years and have different variations like M-CHAT-R (M-CHAT- Revised) and M-CHAT-R/F (M-CHAT- Revised with Follow-up). (Guo et al., 2018; Sangare et al., 2019)
2. **CARS (Childhood Autism Rating Scale)** - It is used to identify autism by looking at development delays in children. The score 1, 2, 3 and 4 indicate a child's behavior as normal, mild, moderate and severe respectively. It includes 15 sections and scores may vary from 15 to 60. The score of more than 36 indicates a severely autistic child (Pratap, 2014).
3. **ADOS (Autism Diagnostic Observation Schedule)** – This is also a screening tool based on machine learning to identify autism and suitable for different ages of patients. The ADOS-R method claimed to speed up the procedure of detecting autism. In this method, feature reduction was performed and implemented on the WEKA tool using a decision tree as a classifier (D P Wall, Kosmicki, Deluca, Harstad, & Fusaro, 2012).
4. **ADI (Autism Diagnostic Interview)** – is a structured interview conducted with parents or caregivers for evaluation of autism or its symptoms. The revised form of tool is known as ADI-R (Zander & Willfors, 2017). The major problem of this tool is that it time-consuming and needs trained staff members who are responsible for conducting the interview.

5. **MRI (Magnetic Resonance Imaging) –** The MRI is an objective way to diagnose autism by evaluating the brain structure. Future research is more inclined towards this method due to its fast and accurate results. The main types of MRIs used in detecting ASD are sMRI, fMRI and rs-fMRI. However, it not a suitable method for toddlers and children below 3, and a crucial task to take their MRI as they may be reluctant to enter the scanner (Pua, Barton, Williams, Craig, & Seal, 2018). The brain connectivity, provided by MRI, is divided into different areas known as the region of interest (ROI) to represent it into various networks. Further, the connectivity pattern of the brain is interpreted using these networks which help to conclude the results.
6. **EEG (Electroencephalogram) –** It is used to check seizure activity. The data is in the form of signals. The autism spectrum disorder is identified by analyzing the psychological signals obtained from different subjects (Ibrahim, Djemal, & Alsuwailem, 2018). With the advancement in technology and machine learning, the EEG has also become automatic and more accurate.

These are most frequently tools used by researchers and clinical experts to detect ASD; however, there are some other tools also like INCLEN (International Clinical Epidemiology Network), ISAA (Indian Scale for Assessment of Autism) which can be used to diagnose ASD.

Challenges With ASD Diagnosis

The medical imaging is more objective to detect ASD in children as compared to screening tools that are subjective. However, this is still a challenging task due to numerous complexities involved in the process as well as data.

The several challenges, shown in figure 4, in this work are explained as follows:

Figure 4. Various challenges with ASD Diagnosis

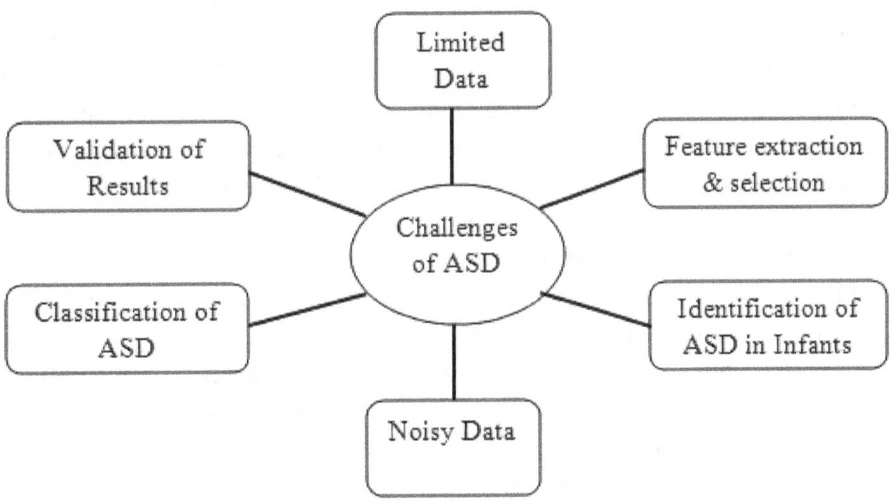

1. **Limited Data, Oversampling and Imbalanced Dataset**- The noticeable challenge of this research is the availability of data. The ABIDE dataset provides data of around 1035 MRI images of various patients of different age groups. But, if the research is done for a particular cohort then the size of data becomes small which may lead to incorrect results. Moreover, the limited dataset for ASD patients causes the class imbalance problem. Some researchers have used under-sampling or over-sampling to solve this problem but it may also affect the actual result.
2. **Validations of Results-** Many researchers have used MRI for detecting ASD and claim about the good accuracy of their results. However, the accuracy ought to be validated by clinical experts who are able to understand MRI and can verify the results. To implement the new system in real life with the same accuracy as achieved on the test set is a challenging task.
3. **Classification of ASD**- ASD is actually a syndrome and just not a disease that can be classified by a binary classifier. Thus, it a huge challenge to classify a patient with neuro disorder in different categories like ADHD (Attention-Deficit/Hyperactivity Disorder) and Asperger syndrome. However, majority of the research studies considered it a binary classification problem only and divided the patients into two categories of ASD and Non-ASD.
4. **Extraction and Selection of Features-** It is important to extract as much as possible features to classify the patient correctly. However, after extracting numerous features, the feature selection method is applied to extract the most relevant features. The selection of features must be done with care so that important features must not be lost. The iterative process can be used to judge the effect of the removal of different features on the performance of the proposed system. Thus, it becomes a crucial task to choose the most relevant and significant features from a large number of extracted features.
5. **Identification of ASD in Infants**- It is not a hard task to take an MRI of children of age 5 years or above but it is a quite challenging task in the case of infants. It is said that the early detection of ASD leads to early prevention but it is very difficult to detect ASD in kids with age less than 3 years. The detection is crucial in case of infants of age less than 12 months. Thus, some different methods must be proposed to detect ASD in children of age less than 36 months.
6. **Noisy Image:** The input image of the brain may contain some noise itself. This noise may occur due to machine problems or due to the movement of the patient. This type of noise may impact the quality of image and hence becomes a challenging task to work with noisy images. Some authors have used noise removal algorithm on images before feature extraction, however, as every small detail in medical images is important so, this step may affect correct results (Thabtah, 2017).

These various challenges make the process of diagnosing ASD a challenging task. With careful analysis, some of the challenges can be avoided like extraction and selection of features, oversampling and undersampling of data, and noise in medical images. However, some other challenges like identifying ASD in infants is still a huge challenge because it is difficult to identify symptoms in infants as well as taking MRI of infants. Moreover, most of the researchers considered ASD as binary classification (ASD or Non-ASD) problem. However, it is difficult to distinguish between different neuro diseases because of their overlapping features. Thus, extending this problem in further classes is still considered as a challenging task.

DISCUSSION

Some researchers used screening tools for detecting autism in children (Zander & Willfors, 2017). While others used images as well as videos and observed the activity of children to detect ASD (Rajagopalan, Dhall, & Goecke, 2013; Rochat et al., 2013). The major findings from this data are facial expression, delay in activity, aggressiveness, repetitive behavior, etc. It is reliable, however, a time-consuming process (Zander & Willfors, 2017). Thus, machine learning has been used with screening tools to fasten the process (Altay & Ulas, 2018). Similarly, machine learning has also been used to find the brain connectivity from MRI data and to diagnose ASD in children (Andriamananjara et al., 2019; Chanel et al., 2016; Mastrovito et al., 2018). It has been investigated by researchers and experts that MRI based autism detection techniques are better in terms of time and accuracy. Moreover, deep learning is used now because of its more promising results. Majority of researchers are using deep learning to detect ASD in less time (Aghdam et al., 2019; Du et al., 2018; Heinsfeld et al., 2018). However, there is a need to integrate these algorithms in the actual clinical environment.

CONCLUSION

ASD is a highly prevalent neurodevelopment disorder that manifests at birth or within 30 months of life. The symptoms may include repetitive behavior, lack of communication and developmental growth of a child. It is necessary to diagnose such disease at an early stage so that some therapies can be provided to the child for the betterment of his life. There are several tools available to diagnose autism and identifying its common symptoms. However, from the last few years, brain imaging is becoming more popular to diagnose such neuro-disorders. The reason behind this trend is more promising results than screening tools as well as these may help to set some standard biomarkers for autism.

Many researchers have proposed methods to detect autism based on MRI using machine or deep learning. However, it is still a challenging task due to small sample size, noise, extracting and selecting significant features. Also, there is need to integrate proposed machine or deep learning based ASD diagnostic algorithm with existing screening tools in actual clinical environment. This would also allow clinical experts to have a better decision-making tool.

FUTURE TRENDS

The traditional research studies have provided various techniques to identify ASD. However, there are still some limitations that need to be overcome in future studies. The main challenge of these kinds of studies is the lack of large datasets. Thus, in the future, the data can be collected from more different sites using big data technologies to improve clinical results which will help in delineating standard biomarkers. Some researchers have tried to combine phenotypic data like age, sex, handedness, IQ and eye status and fMRI data to improve the efficiency of an algorithm. This concept can be further extended to take more instances of MRI images and considering more significant phenotypic data to improve the efficiency of algorithms. The different parameters can be used to evaluate the performance of an algorithm like accuracy, sensitivity, specificity, F1 score, area under curve, etc. However, some researchers have used only one or two parameters to show their results. In the future, more parameters can be used to report results. The improvement in time with system performance can also be investigated in the future. Moreover, the challenges mentioned in the given chapter will also serve as a future direction for the researchers. Therefore, we suggest researchers to develop a better method for accurately detecting ASD by overcoming these challenges.

REFERENCES

Aghdam, M. A., & Sharifi, A. (2018). Combination of rs-fMRI and sMRI Data to Discriminate Autism Spectrum Disorders in Young Children Using Deep Belief Network. *Journal of Digital Imaging*, *31*(6), 895–903. doi:10.100710278-018-0093-8 PMID:29736781

Aghdam, M. A., Sharifi, A., & Pedram, M. M. (2019). Diagnosis of Autism Spectrum Disorders in Young Children Based on Resting-State Functional Magnetic Resonance Imaging Data Using Convolutional Neural Networks. *Journal of Digital Imaging*, *32*(6), 1–20. doi:10.100710278-019-00196-1 PMID:30963340

Altay, O., & Ulas, M. (2018). Prediction of the Autism Spectrum Disorder Diagnosis with Linear Discriminant Analysis Classifier and K-Nearest Neighbor in Children. *6th International Symposium on Digital Forensic and Security (ISDFS),* 1–4. 10.1109/ISDFS.2018.8355354

Andriamananjara, A., Muntari, R., & Crimi, A. (2019). Overlaps in brain dynamic functional connectivity between schizophrenia and autism spectrum disorder. *Scientific American*, *2*, e00019. doi:10.1016/j.sciaf.2018.e00019

Baio, J., Wiggins, L., Christensen, D. L., Maenner, M. J., Daniels, J., Warren, Z., ... Durkin, M. S. (2018). Prevalence of Autism Spectrum Disorder Among Children Aged 8 Years— Autism and Developmental Disabilities Monitoring Network, 11 Sites, United States, 2014. *MMWR. Surveillance Summaries*, *67*(6), 1–23. doi:10.15585/mmwr.ss6706a1 PMID:29701730

Barttfeld, P., Wicker, B., Cukier, S., Navarta, S., Lew, S., Leiguarda, R., & Sigman, M. (2012). State-dependent changes of connectivity patterns and functional brain network topology in autism spectrum disorder. *Neuropsychologia*, *50*(14), 3653–3662. doi:10.1016/j.neuropsychologia.2012.09.047 PMID:23044278

Barua, M. M., & Daley, D. T. C. (n.d.). Autism. *Autism Spectrum Disorders – Rehabilitation Council of India*, 1–36. Retrieved from http://www.rehabcouncil.nic.in/writereaddata/autism.pdf

Bhargavan, R. (2019). Effectiveness of video assisted teaching on knowledge, attitude and practice among primary caregivers of children with Autism Spectrum Disorder Article information. *Advances in Autism*. doi:10.1108/AIA-10-2018-0039

Borràs-Ferrís, L., Pérez-Ramírez, Ú., & Moratal, D. (2019). Link-level functional connectivity neuroalterations in autism spectrum disorder: A developmental resting-state fMRI study. *Diagnostics (Basel)*, *9*(1), 32. doi:10.3390/diagnostics9010032 PMID:30901848

Bos, D. J., Van Raalten, T. R., Oranje, B., Smits, A. R., Kobussen, N. A., Belle, J., & Van. (2014). Developmental differences in higher-order resting-state networks in Autism Spectrum Disorder. *NeuroImage. Clinical*, *4*, 820–827. doi:10.1016/j.nicl.2014.05.007 PMID:24936432

Chanel, G., Pichon, S., Conty, L., Berthoz, S., Chevallier, C., & Grèzes, J. (2016). Classification of autistic individuals and controls using cross-task characterization of fMRI activity. *NeuroImage. Clinical, 10*, 78–88. doi:10.1016/j.nicl.2015.11.010 PMID:26793434

Dekhil, O., Hajjdiab, H., Ayinde, B., Shalaby, A., Switala, A., Sosnin, D., … El-baz, A. (2018). Using Resting State Functional MRI to Build A Personalized Autism Diagnosis System. *2018 IEEE 15th International Symposium on Biomedical Imaging (ISBI 2018)*, 1381–1385.

Di Martino, A., Yan, C. G., Li, Q., Denio, E., Castellanos, F. X., Alaerts, K., ... Milham, M. P. (2014). The autism brain imaging data exchange: Towards a large-scale evaluation of the intrinsic brain architecture in autism. *Molecular Psychiatry, 19*(6), 659–667. doi:10.1038/mp.2013.78 PMID:23774715

Du, Y., Fu, Z., & Calhoun, V. D. (2018). Classification and prediction of brain disorders using functional connectivity: Promising but challenging. *Frontiers in Neuroscience, 12*, 1–29. doi:10.3389/fnins.2018.00525 PMID:30127711

Dvornek, N. C., Ventola, P., & Duncan, J. S. (2018). Combining Phenotypic and Resting-State fMRI Data For Autism Classification with Recurrent Neural Networks. *2018 IEEE 15th International Symposium on Biomedical Imaging (ISBI 2018)*, 725–728.

Eslami, T., Mirjalili, V., Fong, A., Laird, A., & Saeed, F. (2019). *ASD-DiagNet : A hybrid learning approach for detection of Autism Spectrum Disorder using fMRI data.* ArXiv Preprint ArXiv:1904.07577

Geetha, B., Sukumar, C., Dhivyadeepa, E., Reddy, J. K., & Balachandar, V. (2018). Autism in India: A case–control study to understand the association between socio-economic and environmental risk factors. *Acta Neurologica Belgica, 119*(3), 393–401. doi:10.100713760-018-01057-4 PMID:30554347

Guo, C., Luo, M., Wang, X., Huang, S., Meng, Z., Shao, J., & Zhang, X. (2018). Reliability and Validity of the Chinese Version of Modified Checklist for Autism in Toddlers, Revised, with Follow-Up (M-CHAT-R / F). *Journal of Autism and Developmental Disorders*. doi:10.100710803-018-3682-y PMID:30047095

Ha, S., Sohn, I.-J., Kim, N., Sim, H. J., & Cheon, K.-A. (2015). Characteristics of Brains in Autism Spectrum Disorder: Structure, Function and Connectivity across the Lifespan. *Experimental Neurobiology, 24*(4), 273–284. doi:10.5607/en.2015.24.4.273 PMID:26713076

Heinsfeld, A. S., Franco, A. R., Craddock, R. C., Buchweitz, A., & Meneguzzi, F. (2018). Identification of autism spectrum disorder using deep learning and the ABIDE dataset. *NeuroImage. Clinical, 17*, 16–23. doi:10.1016/j.nicl.2017.08.017 PMID:29034163

Hyde, K. K., Novack, M. N., Lahaye, N., Parlett-pelleriti, C., Anden, R., Dixon, D. R., & Linstead, E. (2019). Applications of Supervised Machine Learning in Autism Spectrum Disorder Research : A Review. *Review Journal of Autism and Developmental Disorders, 6*(2), 128–146. doi:10.100740489-019-00158-x

Ibrahim, S., Djemal, R., & Alsuwailem, A. (2018). Electroencephalography (EEG) signal processing for epilepsy and autism spectrum disorder diagnosis. *Biocybernetics and Biomedical Engineering, 38*(1), 16–26. doi:10.1016/j.bbe.2017.08.006

Jain, S. M. (2018). *Detection of Autism using Magnetic Resonance Imaging data and Graph Convolutional Neural Networks Detection of Autism using Magnetic Resonance Imaging data and Graph Convolutional Neural Networks* (Master Dissertation). Rochester Institute of Technology.

Kassraian-Fard, P., Matthis, C., Balsters, J. H., Maathuis, M. H., & Wenderoth, N. (2016). Promises, pitfalls, and basic guidelines for applying machine learning classifiers to psychiatric imaging data, with autism as an example. *Frontiers in Psychiatry*, *7*(Dec). doi:10.3389/fpsyt.2016.00177 PMID:27990125

Katuwal, G. J., Cahill, N. D., Baum, S. A., & Michael, A. M. (2015). The predictive power of structural MRI in Autism diagnosis. *2015 37th Annual International Conference of the IEEE Engineering in Medicine and Biology Society (EMBC)*, 4270–4273. 10.1109/EMBC.2015.7319338

Ker, J., Wang, L., Rao, J., & Lim, T. (2017). Deep Learning Applications in Medical Image Analysis. *IEEE Access : Practical Innovations, Open Solutions*, *6*, 9375–9379. doi:10.1109/ACCESS.2017.2788044

Khosla, M., Jamison, K., Kuceyeski, A., & Mert, R. (2018). *3D Convolutional Neural Networks for Classification of Functional Connectomes. In Deep Learning in Medical Image Analysis and Multimodal Learning for Clinical Decision Support* (pp. 137–145). Cham: Springer.

Kong, Y., Gao, J., Xu, Y., Pan, Y., Wang, J., & Liu, J. (2018). Classification of Autism Spectrum Disorder by Combining Brain Connectivity and Deep Neural Network Classifier. *Neurocomputing*. doi:10.1016/j.neucom.2018.04.080

Litjens, G., Kooi, T., Bejnordi, B. E., Arindra, A., Setio, A., Ciompi, F., ... Clara, I. S. (2017). A Survey on Deep Learning in Medical Image Analysis. *Medical Image Analysis*, *42*, 60–88. doi:10.1016/j.media.2017.07.005 PMID:28778026

Lynch, C. J., Uddin, L. Q., Supekar, K., Khouzam, A., Phillips, J., & Menon, V. (2013). Default mode network in childhood autism: Posteromedial cortex heterogeneity and relationship with social deficits. *Biological Psychiatry*, *74*(3), 212–219. doi:10.1016/j.biopsych.2012.12.013 PMID:23375976

Mastrovito, D., Hanson, C., & Hanson, S. J. (2018). NeuroImage : Clinical Differences in atypical resting-state effective connectivity distinguish autism from schizophrenia. *NeuroImage. Clinical*, *18*(February), 367–376. doi:10.1016/j.nicl.2018.01.014 PMID:29487793

Mertz, L. (2017). Sharing data to solve the autism riddle: An interview with Adriana Di Martino and Michael Milham of ABIDE. *IEEE Pulse*, *8*(6), 6–9. doi:10.1109/MPUL.2017.2750819 PMID:29155370

Nielsen, J. A., Zielinski, B. A., Fletcher, P. T., Alexander, A. L., Lange, N., Bigler, E. D., ... Anderson, J. S. (2013). Multisite functional connectivity MRI classification of autism: ABIDE results. *Frontiers in Human Neuroscience*, *7*(SEP), 1–12. doi:10.3389/fnhum.2013.00599 PMID:24093016

Pereira, F., Mitchell, T., & Botvinick, M. (2009). NeuroImage Machine learning classifiers and fMRI : A tutorial overview. *NeuroImage*, *45*(1), S199–S209. doi:10.1016/j.neuroimage.2008.11.007 PMID:19070668

Plitt, M., Anne, K., & Martin, A. (2015). NeuroImage : Clinical Functional connectivity classification of autism identifies highly predictive brain features but falls short of biomarker standards. *NeuroImage. Clinical*, *7*, 359–366. doi:10.1016/j.nicl.2014.12.013 PMID:25685703

Pratap, A., & Kanimozhiselvi, C. S. (2014). Predictive assessment of autism using unsupervised machine learning models. *International Journal of Advanced Intelligence Paradigms*, *6*(2), 113–121. doi:10.1504/IJAIP.2014.062174

Pua, E. P. K., Barton, S., Williams, K., Craig, J. M., & Seal, M. (2018). Individualised MRI training for paediatric neuroimaging in autism spectrum disorders: A child-focused approach. *bioRxiv*, *61*(03), 462234.

Rajagopalan, S. S., Dhall, A., & Goecke, R. (2013). Self-Stimulatory Behaviours in the Wild for Autism Diagnosis. *Proceedings of the IEEE International Conference on Computer Vision Workshops*, 755–761. 10.1109/ICCVW.2013.103

Razzak, M. I., Naz, S., & Zaib, A. (2018). Deep learning for medical image processing: Overview, challenges and the future. *Lecture Notes in Computational Vision and Biomechanics*, *26*, 323–350. doi:10.1007/978-3-319-65981-7_12

Rochat, M. J., Veroni, V., Bruschweiler-stern, N., Pieraccini, C., Bonnet-brilhault, F., Barthélémy, C., ... Rizzolatti, G. (2013). Neuropsychologia Impaired vitality form recognition in autism. *Neuropsychologia*, *51*(10), 1918–1924. doi:10.1016/j.neuropsychologia.2013.06.002 PMID:23792328

Sangare, M., Toure, H. B., Toure, A., Karembe, A., Dolo, H., Coulibaly, Y. I., ... Geschwind, D. H. (2019). Validation of two parent-reported autism spectrum disorders screening tools M-CHAT-R and SCQ in Bamako, Mali. *eNeurologicalSci*, *15*(March), 1–5. doi:10.1016/j.ensci.2019.100188 PMID:30923752

Sartipi, S., Shayesteh, M. G., & Kalbkhani, H. (2018). Diagnosing of Autism Spectrum Disorder based on GARCH Variance Series for rs-fMRI data. *2018 9th International Symposium on Telecommunications (IST)*, 86–90.

Thabtah, F. (2017). Autism Spectrum Disorder Screening : Machine Learning Adaptation and DSM-5 Fulfillment. *Proceedings of the 1st International Conference on Medical and Health Informatics 2017*, 1–6.

Thabtah, F. (2018). Machine learning in autistic spectrum disorder behavioral research : A review and ways forward. *Informatics for Health & Social Care*, *00*(00), 1–20. doi:10.1080/17538157.2017.1399132 PMID:29436887

Wall, D. P., Dally, R., Luyster, R., Jung, J.-Y., & DeLuca, T. F. (2012). Use of artificial intelligence to shorten the behavioral diagnosis of autism. *PLoS One*, *7*(8), 1–8. doi:10.1371/journal.pone.0043855 PMID:22952789

Wall, D. P., Kosmicki, J., Deluca, T. F., Harstad, E., & Fusaro, V. A. (2012). Use of machine learning to shorten observation-based screening and diagnosis of autism. *Translational Psychiatry*, *2*(4), e100. doi:10.1038/tp.2012.10 PMID:22832900

Xiao, X., Fang, H., Wu, J., Xiao, C., Xiao, T., Qian, L., ... Xiao, Z. (2017). Diagnostic Model Generated by MRI-Derived Brain Features in Toddlers With Autism Spectrum Disorder. *Autism Research*, *10*(4), 620–630. doi:10.1002/aur.1711 PMID:27874271

Yang, X., Sarraf, S., & Zhang, N. (2018). Deep Learning-based framework for Autism functional MRI Image Classification. *Journal of the Arkansas Academy of Science*, *72*(1), 47–52.

Zander, E., Willfors, C., Berggren, S., Coco, C., Holm, A., Jifält, I., ... Bölte, S. (2017). The Interrater Reliability of the Autism Diagnostic Interview-Revised (ADI-R) in Clinical Settings. *Psychopathology, 50*(3), 219–227. doi:10.1159/000474949 PMID:28528329

Zhang, F., Savadjiev, P., Cai, W., Song, Y., Verma, R., Westin, C. F., & O'Donnell, L. J. (2016). Fiber clustering based white matter connectivity analysis for prediction of Autism Spectrum Disorder using diffusion tensor imaging. *Proceedings - International Symposium on Biomedical Imaging,* 564–567. 10.1109/ISBI.2016.7493331

Zhou, Y., Yu, F., & Duong, T. (2014). Multiparametric MRI Characterization and Prediction in Autism Spectrum Disorder Using Graph Theory and Machine Learning. *PLoS One*, *9*(6), 1–10. doi:10.1371/journal.pone.0090405 PMID:24922325

KEY TERMS AND DEFINITIONS

ABIDE (Autism Brain Imaging Data Exchange): ABIDE is a public and multicenter dataset with 1112 existing resting-state functional magnetic resonance (rs-fMRI) imaging datasets with corresponding structural MRI and phenotypic information from 539 individuals with autism spectrum disorders (ASD) and 573 age-matched typical controls (TC).

Autism Spectrum Disorder (ASD): It is a lifelong neurological disorder which causes social impairment like repetitive behavior and communication problem in children.

Blood-Oxygen-Level-Dependent (BOLD): BOLD signals allow us to observe neuro activity. BOLD imaging is a kind of fMRI imaging used to observe activity of the brain.

Deep Learning: Deep learning is a kind of machine learning technique with automatic image interpretation and feature learning facility. The different deep learning algorithms are convolutional neural network (CNN), deep neural network (DNN), recurrent neural network (RNN), genetic adversarial networks (GAN), etc.

fMRI (functional Magnetic Resonance Imaging): Measures brain activity by detecting changes associated with blood oxygenation and the flow that occur in response to neural activity.

Functional Connectivity: Is defined as the temporal correlation between in high amplitude, low-frequency spontaneously generated BOLD signal between voxels or brain regions. It helps to interpret how different brain regions interact with each other to perform any activity.

Machine Learning: Is an application of artificial intelligence (AI) that provides systems the ability to automatically learn and improve from experience without being explicitly programmed.

MRI (Magnetic Resonance Imaging): Is a type of medial image that uses strong magnetic fields and radio waves to produce detailed images of the inside of the body.

rs-fMRI (resting-state functional Magnetic Resonance Imaging): Is a method of functional magnetic resonance imaging (fMRI), which is used in brain mapping to evaluate regional interactions that occur in the absence of stimulus or task.

Schizophrenia (SZ): Is a chronic and severe mental disorder that affects how a person thinks, feels, and behaves. The person with this disease interprets reality abnormally.

Typical Development (TD): Child development is typically defined as a normal progression by which children change as they grow older by acquiring and refining knowledge, behaviors, and skills.

Chapter 16
A Review of Supportive Computational Approaches for Neurological Disorder Identification

Dulani Meedeniya
https://orcid.org/0000-0002-4520-3819
University of Moratuwa, Sri Lanka

Iresha Rubasinghe
University of Moratuwa, Sri Lanka

ABSTRACT

At present there is a growth of physical symptoms with psychological overlays, resulting in neurodevelopment disorders, where both psychiatrist and medical specialties work in collaboration to provide optimal care for the patients. Disorders such as autism spectrum disorder, attention-deficit hyperactivity disorder, Down syndrome, cerebral palsy, sickle cell disease, and Alzheimer disease are more prevalent. These may have a genetic influence and give certain behavioural disturbances due to associated medical issues. The symptoms are observable in early childhood, and they may consist of comorbid medical disorders. This chapter addresses recent studies together with the applied techniques in this context. Further, this chapter shows the limitations, challenges in current practices, and possible future research directions.

INTRODUCTION

Overview of Neurological Disorders

Healthy lifestyles and behaviours are important for the betterment of society. Health informatics is a rapidly evolving area that acquires, analyse and manage biomedical and healthcare data in conjunction with computer engineering to provide a better healthcare service. At present there is a growth of physical

DOI: 10.4018/978-1-7998-3069-6.ch016

symptoms with psychological overlays, resulting in neurodevelopment disorders, where both psychiatrist and medical specialities work in collaboration to provide optimal care for the patients. Disorders such as Autism Spectrum Disorder (ASD), Alzheimer Disease, down syndrome, Attention-Deficit Hyperactivity Disorder (ADHD), cerebral palsy, Sickle Cell Disease (SCD), depression, dyslexia and anxiety are more prevalent (Wilhelm, Schneider, & Friedman, 2006). Neurological disorders directly affect the brain and nerve system and causing development disabilities, which have become one of the major health issues worldwide (WHO, 2016). Some of these disorders are mostly encountered in children and continuing to adulthood that can be a lifelong health problem.

At present, here is an increasing growth in psychophysiological disorders. World statistics have shown that 9.4% of children have diagnosed with ADHD in 2016. The rate of ADHD affected children has increased by more than 50% from 2008 to 2012 (CDC, 2018). According to USA statistics, there is an ASD patient in every 68 children. In a recent study in Sri Lanka, being a developing country, it is found that 10% of the children involved in the study are suffering from ASD. Another study shows that 1 in every 93 children are affected by ASD in Sri Lanka (Rohanachandra, Dahanayake, Rohanachandra, & Wijetunge, 2017). Thus, it requires special attention, awareness and treatments of neurological disorders.

The neurological disorders may have a genetic influence and give certain behavioural disturbances due to associated medical issues. The symptoms such as hyperactivity, impulsivity and inattention are observable in early childhood and they may consist of comorbid medical disorders (Henry et al, 2016). These disorders show a high rate of patterns of such symptoms compared to normal-healthy people (WHO, 2016).

However, the early identification of most chronic disorders is restricted due to the unawareness and expenses in the check-up procedures used for diagnosis. For example, in general, patients visit a medical practitioner only when experiencing significant symptoms. Further, in practice the chronic diseases diagnosis procedure is performed manually by the medical experts by examining the test reports. Thus, although different types of testing criteria exist based on advanced technologies, the manual contribution can be error-prone, expensive or complex, and required expert knowledge.

Most of the neurological disorders are under-diagnosed due to the lack of accurate diagnosis methods. Consequently, there is a high risk of child patients with these disorders, to continue the symptoms to adulthood (WHO, 2016). Therefore, the early detection and identification of neurological disorders are important to prevent severe symptoms and difficulties in executive comorbidity, where a person can have many disorders at the same time. For instance, some of the disorders with a high risk of comorbidity are depression, anxiety, learning disability, repetitive movements and attention issues. Hence, early diagnosis of the neurological disorders will be helpful to minimize the severe impact on patients and to develop good mental health (Henry et al, 2016).

The psychophysiological data and clinical diagnosis measurements involved in the diagnosis of the disorders include computerized tomography scans, Electroencephalography (EEG), eye movement data, functional Magnetic Resonance Imaging (fMRI), child behaviour analysis and anatomical scales such as Quantitative Electroencephalography (Gemmell & Staff, 2005)(Bailey, 2014)(Abreu, Leal, & Figueiredo, 2018). However, manual diagnosis is still challenging due to complex layers with the encapsulated data.

Chronic disorders are the conditions that last more than three months. It may limit daily activities and requires medical attention continuously (Oliver et al, 2016). Generally, these disorders neither can be prevented by vaccines nor cured by medication. At present there is an increase in patients with chronic disorders. The neurological chronic disorders caused due to differences in brain regions than a healthy person. Figure 1 shows an overview of the identification of possible chronic disorders using medical image analysis and the details are discussed in later sections.

Figure 1. Overview of the psychophysiological disorder identification process

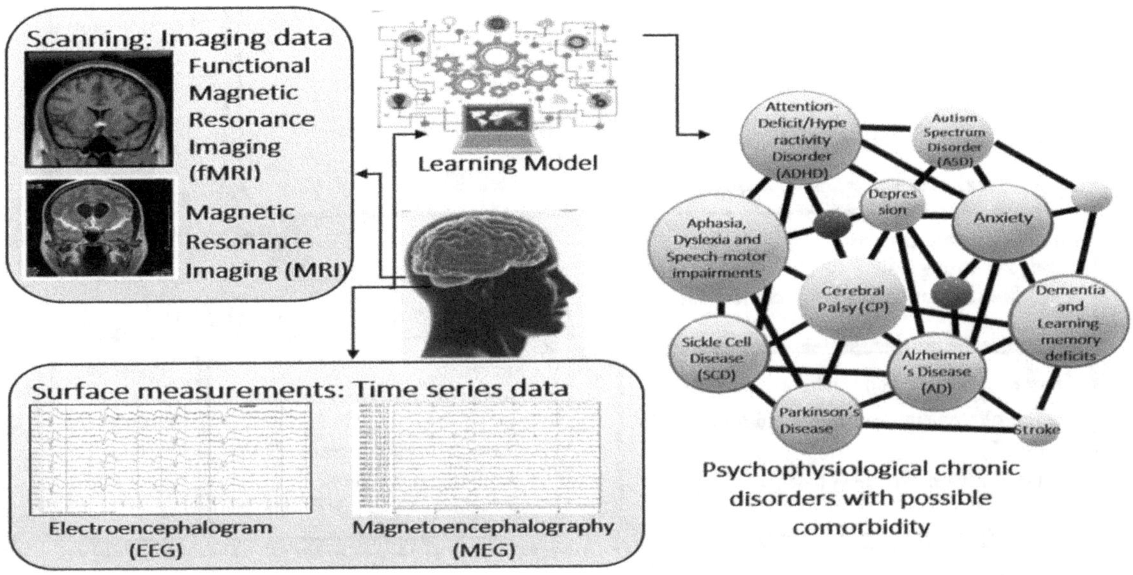

Chapter Structure

The chapter is structured as shown in Figure 2. Section 1 gives an overview of neurological disorders. Section 2 explores the neuroimaging data types in the diagnosis process. The clinical diagnosis test in the current practice is described in Section 3 and the supporting data types are explored in Section 4. Section 5 presents the neuroimaging data pre-processing techniques. Section 6 and Section 7 explores different learning models and implementation frameworks, respectively. Related neurological disorders identification models are described in Section 8. Section 9 describes the evaluation techniques. Finally, Section 10 compares the literature and concludes the review.

Figure 2. Structure of the review process

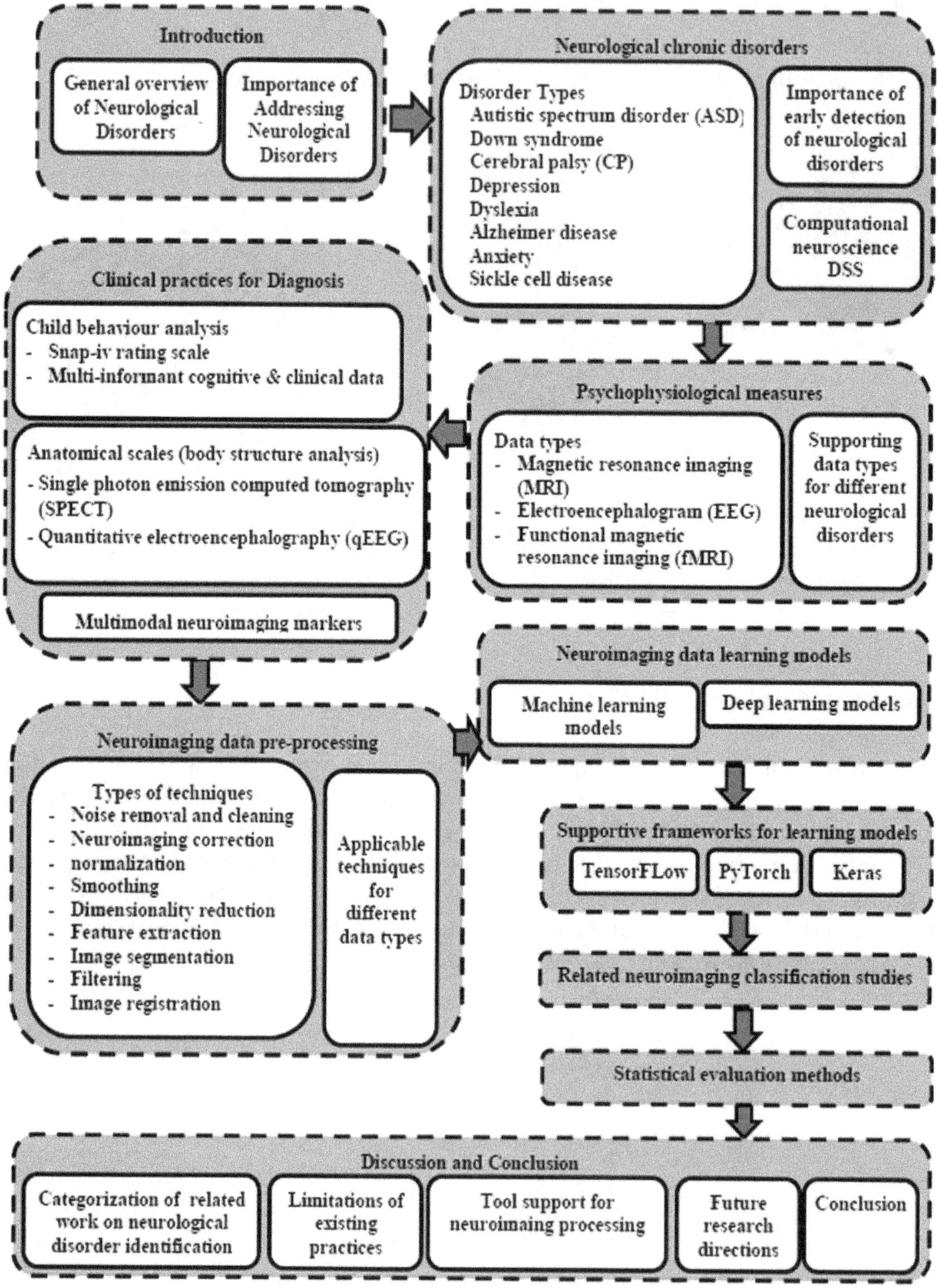

NEUROLOGICAL CHRONIC DISORDERS

Motivation for Neurological Disorder Identification Approaches

In addressing the problematic scenarios in medical science, computer-oriented diagnosis methods have arisen. Machine Learning (ML) and recently Deep Learning (DL) approaches have been rigorously used to build computational models that are capable of diagnosing medical test reports (Deng, 2014) (Siuly & Zhang, 2016). Consequently, many related studies have particularly addressed psychophysiological chronic disease diagnosis using ML and DL based classification approaches. Especially, the use of DL methods has contributed to achieving higher accuracy levels in recent studies, leading the ML techniques closer to artificial intelligence for better decision making (Kuang, Guo, An, Zhao, & He, 2014)(Heinsfeld, Franco, Craddock, Buchweitz, & Meneguzzi, 2018). However, each study has been limited to only one or two psychophysiological chronic diseases. Some studies have addresses ADHD and Autistic Spectrum Disorder (ASD) together, while other studies have been limited to one specific disorder. Therefore, there is a practical challenge to extend the existing results towards clinical usage in practice.

Given a set of neuroimaging test reports such as EEG, MRI, fMRI scan images, it is required to identify the existence of any psychophysiological chronic diseases on them (Brihadiswaran et al., 2019) (de Silva et al., 2019a). Accuracy and performance are crucial to ensure when it is required to diagnose a given input over multiple diseases than checking for a single disease. Therefore, the use of DL methods over ML techniques seems to be more useful. Accordingly, this chapter analyses the existing promising ML, DL methods and related studies.

Types of Neurological Disorders

Autistic Spectrum Disorder (ASD)

Autistic Spectrum Disorder (ASD) affects the communication of a person and shows behavioural issues. Generally, the ASD symptoms with development disorder appear in early childhood. This is also known as a spectrum disorder since has a wide set of variations and types (Jin et al., 2015).

Attention-Deficit/Hyperactivity Disorder (ADHD)

Attention-Deficit/Hyperactivity Disorder (ADHD) is a type of disorder in the brain nervous system that shows attention issues, extreme activity, behaviours without concerning the consequences, which are not normal with respective to the age of the person. Generally, ADHD diagnoses in early childhood, while more common in boys and has a possibility to continue to adulthood (Marcano, Bell, & Beex, 2018). There is no exact cure and can relieve with well-defined therapies and medications. Moreover, these disorders add risk for daily life conditions such as major life changes, thyroid issues and sleeping pattern problems (Bron et al, 2016).

Down Syndrome

Down syndrome is another genetic disorder that causes abnormal cell division due to a defect in a chromosome. Normally, the extra chromosome affects the appearance, thinking ability and learning capability.

This cause physical abnormality such as intellectual disabilities, distinctive facial features and delay in physical growth (Skotko et al., 2017). There is a growing risk of emerging many medical conditions for the people who have Down syndrome. For instance, many children with Down syndrome are born with hearth defects and digestive abnormalities.

Cerebral Palsy (CP)

Cerebral Palsy (CP) is a neurological condition that occurs due to abnormal brain developments. The brain damage can occur before birth, during the delivery or short after birth. The symptoms appear in the early childhood result in a disorder of movements that affects body movements, muscle coordination and balance (Fan, Li, Gilbert, O'Callaghan, & Wijlaars, 2018). Moreover, that can be issued in vision, hearing and speaking as well. Although there is no permanent cure, treatments and therapies will help to overcome the risk situations.

Depression

Another common illness that affects how a person feels, the way of thinking and reacting is depression, which is higher in adults around 65 years old than children and youth. Also, women are more subjected to be depressed than men. Further, depression can occur dues many reasons and it is treatable in most of the cases ("NIMH » Depression," 2018).

Dyslexia

Dyslexia is a reading and learning disability with the issues of language processing. It may not affect the intelligence though can be a lifelong problem. This is identified to be in 1 in every 10 people in the United Kingdom (Tamboer, Vorst, Ghebreab, & Scholte, 2016). Though an exact cause or medication is still not found, it is observed that dyslexia is more often running in families based on genetics.

Alzheimer Disease (AD)

A common type of dementia that affects memory is Alzheimer Disease (AD), and the symptoms can get worse over time. Although AD is not a general effect of aging, the increasing age is a risk factor as the brain cells are failing. Generally, elderly people suffer from AD than children and youth ("Alzheimer's Association," 2018). Also, women are more suffering by AD than men in gender-wise. Further, both depression and AD seem to appear together.

Anxiety

Anxiety is another psychophysiological disorder associated with the continuous feeling of unease for a long time that can affect daily lives. Particularly, anxiety can be an effect of another illness such as panic disorder or phobias (Liu et al., 2015). Although feeling anxiety is normal in life, this can interrupt daily activities. Thus, proper treatments are essential to avoid uncontrollable situations and long-lasting conditions. These symptoms may occur during childhood and continue into adulthood.

Sickle Cell Disease (SCD)

Sickle Cell Disease (SCD) is a disorder in the genetical red blood cells, named haemoglobin. This cause abnormal protein in the red blood cells that transmits oxygen. (Cologner et al., 2017). SCD is observed to be higher in early childhood, where low red blood cells count can be noticed and may result in shortening life expectancy. The most common symptoms include frequent infections, lack of energy, delayed growth, periodic pains, painful swelling and vision issues. This can lead to complications such as organ damage, stroke and blindness. The severity of this life-long illness varies from individual to individual. Although, there are no standard solutions, there are treatments to manage and live with the disease.

Early Detection of Neurological Disorders

Most of the neurological disorders occur due to a genetical influence. Hence, the early detection of a disorder during childhood helps to proceed with the relevant therapies and medications, to control the symptoms. That can minimize the consequences and the severities in the long run. Also, identifying the genes that cause these disorders is beneficial to investigate the scientific patterns of infected genes. On the other hand, the other suspected causes of disorders such as stress levels, eating patterns, lack of physical activities and verbal exercises can be handled properly to minimise the effects, by diagnosis in early childhood (Wilhelm, Schneider, & Friedman, 2006). Thus, a child suffering from a disorder can be trained to lead a much normal lifestyle with the required good practices and medications towards their adulthood. Therefore, the early identification of these psychophysiological conditions is crucial to reduce the consequences, though medical science is still experimenting with permanent solutions.

Computational Neuroscience Decision Support Systems

Decision Support System (DSS) is a software system with a knowledge base, model and interactive user interface. It supports to compile important data with the expert knowledge for the decision-making process (Oliver et al, 2016). Several recent studies have directed towards DSS that facilitate to discriminate pattern in psychophysiological data such as fMRI (Rubasinghe & Meedeniya, 2020))(Ariyarathne et al., 2020), EEG (Haputhanthri et al., 2019), eye moment data (de Silva et al., 2019b) and a combination of different data types in order to identify positive and negative subjects of neurological disorders.

Most of these approaches have used data-pre-processing techniques specific to the considered data type and suggested classifiers that are resulted in high classification accuracies. Majority of the studies have addressed the diagnosis of neurological disorders using ML and DL based classification approaches. The use of DL methods has shown higher accuracy levels. However, each study has been limited to focus only on one or two neurological disorders, mainly ADHD and ASD have been addressed together while other studies have been limited to one disorder. Therefore, there is a practical challenge to extend the existing results towards clinical usage in practice.

PSYCHOPHYSIOLOGICAL MEASURES

Overview of Psychophysiological Metrics

Neuroimaging is the use of various techniques to generate the structure of activities in a brain nerves system (Bowman, 2014). Table 1 summarises the symptoms in neurological disorder types with supportive data types used for the diagnosing process.

Table 1. Summary of psychophysiological chronic diseases

Disease	Symptoms	Data Types Used for Diagnosis
ADHD (Marcano et al., 2018)	Inattention, hyperactivity, impulsivity, lack of ability in time management, unorganized.	EEG, MRI, fMRI, CT scans, eye movement tracking, blood tests.
Autism Spectrum Disorder (ASD) (Jin et al., 2015)	Communication and interaction issues, repetitive behaviors, limited daily functions, restricted interests, inconsistent eye contact.	EEG, MRI, fMRI, eye movement tracking.
Depression ("NIMH» Depression," 2018)	Unreasonable mood swings, changes in appetite, sleeping difficulties, loss of pleasure, suicidal feelings.	EEG, ECT, repetitive transcranial magnetic and vagus nerve stimulation, cognitive ability score, MRI, fMRI, demographics.
Dyslexia (Tamboer et al., 2016)	Difficulty in reading, writing in learning. Word confusions, inability to understand verbal instructions, inconsistent spelling, unorganized,	EEG, MRI, fMRI.
Alzheimer disease ("Alzheimer's association," 2018)	Remembering difficulties, memory loss, disorientation, difficulty in speaking, walking. Confusion.	EEG, MRI, fMRI.
Cerebral Palsy (CP) (Fan et al., 2018)	Movement dysfunction, awkward positions, stiff muscles, floppy muscle tone, difficulty in performing daily activities.	MRI, fMRI.
Anxiety (Liu et al., 2015)	Restless, worried, lack of concentration, sleeping difficulties, heart palpations.	MRI, fMRI.
SCD (Coloigner et al., 2017)	Fatigue, shortness of breath, delayed growth,	EEG, fMRI.
Down syndrome (Skotko et al., 2017)	Poor muscle tone, flattened face, smaller head, slow learning, impulsive, less attention.	EEG, fMRI, blood tests, nuchal translucency test.

Among many, EEG, MRI, fMRI, SPECT and qEEG are found to be more useful in the diagnosis of neurological disorders. Although, different techniques exist, there are major differences between EEG versus MRI/ fMRI. EEG is focused on temporal resolution while MRI and fMRI are for spatial resolution. Thus, some studies have used both data types for the diagnosis of neurological disorders. Considering the related literature ADHD and ASD identification using MRI or fMRI data have been widely addressed. Accordingly, there exist common symptoms such as sleeping issues, lack of concentration and unorganized behaviour in the daily lives of the people with neurological disorders. EEG, MRI and fMRI remain the most commonly used neuroimaging data types associated with these disorders.

Magnetic Resonance Imaging (MRI)

MRI provides structural information in the form of a map of the brain at a given time (Salvatore, 2014). Accordingly, MRI is used to determine the sizes of brain regions to detect abnormalities such as tumours.

Electroencephalogram (EEG)

EEG is used to monitor the electrical activity of the brain. EEG captures the brain wave patterns by placing electrodes on the scalp. These surface measurements, capture the variations of brain activities in response to a given stimulus (Abreu et al., 2018).

Functional Magnetic Resonance Imaging (fMRI)

The primary technology behind Functional Magnetic Resonance Imaging (fMRI) is the same as Magnetic Resonance Imaging (MRI), though fMRI is calculated in determining the number of changes in oxygenated blood (Abreu et al., 2018).

Current Practices of Clinical Diagnosis Measurements

There exist disorder specific and common methodologies to obtain diagnosis purpose measures. The collection of neuroimaging data of a patient such as EEG, MRI, fMRI and CT scans is the most known methodology among the general public. In addition, there exist different dimensional measurements and scales to assess the disorders comprehensively.

Child Behaviour Analysis

Analysing the behavioural aspects of children for the neurological disorder diagnosis is useful in many ways; (1) to understand the physical and physiological consequences, (2) to gain information on whom to be screened further towards accurate diagnosis, (3) to identify the need of preventing the effects of disorders in a way communication to general public easily (Wilhelm et al., 2006). Thus, the necessary society support for children with special care can be secured.

SNAP-IV Rating Scale

One of the earliest clinical practice is the SNAP-IV rating scale. This was derived from the Swanson, Nolan and Pelham (SNAP) survey found in 1983 (Bussing et al., 2008). Also, SNAP-IV consists of items taken from ADHD DSM-IV criteria and DSM-III-R scale, Conners Index Questionnaire and IOWA Conners Questionnaire. This is a rating scale with three levels from 0 to 3 and the final score is calculated by averaging the overall sum. The items to be rated are behavioural aspects such as inattention, forgetfulness, distractibility.

Multi-Informant Cognitive and Clinical Data

Assessing multi-informant cognitive and clinical data is another behavioural approach. A collection of reports from various sources such as a patient's significant others information that elaborates the context data and clinical interview results that provide insight into the patient (Kraemer et al., 2003). However, there is no standard mechanism on integrating different types of data and various methodologies exist in research level.

Anatomical Scales

The anatomical scales assess the patient's bodily structure than behavioural analysis.

Single Photon Emission Computed Tomography (SPECT)

A Single Photon Emission Computed Tomography (SPECT) scan is a type of imaging test that uses gamma rays. It shows the blood circulation to organs and tissues within the body (Gemmell & Staff, 2005). Especially SPECT is applied to monitor blood flow in the brain and differs from MRI or CT scans due to the ability of detecting decreased blood flows in any injured areas of the brain. Moreover, SPECT scans are used in practice to evaluate seizures.

Quantitative Electroencephalography (qEEG)

A general EEG captures the electrical activity of the brain, whereas Quantitative Electroencephalography (qEEG) adds an additional mathematical and statistical analysis layer to that to compare the results parameter wise such that age wise and gender wise (Bailey, 2014). Consequently, qEEG process generates a brain map using the obtained quantitative measurements and comparisons which helps to identify patterns of brain dysfunctions.

Multimodal Neuroimaging Markers

Multimodal neuroimaging markers are used to identify the correlation between disorders and behavioural information. ADHD diagnosis study (Ball et al., 2019), has used multimodal neuroimaging data, multi-informant cognitive data and the clinical information. They had applied multivariate analysis technique to find associations among the used heterogeneous data models. The use of several neuroimaging markers is advantageous in computation. In another ADHD study (Wolfers et al., 2017), a multimodal linked Independent Component Analysis (ICA) method is applied to diffusion and MRI data.

An assessment of autosomal Alzheimer Disease (AD) is done in (Yau et al., 2015) using clinical markers along with MRI neuroimaging data. They have identified the links among amyloidosis, metabolism, general cognition, verbal memory and hippocampal volume in AD patients by following linear mixed models over biomarkers. Another study on AD that has used Statistical parametric mapping (SPM) and voxel-based morphometry (VBM) techniques to assess PiB data have shown that MRI with PiB-PET help for diagnostic prediction and classifications instead of using separately (Jack et al., 2008).

Table 2. Summary of the applicability of pre-processing technique vs data type

Technique		EEG	qEEG	MEG	fMRI	MRI	PET	Ultra-sound	CT scan	SP ECT	ECG
Dimension reduction	Principal Component Analysis (PCA)	√		√	√	√	√	√	√	√	√
	Generalized Linear Model (GLM)	√	√	√	√	√		√	√	√	√
Noise removal	Wavelet transform	√		√	√	√	√	√	√	√	√
	Conventional filters	√		√	√	√					√
	Adaptive filters (change the linear filter coefficients)	√		√	√	√	√	√	√	√	√
	Smoothing filters	√		√	√	√		√	√		√
	Independent Component Analysis (ICA)	√		√	√	√	√	√	√		√
	Histogram equalization	√			√	√	√	√	√		√
Image filtering	Median filter	√		√		√	√	√		√	√
	Fuzzy filter				√	√		√	√		
	Density Estimation Filters	√		√	√			√			
Image correction	Motion correction	√	√	√	√	√	√	√	√	√	√
	Slice timing correction				√						
	Head motion correction	√	√	√	√	√	√	√	√	√	√
	Distortion correction	√	√	√	√	√	√	√	√	√	√
Normalization	Spatial/ Surface (FreeSurfer)			√	√	√				√	
	Histogram-based	√			√	√		√	√		√
	Statistical	√			√	√			√		√
	Volume-based (SPM 5 nonlinear normalization)				√	√	√				√
	Landmark-based (brain area)				√	√					
	Homomorphic Filtering	√			√	√			√		√
Smoothing	Laplacian	√		√	√	√	√	√	√	√	√
	Differencing filter	√		√	√	√		√	√		√
	Spatial smoothing				√	√		√	√		
Segmentation	Shape-based				√	√					
	Atlas-based				√	√			√		
	Time frequency-based (Singular Spectrum)	√									√
	Interactive segmentation (Interactive Graph Cuts)	√			√	√		√	√		√
Feature extraction	Singular Value Decomp.	√		√	√	√	√	√	√	√	√
	Discrete wavelet transforms	√		√	√	√	√	√	√	√	√
	Fast Fourier transform (FFT)	√		√	√	√	√	√	√	√	√
	Max pooling	√	√	√	√	√	√	√	√	√	√
Quality improvement	Contrast Stretching	√			√	√		√	√		√
	Spatial domain methods				√	√					
	Frequency domain methods	√			√						

Even though these approaches of multimodal neuroimaging markers have started to show significant results, still not majority of psychophysiological chronic disorders are involved in literature such as CP and SCD. Hence, there is a research hindrance to be addressed as most of the neurological disorders share common symptoms, that result in patients to have multiple disorders.

Neuroimaging Data Pre-Processing

Image processing can be categorized into digital and medical image processing. The pre-processing of medical images is complex since the majority are 3-dimensional and 4-dimensional modalities. This section presents an overview of generic pre-processing techniques applied on neuroimaging modalities such as MRI, fMRI and EEG. Majority of these can be performed using Python libraries such as scikit-learn, Nilearn, NiBabel, NumPy, Pandas and image processing and learning tools like MATLAB, Weka, ImageJ and OpenCV. Table 2 summarises the pre-processing techniques that are applicable to different data types. Each neuroimaging method has a specific uniqueness and usefulness in different contexts.

Noise Removal and Cleaning

The mostly occurring types of noises in medical images are Gaussian, Salt and Pepper, Speckle, Brownian noises and motion-related noises. Noise represents any unwanted data included in an image (Abreu et al., 2018). For instance, the motion-related noise is regarding the unnecessary head movements in neuroimaging data. The noise exclusion is known by denoising and there are several denoising algorithms such as Principal Component Analysis (PCA), Histogram equalization, wavelet transform, median filter and Independent Component Analysis (ICA). The appropriateness of selecting a denoising technique depends on the type of neuroimaging and the signals contained in them. More specific techniques like Component based noise correction (CompCor), Anatomy-based correlation correction (ANATICOR) and denoising using external recordings are used in BOLD (Blood oxygen-level-dependent) fMRI neuroimage denoising (Caballero-Gaudes and Reynolds, 2017).

Neuroimaging Correction

There can be various forms of motion in a brain image such as rigid body motion and deformable motion that might occur periodically, randomly or continuously. Motion correction is used to estimate the correction of poor resolution. This helps with functional information extraction and statistical analysis (Klette, 2014). The main two types of motion correction in brain images include retrospective and prospective motion correction (Abreu et al., 2018). Motion correction consists of multiple image registration tasks to render the images. Slice-timing correction is used to improve the fMRI analysis when the acquisition speed is slow. Here, the images are interpolated between each other to mitigate the longer time gaps among slices. Moreover, in brain images, geometric distortion occurs due to magnetic field inhomogeneity that affects the accuracy of image registrations. The distortion correction is done by spatial distribution mapping.

Normalization

The regional sections in a brain image are difficult to determine due to their varying shape and size. Normalization is the approach of creating a reference frame and aligning the brain images by the spatial transformation. This may also be known by 'co-registration' due to the similarity in both tasks though normalization is more complex than the co-registration in practice. The reason is normalization is targeting to align data from several subjects whereas in co-registration the focus is on single subjects. However, normalization can be started with co-registration. The landmark-based, surface-based and volume-based templates are used in practice to align the images (Toennies, 2017b). In general, the MNI (Montreal Neurologic Institute) atlases and Talairach are two most popular templates used for MRI and fMRI neuroimages since a long time as Talairach atlas is introduced in 1988 (Brett, Christoff, Cusack and Lancaster, 2001).

Smoothing

Smoothing is useful to average the intensities of voxels in neuroimaging by applying a blurring kernel in practice to enhance the Signal to Noise Ratio (SNR). Thus, the result becomes smooth with hard edges and a low spatial frequency (Larobina & Murino, 2014). The main goal is smoothing is also to eliminate noise as much as possible. Smoothing can be spatial and/ or temporal smoothing. Although spatial smoothing helps to achieve good SNR, it may decrease the image resolutions and images tend to become blurry. Thus, it has a trade-off between SNR and resolution which has to be balanced based on context and requirements. In contrast, temporal smoothing is about smoothing the time series of each pixel in an image which leads to SNR improvement and the removal of higher frequency fluctuations.

Dimensionality Reduction

The medical images like MRI, fMRI, EEG are mostly in high-dimensional 3D and 4D. Hence, it is required to minimise the dimensions for analysis but without affecting the useful data concatenated in them. The Principle Component Analysis (PCA), computation of mean, covariance, NeRV algorithm, LDA-NeRV (Nybo, 2015) and Generalized Linear Model (GLM) are few dimensionality reduction techniques (Pang, Lansdell, & Fairhall, 2016). The non-linear Locally Linear Embedding (LLE) is another algorithm in practice for fMRI time series data reduction (Mannfolk et al., 2010). Dimensionality reduction is helpful in optimization, computation as well as visualizing large amounts of data that have a higher number of features associated with each. For example, most of the existing plotting methods and graphs are two dimensional (2D) which are unable to represent high dimensional data in a human readable manner. Another closely related approach in dimensionality reduction is known as variable selection for pre-processing. That helps to focus to select important features depending on the requirements in the problem domain.

Feature Extraction

The neuroimaging scanner machines also perform a feature extraction phase in acquiring images such as by extracting time-independent activation coefficients in fMRI signals. The feature extraction in neuroimaging is usually a combination of several pre-processing stages such as slicing, noise removal, templating and ROI segmentation. The features to be extracted based on the type of neuroimaging modality and type of disorder or the nature of the addressed problem (Salvatore et al., 2014). For instance, gray scale, texture, shape, voxels are some of the common features in brain images. However, the important features to be extracted depends on the domain. Hence, there exist feature extraction methods like task-specific feature extraction (Jang, Plis, Calhoun and Lee, 2017). The deep learning methods like DBN are used to represent a large number of feature spaces as neurons in layered structures during the process. That allows to assign weights to features, perform computations among weight-feature matrices.

Image Segmentation

Medical image segmentation is performed in a combination of several segmentation algorithms depending on the characteristics of medical image modalities. The edge-based, split and merge techniques, hybrid methods, manual, intensity-based like Fuzzy thresholding and region growing, atlas-based and surface-based like active contours are popular for brain image segmentation (Ahmadvand & Daliri, 2014). Segmentation is useful in neuroimaging for analysis of brain development and even for surgical planning in practice. The goal is to partition an image into meaningful sections in a useful manner but without any overlapping among sections. The base of dividing into partitions can be according to any attributes like edges, colour or pixel/ brain tissue intensity.

Filtering

Filtering is used to for noise reduction, removal and smoothing of neurological data. This can be done in spatial filtering and temporal filtering. Generally, temporal filtering is used to reduce unwanted frequencies in neuroimaging and led to improving the signal-to-noise ratio. The main types are high-pass (removes frequencies below a given threshold), low-pass (removes high-frequency noise) and band-pass (considers a defined frequency range) / band stop (remove specific frequency that reflects only noise) filtering; for instance in EEG signals (Urigüen, and Garcia-Zapirain, 2015). Spatial filtering is used to remove physiological noise. For instance, in fMRI images contain low-frequency drifts that occur due to physiological noise. Hence, high-pass filtering can be used to flatter the noise spectrum. Therefore, the types of frequencies to be removed should be identified, among the set of frequencies such as task-frequency and noise frequency. The prominent image filters that are also applied on medical images include binary thresholding filter, median filter, mean filter and recursive Gaussian filter (Toennies, 2017a).

Image Registration

Image registration adjusts the elements and features of an image with respect to a second image in a way suitable for further processing (Toennies, 2017a). However, it is challenging due to complexities in 2D and 3D image modalities. Hence, image registration itself is a major research direction especially in the domain of medical imaging where the complexities are higher. The automated approaches for SPECT brain image and plantar pressure image registration are addressed in the work in (Toennies, 2017a), where they have applied feature-based and intensity-based methods, since still the automated registration is not in clinical practice. Toennies (2017a) has focused on nuclear medicine images registration. They have discussed the topic in terms of current geometric transformation algorithms, optimization of algorithms, characterizing image modalities using similarity measures and interpolation.

NEUROIMAGING DATA LEARNING MODELS

Classification of Neuroimaging Support Learning Models

The widely used data learning architectures and models for neuroimaging classification includes both Machine learning (ML) and Deep learning (DL) methods. The ML algorithms are in supervised, unsupervised and reinforcement capabilities. DL is known for improving the accuracy of ML applications with the involvement of advanced hardware requirements, specifically, the processing power as ML techniques are lacking the applicability on larger datasets (Deng, 2014). Thus, DL which is a subset of ML, has become a widely used technique in psychophysiological chronic disease identification. Figure 3 summarizes the data learning models used in related studies on neuroimaging data.

Figure 3. Data learning models classification

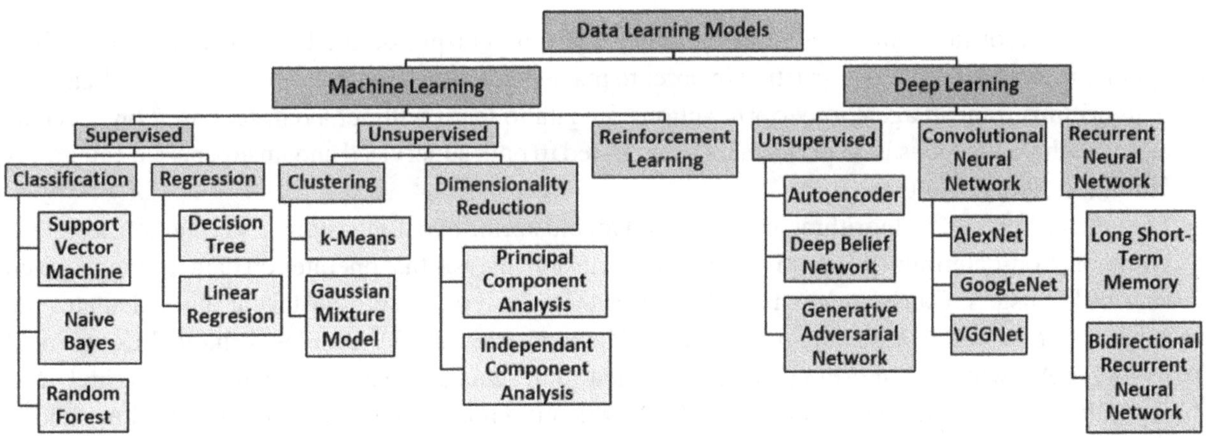

Support Vector Machine (SVM) is a prominent application in literature in machine learning classification. Moreover, Convolutional Neural Networks (CNN), Generative Adversarial Networks (GANs), Deep Belief Network (DBN) and Autoencoders (AE) models in DL have shown significant accuracy and performance results for neuroimaging data in recent studies. The architectures; DBN and CNN are mainly applied in the recent related work on neurological disorder classifications. Further, Max Pooling, backpropagation, Stochastic Gradient Descent (SGD), Batch Normalization, Transfer Learning and Learning Rate Decay are some of the common DL related techniques.

Supervised Machine Learning

Supervised ML algorithms are based on a given set of samples and make predictions by searching for patterns within the labelled data. The supervised ML algorithms are mainly applied for classification and regression. SVM is a widely used ML algorithm, that outputs an optimal hyperplane which categorizes test data, given the labelled training dataset (Tenev et al., 2014). On the other hand, k-Nearest Neighbor (KNN) learning algorithm considers labelled data to learn how to label other data points based on neighbour's vote. Another ML algorithm is Naïve Bayes (NB), which is a Bayes theorem based probabilistic classifier. It assumes independence in predictors. Random Forest (RF) is a collaborative model that considers an average of multiple Decision Trees (DT) and gets an overall best performance by combining all of them (Liaw & Wiener, 2002). DT is an ML algorithm that uses branching methods for matching all the possible outcomes having the applicability to regression as well.

Besides, linear regression and Logistic Regression (LR) are two other regression algorithms (de Vos et al., 2018). Linear regression shows the relationship between two variables and best fits line among all data points whereas LR is a statistical method for binary classification problems to estimate parameters of a logistic model. Moreover, the lasso is a variable selection and a shrinkage method to obtain a subset of predictors in regression analysis. Another regression algorithm; Support Vector Regression (SVR) follows similar principles as SVM. Although SVR is a regression method that finds a model that can explain the output of an input, SVR is also used for classification.

Unsupervised Machine Learning

Unsupervised algorithms are capable of handling data without pre-defined labels and organize into groups of clusters based on their structure in order to make predictions. Besides, Reinforcement Learning (RL) algorithms train an agent to perform actions on data to learn without a dataset based on previous experience where the focus is on performance compared to both supervised and unsupervised categories (Aslanides, Leike, & Hutter, 2017).

The unsupervised ML algorithms are often used for clustering and dimensionality reduction. k-Means is a common, non-deterministic iterative method for cluster analysis that operates on data through a given number of k clusters. Gaussian Mixture Model (GMM) is a type of soft clustering that calculates the probability of data before assigning into clusters (Marcano et al., 2018). Besides, Principal Component Analysis (PCA), which is an orthogonal method that represents a linear combination of original variables and Independent component analysis (ICA), which is a non-orthogonal, computational method to separate a multivariate signal where all components are equally treated are approaches for dimensionality reduction (Case et al., 2017).

Deep Learning Models

Deep learning models can be mainly categorized into unsupervised, Convolution Neural Networks (CNN) and Recurrent Neural Networks, as shown in Figure 3. Autoencoders (AE) is a tye of unsupervised DL model, that use input vectors to compute the output vectors, such that the output is same as input vectors (Heinsfeld et al., 2018)(Sen, Borle, Greiner, & Brown, 2018). Thus, AEs are conceptually simple. The common applications of AE are for feature learning, outlier detection, dimension reduction, speech and image recognition. The compression vs conceptualization dilemma is a mainly known limitation in AE.

Deep Belief Networks (DBN) is a generative graphical model. It consists of Restricted Boltzmann Machines (RBM) layers for pre-learning and a feedforward method for refinement. Boltzmann Machines (BM) is a symmetrically connected network in different variations such as RBM and Deep BM (DBM) (Kuang et al., 2014). The neurons in a BM make stochastic decisions that whether to be on or off and extracts higher level features from raw input vectors. The leading applications of DBNs include the image, face recognition and vocabulary phonetic recognition. For instance, NASA uses for satellite imagery classification. DBNs learn higher level features of a data set in an unsupervised training. However, DBNs may complex to train due to the vanishing gradient.

Generative Adversarial Network (GAN) is a network that trains two models in parallel. It uses a parameter count smaller than normal compared to the amount of data used to train the network (Tran et al., 2017). Generally, GANs are effective at generating data similar to training data. Hence, it is applied for image, sound and video classification tasks. Tending to capture input data style in output images in a coherent manner is a drawback in GANs.

The Convolutional Neural Network (CNN) is a feed-forward network made up of neurons having learnable weights. Generally, a CNN consists of three types of layers; (i) convolution-to filter (ii) pooling-to downsample (iii) fully-connected-to partition. There exist different variations of CNN implementations such as LeNet, AlexNet, ZF Net, GoogLeNet, VGGNet, ResNet and many more (Acharya et al., 2018) (Sarraf & Tofighi, 2016)(Spasov, Passamonti, Duggento, Lio, & Toschi, 2018). The common applications of CNN model are 2D images classifications, self-driving cars, text analytics, optical character recognition, sound analysis, robotics, treatments for visually impaired and 3D datasets; MRI, fMRI data classifications. Comparatively to other models, CNN is widely used due to its high suitability for spatial data, the capability to learn higher-order features in data via convolutions and is found more useful when having more structure to input data. Nevertheless, powerful hardware accelerations like GPU are essential for better performance.

Supportive Implementation Frameworks for Learning Models

There exist a variety of ML and DL implementation frameworks in the form of open source libraries as well as software tools. The programming language Python is leading most of them due to its comparatively higher capabilities in complex mathematical computations. Accordingly, the most popular ML and DL supportive open source frameworks TensorFlow, PyTorch and Keras are all written in Python. Moreover, the software tools; MATLAB, Weka and R Studio supports the implementations of data learning models.

TensorFlow

TensorFlow is a widely used, Python based, open source software library interface developed at Google's AI for ML algorithms. It is flexible to be used within a range of hardware and computational power from CPUs to TPUs, irrespective of the device type. The Deep Probabilistic Programming Language (DPPL) Edward is built on top of TensorFlow (Tran et al., 2017).

PyTorch

Another open source ML library in Python is PyTorch, developed by the artificial intelligent research group of Facebook (Paszke et al., 2017). In considering the community support, TensorFlow is ahead of PyTorch since this is relatively newer than the former.

Keras

Keras is a higher level, open source DL API developed by a Google engineer in Python that runs on TensorFlow with user friendliness, modularity and extensibility (Chollet, 2015). Keras is behind the

TensorFlow and PyTorch in terms of performance and hence ideal for relatively smaller datasets. However, Keras provides easy debugging with rapid prototyping due to its simple architecture.

Figure 4. ADHD classification model architecture (Kuang et al., 2014)

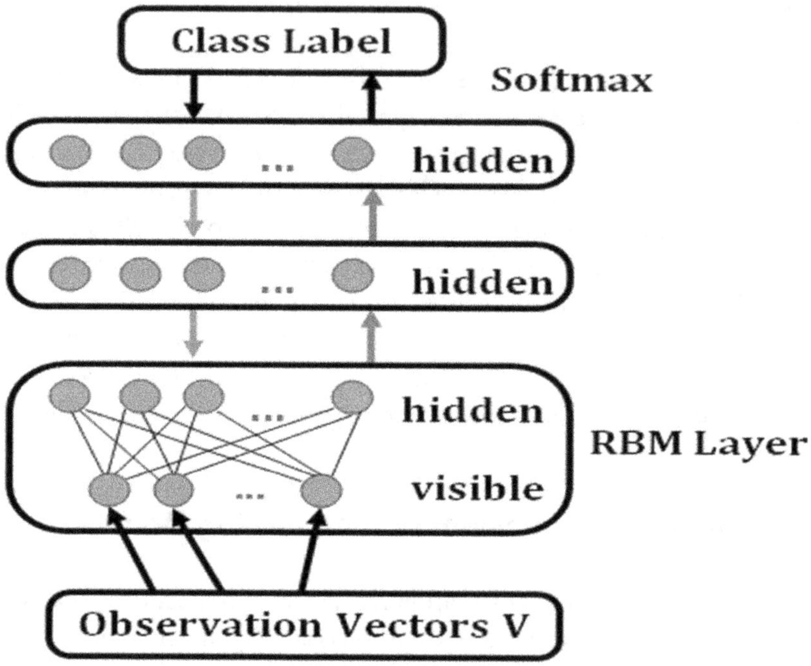

RELATED NEUROIMAGING CLASSIFICATION STUDIES

Research Model 1

The work presented in (Kuang et al., 2014) is a DL based ADHD classification model. They have adapted the DBN architecture consists of Gaussian-Bernoulli RBM having 3 hidden layers and Softmax regression for predicting the ADHD status and subtype in a given dataset. The resting state fMRI data has obtained from ADHD-200 dataset, followed by FFT and max-pooling techniques for pre-processing. Figure 4 shows the composition of DBN with 3-layered RBM and Softmax. The upward and downward arrows between the hidden layers denote generative and fine-tuning processes, respectively. Each RBM is a 2-layered undirected graphical model, where the visible units to denote the observations and hidden units represent the features. The DBN is trained as a stack of RBMs and Softmax has performed the fine-tuning. Further, they have conducted the classification with neural networks (NN) with one hidden layer for ML classification and the results of the DBN model has shown discrimination with higher accuracy. Also, NN has shown better results over the DBN model in some datasets. However, it is limited for examining a region of the brain, which can be extended towards the entire brain.

Research Model 2

A DL classification model for ASD based on brain activation patterns is discussed using Autoencoders (AE) (Heinsfeld et al., 2018). They have selected the denoising AE architecture, which is a category of UPN in DNN architecture categorization and Softmax for model training. The resting state fMRI dataset of 505 ASD participants and 530 normal people with gender distribution obtained from ABIDE database are used for applying the model's classification. Figure 5 illustrates the way learning from AEs is transferred to the classifier with Softmax.

Figure 5. Transfer learning from autoencoders (Heinsfeld et al., 2018)

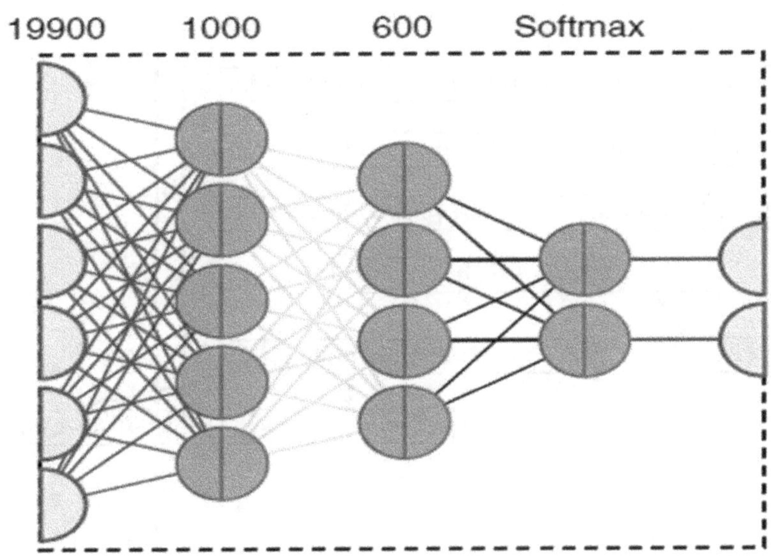

Additionally, they have conducted the classification using supervised ML classifiers; SVM and RF. Then the outcomes of the learning models are compared by 10-fold cross-validation. The results have shown higher accuracy and sensitivity for the DL model and the second-best results for SVM. However, SVM models have performed in less time, while DL model has consumed more time since DL architectures require high processing power.

Research Model 3

The related work (Sarraf & Tofighi, 2016) has conducted an AD classification using the CNN architecture in DL based on WB voxel-level features on resting-state fMRI and MRI data. They have applied the LeNet-5 CNN implementation with Softmax and max-pooling as shown in Figure 6 along with 5-fold cross validation for classifier performance evaluation. Accordingly, the results signify a high accuracy of 96%. Further, they have experimented using SVM and has shown that the CNN model has outperformed SVM accuracy. Additionally, this work has distinguished the useful features in the context. However, the used dataset is with a small data combination of 28 AD patients from the ADNI database and 15 healthy controls, which is a limitation to generalize the classification results accuracy.

Figure 6. LeNet-5 network model implementation (Sarraf & Tofighi, 2016)

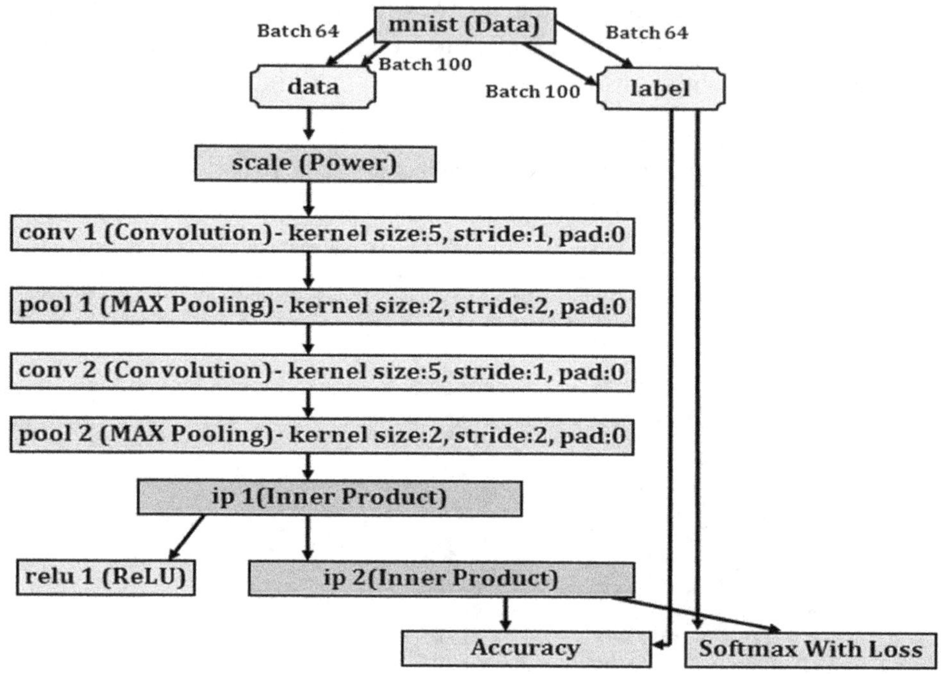

Figure 7. Schematic diagram of classification framework (Liu et al., 2015)

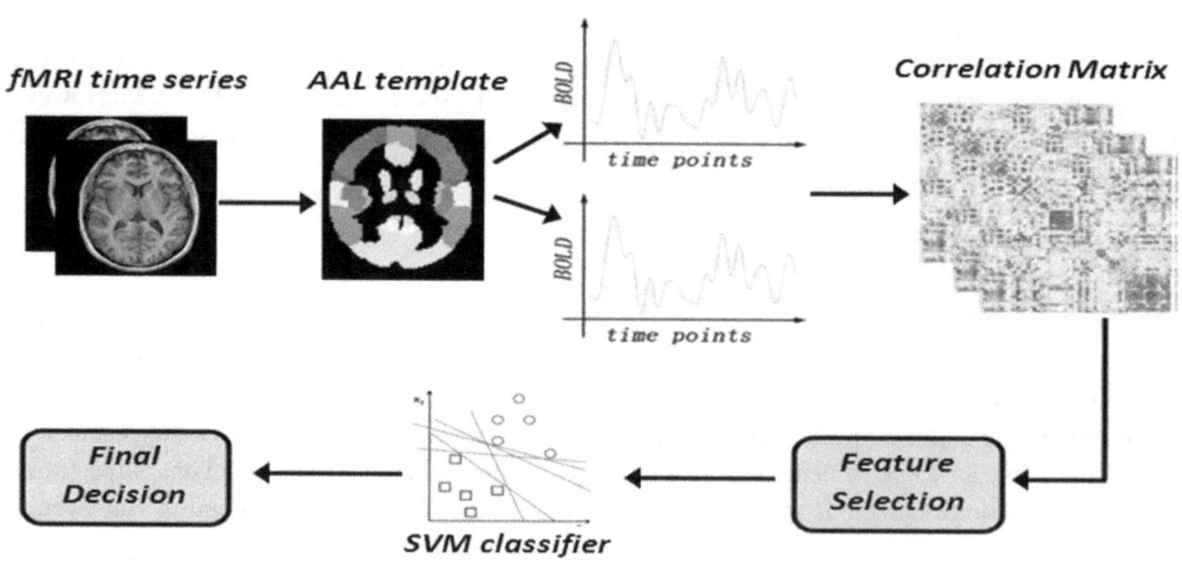

Research Model 4

Among the anxiety disorder classification related studies, a SAD classification multivariate pattern analysis (MVPA) framework is presented (Liu et al., 2015), as shown in Figure 7 using ML linear and non-linear SVM classifiers.

They have used the fMRI data with the focus on whole-brain functional connectivity. Firstly, the resting state fMRI data are partitioned into 116 regions via the Automated Anatomical Labeling (AAL) template in this framework. Secondly, parsed through a correlation matrix towards feature selection and given to the SVM classifier. The results were compared with both linear and nonlinear kernels using RBF and have shown that linear SVM reduces overfitting than nonlinear SVM. However, they have used a small dataset with 20 SAD patients and 20 healthy controls, which is a major limitation to confirm the findings.

Research Model 5

Another EEG based study is presented by Acharya et al. (2018). They have used DL architecture CNN with 13 layers and backpropagation followed by semi-manual feature selection for the classification of depression versus healthy people (Acharya et al., 2018). They have used a small EEG dataset of 15 depressed patients and 15 healthy controls with the batch size of training samples as 5 for backpropagation algorithm. Figure 8 depicts the high-level architecture for a clinical setting in practice with the proposed model hosted in the cloud. The results of this model have shown a higher accuracy level of 93% and have identified the brain region characteristics in depressed and healthy people. However, the use of the small dataset without a proper gender, the age distribution is a limitation in this work to generalize the results.

Figure 8. 13-layered CNN model into the clinical setting (Acharya et al., 2018)

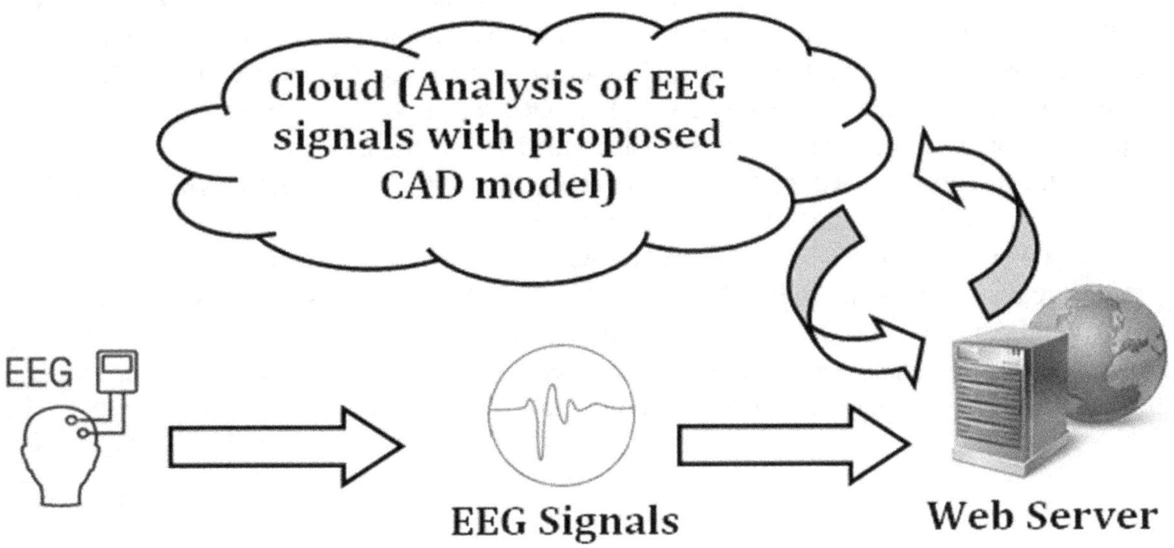

Table 3. Validation methods

Validation Method	Description	Related Work
K-fold cross-validation	Splitting in a way k-1 data is used as a training set while remaining is test set.	(Tenev et al., 2014)(Heinsfeld et al., 2018)(Chen et al., 2016)(Li, Sharma, Meng, Purushwalkam, & Gowen, 2017)(Tamboer et al., 2016)(Płoński et al., 2017) (Khedher et al., 2017)(de vos et al., 2018)
Loocv	All data except one record is used for training set while excluded one as testing data and repeated for n time if have n data items in total.	(Heinsfeld et al., 2018)(Chen et al., 2016)(Li et al., 2017)(Sacchet, Prasad, Foland-ross, Thompson, & Gotlib, 2015)(Rosa et al., 2015)(Płoński et al., 2017)
Bootstrapping	Randomly selected training set with replacement such that the k in k-fold method differs from the fold to fold.	(Galgani, Sun, Lanzi, & Leigh, 2009)
Random sampling	The test set is randomly selected, while remaining as training data.	(Bi, Wang, Shu, Sun, & Xu, 2018)

Further, feature selection is a key activity for the success of a classification model since there can be less significant and even redundant features. Hence, the identification of the most important and effective features from dermoscopic images is one of the domains addressed in the literature (Toennies, 2017a). They have explored the usage of colour and shape features for better classification accuracy involving three different image databases for experiments. Moreover, they have shown the inapplicability of ABCD rule as a rule of thumb and the use of furrows and ridges as features for some skin lesion classifications.

Evaluation Techniques

In the health care domain, it is important to ensure the trustworthiness of any novel solution. Hence, it is a must for computerized health care solutions to conduct evaluations on the proposed systems. Therefore, all the ML and DL related classification solutions that have addressed psychophysiological chronic disorders also provide their solutions with a given evaluation methodology and corresponding results. The accuracy measures such as precision, recall, F1, ROC, and performance metrics such as sensitivity and specificity are mainly in usage for classification model evaluations.

Among the discussed related works, (Acharya et al., 2018), (Liu et al., 2015), (Kuang et al., 2014), (Heinsfeld et al., 2018), (Sarraf & Tofighi, 2016) have used accuracy, sensitivity and specificity for results validation. Table 3 lists the validation techniques widely applied in the recent related work regarding ML and DL classifications on EEG/ MRI/ fMRI data. Most of the work has applied k-fold cross validation as 10-fold, 5-fold and LOOCV together while other techniques are slightly used. These techniques are based on the error rate data of the model. However, other techniques such as holdout validation, precision-recall method, bagging that can be applied based on context and dataset type.

Table 4. Psychophysiological chronic disease related work analysis

Related Work	Disease					Classification Technique					
	ADHD	**ASD**	**AD**	**Depression**	**Dyslexia**	**SVM**	**RF**	**NB**	**LR**	**CNN**	**DBN**
(Acharya et al., 2018)				√						√	
(Bi et al., 2018)		√				√					
(Chen et al., 2016)		√				√					
(De vos et al., 2018)			√						√		
(Ariyarathne et al., 2020)	√									√	
(Duda, Ma, Haber, & Wall, 2016)	√	√				√	√		√		
(Ghiassian, Greiner, Jin, & Brown, 2013)	√	√				√					
(Haputhanthri et al., 2019)		√					√		√		
(Kuang et al., 2014)	√										√
(Khedher et al., 2017)			√			√					
(Li et al., 2017)		√				√		√			
(Płoński et al., 2017)					√	√	√		√		
(Rosa et al., 2015)				√		√					
(Rubasinghe et al., 2019)	√									√	
(Sacchet et al., 2015)				√		√					
(Sarraf & tofighi, 2016)			√							√	
(Sen et al., 2018)	√	√				√					
(Spasov et al., 2018)			√							√	
(Tamboer et al., 2016)					√	√					
(Tenev et al., 2014)	√					√					

DISCUSSION

Limitations in Current Practices

Some of the related studies have applied more than one ML and/or DL techniques as summarized in Table 4. Most of the psychophysiological disease classifications have applied the ML SVM classifier in linear and non-linear kernels with high accuracy and performance results, but for smaller data sets.

In addition, some have applied SVM along with RF, NB and LR by showing SVM performs better than them. However, DL architectures; DBN, CNN and autoencoders that have been applied in the recent related works have shown improved accuracy with advanced hardware and processing power requirements. Another commonality in these studies is having a limited focus on one or two diseases (Brihadiswaran et al., 2019) (de Silva et al., 2019a).

Furthermore, Table 5 summarises some bio images pre-processing and analysis tools available in the literature and state-of-the-art tools that are used on EEG/ fMRI/ MRI data. Besides, all these tools are powerful with many features than listed in Table 5. Apart from these, most of the classification, clustering supportive tools such as MATLAB, WEKA, TensorFlow etc. provide their inbuilt functions for pre-processing and analysis tasks.

Table 5. Neuroimaging pre-processing and analysis tools

Tool	Segmentation	Smoothing	Registration	Time-Frequency Decomposition	Filtering
Afni (analysis of functional neuroimaging) (Keehn, Nair, Lincoln, Townsend, & Müller, 2016)	√	√	√	√	√
Ants (advanced normalization tools) (Spasov et al., 2018)	√		√	√	√
ADHD-care (de Silva et al., 2019b) (Ariyarathne et al., 2020)		√	√		
ASDGenus (channel optimised classification) (Haputhanthri et al., 2019)		√		√	√
Eeglab (Matlab toolbox)(Billeci et al., 2017)				√	
Fmriprep ("fmriprep", 2019)	√	√	√	√	√
Freesurfer (Płoński et al., 2017)	√	√	√	√	√
Knime (Konstanz Information Miner)	√	√		√	√
Loni ("usc", 2019)	√		√		
SPM (Salford Predictive Modeler) (Sato et al., 2015)(Rosa et al., 2015) (Khedher et al., 2017) (Liu et al., 2015)	√	√	√		

FUTURE RESEARCH DIRECTIONS

In recent related studies, it is noticeable that mostly they have been focused only on one disorder at a time (de Silva et al., 2019a). Although the use of ML and DL approaches has mainly contributed to improving the accuracy levels, some of the studies have been conducted only on smaller datasets (Haputhanthri et al., 2019). Thus, their applicability in practice is limited. Therefore, there is a requirement for a generic framework that combines disorder-specific computational solutions, towards the diagnosis of many psychophysiological chronic diseases.

A review study (Toennies, 2017a) suggests the evolution of features, computational models to detect the existence patterns, novel feature selection and evaluation techniques for classifiers would create a positive impact. Thus, it is important to improve the neuroimaging feature selection techniques and characterize the heterogeneity aspects of different neurological disorders to obtain accurate classification results. Another review Brihadiswaran et al., 2019), has shown the requierment of a generic DSS to handle different data types using optimized techniques, that is applicable in practice. In order to support the biomarker for the treatments, there is a need for a generic approach to acquire, process and analyse similar data types.

Lack of performance and efficiency are challenges in neuroimaging processing and classification. Thus, improving neurological disorder identification approaches to satisfy the higher accuracy, sensitivity, specificity and reliability is another possible research direction. Further, case studies can be conducted by addressing both behavioural analysis and computational models together. This will be useful for a comparative analysis for the utilization of techniques to determine a given neurological disorder.

CONCLUSION

Neurological chronic disorders that are concerned with both mental and physical processes have gained attention in medical science, since they affect a person's daily lifestyle. Different types of behavioural analysis and psychophysiological measures are used to support the diagnosis process. There are common symptoms among many of the psychophysiological disorders and the neuroimaging metrics such as EEG, MRI, fMRI are commonly used in the diagnosis process. On the other hand, different learning models have rigorously applied in every domain with significant accuracy and performance values by reducing human effort. This chapter has addressed different approaches to the identification of psychophysiological chronic diseases. The existing recent literature is explored and analyzed in this chapter, considering their context, the methodology followed, techniques and tools used. The major commonalities in them are being limited to address one or two diseases, using a smaller dataset without proper gender, age distributions, and lesser application of learning techniques. Thus, learning models with the use of artificial intelligence is still open for the application in this context of psychophysiological chronic disease identification process, as the few studies that used deep learning methods have shown high accuracy levels compared to machine learning methods. Finally, this chapter has identified the existing limitations, challenges and suggested future possible research directions.

ACKNOWLEDGMENT

The author acknowledges the support received from the Senate Research Committee Grant SRC/LT/2019/18, University of Moratuwa, Sri Lanka for this research study.

REFERENCES

Abreu, R., Leal, A., & Figueiredo, P. (2018). EEG-Informed fMRI: A Review of Data Analysis Methods. *Frontiers in Human Neuroscience*, *12*, 29. doi:10.3389/fnhum.2018.00029 PMID:29467634

Acharya, U. R., Oh, S. L., Hagiwara, Y., Tan, J. H., Adeli, H., & Subha, D. P. (2018). Automated EEG-based screening of depression using deep convolutional neural network. *Computer Methods and Programs in Biomedicine*, *161*, 103–113. doi:10.1016/j.cmpb.2018.04.012 PMID:29852953

Ahmadvand, A., & Daliri, M. R. (2014). Brain MR Image Segmentation Methods and Applications. *OMICS Journal of Radiology*, *02*(04), 1–3. doi:10.4172/2167-7964.1000e130

Alzheimer's Association. (2018). Retrieved December 4, 2018, from https://www.alz.org/alzheimers-dementia/what-is-alzheimers

Ariyarathne, G., de Silva, S., Dayarathna, S., Meedeniya, D., & Jayarathna, S (2020). ADHD Identification using CNN with Seed-based Correlation Approach for fMRI Data. In *9th International Conference on Software and Computer Applications (ICSCA 2020)*. ACM. (pp. 31-35)

Aslanides, J., Leike, J., & Hutter, M. (2017). *Universal Reinforcement Learning Algorithms: Survey and Experiments*. Academic Press.

Bailey, T. (2014). Diagnosing and Treating Developmental Disorders with qEEG and Neurotherapy. In *Clinical Neurotherapy* (pp. 321–355). Elsevier. doi:10.1016/B978-0-12-396988-0.00013-1

Ball, G., Malpas, C. B., Genc, S., Efron, D., Sciberras, E., Anderson, V., ... Silk, T. J. (2019). Multimodal Structural Neuroimaging Markers of Brain Development and ADHD Symptoms. *The American Journal of Psychiatry*, *176*(1), 57–66. doi:10.1176/appi.ajp.2018.18010034 PMID:30220220

Bi, X., Wang, Y., Shu, Q., Sun, Q., & Xu, Q. (2018). Classification of Autism Spectrum Disorder Using Random Support Vector Machine Cluster. *Frontiers in Genetics*, *9*, 18. doi:10.3389/fgene.2018.00018 PMID:29467790

Billeci, L., Narzisi, A., Tonacci, A., Sbriscia-Fioretti, B., Serasini, L., Fulceri, F., ... Muratori, F. (2017). An integrated EEG and eye-tracking approach for the study of responding and initiating joint attention in Autism Spectrum Disorders. *Scientific Reports*, *7*(1), 13560. doi:10.103841598-017-13053-4 PMID:29051506

Bowman, F. D. (2014). Brain Imaging Analysis. *Annual Review of Statistics and Its Application*, *1*(1), 61–85. doi:10.1146/annurev-statistics-022513-115611 PMID:25309940

Brett, M., Christoff, K., Cusack, R., & Lancaster, J. (2001). Using the talairach atlas with the MNI template. *NeuroImage*, *13*(6), 85. doi:10.1016/S1053-8119(01)91428-4

Brihadiswaran, G., Haputhanthri, D., Gunathilaka, S., Meedeniya, D., & Jayarathna, S. (2019). A Review of EEG-based Classification for Autism Spectrum Disorder. *Journal of Computational Science*, *15*(8), 1161–1183. doi:10.3844/jcssp.2019.1161.1183

Bron, T. I., Bijlenga, D., Kooij, J. J., Vogel, S. W. N., Wynchank, D., Beekman, A. T. F., & Penninx, B. W. J. H. (2016). Attention-deficit hyperactivity disorder symptoms add risk to circadian rhythm sleep problems in depression and anxiety. *Journal of Affective Disorders*, *200*, 74–81. doi:10.1016/j.jad.2016.04.022 PMID:27128360

Bussing, R., Fernandez, M., Harwood, M., Wei Hou, W., Garvan, C. W., Eyberg, S. M., & Swanson, J. M. (2008). Parent and teacher SNAP-IV ratings of attention deficit hyperactivity disorder symptoms: Psychometric properties and normative ratings from a school district sample. *Assessment*, *15*(3), 317–328. doi:10.1177/1073191107313888 PMID:18310593

Caballero-Gaudes, C., & Reynolds, R. C. (2017). Methods for cleaning the BOLD fMRI signal. *NeuroImage, 154*, 128–149. doi:10.1016/j.neuroimage.2016.12.018 PMID:27956209

Case, M., Zhang, H., Mundahl, J., Datta, Y., Nelson, S., Gupta, K., & He, B. (2017). Characterization of functional brain activity and connectivity using EEG and fMRI in patients with sickle cell disease. *NeuroImage. Clinical, 14*, 1–17. doi:10.1016/j.nicl.2016.12.024 PMID:28116239

CDC. (2018). *Centers for Disease Control and Prevention, Data and Statistics About ADHD.* Retrieved March 4, 2019, from https://www.cdc.gov/ncbddd/adhd/data.html

Chen, H., Duan, X., Liu, F., Lu, F., Ma, X., Zhang, Y., ... Chen, H. (2016). Multivariate classification of autism spectrum disorder using frequency-specific resting-state functional connectivity—A multicenter study. *Progress in Neuro-Psychopharmacology & Biological Psychiatry, 64*, 1–9. doi:10.1016/j.pnpbp.2015.06.014 PMID:26148789

Chollet, F. (2015). *Keras.* Retrieved January 3, 2019, from https://keras.io/

Coloigner, J., Kim, Y., Bush, A., Choi, S., Balderrama, M. C., Coates, T. D., ... Wood, J. C. (2017). Contrasting resting-state fMRI abnormalities from sickle and non-sickle anemia. *PLoS One, 12*(10), e0184860. doi:10.1371/journal.pone.0184860 PMID:28981541

de Silva, S., Dayarathna, S., Ariyarathne, G., Meedeniya, D., & Jayarathna, S. (2019a). A Survey of Attention Deficit Hyperactivity Disorder Identification Using Psychophysiological Data. *International Journal of Online and Biomedical Engineering, 15*(13), 61–76. doi:10.3991/ijoe.v15i13.10744

de Silva, S., Dayarathna, S., Ariyarathne, G., Meedeniya, D., Jayarathna, S., Michalek, A. M. P., & Jayawardena, G. (2019b). A Rule-Based System for ADHD Identification using Eye Movement Data. In *Moratuwa Engineering Research Conference (MERCon)*, (pp. 538-543), IEEE. 10.1109/MERCon.2019.8818865

de Vos, F., Koini, M., Schouten, T. M., Seiler, S., van der Grond, J., Lechner, A., ... Rombouts, S. A. R. B. (2018). A comprehensive analysis of resting state fMRI measures to classify individual patients with Alzheimer's disease. *NeuroImage, 167*, 62–72. doi:10.1016/j.neuroimage.2017.11.025 PMID:29155080

Deng, L. (2014). Deep Learning: Methods and Applications. *Foundations and Trends® in Signal Processing, 7*(3–4), 197–387. doi:10.1561/2000000039

Duda, M., Ma, R., Haber, N., & Wall, D. P. (2016). Use of machine learning for behavioral distinction of autism and ADHD. *Translational Psychiatry, 6*(2), 732. doi:10.1038/tp.2015.221 PMID:26859815

Fan, H., Li, L., Gilbert, R., O'Callaghan, F., & Wijlaars, L. (2018). A machine learning approach to identify cases of cerebral palsy using the UK primary care database. *Lancet, 392*, S33. doi:10.1016/S0140-6736(18)32077-4

Galgani, F., Sun, Y., Lanzi, P. L., & Leigh, J. (2009). Automatic analysis of eye tracking data for medical diagnosis. In *2009 IEEE Symposium on Computational Intelligence and Data Mining* (pp. 195–202). IEEE. 10.1109/CIDM.2009.4938649

Gemmell, H. G., & Staff, R. T. (2005). Single Photon Emission Computed Tomography (SPECT). In Practical Nuclear Medicine (pp. 21–33). London: Springer. doi:10.1007/1-84628-018-4_2

Ghiassian, S., Greiner, R., Jin, P., & Brown, M. R. G. (2013). *Learning to Classify Psychiatric Disorders based on fMR Images: Autism vs Healthy and ADHD vs Healthy*. Academic Press.

Haputhanthri, D., Brihadiswaran, G., Gunathilaka, S., Meedeniya, D., Jayarathna, S., Jaime, M., & Jayawardena, Y. (2019). An EEG based Channel Optimized Classification Approach for Autism Spectrum Disorder. In *Moratuwa Engineering Research Conference (MerCon),* (pp. 123-128). IEEE. 10.1109/MERCon.2019.8818814

Heinsfeld, A. S., Franco, A. R., Craddock, R. C., Buchweitz, A., & Meneguzzi, F. (2018). Identification of autism spectrum disorder using deep learning and the ABIDE dataset. *NeuroImage. Clinical, 17*, 16–23. doi:10.1016/j.nicl.2017.08.017 PMID:29034163

Henry, J., von Hippel, W., Molenberghs, P., Lee, T., & Sachdev, P. S. (2016). Clinical assessment of social cognitive function in neurological disorders. *Nature Reviews. Neurology, 12*(1), 28–39. doi:10.1038/nrneurol.2015.229 PMID:26670297

Jack, C. R. Jr, Lowe, V. J., Senjem, M. L., Weigand, S. D., Kemp, B. J., Shiung, M. M., ... Petersen, R. C. (2008). 11C PiB and structural MRI provide complementary information in imaging of Alzheimer's disease and amnestic mild cognitive impairment. *Brain, 131*(3), 665–680. doi:10.1093/brain/awm336 PMID:18263627

Jang, H., Plis, S. M., Calhoun, V. D., & Lee, J. H. (2017). Task-specific feature extraction and classification of fMRI volumes using a deep neural network initialized with a deep belief network: Evaluation using sensorimotor tasks. *NeuroImage, 145*, 314–328. doi:10.1016/j.neuroimage.2016.04.003 PMID:27079534

Jin, Y., Wee, C. Y., Shi, F., Thung, K. H., Ni, D., Yap, P. T., & Shen, D. (2015). Identification of infants at high-risk for autism spectrum disorder using multiparameter multiscale white matter connectivity networks. *Human Brain Mapping, 36*(12), 4880–4896. doi:10.1002/hbm.22957 PMID:26368659

Keehn, B., Nair, A., Lincoln, A. J., Townsend, J., & Müller, R. A. (2016). Under-reactive but easily distracted: An fMRI investigation of attentional capture in autism spectrum disorder. *Developmental Cognitive Neuroscience, 17*, 46–56. doi:10.1016/j.dcn.2015.12.002 PMID:26708773

Khedher, L., Illán, I. A., Górriz, J. M., Ramírez, J., Brahim, A., & Meyer-Baese, A. (2017). Independent Component Analysis-Support Vector Machine-Based Computer-Aided Diagnosis System for Alzheimer's with Visual Support. *International Journal of Neural Systems, 27*(03), 1650050. doi:10.1142/S0129065716500507 PMID:27776438

KletteR. (2014). *Image Processing*. doi:10.1007/978-1-4471-6320-6_2

Kraemer, H. C., Measelle, J. R., Ablow, J. C., Essex, M. J., Boyce, W. T., & Kupfer, D. J. (2003). A New Approach to Integrating Data From Multiple Informants in Psychiatric Assessment and Research: Mixing and Matching Contexts and Perspectives. *The American Journal of Psychiatry, 160*(9), 1566–1577. doi:10.1176/appi.ajp.160.9.1566 PMID:12944328

Kuang, D., Guo, X., An, X., Zhao, Y., & He, L. (2014). *Discrimination of ADHD Based on fMRI Data with Deep Belief Network*. Cham: Springer. doi:10.1007/978-3-319-09330-7_27

Larobina, M., & Murino, L. (2014). Medical image file formats. *Journal of Digital Imaging*, *27*(2), 200–206. doi:10.100710278-013-9657-9 PMID:24338090

Li, B., Sharma, A., Meng, J., Purushwalkam, S., & Gowen, E. (2017). Applying machine learning to identify autistic adults using imitation: An exploratory study. *PLoS One*, *12*(8), e0182652. doi:10.1371/journal.pone.0182652 PMID:28813454

Liaw, A., & Wiener, M. (2002). Classification and regression by randomForest. *R News*, *2*, 18–22.

Liu, F., Guo, W., Fouche, J.-P., Wang, Y., Wang, W., Ding, J., ... Chen, H. (2015). Multivariate classification of social anxiety disorder using whole brain functional connectivity. *Brain Structure & Function*, *220*(1), 101–115. doi:10.100700429-013-0641-4 PMID:24072164

Mannfolk, P., Wirestam, R., Nilsson, M., Ståhlberg, F., & Olsrud, J. (2010). Dimensionality reduction of fMRI time series data using locally linear embedding. *Magma (New York, N.Y.)*, *23*(5–6), 327–338. doi:10.100710334-010-0204-0 PMID:20229085

Marcano, J. L., Bell, M. A., & Beex, A. A. (2018). Classification of ADHD and non-ADHD subjects using a universal background model. *Biomedical Signal Processing and Control*, *39*, 204–212. doi:10.1016/j.bspc.2017.07.023 PMID:31186670

NIMH Depression. (2018). Retrieved December 4, 2018, from https://www.nimh.nih.gov/health/topics/depression/index.shtml

Nybo, K. (2015). *Dimensionality reduction methods for fMRI analysis and visualization* (Thesis). Aslto University.

Oliver, D. J., Borasio, G. D., Caraceni, A., de Visser, M., Grisold, W., Lorenzl, S., ... Voltz, R. (2016). A consensus review on the development of palliative care for patients with chronic and progressive neurological disease. *European Journal of Neurology*, *23*(1), 30–38. doi:10.1111/ene.12889 PMID:26423203

Pang, R., Lansdell, B. J., & Fairhall, A. L. (2016). Dimensionality reduction in neuroscience. *Current Biology*, *26*(14), R656–R660. doi:10.1016/j.cub.2016.05.029 PMID:27458907

Paszke, A., Chanan, G., Lin, Z., Gross, S., Yang, E., Antiga, L., & Devito, Z. (2017). Automatic differentiation in PyTorch. *31st Conference on Neural Information Processing Systems*, 1–4. 10.1017/CBO9781107707221.009

Płoński, P., Gradkowski, W., Altarelli, I., Monzalvo, K., van Ermingen-Marbach, M., Grande, M., ... Jednoróg, K. (2017). Multi-parameter machine learning approach to the neuroanatomical basis of developmental dyslexia. *Human Brain Mapping*, *38*(2), 900–908. doi:10.1002/hbm.23426 PMID:27712002

Rohanachandra, Y. M., Dahanayake, D. M. A., Rohanachandra, L. T., & Wijetunge, G. S. (2017). Knowledge about diagnostic features and comorbidities of childhood autism among doctors in a tertiary care hospital. *Sri Lanka Journal of Child Health*, *46*(1), 29. doi:10.4038ljch.v46i1.8093

Rosa, M. J., Portugal, L., Hahn, T., Fallgatter, A. J., Garrido, M. I., Shawe-Taylor, J., & Mourao-Miranda, J. (2015). Sparse network-based models for patient classification using fMRI. *NeuroImage*, *105*, 493–506. doi:10.1016/j.neuroimage.2014.11.021 PMID:25463459

Rubasinghe, I. D., & Meedeniya, D. A. (2020). Automated Neuroscience Decision Support Framework. In Deep Learning Techniques for Biomedical and Health Informatics. Academic Press. doi:10.1016/B978-0-12-819061-6.00013-6

Sacchet, M. D., Prasad, G., Foland-Ross, L. C., Thompson, P. M., & Gotlib, I. H. (2015). Support Vector Machine Classification of Major Depressive Disorder Using Diffusion-Weighted Neuroimaging and Graph Theory. *Frontiers in Psychiatry*, *6*, 21. doi:10.3389/fpsyt.2015.00021 PMID:25762941

Salvatore, C., Cerasa, A., Castiglioni, I., Gallivanone, F., Augimeri, A., Lopez, M., ... Quattrone, A. (2014). Machine learning on brain MRI data for differential diagnosis of Parkinson's disease and Progressive Supranuclear Palsy. *Journal of Neuroscience Methods*, *222*, 230–237. doi:10.1016/j.jneumeth.2013.11.016 PMID:24286700

Sarraf, S., & Tofighi, G. (2016). *Classification of Alzheimer's Disease using fMRI Data and Deep Learning Convolutional Neural Networks*. arXiv:1603.0863

Sato, J. R., Moll, J., Green, S., Deakin, J. F. W., Thomaz, C. E., & Zahn, R. (2015). Machine learning algorithm accurately detects fMRI signature of vulnerability to major depression. *Psychiatry Research: Neuroimaging*, *233*(2), 289–291. doi:10.1016/j.pscychresns.2015.07.001 PMID:26187550

Sen, B., Borle, N. C., Greiner, R., & Brown, M. R. G. (2018). A general prediction model for the detection of ADHD and Autism using structural and functional MRI. *PLoS One*, *13*(4), e0194856. doi:10.1371/journal.pone.0194856 PMID:29664902

Siuly, S., & Zhang, Y. (2016). Medical Big Data: Neurological Diseases Diagnosis Through Medical Data Analysis. *Data Science and Engineering.*, *1*(2), 54–64. doi:10.100741019-016-0011-3

Skotko, B. G., Macklin, E. A., Muselli, M., Voelz, L., McDonough, M. E., Davidson, E., ... Rosen, D. (2017). A predictive model for obstructive sleep apnea and Down syndrome. *American Journal of Medical Genetics. Part A*, *173*(4), 889–896. doi:10.1002/ajmg.a.38137 PMID:28124477

Spasov, S. E., Passamonti, L., Duggento, A., Lio, P., & Toschi, N. (2018). A Multi-modal Convolutional Neural Network Framework for the Prediction of Alzheimer's Disease. In *2018 40th Annual International Conference of the IEEE Engineering in Medicine and Biology Society (EMBC)* (pp. 1271–1274). IEEE. 10.1109/EMBC.2018.8512468

Tamboer, P., Vorst, H. C. M., Ghebreab, S., & Scholte, H. S. (2016). Machine learning and dyslexia: Classification of individual structural neuro-imaging scans of students with and without dyslexia. *NeuroImage. Clinical*, *11*, 508–514. doi:10.1016/j.nicl.2016.03.014 PMID:27114899

Tenev, A., Markovska-Simoska, S., Kocarev, L., Pop-Jordanov, J., Müller, A., & Candrian, G. (2014). Machine learning approach for classification of ADHD adults. *International Journal of Psychophysiology*, *93*(1), 162–166. doi:10.1016/j.ijpsycho.2013.01.008 PMID:23361114

Toennies, K. D. (2017a). *Guide to Medical Image Analysis*. London: Springer London; doi:10.1007/978-1-4471-7320-5

Toennies, K. D. (2017b). *Registration and Normalization*. doi:10.1007/978-1-4471-7320-5_10

Tran, D., Hoffman, M. D., Saurous, R. A., Brevdo, E., Murphy, K., & Blei, D. M. (2017). Deep Probabilistic Programming. *International Conference on Learning Representations.*

Urigüen, J. A., & Garcia-Zapirain, B. (2015). EEG artefact removal-state-of-the-art and guidelines. *Journal of Neural Engineering*, *12*(3), 031001. doi:10.1088/1741-2560/12/3/031001 PMID:25834104

WHO. (2016). *World Health Organization Report, Neurological Disorders: Public Health Challenges.* https://www.who.int/mental_health/neurology/neurological_disorders_report_web.pdf

Wilhelm, F. H., Schneider, S., & Friedman, B. H. (2006). Psychophysiological Assessment. Clinician's Handbook of Child Behavioral Assessment, 201–231. doi:10.1016/B978-012343014-4/50010-1

Wolfers, T., Arenas, A. L., Onnink, A. M. H., Dammers, J., Hoogman, M., Zwiers, M. P., ... Beckmann, C. F. (2017). Refinement by integration: Aggregated effects of multimodal imaging markers on adult ADHD. *Journal of Psychiatry & Neuroscience*, *42*(6), 386–394. doi:10.1503/jpn.160240 PMID:28832320

Yau, W. Y. W., Tudorascu, D. L., McDade, E. M., Ikonomovic, S., James, J. A., Minhas, D., ... Klunk, W. E. (2015). Longitudinal assessment of neuroimaging and clinical markers in autosomal dominant Alzheimer's disease: A prospective cohort study. *Lancet Neurology*, *14*(8), 804–813. doi:10.1016/S1474-4422(15)00135-0 PMID:26139022

ADDITIONAL READING

Hesamian, M. H., Jia, W., He, X., & Kennedy, P. (2019). Deep Learning Techniques for Medical Image Segmentation: Achievements and Challenges. *Journal of Digital Imaging*, *32*(4), 1–15. doi:10.100710278-019-00227-x PMID:31144149

Iqbal, T., & Ali, H. (2018). Generative Adversarial Network for Medical Images (MI-GAN). *Journal of Medical Systems*, *42*(11), 231. doi:10.100710916-018-1072-9 PMID:30315368

Laukamp, K. R., Thiele, F., Shakirin, G., Zopfs, D., Faymonville, A., Timmer, M., ... Borggrefe, J. (2019). Fully automated detection and segmentation of meningiomas using deep learning on routine multiparametric MRI. *European Radiology*, *29*(1), 124–132. doi:10.100700330-018-5595-8 PMID:29943184

Lee, J.-G., Jun, S., Cho, Y.-W., Lee, H., Kim, G. B., Seo, J. B., & Kim, N. (2017). Deep Learning in Medical Imaging: General Overview. *Korean Journal of Radiology*, *18*(4), 570–584. doi:10.3348/kjr.2017.18.4.570 PMID:28670152

Maier, A., Syben, C., Lasser, T., & Riess, C. (2019). A gentle introduction to deep learning in medical image processing. *Zeitschrift fur Medizinische Physik*, *29*(2), 86–101. doi:10.1016/j.zemedi.2018.12.003 PMID:30686613

Shen, D., Wu, G., & Suk, H.-I. (2017). Deep Learning in Medical Image Analysis. *Annual Review of Biomedical Engineering*, *19*(1), 221–248. doi:10.1146/annurev-bioeng-071516-044442 PMID:28301734

Wang, G., Li, W., Zuluaga, M. A., Pratt, R., Patel, P. A., Aertsen, M., ... Vercauteren, T. (2018). Interactive Medical Image Segmentation Using Deep Learning With Image-Specific Fine Tuning. *IEEE Transactions on Medical Imaging*, *37*(7), 1562–1573. doi:10.1109/TMI.2018.2791721 PMID:29969407

Zhou, Z., Wang, Y., Guo, Y., Qi, Y., & Yu, J. (2019). Image Quality Improvement of Hand-held Ultrasound Devices with a Two-stage Generative Adversarial Network. *IEEE Transactions on Biomedical Engineering*, 1–1. doi:10.1109/TBME.2019.2912986 PMID:31021759

KEY TERMS AND DEFINITIONS

Convolutional Network: A type of deep neural networks in deep learning that consists of several convolutional layers.

Generative Adversarial Network: A category of deep learning neural networks that are composed of two competitive neural networks together.

Optimization: The process of finding the best and optimal solution in machine learning algorithms.

Probabilistic Programming: The paradigm of programming probabilistic models to inference automatically using specially developed programming languages.

Psychophysiological: A subcategory of physiology in terms of both mental and physical health together.

Segmentation: The process of partitioning an image into segments based on certain criteria to simplify an image in a useful manner to ease the further required analysis.

Stochastic Gradient Descent: An iterative optimization method with random sample selection to obtain gradients.

Validation: Validating a machine learning model to evaluate a trained model using a test data set once a model is trained using a training data set.

Chapter 17
Big Data-Based System:
A Supportive Tool in Autism Spectrum Disorder Analysis

Tanu Wadhera
https://orcid.org/0000-0002-7646-2303
Dr. B. R. Ambedkar National Institute of Technology, Jalandhar, India

Deepti Kakkar
https://orcid.org/0000-0002-9681-1291
Dr. B. R. Ambedkar National Institute of Technology, Jalandhar, India

ABSTRACT

In the health domain, the move of generating big data is opening new methodologies in detection as well as prediction of various diseases and disorders. The first phase of the present chapter has provided insights into the role of big data analytics in the detection of one such neuro-disorder, that is, autism spectrum disorder (ASD). The data lake concept has provided a direction to resolve the issue by providing a common platform for storing tremendous amount of data in all formats (structured, unstructured, or raw). However, if the entire data have potential value, the data lakes need to be strategically designed as otherwise it can lead to data swamps. Therefore, in the second phase, data lake based on Hadoop architecture and Apache Spark engine has been provided for the analysis of the health data. The proposed system has resolved the data storage issue, management, and analytics on a single platform. Hence, the novelty of the chapter is that it is pointing towards the faster exploration as well as management of data so that the timely generation of hypothesis can help in analyzing ASD.

INTRODUCTION

Big data is the information hub with data collection from different sources and allows working on huge samples of the data that can determine the results even due to minute variations in the factors. This hub provides various options for pooling and exploring the different aspects of data in order to manage as well as predict the therapeutic outcomes. Hence, the data have unprecedented generation volume, veloc-

DOI: 10.4018/978-1-7998-3069-6.ch017

ity, and variety (Sarkar, 2017). The term 'volume' indicates the huge amount of data originating from sensors, recording machines, internet and healthcare data. 'Velocity' refers to generation, retrieval and speed of the data and 'variety' refers to the different types and formats of data that are generated such as structured, unstructured or real-time data and used for various purposes, such as big data analytics. The term veracity was added to big data for the healthcare domain referring to the trustworthiness, quality, accuracy and precision of the data (Feldman, Martin & Skotnes, 2012). The storage, processing, analysis and retrieval of such type of data need a more sophisticated environment and infrastructure and big data technology is providing an efficient platform for these data sets. The big data analytics approach takes the information collection concept to a completely different and new level and is being effectively used in a number of sectors such as information technology, customer care services, and risk management in fields such as business, astronomy and forecasting and in the healthcare sector (Andreu-Perez et al., 2015). In healthcare system, the patient data is heterogeneous, involves incomplete and imprecise observations derived from various sources such as diagnosis, treatment, injury, and mental impairments. It can be structured data such as signals, phenotypes, omics, International Classification of Diseases (ICD) codes and unstructured data such as clinical prescriptions, imaging, electronic health records and environmental factors (Cyganek et al., 2016, Dinov, 2016, Tanu &Kakkar, 2018a, Wang, Kung, & Byrd, 2018). In 2020, the worldwide digital healthcare data is expected to cross 25000 petabytes from 500 petabytes (2012 record) (Sun, J., & Reddy, 2013). In case of neurological disorders, especially ASD, the heterogeneity of the disorder demands that the data needs to be big not only in volume (sample size) but also in availability (open access) and depth (multiple amounts of data from the same individual). This database can be utilized in identification, prognosis, and diagnosis as well as in the treatment of the disorder. One of the studies provided an oracle-based computational model deploying big data for treating the ASD (Mani, Berkovich, & Liao, 2014). This model inserts new information into the brain of autistic individuals to understand the information-processing in their brain and improve their behavior.

Autism Spectrum Disorder (ASD) is a developmental disorder majorly targeting social communication and interaction domain and leading to restricted & repetitive behavior in individuals. In the world, almost 1-2% of the population suffers from ASD (Lombardo, Lai & Baron-Cohen, 2018). The seriousness of the disorder sounds from the percentage affecting the children worldwide. It is no more a western disease, as in India the number of ASD affected individuals is roughly 23 after 10,000 (Tanu and Kakkar, 2018b). The diagnostic age for the disorder is 2.5–3 years and at that time the disorder gets fully developed, leaving very minimum possibility of retracing the symptoms. These figures indicate that the experts/clinicians need to be vigilant in detecting and monitoring ASD suspected or affected individuals in order to reduce the diagnostic age. But, it is not possible, for the clinicians, to consider the entire amount of data, especially unstructured, to diagnose the individual properly at the proper time. There is a need to develop new strategies or systems that can diagnose the disorder and monitor health care effectively and cheaply (Weil, 2014). Moreover, to analyze the structured data such as brain signals or images, Machine Learning (ML) algorithms also demand a huge variety of data for training and testing. As if the training will be done on large datasets, only then the disorder can be tested efficiently. Since the disorder symptoms and deficits prevail unevenly, big data can make it possible to identify assistive personalized diagnostic and treatment methodologies (Raghupathi and Raghupathi, 2014). For big data based healthcare applications, the integration and exchange of the various heterogeneous datasets is an important requirement.

Challenges in Existing Methodologies

In identifying, treating and monitoring ASD and other neurological disorders a lot more statistical such as screening scales, signaling and imaging techniques such as Electroencephalogram (EEG), Magnetic Resonance Imaging (MRI) or functional Magnetic Resonance Imaging (fMRI) and the technology based methods viz. eye trackers or motion detection sensors are utilized (Fukuyama et al., 2017, Tanu and Kakkar, 2018b) are prevailing. These techniques provide different ways for detecting disorder, but even then ASD detection is a challenging process. Some of the challenges that still exist and have become the reason for the delay in diagnosis process are listed below.

1. *Manual Analysis*: The physicians/experts generally make the diagnosis and treatment decisions according to their judgment. It is not only a time-consuming but erroneous process since the disorder is not homogeneous in nature. In order to deal with the heterogeneity, a huge amount of data is required and manual analysis of such vast data is a difficult process.
2. *Lack in Cutting-edge Technology:* Although ML algorithms are entering the diagnostic filed at very high frequency, there are significant challenges in deploying and scaling ML algorithms. These benefits of the algorithms are in proportion to the data- more the data, the better the ML algorithms accuracy. There is a need to collect data from different sources as well as store data durable as one cannot know in advance how much data and when the data is required. The storage space should have a disposable infrastructure as when the data is no more required for training purpose then it can be easily disposed. In addition, the computational and storage data also needs to be decoupled so that the required workloads get run whenever required.
3. *Poor Dataset*: The study of small sample sets for concluding the disorder nature is the major problem in carrying out the ASD diagnosis. Although the triad of core symptoms (impaired social communication, interaction, and restricted and repetitive behavior) defines and detects the disorder, but the co-morbidities and symptom variations among the individuals make it hard to understand the disorder. The accuracy and efficiency of disorder detection need a large dataset which ASD lacks.
4. *Single Approach Based Computer-aided Diagnostic (CAD) Systems:* The CAD systems are providing a helping hand to the experts and assist them in identifying disorders by automatically interpreting the data on the basis of the evidences from past clinical data (Siuly & Zhang, 2016). But, the proposed CAD systems are oriented towards a single methodology only such as analyzing the EEG signals using fast-Fourier transform & power spectral density (Sudirman et al., 2010) or Fisher's linear discriminant (Alhaddad et al., 2012) or k-nearest neighbors (Sheikhani et al., 2008) and various others.
5. *Ongoing Process:* The diagnosis of ASD is an ongoing process because the studies have found the dysfunctionalities in ASD individuals on the basis of only one marker, one abnormality, one gene, and various other singular parameters. Due to this, it is very difficult to improve these findings further as it becomes difficult to replicate the same results. The studies conduct their own experiments every time and conclude them accordingly, making the ASD analysis an unstable process.
6. *Lack in Accumulating Uniform ASD Cohorts*: The different studies have their own defined sample sets and the results reporting any marker or trademark for ASD identification are corresponding to that set. These studies instead of decoding disorder nature further add nonuniformity in disorder

definition. There is a need of standard, large and enrich database that can define the multi-levels of heterogeneity more precisely and uniformly.

These challenges clearly show that ASD analysis is not an easy process and cannot be done using a single domain data. A platform that can provide data from all the domains, if needed, in a single unit can provide the optimum solution. Thus, the chapter has provided a solution by utilizing a big data based approach instead of traditional approaches in making an analytic system. In the first section, the different sources for acquiring the data and knowledge of ASD are provided. In later sections, the analytic system for processing and storing the data, generated by all the listed sources, on a single platform is framed.

Big Data in ASD

The detection methodologies and diagnostic techniques demand 'big', 'deep' and 'open' data for enhancing the identification of the disorder. The vast information from various clinics, healthcare systems, & realtime monitoring units can detect and predict the disorder more precisely and faster as compared to handcrafted databases. The different sources from which the knowledge of ASD can be acquired to contribute to the big amount of data are shown in tabular form in Table 1. Although all the healthcare data are stored as structured data, but the insufficiency of golden standards in collecting ASD data has lead to a number of semi or unstructured data. One of the recent studies has provided a review of all the data required for describing ASD heterogeneity (Tanu & Kakkar, 2018c).

Table 1. Different sources and type of data of ASD subjects

Data Type	Sources	References
Structured Data	Electronic Health Record (EHR), Imaging data such as MRI or fMRI, Bio-signaling data such as EEG or EMG.	Chaddad et al., 2017, Zhao et al., 2016
Semi-structured Data	Home care sensors such as iproc stress sensor, eye tracker, Skin conductance response, social media and internet data	Fukuyama et al., 2017, Northrup, Lantz, & Hamlin, 2016, Sasson & Elison, 2012, Tanu & Kakkar, 2018b
Unstructured Data	Textual notes of experts/clinicians, screening scale output, images of ASD individuals, home-based videos for diagnosis	Clifford, Young & Williamson, 2007, Haglund et al., 2016

The different markers that help in building the structured, unstructured and semi-structured data in ASDare explained as:

1. *Neurological Markers:* The imaging and bio-signaling modalities, their acquisition timings, saving formats, and resolutions generate the data that can cover all the Vs of the big data. The different database sources available are ABIDE (Di Martino et al., 2017), National Database for Autism Research (NDAR; Hall et al., 2012) and various other self-captured datasets helped in finding the different markers such as anatomical abnormalities, hippocampus and amygdala dysfunction,

cerebellum volume deficits, abnormal activation of brain hemispheres, Audio Brainstem Response (ABR) and Visual Evoked Potential (VEP) (Miron et al., 2015, Sayorwan et al., 2018), low heart rate, high electrodermal response (Cotter et al., 2017, Fukuyama et al., 2017, Song, Liu, and Kong, 2016) that can help in detecting ASD. Recently, Apache spark engine has been utilized in finding the group-wise consistent spatial features of brain connectivity map from fMRI data in ASD individuals (Zhao et al., 2016).

2. *Genetic and Environmental Markers:* The variations in the genetic factors can help in detecting approximately 5-40% of ASD population and near about 10% of the affected individuals have been identified through their genetic conditions (Carter & Scherer, 2013). The genetic databases such as Simons Foundation Autism Research Initiative (SFARI; Consortium, 2012) and National Institute for Mental Health (NIMH) helped in examining the nucleotide variations or mutations, copy number variants, chromosomal deletions, protein-coding genome regions, cytogenetic abnormalities, fragile X mutations and other genetic factors leading to ASD (Yuen et al., 2015). Recently, a study found 18 new candidates causing genetic variations that lead to the risk of ASD in the individuals (Yuen et al., 2017). The database is getting enriched and the traditional technologies used in determining the genetic markers includes karyotyping, targeted gene and whole-exome sequencing, chromosomal micro-array and Bioinformatics analysis (Tammimies et al., 2015, Yuen et al., 2015). The interaction between genetics and exposure to environmental toxicants leads to epigenetic markers in ASD (Loke, Hannan, & Craig, 2015). The collection of these markers indicates that ASD is a genetically heterogeneous disorder and demands a cuttingedge technology for better detection.
3. *Inheritable Markers:* The evidences of re-occurrence from the families (12.9-18.7%) and the twins (70-90%) demonstrate that the disorder is inheritable (Yuen et al., 2015, Sealey et al., 2016). The epigenetic differences, caused by variations in the gene expressions, diet and environmental factors, play a crucial role in the transgenerational inheritance of the ASD markers (Eshraghi et al., 2018). It has been reported that in twins if one child is ASD affected then there is a 90% chance that the other will also be suffering from ASD. Also, a recent study investigated that if parents have any neurodevelopmental disorder such as ASD then their child, even though not fully affected by ASD, but tend to have any of its core traits such as restricted interest and repetitive behavior (Evans et al., 2017). There are no proper dataset or any format for keeping the record of this important information and hence, demands a system that can consider the contribution of this unstructured and raw information in ASD.
4. *Behavioral, Developmental and Cognitive Markers:* These markers appropriately distinguish ASD from the normal individuals at an age of 12-18 months and add less heterogeneity to ASD markers (Miles, 2015). These include language impairment and vocal atypicalities, repetitive activities such as hand-flapping, motor-movements, rocking and repetition of some noise, imaginative impairment, no reaction to pain and risk, whirling and various others. The visual & attention disengagement, perception of eye gazes & social cues deficits, empathy impairment, gaze shifting problem, lack of processing things globally, prediction impairment are some of the markers pointing towards the cognitive impairment in ASD (Bedford et al., 2017, Cotter et al., 2017, Sinha et al., 2014). The screening and diagnostic scales, modern technology based tools such as eye trackers or motion detectors and psychophysical measures help in building the database related to these markers.
5. *Diagnostic Systems:* The ASD diagnostic label was firstly given in *Diagnostic and Statistical Manual of Mental Disorders, Third Edition* (DSM-III; American Psychiatric Association, 1980). After that, the terminologies such as autism, Pervasive Developmental Disorder-Not Otherwise

Specified (PDD-NOS) and Asperger's Syndrome (AS) were included in DSM-IV, Text Revision (APA, 2000). These three terms are now combined under the ASD umbrella and sensory idiosyncratic responses are considered with ASD core symptoms in new edition DSM-5® (APA, 2013). The advancements in the diagnostic concept, due to growth in different versions of the diagnostic systems such as ICD-10, DSM-III-R, DSM-IV and DSM-5, enhances and broadens the heterogeneity of the disorder at the definition, detection and intervention levels.

In addition to these markers, various other morphological deviations (less than 5% of individuals) and mental-health co-morbidities exist in ASD affected individuals (Tammimies et al., 2015). Also, the information about intervention approaches, medical co-morbidities, outcomes and response to treatment, affected child's feedback and progress, record keeping, doctor's textual reports, and patient history can be combined with the diagnostic markers to increase the accuracy of disorder detection and prediction. These sources, on integration, as shown in Fig. 1 can provide a plethora of the ASD features that can improve the diagnostic methodologies. The non-uniformity of the data shows that ASD diagnosis is not a type of one-size-fits-all methodology, but demands a methodology that can combine heterogeneous data for detection and treatment.

Figure 1. Big Data Sources

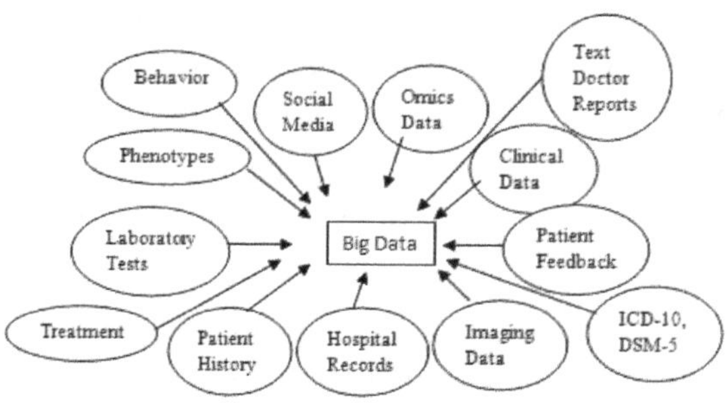

The growing initiatives in the field of big data are not only improving the existing databases, which are 33 in number as reported, but also generating the new ones such as MSSNG (Al-jawahiri & Milne, 2017). The dependency on different sources of information promotes awareness among the people, increases engagement with disordered individuals and enhances the clinical diagnostic standards. However, the collection of data and forming heterogeneous datasets cannot solve the purpose of diagnosis. The struggle to explore the data such as what is the data format, data source, usability and schema. In addition, the massive amount of data needs to be processed efficiently and parallely with less number of computations.

In such situations, Data Lake can provide a relief to all the pain points. One can store any amount of data without thinking about the source and structure and can run the different analytical engines such as Hadoop or Apache Spark (https://spark.apache.org) for programming and processing the large datasets (Da Silva Morais, 2015). Various other advantages of Data Lake are: (i) storage of real-time, nonrelational and relational data, (ii) provides storage at low cost and fast query result, and (iii) data can be stored in any schema. For data analysis, Hadoop engine can provide the distributed and parallel processing of large data sets using programming models, but it's complicated installation process, not user friendly environment, low memory efficiency, high dependency on the hardware structure were some of the difficulties that demand for other analytical engines. The platform such as Apache Spark is fast, supporting more programming languages, less dependent on hardware, handling streaming and real-time data, more memory efficient in comparison to Hadoop (Freeman et al., 2014). Spark engine is a cluster computing and supports in-memory processing for carrying out large-scale tasks speedily, interactively and iteratively as compared to batch (map reduce), stream (Apache Storm) or graph processing (Apache Giraph) tools. Its numerous libraries and wide range of tools – ML lib, SparkR, PySpark, GarphX make the processing, optimizing particular problem and expressing of learning based algorithms much easier (Boubela et al., 2016). In cognitive neuroscience, it is useful as it has the capability to implement the distributed algorithms using statistical modelling approaches such as linear regression or Principal Component Analysis (PCA). On the basis of these advantages and applications, an Apache Spark based analytics system is proposed and discussed in following section.

PROPOSED APPROACH AND METHDOLOGY

As discussed above, an Apache Spark engine has numerous advantages but has data management problem. In order to manage data it has to depend upon the external data storage units such as Hadoop or other technologies. The data storage issue of Apache Spark has been resolved with the usage of Data Lake within the engine. The novelty of the proposed system is that it is a dual approach system that can manage the massive data and can be used as a generalized model for analyzing the disorder. The system has capability to resolve the complexity of the data as it can process such a big amount of data and enclose the data in a proper format ranging from demographic to clinical information. The proposed system can assist clinicians and neurologists in making more-informed decisions regarding disorder nature and carrying out analysis using a massive amount of data.

In order to diagnose ASD, the disordered-specific network needs to be compared with the neurotypical networks. The comparison is possible if the data is collected, from the sources discussed in the above section, for both the subjects (ASD and neurotypical). In this scenario, a very large amount of the data will get generated and processing this data traditionally is not possible. For example, if the subjects are compared on the basis of brain signals then the data will appear in form of MRI or fMRI signals. This data is very huge, complex, non-stationary, non-linear and represent multiple information patterns of the brain. The direct comparison of the signals is not a solution to understand their physical dynamics and brain disorders. Various decomposition algorithms such as Empirical Mode Decomposition (EMD) or Support Vector Machine (SVM) are used in processing brain signals, but they require a lot of computations and are very complex (Li et al., 2013). The efficient decomposition and analysis of massive brain signals demand parallel processing such as combining the traditional approaches with parallel processing of big data technology. One of the studies has utilized parallel Ensemble EMD (combining EEMD with Big data processing technology called Hadoop) and showed an improvement in the processing performance of fMRI signals (Wang et al., 2012). So, in order to compare the signals of both groups minutely, the data need to be represented in scattered blocks linearly so that by combining these blocks the data can be regenerated. This type of distributed computing is the potential solution rather than relying on single-workstations. In this way, using parallel processing engines such as Apache Spark, the machine learning algorithms can compare the large volumes of data in a compact form and can also reconstruct the signal faithfully. As shown in Figure 2, an Apache Spark system examines the data in order to uncover the unknown patterns and markers of the disorders and its sub-types. The block diagram is for any client generated query and explained the way in which the query is being processed.

Data Source and Collection Layer

There are multitude information systems for capturing the information about the patient and some of the sources are listed in Figure 1. The data and information collected from the different sources will be in diverse form, at different frequencies, in structured and un-structured form. The data not only captures the past information, but also current reports, medication and feedback. In ASD individuals, the data needs to be captured at regular intervals of time such as after one month or three month gap the patient needs another seating with clinicians/neurologists. The big data approach considers the association between the data and the information collected and completeness of patient disorder cycle. The data completeness is the key of big data as the emerging variation in the diagnostic approaches.

Data Lake

The data collected from different sources is fed into data lake in its native form. It is a storage area for depositing every type of data in its raw form, structured, semi-structured or unstructured form. The large amount of data is stored without any size limitation that enhances the data analysis performance. It is a low cost data repository system and supports all types of data formats for carrying out compression and encryption. The data and queries can be prepared and encrypted in a suitable format, configured and reconfigured as per requirement in less time. It offers schema-on-read which means that when the data is needed, only then it is processed and given a particular shape and structure. The data from the lake can be directly pulled by the user for processing, analyzing, deriving new insights or keeping in the storage units without knowing its format. The data from data lake can be analyzed using two different ways:

1. It is the proposed approach such that the data can be analyzed directly by feeding the data to the Apache Spark engine. In this scenario, there is no need of using other's management systems. But this is possible only by designing a proper Application Programming Interfaces (APIs) that can read the all the types of data directly without knowing about its structure and any in-between processing. These designed APIs need to have the potential in adding insights to the data whenever the data gets accumulated in data lake from new sources. For example, for analyzing the timeseries data spark provides spark-ts library. If there is a need to store data then the available storage systems can be used for storing only the most frequently used and the repetitive data. For example, row matrix is used to store time series data column wise (Boubela et al., 2016). This would be advantageous as the data will be available easily for analysis purposes and the need of fetching it in its raw form will be reduced.
2. The second option is the traditional option where one can store the data in proper format which can be pulled from different storage systems when required. Spark offers a number of options for storing the large data. The local storage system can be used for storing, reading and writing files. The HDFS option can also be used which is available with Hadoop. The traditional RDBMS sources such as SQL including oracle or MySQL server are used for storing the structured and complex data in tabular form. The data in SQL need to follow the identical structure otherwise it can disrupt the

entire system. On the other hand, the No SQL databases such as Cassandra, HBase and MongoDB do not pose such restrictions and can handle data of any format. These open-source and distributed data management systems can be used to handle massive data in unstructured formats. The data can also be stored in the cloud using a S3 bucket which is cheap, scalable and high speed method for data backup and retrieval.

a. *Ingestion Layer:* It takes care of data that it is in the right shape and format for proper storage. It acts as a passage for moving the data from the source to the storage and analysis system. The data can be ingested using batch-processing (data is ingested batchwise at periodic intervals) or real-time streaming. The ingestion layer is implemented with Apache Kafka which is Apache Kafka (a scalable message broker) to provide high-throughput, fault-tolerance, and real-time data processing. For example, for ingesting doctor's notes or EHR (Ross, Wei, & Ohno-Machado, 2014) data to bring them in standard form the HL7 / Fast Healthcare Interoperability Resources (FHIR) protocol can be used.

Figure 2. Apache Spark Engine with Hadoop-based Data Lake Based Analytic System for ASD

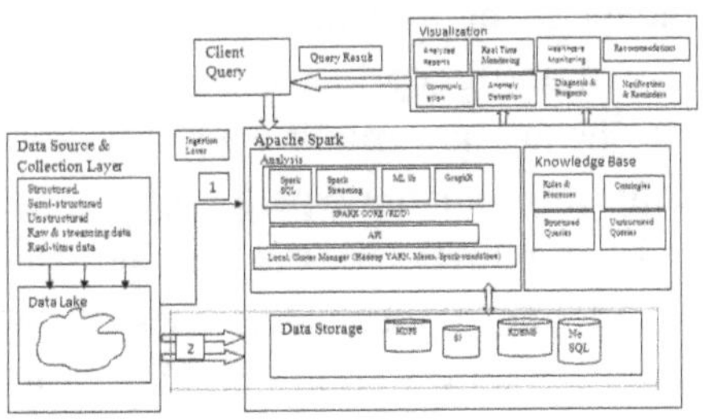

b. *Apache Spark Analytic System:* It is a general purpose cluster computing algorithm working on the principal of dispersing the data across the different clusters and processing them in parallel. It consists of a central coordinator called driver and different executors. It includes high-level APIs such as Scala, R, and Java for using it interactively (Boubela et al., 2016).
   i. *Cluster Manager: T*he cluster manager is the framework over which the Apache Spark is framed and through which a Spark application is launched on the machines. The cluster is accessed by spark using the spark context (a spark application). There are a number of other cluster managers which Spark supports such as Local cluster, Mesos, Hadoop YARN and even spark-standalone scheduler (inbuilt) in case any of the external one fails. The spark-standalone enables the users to launch their own private Spark cluster.
   ii. *Spark Core:* The core can process and access the data by reading it from the storage systems. The entry for interaction with the spark core is provided by the spark context. Besides this, spark context helps in representing the connection with the spark cluster and distributing the jobs. The fundamental unit of data is called as Resilient Distributed Data (RDD) which performs a parallel operation by distributing the data across cluster nodes. Most of the data collected for ASD diagnosis are unstructured and raw in nature and hence, RDDs can easily handle these datasets using low-level transformations. Spark provides another two abstractions (data set and data frame) to deal with structured and

semi-structured data. RDD is read-only, distributed, fault-tolerant and the main logical unit. It is re-usable and can share data among multiple computational jobs involving regression, clustering or various other tasks.

iii. *Analysis Libraries:* The analysis tools in spark allow performing the data processing along with the analysis of data. It provides a very fast and parallelized platform for carrying out the operations on single as well as on thousands of nodes. The integration of the various libraries on a single platform and in one framework can provide new opportunities for analyzing the data and even not so massive signals such as EEG. In healthcare systems the brain signals can be analyzed by generating the covariance matrix, sparse similarity matrix (Zhao et al., 2016), cluster computing (Freeman et al., 2014) or single value decomposition of the signals and then processing them using the spark engine.

- *ML lib:* The machine learning algorithms boost the disorder predictive factors and fit different models to help experts in finding the disordered individual among the undiagnosed. It can recommend, diagnose and monitors on the basis of massive structured and unstructured data using the different classifiers such as SVM, Random forests, K-Means clustering and similarity measure algorithms such as Dimension Independent Matrix Square using MapReduce (Meng at al., 2016, Zhao et al., 2016) and deep learning algorithms. Besides, computations, alerts, notification and healthcare monitoring are done through SparkML. Information retrieval is done through the Spark SQL and SPARQL, where Spark GraphX works as the visual analytics of the queried data. This library helps in extracting the different features of the raw data by scaling, converting or using other transformation techniques and supports pipelining in operations. The different extractors used by MLlib are Term Frequency-Inverse Document Frequency (TF-IDF), Word2VecModel, CountVectorizer and transformers available are tokenizer, binarizer, stringindexer, polynomial expansion, PCA, one hot encoder and various others. After the transformation, the required features are selected from the large pool of the features. This feature selector using vector slicer, integer or string indices or various other selectors lead to a new vector representing the subset of the features or a new feature set. At last, the Locality Sensitive Hashing (LSH) algorithm help in reducing the dimensionality of the feature vector using other algorithms such as Bucketed Random Projection for Euclidean Distance.
- GraphX: It is a graph computation engine that enables users to process the queried data graphically and provides its visual analytics. The different Visualization tools used for effective understanding of data are rCharts, matplotlib, and ggplot2.
- Spark SQL: The SQL or HQL queries of the users/clients for processing structured or semi-structured data are handled using Spark SQL. Basically, it helps in retrieving the information.

Besides these, the other applications supported by Spark are SparkR (analyzing large datasets), Spark streaming (for real-time data) and many others.

iv. Knowledge-Base Rules: The hybrid spark architecture has a rule engine and an ontology reasoner. The ontologies generated using ontology reasoners such as Pellet or TrOWL provides automated reasoning to support decision-making. These additional features provide an aid to machine learning algorithms in making highly uncertain clinical decisions. The processes and reasoners can pull the clinical knowledge from biomedical ontologies and Clinical Practice Guidelines (CPGs) and the rule producers converts CPGs into some feasible rules in integration with clinical events. The integration of possible rules, reasoners and processes is done using different disciplines such as Neural-Symbolic Integration combines deep neural networks with reasoning ontologies such as OWL. This neural network based combination helps in inferring various clinical facts and in improving the interpretability of prediction models.

v. *Visualization & Interpretation by the Client:* Finally, the data is visualized and interpreted using different tools to solve any of the queries related to the patient. The generated information can resolve the present query or can be used as reference for another patient's diagnosis. The data can be sent to other servers for tele-health sector or can be used for generating reports. The reminders and notifications regarding an important event or any alert information related to affected individuals can be sent to the people concerned with them. The data can be used for real-time processing or for diagnosis and prognosis purposes.

In this way the query of the client is resolved and the data can be interpreted by visualizing and solving the problem found in the individual. The Apache Spark engine to which the query is fed can itself act as the master node and can distribute the query on various other nodes. The analytic system presented here has the potential to understand every facet of the disorder from onset to the present condition of individuals and can relate the observations to treatment and intervention. Hence, 'big and 'open' data aims to create, integrate and then analyze the large datasets in order to provide insights into disorder complexities.

DISCUSSION

Big Data is primitively used in predictive analytics, finding new insights in clinical databases, and integrating the patient data for providing a platform for better diagnosis and treatment. These big data based predictive systems also help the patients by identifying the improvement demanding areas such as intervention, early identification, health monitoring, support in clinical decisions and disorder surveillance. In ASD, the heterogeneous and massive data provide the 360 degree information of the disordered individuals. In the first phase of the chapter, the different sources from which the data related to ASD can be accumulated have been provided. The sources have clearly shown the heterogeneity, different platforms and formats for accumulating the data. These sources provide the range of ASD symptoms and the extent to which one needs to collect data to detect the disorder. This vast information would be of use only if the data is linked securely, transformed into practical knowledge, analyzed for identifying new patterns & improving healthcare and finding the right approach for affected individuals.

In the second phase, an analytic system has been presented for analyzing the data collected from different sources to provide knowledge of ASD. The framework presented in this chapter has merged different data analysis and computational approaches on a single platform. The analytic system has the potential to support clinicians in distinguishing the ASD from neurotypical subjects, stratifying ASDs into subtypes by finding the differences as well as commonalities in the given data and then doing the group-wise comparison among the affected individuals. The system focuses on developing new APIs that can analyze the data directly from colossal repositories and data lakes rather than depending upon the data management system. This step is advantageous as the data will be prepared and processed at the time of the requirement. The data which is being used frequently by the physicians can be stored, if required, for faster processing. The availability of different data analysis methods and combining them with the knowledge base can provide the correlation between the data and analyze it more efficiently. The proposed system, if implemented, has the capability to assist clinicians and neurologists in making more informed decisions regarding disorder nature and analyzing massive amount of data. The research using big data methodologies is limited on health fronts as this demands high effort for the first time analysis and lacks in providing proper interfaces to different data formats. The supportive system provided in this chapter also demands proper APIs for extracting data directly from the data lake to make this system a supportive tool.

The capability of big data to scrutinize the disorder markers on single platform rather than looking at disorder patterns individually can identify the individual who is at risk of ASD or sub-level of the individual on the spectrum. It would be beneficial to replicate the findings for further investigations on the basis of reliable and conclusive results provided by different big data based studies. The collection of massive datasets is not what ASD demands, but the characteristics of big data such as deep, open are required for dealing with this non-uniform disorder. This type of voluminous data has the potential to enlist the proper markers of the disorder that can be fixed & retraced by prescribing the proper treatment. The data availability can even eliminate those age barriers for diagnosis and can provide faster access to diagnosis as well as intervention. The high computational speed, low cost and parallel processing of data can analyze the data very fast at early ages and thus, can reduce the diagnostic age. Although, in healthcare domain the big data analytics is in its infancy, but it offers a promising direction in analyzing the health related data. The 'big data' can be seen as the new standard that can provide information about the potential risks causing ASD. Hence, the key to decompose the multi-level heterogeneity of ASD is big data.

FUTURE STUDIES

In future, if proper APIs and other requisites get fulfilled properly, then Apache Spark can be proved as a boon in the healthcare domain. There is a need to work on efficient use of data management systems and repositories to improve the healthcare units and lower the cost. The present and past findings need to be fused using analytic engines in combination of knowledge based rules to shape the future of health monitoring units. The provision for entertaining more data complexities is required for adding more opportunities to big data analytics and for yielding better outcomes. There is a need to do more work on the structure and terminology of medical data for developing the ontology-savvy healthcare units. More work needs to be done on deep learning algorithms in order to make the ASD diagnostics faster, more timely, more accurate, cheaper and more accessible. The data abundance is the driving factor and should be employed in any possible way for understanding ASD in a better way rather than testing few hypotheses against small datasets.

REFERENCES

Al-jawahiri, R., & Milne, E. (2017). Resources available for autism research in the big data era: A systematic review. *PeerJ*, *5*, e2880. doi:10.7717/peerj.2880 PMID:28097074

Alhaddad, M. J., Kamel, M. I., Malibary, H. M., Ebtehal, A., Thabit, K., Dahlwi, F., & Hadi, A. A. (2012). Diagnosis autism by fisher linear discriminant analysis FLDA via EEG. *Int J Bio-Sci Bio-Technol*, *4*(2), 45–54.

American Psychiatric Association. (1980). Diagnostic and Statistical Manual of Mental Disorders, 3rd Edition (DSM-III). Washington, DC: American Psychiatric Association.

American Psychiatric Association. (2000). *DSM-IV-TR: Diagnostic and statistical manual of mental disorders, text revision* (Vol. 75). Washington, DC: American Psychiatric Association.

American Psychiatric Association. (2013). *Diagnostic and statistical manual of mental disorders (DSM-5®)*. American Psychiatric Pub.

Andreu-Perez, J., Poon, C. C., Merrifield, R. D., Wong, S. T., & Yang, G. Z. (2015). Big data for health. *IEEE Journal of Biomedical and Health Informatics*, *19*(4), 1193–1208. doi:10.1109/JBHI.2015.2450362 PMID:26173222

Bacon, E. C., Dufek, S., Schreibman, L., Stahmer, A. C., Pierce, K., & Courchesne, E. (2014). Measuring outcome in an early intervention program for toddlers with autism spectrum disorder: Use of a curriculum-based assessment. *Autism Research and Treatment*, *2014*, 2014. doi:10.1155/2014/964704 PMID:24711926

Bedford, R., Gliga, T., Shephard, E., Elsabbagh, M., Pickles, A., Charman, T., & Johnson, M. H. (2017). Neurocognitive and observational markers: Prediction of autism spectrum disorder from infancy to mid-childhood. *Molecular Autism*, *8*(1), 49. doi:10.118613229-017-0167-3 PMID:29018511

Boubela, R. N., Kalcher, K., Huf, W., Našel, C., & Moser, E. (2016). Big data approaches for the analysis of large-scale fMRI data using apache spark and GPU processing: A demonstration on resting-state fMRI data from the human connectome project. *Frontiers in Neuroscience*, *9*, 492. doi:10.3389/fnins.2015.00492 PMID:26778951

Carter, M. T., & Scherer, S. W. (2013). Autism spectrum disorder in the genetics clinic: A review. *Clinical Genetics*, *83*(5), 399–407. doi:10.1111/cge.12101 PMID:23425232

Chaddad, A., Desrosiers, C., Hassan, L., & Tanougast, C. (2017). Hippocampus and amygdala radiomic biomarkers for the study of autism spectrum disorder. *BMC Neuroscience*, *18*(1), 52. doi:10.118612868-017-0373-0 PMID:28821235

Clifford, S., Young, R., & Williamson, P. (2007). Assessing the early characteristics of autistic disorder using video analysis. *Journal of Autism and Developmental Disorders*, *37*(2), 301–313. doi:10.100710803-006-0160-8 PMID:17031450

Cotter, J., Granger, K., Backx, R., Hobbs, M., Looi, C. Y., & Barnett, J. H. (2017). Social cognitive dysfunction as a clinical marker: A systematic review of meta-analyses across 30 clinical conditions. *Neuroscience and Biobehavioral Reviews*. PMID:29175518

Cyganek, B., Graña, M., Krawczyk, B., Kasprzak, A., Porwik, P., Walkowiak, K., & Woźniak, M. (2016). A Survey of Big Data Issues in Electronic Health Record Analysis. *Applied Artificial Intelligence*, *30*(6), 497–520. doi:10.1080/08839514.2016.1193714

Da Silva Morais, T. (2015, January). Survey on frameworks for distributed computing: Hadoop, Spark and Storm. In *Proceedings of the 10th Doctoral Symposium in Informatics Engineering-DSIE* (*Vol. 15*). Academic Press.

Di Martino, A., O'Connor, D., Chen, B., Alaerts, K., Anderson, J. S., Assaf, M., ... Blanken, L. M. (2017). Enhancing studies of the connectome in autism using the autism brain imaging data exchange II. *Scientific Data*, *4*(1), 170010. doi:10.1038data.2017.10 PMID:28291247

Dinov, I. D. (2016). Volume and value of big healthcare data. *Journal of Medical Statistics and Informatics*, *4*(1), 4. doi:10.7243/2053-7662-4-3 PMID:26998309

Eshraghi, A. A., Liu, G., Kay, S. I. S., Eshraghi, R. S., Mittal, J., Moshiree, B., & Mittal, R. (2018). Epigenetics and Autism Spectrum Disorder: Is There a Correlation? *Frontiers in Cellular Neuroscience*, *12*, 78. doi:10.3389/fncel.2018.00078 PMID:29636664

Evans, D. W., Uljarević, M., Lusk, L. G., Loth, E., & Frazier, T. (2017). Development of two dimensional measures of restricted and repetitive behavior in parents and children. *Journal of the American Academy of Child and Adolescent Psychiatry*, *56*(1), 51–58. doi:10.1016/j.jaac.2016.10.014 PMID:27993229

Feldman, B., Martin, E. M., & Skotnes, T. (2012). Big data in healthcare hype and hope. *October 2012. Dr. Bonnie, 360.*

Freeman, J., Vladimirov, N., Kawashima, T., Mu, Y., Sofroniew, N. J., Bennett, D. V., ... Ahrens, M. B. (2014). Mapping brain activity at scale with cluster computing. *Nature Methods*, *11*(9), 941–950. doi:10.1038/nmeth.3041 PMID:25068736

Fukuyama, H., Kumagaya, S. I., Asada, K., Ayaya, S., & Kato, M. (2017). Autonomic versus perceptual accounts for tactile hypersensitivity in autism spectrum disorder. *Scientific Reports*, *7*(1), 8259. doi:10.103841598-017-08730-3 PMID:28811601

Haglund, N., Dahlgren, S., Källén, K., Gustafsson, P., & Råstam, M. (2016). The Observation Scale for Autism (OSA): A New Screening Method to Detect Autism Spectrum Disorder before Age Three Years. *Journal of Intellectual Disability-Diagnosis and Treatment*, *3*(4), 230–237. doi:10.6000/2292-2598.2015.03.04.9

Hall, D., Huerta, M. F., McAuliffe, M. J., & Farber, G. K. (2012). Sharing heterogeneous data: The national database for autism research. *Neuroinformatics*, *10*(4), 331–339. doi:10.100712021-012-9151-4 PMID:22622767

Kakkar, D. (2018, January). A Study on Machine Learning Based Generalized Automated Seizure Detection System. In *2018 8th International Conference on Cloud Computing, Data Science & Engineering (Confluence)* (pp. 769-774). IEEE.

Kakkar, D. (2019). Diagnostic Assessment Techniques and Non-Invasive Biomarkers for Autism Spectrum Disorder. *International Journal of E-Health and Medical Communications*, *10*(3), 79–95. doi:10.4018/IJEHMC.2019070105

Karimi, P., Kamali, E., Mousavi, S. M., & Karahmadi, M. (2017). Environmental factors influencing the risk of autism. *Journal of Research in Medical Sciences, 22*.

Li, S., Zhou, W., Yuan, Q., Geng, S., & Cai, D. (2013). Feature extraction and recognition of ictal EEG using EMD and SVM. *Computers in Biology and Medicine*, *43*(7), 807–816. doi:10.1016/j.compbiomed.2013.04.002 PMID:23746721

Loke, Y. J., Hannan, A. J., & Craig, J. M. (2015). The role of epigenetic change in autism spectrum disorders. *Frontiers in Neurology*, *6*, 107. doi:10.3389/fneur.2015.00107 PMID:26074864

Lombardo, M. V., Lai, M. C., & Baron-Cohen, S. (2018). Big data approaches to decomposing heterogeneity across the autism spectrum. *bioRxiv*, 278788.

Mani, G., Berkovich, S., & Liao, D. (2014, August). Adaptive and Interactive Design Based on Big Data Computational Model for Treating Autism. In *Computing for Geospatial Research and Application (COM. Geo), 2014 Fifth International Conference on* (pp. 121-122). IEEE. 10.1109/COM.Geo.2014.7

Meng, X., Bradley, J., Yavuz, B., Sparks, E., Venkataraman, S., Liu, D., ... Xin, D. (2016). Mllib: Machine learning in apache spark. *Journal of Machine Learning Research*, *17*(1), 1235–1241.

Miles, J. H. (2015). Complex autism spectrum disorders and cutting-edge molecular diagnostic tests. *Journal of the American Medical Association*, *314*(9), 879–880.

Miron, O., Ari-Even Roth, D., Gabis, L. V., Henkin, Y., Shefer, S., Dinstein, I., & Geva, R. (2015). Prolonged auditory brainstem responses in infants with autism. *Autism Research*, *9*(6), 689–695. doi:10.1002/aur.1561 PMID:26477791

Northrup, C. M., Lantz, J., & Hamlin, T. (2016). Wearable stress sensors for children with autism spectrum disorder with in situ alerts to caregivers via a mobile phone. *Proceedings, 2*(1), e9.

Raghupathi, W., & Raghupathi, V. (2014). Big data analytics in healthcare: Promise and potential. *Health Information Science and Systems*, *2*(1), 3. doi:10.1186/2047-2501-2-3 PMID:25825667

Ross, M. K., Wei, W., & Ohno-Machado, L. (2014). "Big data" and the electronic health record. *Yearbook of Medical Informatics*, *9*(1), 97–104. doi:10.15265/IY-2014-0003 PMID:25123728

Sarkar, B. K. (2017). Big data for secure healthcare system: A conceptual design. *Complex & Intelligent Systems*, *3*(2), 133–151. doi:10.100740747-017-0040-1

Sasson, N. J., & Elison, J. T. (2012). Eye tracking young children with autism. *Journal of Visualized Experiments*, *§§§*, 61. PMID:22491039

Sayorwan, W., Phianchana, N., Permpoonputtana, K., & Siripornpanich, V. (2018). A Study of the Correlation between VEP and Clinical Severity in Children with Autism Spectrum Disorder. *Autism Research and Treatment, 2018*, 2018. doi:10.1155/2018/5093016 PMID:29568651

Sealey, L. A., Hughes, B. W., Sriskanda, A. N., Guest, J. R., Gibson, A. D., Johnson-Williams, L., ... Bagasra, O. (2016). Environmental factors in the development of autism spectrum disorders. *Environment International, 88*, 288–298. doi:10.1016/j.envint.2015.12.021 PMID:26826339

Sheikhani, A., Behnam, H., Mohammadi, M. R., Noroozian, M., & Golabi, P. (2008) Connectivity analysis of quantitative electroencephalogram background activity in autism disorders with short time fourier transform and coherence values. Congress on image and signal processing, 207–212. doi:10.1109/CISP.2008.595

Simons, VIP Consortium. (2012). Simons Variation in Individuals Project (Simons VIP): A genetics-first approach to studying autism spectrum and related neurodevelopmental disorders. *Neuron, 73*(6), 10631067. PMID:22445335

Sinha, P., Kjelgaard, M. M., Gandhi, T. K., Tsourides, K., Cardinaux, A. L., Pantazis, D., ... Held, R. M. (2014). Autism as a disorder of prediction. *Proceedings of the National Academy of Sciences, 111*(42), 15220-15225.

Siuly, S., & Zhang, Y. (2016). Medical big data: Neurological diseases diagnosis through medical data analysis. *Data Science and Engineering, 1*(2), 54–64. doi:10.100741019-016-0011-3

Song, R., Liu, J., & Kong, X. J. (2016). Autonomic Dysfunction and Autism: Subtypes and Clinical Perspectives. *North American Journal of Medicine & Science, 9*(4).

Sudirman, R., Saidin, S., & Safri, N. M. (2010). Study of electroencephalography signal of Autism and down syndrome children using FFT. In *IEEE symposium on industrial electronics and applications* (pp. 401–406). ISIEA. doi:10.1109/ISIEA.2010.5679434

Sun, J., & Reddy, C. K. (2013, August). Big data analytics for healthcare. In *Proceedings of the 19th ACM SIGKDD international conference on Knowledge discovery and data mining* (pp. 1525-1525). ACM.

Tammimies, K., Marshall, C. R., Walker, S., Kaur, G., Thiruvahindrapuram, B., Lionel, A. C., ... Woodbury-Smith, M. (2015). Molecular diagnostic yield of chromosomal microarray analysis and wholeexome sequencing in children with autism spectrum disorder. *Journal of the American Medical Association, 314*(9), 895–903. doi:10.1001/jama.2015.10078 PMID:26325558

Tanu, T., & Kakkar, D. (2018). *Strengthening risk prediction using statistical learning in children with autism spectrum disorder*. Advances in Autism.

The Apache Software Foundation. (2015). *Apache Spark*. Available online at: https://spark.apache.org/

Wadhera, T., & Kakkar, D. (2019). Eye Tracker: An Assistive Tool in Diagnosis of Autism Spectrum Disorder. In Emerging Trends in the Diagnosis and Intervention of Neurodevelopmental Disorders (pp. 125-152). IGI Global.

Wang, L., Chen, D., Ranjan, R., Khan, S. U., KolOdziej, J., & Wang, J. (2012, December). Parallel processing of massive EEG data with MapReduce. In *Parallel and Distributed Systems (ICPADS), 2012 IEEE 18th International Conference on* (pp. 164-171). IEEE.

Wang, Y., Kung, L., & Byrd, T. A. (2018). Big data analytics: Understanding its capabilities and potential benefits for healthcare organizations. *Technological Forecasting and Social Change*, *126*, 3–13. doi:10.1016/j.techfore.2015.12.019

Weil, A. R. (2014). *Big data in health: a new era for research and patient care*. Academic Press.

Yuen, R. K., Merico, D., Bookman, M., Howe, J. L., Thiruvahindrapuram, B., Patel, R. V., ... Pellecchia, G. (2017). Whole genome sequencing resource identifies 18 new candidate genes for autism spectrum disorder. *Nature Neuroscience*, *20*(4), 602–611. doi:10.1038/nn.4524 PMID:28263302

Yuen, R. K., Thiruvahindrapuram, B., Merico, D., Walker, S., Tammimies, K., Hoang, N., ... Gazzellone, M. J. (2015). Whole-genome sequencing of quartet families with autism spectrum disorder. *Nature Medicine*, *21*(2), 185–191. doi:10.1038/nm.3792 PMID:25621899

Zhao, Y., Chen, H., Li, Y., Lv, J., Jiang, X., Ge, F., ... Zhao, S. (2016). Connectome-scale group-wise consistent resting-state network analysis in autism spectrum disorder. *NeuroImage. Clinical*, *12*, 23–33. doi:10.1016/j.nicl.2016.06.004 PMID:27358766

Compilation of References

Abdulkader, S. N., Atia, A., & Mostafa, M. S. M. (2015). Brain computer interfacing: Applications and challenges. *Egyptian Informatics Journal, 16*(2), 213–230. doi:10.1016/j.eij.2015.06.002

Abirami, S. P., Kousalya, G., & Karthick, R. (2018). Identification and exploration of facial expression in children with ASD in a contact less environment. *Journal of Intelligent & Fuzzy Systems, 36*(3), 2025–2032.

Abreu, R., Leal, A., & Figueiredo, P. (2018). EEG-Informed fMRI: A Review of Data Analysis Methods. *Frontiers in Human Neuroscience, 12*, 29. doi:10.3389/fnhum.2018.00029 PMID:29467634

Acharya, U. R., Oh, S. L., Hagiwara, Y., Tan, J. H., Adeli, H., & Subha, D. P. (2018). Automated EEG-based screening of depression using deep convolutional neural network. *Computer Methods and Programs in Biomedicine, 161*, 103–113. doi:10.1016/j.cmpb.2018.04.012 PMID:29852953

Adjorlu, A., Høeg, E. R., Mangano, L., & Serafin, S. (2017, October). Daily Living Skills Training in Virtual Reality to Help Children with Autism Spectrum Disorder in a Real Shopping Scenario. In *Mixed and Augmented Reality (ISMAR-Adjunct), 2017 IEEE International Symposium on* (pp. 294-302). IEEE. 10.1109/ISMAR-Adjunct.2017.93

Adrien, J. L., Lenoir, P., Martineau, J., Perrot, A., Hameury, L., Larmande, C., & Sauvage, D. (1993). Blind ratings of early symptoms of autism based upon family home movies. *J AM Acad of Child Adoles Psychiatry, 32*(3), 617–626. doi:10.1097/00004583-199305000-00019 PMID:7684363

Afshar, P., Khambhati, A., Stanslaski, S., Carlson, D., Jensen, R., Dani, S., ... Denison, T. (2013). A translational platform for prototyping closed-loop neuromodulation systems. *Frontiers in Neural Circuits, 6*, 117. doi:10.3389/fncir.2012.00117 PMID:23346048

Aghdam, M. A., & Sharifi, A. (2018). Combination of rs-fMRI and sMRI Data to Discriminate Autism Spectrum Disorders in Young Children Using Deep Belief Network. *Journal of Digital Imaging, 31*(6), 895–903. doi:10.100710278-018-0093-8 PMID:29736781

Aghdam, M. A., Sharifi, A., & Pedram, M. M. (2019). Diagnosis of Autism Spectrum Disorders in Young Children Based on Resting-State Functional Magnetic Resonance Imaging Data Using Convolutional Neural Networks. *Journal of Digital Imaging, 32*(6), 1–20. doi:10.100710278-019-00196-1 PMID:30963340

Agnihotri, S., Gaur, P., Bhattacharya, S., Kant, S., & Pandey, S. (2018). Benefits of Yoga in Respiratory Diseases. *Indian J. Pharm. Biol. Res, 6*(4), 10-13.

Agree, E. M. (2014). The potential for technology to enhance independence for those aging with a disability. *Disability and Health Journal, 7*(1), S33–S39.

Ahmadvand, A., & Daliri, M. R. (2014). Brain MR Image Segmentation Methods and Applications. *OMICS Journal of Radiology, 02*(04), 1–3. doi:10.4172/2167-7964.1000e130

Ajmera, S., Sundar, S., Amirtha, G. B., Bhavanani, A. B., Dayanidy, G., & Ezhumalai, G. (2018). A comparative study on the effect of music therapy alone and a combination of music and yoga therapies on the psycho-physiological parameters of cardiac patients posted for angiography. *J Basic ClinAppl Health Sci*, *2*(1), 163–171. doi:10.5005/jp-journals-10082-01145

Alabbas, N. A., & Miller, D. E. (2019). Challenges and assistive technology during typical routines: Perspectives of caregivers of children with autism spectrum disorders and other disabilities. *International Journal of Disability Development and Education*, *66*(3), 273–283. doi:10.1080/1034912X.2019.1578864

Alexander, G. K., Innes, K. E., Selfe, T. K., & Brown, C. J. (2013). "more than I expected": Perceived benefits of yoga practice among older adults at risk for cardiovascular disease. *Complementary Therapies in Medicine*, *21*(1), 14–28. doi:10.1016/j.ctim.2012.11.001 PMID:23374201

Alhaddad, M. J., Kamel, M. I., Malibary, H. M., Ebtehal, A., Thabit, K., Dahlwi, F., & Hadi, A. A. (2012). Diagnosis autism by fisher linear discriminant analysis FLDA via EEG. *Int J Bio-Sci Bio-Technol*, *4*(2), 45–54.

Ali, Z., & Bhaskar, S. B. (2016). Basic statistical tools in research and data analysis. *Indian Journal of Anaesthesia*, *60*(9), 662. doi:10.4103/0019-5049.190623 PMID:27729694

Al-jawahiri, R., & Milne, E. (2017). Resources available for autism research in the big data era: A systematic review. *PeerJ*, *5*, e2880. doi:10.7717/peerj.2880 PMID:28097074

Al-Khalifa, H. S., & George, R. P. (2010). Eye Tracking and e-Learning: Seeing Through Your Students' Eyes. *eLearn*, *2010*(6).

Allen, S., & Anita, M. (2014). Yoga: Therapy for Children on the Autism Spectrum. *Academic Exchange Quarterly Summer*, *18*(2).

Allen, A., Schlosser, R., Brock, K., & Shane, H. (2017). The effectiveness of aided augmented input techniques for persons with developmental disabilities: A systematic review. *Augmentative and Alternative Communication*, *33*(3), 1–11. doi:10.1080/07434618.2017.1338752 PMID:28633531

Alper, S., & Raharinirina, S. (2006). Assistive Technology for Individuals with Disabilities: A Review and Synthesis of the Literature. *Journal of Special Education Technology*, *21*(2), 47–64.

Altanis, G., Boloudakis, M., Retalis, S., & Nikou, N. (2013). Children with motor impairments play a kinect learning game: First findings from a pilot case in an authentic classroom environment. *J Interact Design Architect*, *19*, 91–104.

Altay, B., & Demirkan, H. (2014). Inclusive design: Developing students' knowledge and attitude through empathic modelling. *International Journal of Inclusive Education*, *18*(2), 196–217. doi:10.1080/13603116.2013.764933

Altay, O., & Ulas, M. (2018). Prediction of the Autism Spectrum Disorder Diagnosis with Linear Discriminant Analysis Classifier and K-Nearest Neighbor in Children. *6th International Symposium on Digital Forensic and Security (ISDFS)*, 1–4. 10.1109/ISDFS.2018.8355354

Alzheimer's Association. (2018). Retrieved December 4, 2018, from https://www.alz.org/alzheimers-dementia/what-is-alzheimers

Aman, M., Farmer, C., Hollway, J., & Arnold, L. (2008). Treatment of Inattention, Overactivity, and Impulsiveness in Autism Spectrum Disorders. *Child and Adolescent Psychiatric Clinics of North America*, *17*, 713–738. PMID:18775366

American Psychiatric Association. (1980). Diagnostic and Statistical Manual of Mental Disorders, 3rd Edition (DSM-III). Washington, DC: American Psychiatric Association.

American Psychiatric Association. (1994). *Diagnostic and Statistical Manual of Mental Disorders: DSM-IV*. Washington, DC: American Psychiatric Association.

American Psychiatric Association. (2000). *Diagnostic and Statistical Manual of Mental Disorders* (Fourth Edition Text Revision). Washington, DC: American Psychiatric Association.

American Psychiatric Association. (2000). *DSM-IV-TR: Diagnostic and statistical manual of mental disorders, text revision* (Vol. 75). Washington, DC: American Psychiatric Association.

American Psychiatric Association. (2013). *Diagnostic and statistical manual of mental disorders* (5th ed.). Arlington, VA: American Psychiatric Publishing.

American Psychiatric Association. (2013). *Diagnostic and statistical manual of mental disorders (DSM-5®)*. American Psychiatric Pub.

American Psychiatric Association. (2013). *Diagnostic and Statistical Manual of Mental Disorders (DSM-V)* (5th ed.). Washington, DC: American Psychiatric Association Publishing.

American Psychological Association. (1993). *Promotion and dissemination of psychological procedures*. An unpublished task force report for Division 12. Washington, DC: American Psychological Association.

Anagün, Ş. (2018). Teachers' Perceptions about the Relationship between 21st Century Skills and Managing Constructivist Learning Environments. *International Journal of Instruction*, *11*(4), 825–840. doi:10.12973/iji.2018.11452a

Andreu-Perez, J., Poon, C. C., Merrifield, R. D., Wong, S. T., & Yang, G. Z. (2015). Big data for health. *IEEE Journal of Biomedical and Health Informatics*, *19*(4), 1193–1208. doi:10.1109/JBHI.2015.2450362 PMID:26173222

Andrew, D. P., Jason, T. N., & Karen, S. R. (2016). How does difficulty communicating affect the social relationships of older adults? An Exploration using data from a National Survey. *Journal of Communication Disorders*, *62*, 131–146. doi:10.1016/j.jcomdis.2016.06.002 PMID:27420152

Andriamananjara, A., Muntari, R., & Crimi, A. (2019). Overlaps in brain dynamic functional connectivity between schizophrenia and autism spectrum disorder. *Scientific American*, *2*, e00019. doi:10.1016/j.sciaf.2018.e00019

APB (Association of Applied Psychophysiology and Biofeedback). (2003). *Ethical principles of applied psychophysiology and biofeedback*. Wheat Ridge, CO: Association for Applied Psychophysiology and Biofeedback.

Archambault, S. G., & Masunaga, J. (2015). Curriculum mapping as a strategic planning tool. *Journal of Library Administration*, *55*(6), 503–519. doi:10.1080/01930826.2015.1054770

Arking, D. E., Cutler, D. J., Brune, C. W., Teslovich, T. M., West, K., Ikeda, M., & … . (2008). A common genetic variant in the neurexin superfamily member CNTNAP2 increases familial risk of autism. *American Journal of Human Genetics*, *82*, 160–164. PMID:18179894

Arora, N. K., Nair, M. K. C., Gulati, S., Deshmukh, V., Mohapatra, A., Mishra, D., ... Murthy, G. V. S. (2018). Neurodevelopmental disorders in children aged 2–9 years: Population-based burden estimates across five regions in India. *PLoS Medicine*, *15*(7), e1002615. doi:10.1371/journal.pmed.1002615 PMID:30040859

Artchoudane, S., Bhavanani, A. B., Ramanathan, M., & Mariangela, A. (2019). Yoga as a therapeutic tool in autism: A detailed review. *Yoga Mimamsa, 51,* 3-16. Doi:10.4103/ym.ym_3_19

Artchoudane, S., Ranganadin, P., Bhavanani, A. B., Ramanathan, M., & Madanmohan, T. (2018). Effect of adjuvant Yoga therapy on pulmonary function and Quality of life among patients with Chronic Obstructive Pulmonary Disease: A randomized control trial. *J Basic ClinAppl Health Sci, 2*(3), 117-122.

Arthanat, S., Curtin, C., & Knotak, D. (2013). Comparative observations of learning engagement by students with developmental disabilities using an iPad and computer: A pilot study. *Assistive Technology, 25*(4), 204–213. doi:10.1080/10400435.2012.761293 PMID:24620703

Aslanides, J., Leike, J., & Hutter, M. (2017). *Universal Reinforcement Learning Algorithms: Survey and Experiments.* Academic Press.

Aslan, S. (2015). Is learning by teaching effective in gaining 21st Century Skills? The views of pre-service science teachers. *Educational Sciences: Theory and Practice, 15*(6), 1441–1457. doi:10.12738/estp.2016.1.019

Asli, G., Melek, C., Ozgur, B., & Kuscu, N.K. (2012). Sudden Death of a Pregnant Woman in Third Trimester with No Risk Factor. *Case Reports in Obstetrics and Gynecology.* . doi:10.1155/2012/951480

Asperger, H. (1944). Die "autistichen Psychopathen" im Kindersalter. *Archiv für Psychiatrie und Nervenkrankheiten, 117*(1), 76–136. doi:10.1007/BF01837709

Autism & Uni. (2019). Accessed at http://www.autism-uni.org/

Aziz, M. Z., Abdullah, S. A., Adnan, S. F., & Mazalan, L. (2014). Educational App for Children with Autism Spectrum Disorders (ASDs). *Procedia Computer Science, 42*, 70–77. doi:10.1016/j.procs.2014.11.035

Bacon, E. C., Dufek, S., Schreibman, L., Stahmer, A. C., Pierce, K., & Courchesne, E. (2014). Measuring outcome in an early intervention program for toddlers with autism spectrum disorder: Use of a curriculum-based assessment. *Autism Research and Treatment, 2014*, 2014. doi:10.1155/2014/964704 PMID:24711926

BaHammam, A. S., Nashwan, S., Hammad, O., Sharif, M. M., & Pandi-Perumal, S. R. (2013). Objective assessment of drowsiness and reaction time during intermittent Ramadan fasting in young men: A case-crossover study. *Behavioral and Brain Functions, 9*(1), 32. doi:10.1186/1744-9081-9-32 PMID:23937904

Bailey, R. L., Parette, H. P. Jr, Stoner, J. B., Angell, M. E., & Carroll, K. (2006). Family members' perceptions of augmentative and alternative communication device use. *Language, Speech, and Hearing Services in Schools, 37*(1), 50–60. doi:10.1044/0161- 1461(2006/006) PMID:16615749

Bailey, R. L., Stoner, J. B., Parette, H. P., & Angell, M. E. (2006). AAC team perceptions: Augmentative and alternative communication device use. *Education and Training in Developmental Disabilities, 41*(2), 139.

Bailey, T. (2014). Diagnosing and Treating Developmental Disorders with qEEG and Neurotherapy. In *Clinical Neurotherapy* (pp. 321–355). Elsevier. doi:10.1016/B978-0-12-396988-0.00013-1

Baio, J., Wiggins, L., Christensen, D. L., Maenner, M. J., Daniels, J., Warren, Z., ... Durkin, M. S. (2018). Prevalence of Autism Spectrum Disorder Among Children Aged 8 Years— Autism and Developmental Disabilities Monitoring Network, 11 Sites, United States, 2014. *MMWR. Surveillance Summaries, 67*(6), 1–23. doi:10.15585/mmwr.ss6706a1 PMID:29701730

Balan, O., Moldoveanu, A., Moldoveanu, F., Morar, A., & Asavei, V. (2013). Assistive IT for Visually Imapired People. *Journal of Information Systems & Operations Management, 7*(2), 391–404.

Ball, G., Malpas, C. B., Genc, S., Efron, D., Sciberras, E., Anderson, V., ... Silk, T. J. (2019). Multimodal Structural Neuroimaging Markers of Brain Development and ADHD Symptoms. *The American Journal of Psychiatry, 176*(1), 57–66. doi:10.1176/appi.ajp.2018.18010034 PMID:30220220

Ballin, L., Balandin, S., & Stancliffe, R. J. (2012). The speech-generating device (SGD) mentoring program: Training adults who use an SGD to mentor. *Augmentative and Alternative Communication, 28*(4), 254–265. doi:10.3109/07434618.2012.708880 PMID:23256857

Baranek, G. (1999). Autism during infancy: A retrospective video analysis of sensory-motor and social behaviours at 9–12 months of age. *Journal of Autism and Developmental Disorders*, *9*(29), 213–224. PMID:10425584

Barea, R., Boquete, L., Mazo, M., & López, E. (2002). System for assisted mobility using eye movements based on electrooculography. *IEEE Transactions on Neural Systems and Rehabilitation Engineering*, *10*(4), 209–218. doi:10.1109/TNSRE.2002.806829 PMID:12611358

Barkley, R. A.(1992). *Is EEG biofeedback treatment effective for ADHD children?* ChaADDer Box.

Barlow, D. H., Nock, M., & Hersen, M. (2009). *Single-case experimental designs: Strategies for studying behavior change* (3rd ed.). New York: Ally & Bacon.

Baron-Cohen, S., Ring, H. A., Bullmore, E. T., Wheelwright, S., Ashwin, C., & Williams, S. C. R. (2000). The amygdala theory of autism. *Neuroscience and Biobehavioral Reviews*, *24*(3), 355–364. doi:10.1016/S0149-7634(00)00011-7 PMID:10781695

Barrio, B., Miller, D., Ojeme, C., & Tamakloe, D. (2019). Teachers' and parents' knowledge about disabilities and inclusion in Nigeria. *Journal of International Special Needs Education*, *22*(1), 14–24. doi:10.9782/17-00010

Bartak, L., Rutter, M., & Cox, A. (1975). A comparative study of infantile autism and specific development receptive language disorder. I. The children. *The British Journal of Psychiatry*, *126*(2), 149–159. doi:10.1192/bjp.126.2.127 PMID:1131465

Bartlett, M., Otis-Wilborn, A., & Sim, N. J. (2015). CCSS: Rigor or righteousness in special education. *Journal of Reading Education*, (3), 23.

Barttfeld, P., Wicker, B., Cukier, S., Navarta, S., Lew, S., Leiguarda, R., & Sigman, M. (2012). State-dependent changes of connectivity patterns and functional brain network topology in autism spectrum disorder. *Neuropsychologia*, *50*(14), 3653–3662. doi:10.1016/j.neuropsychologia.2012.09.047 PMID:23044278

Barua, M. M., & Daley, D. T. C. (n.d.). Autism. *Autism Spectrum Disorders – Rehabilitation Council of India*, 1–36. Retrieved from http://www.rehabcouncil.nic.in/writereaddata/autism.pdf

Barua, M., Kaushik, J. S., & Gulati, S. (2017). Legal provisions, educational services and health care across the lifespan for autism spectrum disorders in India. *Indian Journal of Pediatrics*, *84*(1), 76–82. doi:10.100712098-016-2261-5 PMID:27917445

Bates, R., Istance, H., Oosthuizen, L., & Majaranta, P. (2005). Survey of de-facto standards in eye tracking. COGAIN conf. on comm. by gaze inter.

Bauman, M. L., & Kemper, T. L. (2005). Neuroanatomic observations of the brain in autism: A review and future directions. *International Journal of Developmental Neuroscience*, *23*(2-3), 183–187. doi:10.1016/j.ijdevneu.2004.09.006 PMID:15749244

Bax, M., Goldstein, M., Rosenbaum, P., Leviton, A., Paneth, N., Dan, B., ... Damiano, D. (2005). Proposed definition and classification of cerebral palsy, April 2005. *Developmental Medicine and Child Neurology*, *47*(8), 571–576. doi:10.1017/S001216220500112X PMID:16108461

Baxter, A. J., Brugha, T. S., Erskine, H. E., Scheurer, R. W., Vos, T., & Scott, J. G. (2015). The epidemiology and global burden of autism spectrum disorders. *Psychological Medicine*, *45*, 601–613. PMID:25108395

Beck, A. R., Stoner, J. B., Bock, S. J., & Parton, T. (2008). Comparison of PECS and the use of a VOCA: A replication. *Education and Training in Developmental Disabilities*, *43*, 198–216.

Bedford, R., Gliga, T., Shephard, E., Elsabbagh, M., Pickles, A., Charman, T., & Johnson, M. H. (2017). Neurocognitive and observational markers: Prediction of autism spectrum disorder from infancy to mid-childhood. *Molecular Autism*, *8*(1), 49. doi:10.118613229-017-0167-3 PMID:29018511

Bedrosian, J. (1999). Efficacy research issues in AAC: Interactive storybook reading. *Augmentative and Alternative Communication*, *15*(1), 45–55. doi:10.1080/07434619912331278565

Bennett, B. E., Bryant, B. K., VandenBos, G. R., & Greenwood, A. (1990). *Professional liability and risk management*. Washington, DC: American Psychological Association. doi:10.1037/11102-000

Benssassi, E. M., Gomez, J., Boyd, L. A. E., Hayes, G. R., & Ye, J. (2018). Wearable assistive technologies for autism: Opportunities and challenges. *IEEE Pervasive Computing*, *17*(2), 11–21. doi:10.1109/MPRV.2018.022511239

Berkman, L. F., & Glass, T. (2000). Social integration, social networks, social support, and health. In L. F. Berkman & I. Kawachi (Eds.), *Social epidemiology*. Oxford, UK: Oxford University Press.

Berkman, L. F., Glass, T., Brissette, I., & Seeman, T. E. (2000). From social integration to health: Durkheim in the new millennium. *Social Science & Medicine*, *51*(6), 843–857. doi:10.1016/S0277-9536(00)00065-4 PMID:10972429

Bernardi, L., Sleight, P., Bandinelli, G., Cencetti, S., Fattorini, L., Wdowczyc-Szulc, J., & Lagi, A. (2001). Effect of rosary prayer and yoga mantras on autonomic cardiovascular rhythms: Comparative study. *BMJ (Clinical Research Ed.)*, *323*(7327), 1446–1449. doi:10.1136/bmj.323.7327.1446 PMID:11751348

Betts, D. E., & Betts, S. W. (2006). *Yoga for children with autism spectrum disorders*. Jessica Kingley Publishers.

Beukelman, D. R., & Mirenda, P. (1998). *Augmentative and alternative communication: Management of severe communication disorders in children and adults* (2nd ed.). Baltimore: Paul H. Brookes.

Beukelman, D., & Mirenda, P. (1998). *Augmentative and alternative communication: Supporting children and adults with complex communication needs* (3rd ed.). Baltimore: Brookes.

Beukelman, D., & Mirenda, P. (2005). *Augmentative and alternative communication: Management of severe communication impairments* (3rd ed.). Baltimore: Brookes.

Beutler, L. E., & Davidson, E. H. (1995). What standards should we use? In S. C. Hayes & V. M. Follette (Eds.), *Scientifi c standards of psychological practice: Issues and recommendations*. Academic Press.

Beymer, D., & Flickner, M. (2003, June). Eye gaze tracking using an active stereo head. In *2003 IEEE Computer Society Conference on Computer Vision and Pattern Recognition Proceedings*, *2*, II-451.

Bhargavan, R. (2019). Effectiveness of video assisted teaching on knowledge, attitude and practice among primary caregivers of children with Autism Spectrum Disorder Article information. *Advances in Autism*. doi:10.1108/AIA-10-2018-0039

Bhat, A., Landa, R., & Galloway, J. (2011). Current perspectives on motor functioning in infants, children, and adults with autism spectrum disorders. *Physical Therapy*, *91*, 1116–1129. PMID:21546566

Bhat, S., Acharya, U. R., Adeli, H., Bairy, G. M., & Adeli, A. (2014). Autism: Cause factors, early diagnosis and therapies. *Reviews in the Neurosciences*, *25*(6), 841–850. doi:10.1515/revneuro-2014-0056 PMID:25222596

Bhavanani, A. B. (2013). A closing word. In *Yoga Chikitsa: Application of yoga as a therapy* (1st ed.). Pondicherry, India: Dhivyananda Creations.

Bhavanani, A. B. (2017). Role of yoga in prevention and management of lifestyle disorders. *Yoga Mimamsa*, *49*(2), 42–47. doi:10.4103/ym.ym_14_17

Bhavanani, A. B., & Udupa, K. (2011). A comparative study of slow and fast suryanamaskar on physiological function. *International Journal of Yoga*, *4*(2), 71–77. doi:10.4103/0973-6131.85489 PMID:22022125

Bhuiyan, N. (2017). *Survey on prescription pattern of eye diseases & eye related drugs*. Academic Press.

Bigelow, K. E. (2012). Designing for Success. *Developing Engineers Who Consider Universal Design Principles.*, *25*(3), 211–225.

Billeci, L., Narzisi, A., Tonacci, A., Sbriscia-Fioretti, B., Serasini, L., Fulceri, F., ... Muratori, F. (2017). An integrated EEG and eye-tracking approach for the study of responding and initiating joint attention in Autism Spectrum Disorders. *Scientific Reports*, *7*(1), 13560. doi:10.103841598-017-13053-4 PMID:29051506

Binger, C. (2008). Grammatical morpheme intervention issues for students who use AAC. *Perspectives on Augmentative and Alternative Communication*, *17*(2), 62–68. doi:10.1044/aac17.2.62

Binger, C., & Kent-Walsh, J. (2012). Selecting skills to teach communication partners: Where do I start? *Perspectives on Augmentative and Alternative Communication*, *21*, 126–134.

Binger, C., & Light, J. (2006). Demographics-of-preschoolers-who-require-augmentative-and-alternativecommunication. *Language, Speech, and Hearing Services in Schools*, *37*, 200–208. PMID:16837443

Binger, C., & Light, J. (2007). The effect of aided AAC modeling on the expression of multi-symbol messages by preschoolers who use AAC. *Augmentative and Alternative Communication*, *23*, 30–43. doi:10.1080/07434610600807470 PMID:17364486

Binorkar, S. V. (2014). Yoga – The Non-Pharmaceutical Approach for Lifestyle Disorders. *Journal of Yoga & Physical Therapy*, *4*(04), e116. doi:10.4172/2157-7595.1000e116

Birbaumer, N. (2007). *A brain computer interface for restoration of movement following stroke*. Neuro Connections.

Bi, X., Wang, Y., Shu, Q., Sun, Q., & Xu, Q. (2018). Classification of Autism Spectrum Disorder Using Random Support Vector Machine Cluster. *Frontiers in Genetics*, *9*, 18. doi:10.3389/fgene.2018.00018 PMID:29467790

Blain, S., McKeever, P., & Chau, T. (2010). Bedside computer access for an individual with severe and multiple disabilities: A case study. *Disability and Rehabilitation. Assistive Technology*, *5*(5), 359–369. doi:10.3109/17483100903323275 PMID:20131978

Blomkvist, J., & Holmlid, S. (2010). Service prototyping according to practitioners. In *Proceedings of 2nd Service Design and Service Innovation conference, ServDes.2010. Linköping Electronic Conference Proceedings, 60*. Linköping, Sweden: Linköping University Electronic Press.

Bock, S. J., Stoner, J. B., Beck, A. R., Hanley, L., & Prochnow, J. (2005). Increasing functional communication in non-speaking preschool children: Comparison of PECS and VOCA. *Education and Training in Developmental Disabilities*, *40*, 264–278.

Bone, D., Bishop, S. L., Black, M. P., Goodwin, M. S., Lord, C., & Narayanan, S. S. (2016). Use of machine learning to improve autism screening and diagnostic instruments: Effectiveness, efficiency, and multi-instrument fusion. *Journal of Child Psychology and Psychiatry, and Allied Disciplines*, *57*(8), 927–937. doi:10.1111/jcpp.12559 PMID:27090613

Bone, D., Goodwin, M. S., Black, M. P., Lee, C. C., Audhkhasi, K., & Narayanan, S. (2014). Applying machine learning to facilitate autism diagnostics: Pitfalls and promises. *Journal of Autism and Developmental Disorders*, 1121–1136. PMID:25294649

Bone, D., Lee, C. C., Black, M. P., Williams, M. E., Lee, S., Levitt, P., & Narayanan, S. (2015). The psychologist as an interlocutor in autism spectrum disorder assessment: Insights from a study of spontaneous prosody. *Journal of Speech, Language, and Hearing Research: JSLHR*, *57*(4), 1162–1177. doi:10.1044/2014_JSLHR-S-13-0062 PMID:24686340

Bopp, K. D., Brown, K. E., & Mirenda, P. (2004). Article. *American Journal of Speech-Language Pathology*, *13*, 5–19. PMID:15101810

Borgestig, M., Falkmer, T., & Hemmingsson, H. (2013). Improving computer usage for students with physical disabilities through a collaborative approach: A pilot study. *Scandinavian Journal of Occupational Therapy*, *20*(6), 463–470. doi: 10.3109/11038128.2013.837506 PMID:24041227

Borgestig, M., Sandqvist, J., Ahlsten, G., Falkmer, T., & Hemmingsson, H. (2017). Gaze- based assistive technology in daily activities in children with severe physical impairments–An intervention study. *Developmental Neurorehabilitation*, *20*(3), 129–141. doi:10.3109/17518423.2015.1132281 PMID:26930111

Borg, J., Lindström, A., & Larsson, S. (2011). Assistive technology in developing countries: A review from the perspective of the Convention on the Rights of Persons with Disabilities. *Prosthetics and Orthotics International*, *35*(1), 20–29. doi:10.1177/0309364610389351 PMID:21515886

Borràs-Ferrís, L., Pérez-Ramírez, Ú., & Moratal, D. (2019). Link-level functional connectivity neuroalterations in autism spectrum disorder: A developmental resting-state fMRI study. *Diagnostics (Basel)*, *9*(1), 32. doi:10.3390/diagnostics9010032 PMID:30901848

Borsos, Z., & Gyori, M. (2017). *Can automated facial expression analysis show differences between autism and typical functioning?* Doi:10.3233/978-1-61499-798-6-797

Bos, D. J., Van Raalten, T. R., Oranje, B., Smits, A. R., Kobussen, N. A., Belle, J., & Van. (2014). Developmental differences in higher-order resting-state networks in Autism Spectrum Disorder. *NeuroImage. Clinical*, *4*, 820–827. doi:10.1016/j.nicl.2014.05.007 PMID:24936432

Bosl, W., Tierney, A., Tager-Flusberg, H., & Nelson, C. (2011). EEG complexity as a biomarker for autism spectrum disorder risk. *BMC Medicine*, *9*(1), 18. doi:10.1186/1741-7015-9-18 PMID:21342500

Boubela, R. N., Kalcher, K., Huf, W., Našel, C., & Moser, E. (2016). Big data approaches for the analysis of large-scale fMRI data using apache spark and GPU processing: A demonstration on restingstate fMRI data from the human connectome project. *Frontiers in Neuroscience*, *9*, 492. doi:10.3389/fnins.2015.00492 PMID:26778951

Boucenna, S., Narzisi, A., Tilmont, E., Muratori, F., Pioggia, G., Cohen, D., & Chetouani, M. (2014). Interactive technologies for autistic children: A review. *Cognitive Computation*, *6*(4), 722–740. doi:10.100712559-014-9276-x

Boutsika, E. (2014). Kinect in education: A proposal for children with autism. *Procedia Computer Science*, *27*, 123–129. doi:10.1016/j.procs.2014.02.015

Bowman, F. D. (2014). Brain Imaging Analysis. *Annual Review of Statistics and Its Application*, *1*(1), 61–85. doi:10.1146/annurev-statistics-022513-115611 PMID:25309940

Bozkurt, G., Uysal, G., & Duzkaya, D. S. (2019). Examination of care burden and stress coping styles of parents of children with autism spectrum disorder. *Journal of Pediatric Nursing, 47*, 142-147.

Bradshaw, J. (2013). The use of augmentative and alternative communication apps for the iPad, iPod and iPhone: An overview of recent developments. *Tizard Learning Disability Review*, *18*(1), 31–37. doi:10.1108/13595471311295996

Brady, N. (2000). Improved comprehension of object names following voice output communication aid use: Two case studies. *Augmentative and Alternative Communication*, *16*(3), 197–204. doi:10.1080/07434610012331279054

Brett, M., Christoff, K., Cusack, R., & Lancaster, J. (2001). Using the talairach atlas with the MNI template. *NeuroImage, 13*(6), 85. doi:10.1016/S1053-8119(01)91428-4

Brihadiswaran, G., Haputhanthri, D., Gunathilaka, S., Meedeniya, D., & Jayarathna, S. (2019). A Review of EEG-based Classification for Autism Spectrum Disorder. *Journal of Computational Science, 15*(8), 1161–1183. doi:10.3844/jcssp.2019.1161.1183

Bringas, J. A. S., León, M. A. C., Cota, I. E., & Carrillo, A. L. (2016, October). Development of a videogame to improve communication in children with autism. In *Learning Objects and Technology (LACLO), Latin American Conference on* (pp. 1-6). 10.1109/LACLO.2016.7751751

Brinker, T. J., Hekler, A., Utikal, J. S., Grabe, N., Schadendorf, D., Klode, J., ... von Kalle, C. (2018). Skin cancer classification using convolutional neural networks: Systematic review. *Journal of Medical Internet Research, 20*(10), e11936. doi:10.2196/11936 PMID:30333097

Brolly, X. L., & Mulligan, J. B. (2004, June). Implicit calibration of a remote gaze tracker. In *2004 Conference on Computer Vision and Pattern Recognition Workshop* (pp. 134-134). IEEE. 10.1109/CVPR.2004.366

Bron, T. I., Bijlenga, D., Kooij, J. J., Vogel, S. W. N., Wynchank, D., Beekman, A. T. F., & Penninx, B. W. J. H. (2016). Attention-deficit hyperactivity disorder symptoms add risk to circadian rhythm sleep problems in depression and anxiety. *Journal of Affective Disorders, 200*, 74–81. doi:10.1016/j.jad.2016.04.022 PMID:27128360

Brown, R. I., Schalock, R. L., & Brown, I. (2009). Quality of life: Its application to persons with intellectual disabilities and their families-introduction and overview. *Journal of Policy and Practice in Intellectual Disabilities, 6*(1), 2–6. doi:10.1111/j.1741-1130.2008.00202.x

Brown, T., & Wyatt, J. (2010). Design thinking for social innovation. *Development Outreach, 12*(1), 29–43. doi:10.1596/1020-797X_12_1_29

Bruner, J. (1986). *Actual minds, possible worlds*. Cambridge, MA: Harvard University Press.

Brunero, F., Venerosi, A., Chiarotti, F., & Arduino, G. M. (2019). Are touch screen technologies more effective than traditional educational methods in children with autism spectrum disorders? A pilot study. *Annali dell'Istituto Superiore di Sanita, 55*, 151–160. PMID:31264638

Budzynski, T. H., Budzynski, H. K., Evans, J. R., & Abarbanel, A. (Eds.). (2009). *Introduction to quantitative EEG and neurofeedback: Advanced theory and applications*. Academic Press.

Buie, A. T., Campbell, D. B., Hyman, S. L., & Jirapinyo, P. (2010). Evaluation, Diagnosis, and Treatment of Gastrointestinal disorders in Individuals with ASDs: A consensus report. *Pediatrics, 125*(Supplement 1), S1–S18. doi:10.1542/peds.2009-1878C PMID:20048083

Buitrago, J. A., Bolaños, A. M., & Caicedo Bravo, E. (2019). A motor learning therapeutic intervention for a child with cerebral palsy through a social assistive robot. *Disability and Rehabilitation. Assistive Technology*, 1–6. doi:10.1080/17483107.2019.1578999 PMID:30806105

Bussing, R., Fernandez, M., Harwood, M., Wei Hou, W., Garvan, C. W., Eyberg, S. M., & Swanson, J. M. (2008). Parent and teacher SNAP-IV ratings of attention deficit hyperactivity disorder symptoms: Psychometric properties and normative ratings from a school district sample. *Assessment, 15*(3), 317–328. doi:10.1177/1073191107313888 PMID:18310593

Caballero-Gaudes, C., & Reynolds, R. C. (2017). Methods for cleaning the BOLD fMRI signal. *NeuroImage, 154*, 128–149. doi:10.1016/j.neuroimage.2016.12.018 PMID:27956209

Caffò, A. O., Hoogeveen, F., Groenendaal, M., Perilli, V., Damen, M., Stasolla, F., ... Bosco, A. (2014). Comparing two different orientation strategies for promoting indoor traveling in people with Alzheimer's disease. *Research in Developmental Disabilities*, *35*(2), 572–580. doi:10.1016/j.ridd.2013.12.003 PMID:24380786

Căleanu, C. D. (2013, May). Face expression recognition: A brief overview of the last decade. In *2013 IEEE 8th International Symposium on Applied Computational Intelligence and Informatics (SACI)* (pp. 157-161). IEEE. 10.1109/SACI.2013.6608958

Calhoun, M., Longworth, M., & Chester, V. L. (2011). Gait patterns in children with autism. *Clinical Biomechanics (Bristol, Avon)*, *26*(2), 200–206. doi:10.1016/j.clinbiomech.2010.09.013 PMID:20934239

Campbell, J. E., & Mears, K. M. (2009). *Habilitative treatments for children with ASDs: Speech and occupational therapy, assistive technology*. doi:10.1017/CBO9780511978616.010

Campbell, D. B., Sutcliffe, J. S., Ebert, P. J., Militerni, R., Bravaccio, C., Trillo, S., & … . (2006). A genetic variant that disrupts *MET* transcription is associated with autism. *Proceedings of the National Academy of Sciences of the United States of America*, *10*, 16834–16839. PMID:17053076

Carlsson, M., Hagberg, G., & Olsson, I. (2003). Clinical and aetiological aspects of epilepsy in children with cerebral palsy. *Developmental Medicine and Child Neurology*, *45*(6), 371–376. doi:10.1111/j.1469-8749.2003.tb00415.x PMID:12785437

Caron, J., & Light, J. (2016). "Social media has opened a world of 'open communication:'" Experiences of adults with cerebral palsy who use augmentative and alternative communication and social media. *Augmentative and Alternative Communication*, *32*(1), 25–40. doi:10.3109/07434618.2015.1052887 PMID:26056722

Carper, R., & Courchesne, E. (2005). Localized enlargement of the frontal lobe in autism. *Biological Psychiatry*, *57*, 126–133. PMID:15652870

Carter, M. (2003). Communicative spontaneity of children with high support needs who use augmentative and alternative communication systems II: Antecedents and effectiveness of communication. *Augmentative and Alternative Communication*, *19*(3), 155–169. doi:10.1080/0743461031000112025

Carter, M. T., & Scherer, S. W. (2013). Autism spectrum disorder in the genetics clinic: A review. *Clinical Genetics*, *83*(5), 399–407. doi:10.1111/cge.12101 PMID:23425232

Carter, M., & Grunsell, J. (2001). The behaviour chain interruption strategy: A review of research and discussion of future directions. *Research and Practice for Persons with Severe Disabilities*, *26*(1), 37–49. doi:10.1177/1540796919828082

Casanova, M. F., Buxhoeveden, D., Switala, A., & Roy, E. (2002). Minicolumn pathology in autism. *Neurology*, *58*, 428–432. PMID:11839843

Case, M., Zhang, H., Mundahl, J., Datta, Y., Nelson, S., Gupta, K., & He, B. (2017). Characterization of functional brain activity and connectivity using EEG and fMRI in patients with sickle cell disease. *NeuroImage. Clinical*, *14*, 1–17. doi:10.1016/j.nicl.2016.12.024 PMID:28116239

CDC. (2018). *Centers for Disease Control and Prevention, Data and Statistics About ADHD*. Retrieved March 4, 2019, from https://www.cdc.gov/ncbddd/adhd/data.html

Chaddad, A., Desrosiers, C., Hassan, L., & Tanougast, C. (2017). Hippocampus and amygdala radiomic biomarkers for the study of autism spectrum disorder. *BMC Neuroscience*, *18*(1), 52. doi:10.118612868-017-0373-0 PMID:28821235

Chalkiadaki, A. (2018). A systematic literature review of 21st century skills and competencies in primary education. *International Journal of Instruction*, *11*(3), 1–16. doi:10.12973/iji.2018.1131a

Champa, H. N. & AnandaKumar, K. R. (2010, August). Automated human behavior prediction through handwriting analysis. In *2010 First International Conference on Integrated Intelligent Computing* (pp. 160-165). IEEE.

Chanel, G., Pichon, S., Conty, L., Berthoz, S., Chevallier, C., & Grèzes, J. (2016). Classification of autistic individuals and controls using cross-task characterization of fMRI activity. *NeuroImage. Clinical*, *10*, 78–88. doi:10.1016/j.nicl.2015.11.010 PMID:26793434

Charyulu, K. V. (1999). *Environment Education.* New Delhi, India: Neelkamal Publishers.

Chattha, R., Raghuram, N., Venkatram, P., & Hongasandra, N. R. (2008). Treating the climacteric symptoms in Indian women with an integrated approach to yoga therapy: A randomized control study. *Menopause (New York, N.Y.)*, *15*(5), 862–870. doi:10.1097/gme.0b013e318167b902 PMID:18463543

Chawarska, K., Paul, R., Klin, A., Hannigen, S., Dichtel, L. E., & Volkmar, F. (2007). Parental recognition of developmental problems in toddlers with autism spectrum disorders. *Journal of Autism and Developmental Disorders*, *37*(1), 62–72. PMID:17195921

Chen, C. H., Chou, Y., & Huang, C. Y. (2016). An Augmented-Reality-Based Concept Map to Support Mobile Learning for Science. *The Asia-Pacific Education Researcher*, *25*(4), 567–578. doi:10.100740299-016-0284-3

Chen, H., Duan, X., Liu, F., Lu, F., Ma, X., Zhang, Y., ... Chen, H. (2016). Multivariate classification of autism spectrum disorder using frequency-specific resting-state functional connectivity—A multi-center study. *Progress in Neuro-Psychopharmacology & Biological Psychiatry*, *64*, 1–9. doi:10.1016/j.pnpbp.2015.06.014 PMID:26148789

Chen, J. L., Leader, G., Sung, C., & Leahy, M. (2015). Trends in employment for individuals with autism spectrum disorder: A review of the research literature. *Research Journal of Autism and Developmental Disorders*, *2*(2), 115–127. doi:10.100740489-014-0041-6

Chenowith, N. H. (2014). Culturally responsive pedagogy and cultural scaffolding in literacy education. *Ohio Reading Teacher*, *44*(1), 35–40.

Chen, W. (2012). Multitouch tabletop technology for people with autism spectrum disorder: A review of the literature. *Procedia Computer Science*, *14*, 198–207. doi:10.1016/j.procs.2012.10.023

Chiang, H. M. (2009). Naturalistic observations of elicited expressive communication of children with autism: An analysis of teacher instructions. *Autism*, *13*(2), 165–178. doi:10.1177/1362361308098513 PMID:19261686

Choi, C., & O'Brien, M. (2019). The impact of familism on future care planning for Korean parents caring for their children living with disabilities. *Asia Pacific Journal of Social Work and Development*, 1–14.

Chollet, F. (2015). *Keras*. Retrieved January 3, 2019, from https://keras.io/

Christensen, D. L., Baio, J., & Van Naarden Braun, K. (2016). Prevalence and characteristics of autism spectrum disorder among children aged 8 years—autism and developmental disabilities monitoring network, 11 sites, United States, 2012. *MMWR. Surveillance Summaries*, *65*, 1–23. PMID:27031587

Christiansen, C. H. (1999, November). Defining Lives: Occupation as Identity: An Essay on Competence, Coherence, and the Creation of Meaning. *The American Journal of Occupational Therapy*, *53*(6), 547–558. doi:10.5014/ajot.53.6.547 PMID:10578432

Chu, W., Xue, H., Yao, C., & Cai, D. (2018). Sparse Coding Guided Spatiotemporal Feature Learning for Abnormal Event Detection in Large Videos. *IEEE Transactions on Multimedia*, *21*(1), 246–255. doi:10.1109/TMM.2018.2846411

Clarke, H., McConachie, K., Price, P., & Wood, M. (2001). Views of young people using augmentative and alternative communication systems. *International Journal of Language & Communication Disorders*, *36*(1), 107–115. doi:10.1080/13682820150217590 PMID:11221427

Clarke, M., & Kirton, A. (2003). Patterns of interaction between children with physical disabilities using augmentative and alternative communication systems and their peers. *Child Language Teaching and Therapy*, *19*(2), 135–151. doi:10.1191/0265659003ct248oa

Clarke, M., & Price, K. (2012). Augmentative and alternative communication for children with cerebral palsy. *Paediatrics & Child Health*, *22*(9), 367–371. doi:10.1016/j.paed.2012.03.002

Clarke, M., & Wilkinson, R. (2008). Interaction between children with cerebral palsy and their peers 2: Understanding initiated VOCA-mediated turns. *Augmentative and Alternative Communication*, *24*(1), 3–15. doi:10.1080/07434610701390400 PMID:18256962

Clark, K. R. (2018). Learning theories: Constructivism. *Radiologic Technology*, *90*(2), 180–182. Retrieved from http://www.radiologictechnology.org/content/90/2/180.full.pdf+html PMID:30420576

Clay, V., König, P., & König, S. U. (2019). *Eye tracking in virtual reality*. Academic Press.

Clifford, S., Young, R., & Williamson, P. (2007). Assessing the early characteristics of autistic disorder using video analysis. *Journal of Autism and Developmental Disorders*, *37*(2), 301–313. doi:10.100710803-006-0160-8 PMID:17031450

Cloete, T. L., Wilson, W. J., Petersen, L., & Kathard, H. (2015). Identifying a context-effective school hearing screening test: An emic/etic framework. *International Journal of Audiology*, *54*(9), 605–612. doi:10.3109/14992027.2015.1014575 PMID:25766492

Coben, R. (2006, October). *Hemoencephalography for autistic spectrum disorder*. In The14th Annual Conference of the International Society for Neuronal Regulation, Atlanta, GA.

Cochrane, K. (2010). *Comprehensive neurofeedback training in the context of psychotherapy for transformational change* (Doctoral dissertation). International University for Graduate Studies.

Cockerill, H., Elbourne, D., Allen, E., Scrutton, D., Will, E., McNee, A., ... Baird, G. (2014). Speech, communication and use of augmentative communication in young people with cerebral palsy: The SH & PE population study. *Child: Care, Health and Development*, *40*(2), 149–157. doi:10.1111/cch.12066 PMID:23656274

Cohan, A., & Howlett, C. F. (2017). Global conflicts shattered world peace: John Dewey's influence on peace educators and practitioners. *Education and Culture*, *33*(1), 59–88. doi:10.5703/educationculture.33.1.0059

Cohen, S. (2004). Social relationships and health. *The American Psychologist*, *59*(8), 676–684. doi:10.1037/0003-066X.59.8.676 PMID:15554821

Cohen, S., Conduit, R., Lockley, S. W., Rajaratnam, S. M., & Cornish, K. M. (2014). The relationship between sleep and behavior in autism spectrum disorder (ASD): A review. *Journal of Neurodevelopmental Disorders*, *6*(1), 44. doi:10.1186/1866-1955-6-44 PMID:25530819

Colker, R. (1999). Americans with disabilities act: A windfall for defendants. *Harvard Civil Rights-Civil Liberties Law Review*, 34–99.

Coloigner, J., Kim, Y., Bush, A., Choi, S., Balderrama, M. C., Coates, T. D., ... Wood, J. C. (2017). Contrasting resting-state fMRI abnormalities from sickle and non-sickle anemia. *PLoS One*, *12*(10), e0184860. doi:10.1371/journal.pone.0184860 PMID:28981541

Colque, Caetano, Lustosa de Andrade, & Schwartz. (2016). Histograms of Optical Flow Orientation and Magnitude and Entropy to Detect Anomalous Events in Videos. *IEEE Transactions on Circuits and Systems for Video Technology, 27*, 673–682.

Cook, A. M., & Polgar, J. M. (2014). *Assistive technologies: Principles and practice* (4th ed.). St. Louis, MO: Elsevier Health Sciences.

Cook, A. M., & Polgar, J. M. (2014). *Essentials of Assistive Technologies-E-Book*. Elsevier Health Sciences.

Cook, R., Tessier, A., Klein, M., & Armbruster, V. (2000). Nurturing communication skills. In R. E. Cook, A. Tessier, & M. D. Klein (Eds.), *Adapting early childhood curricula for children in inclusive settings* (5th ed., pp. 290–339). Englewood Cliffs, NJ: Merrill.

Coons, K., & Watson, S. (2013). Conducting Research with Individuals Who Have Intellectual Disabilities: Ethical and Practical Implications for Qualitative Research. *Journal on Developmental Disabilities, 19*(2), 14–24.

Copley, J., & Ziviani, J. (2004). Barriers to the use of assistive technology for children with multiple disabilities. *Occupational Therapy International, 11*(4), 229–243. doi:10.1002/oti.213 PMID:15771212

Copley, J., & Ziviani, J. (2007). Use of a team-based approach to assistive technology assessment and planning for children with multiple disabilities: A pilot study. *Assistive Technology, 19*(3), 109–127. doi:10.1080/10400435.2007.10131869 PMID:17937054

Copple, K., Koul, R., Banda, D., & Frye, E. (2015). An examination of the effectiveness of video modelling intervention using a speech-generating device in preschool children at risk for autism. *Developmental Neurorehabilitation, 18*(2), 104–112. doi:10.3109/17518423.2014.880079 PMID:24564246

Cotter, J., Granger, K., Backx, R., Hobbs, M., Looi, C. Y., & Barnett, J. H. (2017). Social cognitive dysfunction as a clinical marker: A systematic review of meta-analyses across 30 clinical conditions. *Neuroscience and Biobehavioral Reviews*. PMID:29175518

Courchesne, E., Redcay, E., Morgan, J. T., & Kennedy, D. P. (2005). Autism at the beginning: Microstructural and growth abnormalities underlying the cognitive and behavioural phenotype of autism. *Development and Psychopathology, 17*(3), 577–597. PMID:16262983

Craddock, D., O'Halloran, C., Borthwick, A., & McPherson, K. (2006). Interprofessional education in health and social care: Fashion or informed practice? *Learning in Health and Social Care, 5*(4), 220–242. doi:10.1111/j.1473-6861.2006.00135.x

Crawford, M. R., & Schuster, J. W. (1993). Using microswitches to teach toy use. *Journal of Developmental and Physical Disabilities, 5*(4), 349–368. doi:10.1007/BF01046391

Critchley, H. D., Elliott, R., & Mathias, C. J. (2000). Neural activity relating to the generation and representation of galvanic skin conductance response: A functional magnetic imaging study. *The Journal of Neuroscience, 20*, 3033–3040. PMID:10751455

Croso, C. (2013). Human rights are the key to the world we want. *Adult Education and Development, 80*, 78–85. Retrieved from http://www.iiz-dvv.de/en/adult-education-and-development/editions/aed-802013-post-2015/articles/human-rights-are-the-key-to-the-world-we-want/

Crutchfield, B. (2016). *ADA and the Internet: ADA Settlements-Fitting Accessibility Compliance into Your Product Lifecycle*. SSB Bart Group.

Culp, D. M., & Carlisle, M. (1988). *Partners in augmentative communication training (PACT): A resource guide for interaction facilitation training for children*. Tucson: Communication Skill Builders.

Cyganek, B., Graña, M., Krawczyk, B., Kasprzak, A., Porwik, P., Walkowiak, K., & Woźniak, M. (2016). A Survey of Big Data Issues in Electronic Health Record Analysis. *Applied Artificial Intelligence*, *30*(6), 497–520. doi:10.1080/08839514.2016.1193714

Da Silva Morais, T. (2015, January). Survey on frameworks for distributed computing: Hadoop, Spark and Storm. In *Proceedings of the 10th Doctoral Symposium in Informatics Engineering-DSIE* (*Vol. 15*). Academic Press.

Dada, S., & Alant, E. (2009). The effect of aided language stimulation on vocabulary acquisition in children with little or no functional speech. *American Journal of Speech-Language Pathology*, *18*(1), 50–64. doi:10.1044/1058-0360(2008/07-0018) PMID:19106207

Daley, T. C., Singhal, N., & Krishnamurthy, V. (2013). Ethical considerations in conducting research on autism spectrum disorders in low and middle income countries. *Journal of Autism and Developmental Disorders*, *43*(9), 2002–2014. doi:10.100710803-012-1750-2 PMID:23283629

Daley, T. C., Weisner, T., & Singhal, N. (2014). Adults with autism in India: A mixed-method approach to make meaning of daily routines. *Social Science & Medicine*, *116*, 142–149. doi:10.1016/j.socscimed.2014.06.052 PMID:24998867

Dalwai, S., Ahmed, S., Udani, V., Mundkar, N., Kamath, S. S., & Nair, M. K. C. for the National Consultation Meeting for developing IAP guidelines on Neuro Developmental disorders under the aegis of IAP Childhood Disability Group and the Committee on Child Development and Neurodevelopmental disorders (2017). Consensus statement of the Indian Academy of Pediatrics on evaluation and management of autism spectrum disorders. *Indian Pediatr, 54*, 385-393.

Dam, R., & Siang, T. (2019). *5 Stages in the Design Thinking Process.* Access at https://www.interaction-design.org/literature/article/5-stages-in-the-design-thinking-process on 12/07/2019

Daniels, J. L., Forssen, U., Hultman, C. M., Cnattingius, S., Savitz, D. A., Feychting, M., & Sparen, P. (2008). Parental Psychiatric Disorders Associated with Autism Spectrum Disorders. *Paediatrics*, *121*, 1357–1362. PMID:18450879

Dautenhahn, K., & Billard, A. (2002). Games children with autism can play with Robota, a humanoid robotic doll. In Universal access and assistive technology (pp. 179-190). doi:10.1007/978-1-4471-3719-1_18

David, D. O., Costescu, C. A., Matu, S., Szentagotai, A., & Dobrean, A. (in press). Effects of a robot-enhanced intervention for children with ASD on teaching turn-taking skills. *Journal of Educational Computing Research.* doi:10.1177/0735633119830344

Dawson, G., & Osterling, J. (1997). Early intervention in autism. In M. Guralnick (Ed.), *The effectiveness of early intervention* (pp. 307–326). Baltimore, MD: Brookes.

DC, D. (1999). *Military Standard: Human Engineering Design Criteria for Military Systems, Equipment and facilities.* Lockheed Human Factors Engineering Group.

De Pace, C., & Stasolla, F. (2014). Promoting Environmental Control, Social Interaction, and Leisure/Academy Engagement Among People with Severe/Profound Multiple Disabilities Through Assistive Technology. In G. Kouroupetroglou (Ed.), Assistive Technologies and Computer Access for Motor Disabilities (pp. 285–319). Hershey, PA: IGI Global. doi:10.4018/978-1-4666-4438-0.ch010

de Silva, S., Dayarathna, S., Ariyarathne, G., Meedeniya, D., & Jayarathna, S. (2019a). A Survey of Attention Deficit Hyperactivity Disorder Identification Using Psychophysiological Data. *International Journal of Online and Biomedical Engineering*, *15*(13), 61–76. doi:10.3991/ijoe.v15i13.10744 de Silva, S., Dayarathna, S., Ariyarathne, G., Meedeniya, D., & Jayarathna, S. (2020). ADHD Identification using CNN with Seed-based Correlation Approach for fMRI Data. In *9th International Conference on Software and Computer Applications (ICSCA 2020)*. ACM.

de Silva, S., Dayarathna, S., Ariyarathne, G., Meedeniya, D., Jayarathna, S., Michalek, A. M. P., & Jayawardena, G. (2019b). A Rule-Based System for ADHD Identification using Eye Movement Data. In *Moratuwa Engineering Research Conference (MERCon)*, (pp. 538-543), IEEE. 10.1109/MERCon.2019.8818865

de Vos, F., Koini, M., Schouten, T. M., Seiler, S., van der Grond, J., Lechner, A., ... Rombouts, S. A. R. B. (2018). A comprehensive analysis of resting state fMRI measures to classify individual patients with Alzheimer's disease. *NeuroImage*, *167*, 62–72. doi:10.1016/j.neuroimage.2017.11.025 PMID:29155080

DeCoste, D. C. (1997). T: programs for children who employ AAC systems due to severe speech and physical disabilities continues to present a monumental challenge to professionals. The reason is simple yet confounding: unable to speak or to manipulate pencil and paper, these children have difficulty developing and demonstrating their ability to read and write through convention. The Handbook of Augmentative and Alternative Communication, 283.

DeHart, J. D. (2019). Two Birds, One Stone: Exploring complex writing through poetry. *Knowledge Quest*, *47*(5), E1–E4.

Dehkordi, S. R. & Riaza. M. R. (2014). *Using Mobile Game Application to Teach Children with Autism Spectrum Disorder (ASD) Multiple Cues Responding: A Pilot Study*. doi:10.1109/IUSER.2014.7002705

Dekhil, O., Hajjdiab, H., Ayinde, B., Shalaby, A., Switala, A., Sosnin, D., … El-baz, A. (2018). Using Resting State Functional MRI to Build A Personalized Autism Diagnosis System. *2018 IEEE 15th International Symposium on Biomedical Imaging (ISBI 2018)*, 1381–1385.

Demos, J. N. (2005). *Getting started with neurofeedback*. New York: W. W. Norton & Company.

Deng, L. (2014). Deep Learning: Methods and Applications. *Foundations and Trends® in Signal Processing, 7*(3–4), 197–387. doi:10.1561/2000000039

Deruyter, F., McNaughton, D., Caves, K., Bryen, D. N., & Williams, M. B. (2007). Enhancing AAC connections with the world. *Augmentative and Alternative Communication*, *23*(3), 258–270. doi:10.1080/07434610701553387 PMID:17701744

Dewey, J., & Jackson, P. W. (1990). *The school and society and the child and the curriculum a centennial publication*. Chicago, IL: The University of Chicago Press.

Dhillon, H. S., Singla, R., Rekhi, N. S., & Jha, R. (2009, August). EOG and EMG based virtual keyboard: A brain-computer interface. In *2009 2nd IEEE International Conference on Computer Science and Information Technology* (pp. 259-262). IEEE. 10.1109/ICCSIT.2009.5234951

Dhir, H. (2019). Planning curriculum for teaching thinking skills needed for 21st century education. In Handbook of research on critical thinking and teacher education pedagogy (pp. 107-133). doi:1 doi:0.4018/978-1-5225-7829-1.ch007

Di Martino, A., O'Connor, D., Chen, B., Alaerts, K., Anderson, J. S., Assaf, M., ... Blanken, L. M. (2017). Enhancing studies of the connectome in autism using the autism brain imaging data exchange II. *Scientific Data*, *4*(1), 170010. doi:10.1038data.2017.10 PMID:28291247

Di Martino, A., Yan, C. G., Li, Q., Denio, E., Castellanos, F. X., Alaerts, K., ... Milham, M. P. (2014). The autism brain imaging data exchange: Towards a large-scale evaluation of the intrinsic brain architecture in autism. *Molecular Psychiatry*, *19*(6), 659–667. doi:10.1038/mp.2013.78 PMID:23774715

Diamond, A., & Lee, K. (2011). Interventions shown to aid executive function development in children 4-12 years Old. *Science*, *19*(6045), 959–964. doi:10.1126cience.1204529 PMID:21852486

Didehbani, N., Allen, T., Kandalaft, M., Krawczyk, D., & Chapman, S. (2016). Virtual reality social cognition training for children with high functioning autism. *Computers in Human Behavior, 62*, 703–711. doi:10.1016/j.chb.2016.04.033

Dinov, I. D. (2016). Volume and value of big healthcare data. *Journal of Medical Statistics and Informatics, 4*(1), 4. doi:10.7243/2053-7662-4-3 PMID:26998309

Dinov, M., & Leech, R. (2017). Tracking and optimizing human performance using deep reinforcement learning in closed-loop behavioral-and neurofeedback: A proof of concept. *bioRxiv*, 225995.

Dixon, D. (2011). The future of apps in the classroom. *ASHA Leader, 16*(12), 30–30. doi:10.1044/leader.SCM.16122011.30

Doijad, V. P., & Surdi, A. D. (2012). Effect of short term yoga practice on pulmonary function tests. *Indian Journal of Basic and Applied Medical Research, 3*(1), 226–230.

Donofrio, M. T., Bremer, Y. A., Schieken, R. M., Gennings, C., Morton, L. D., Eidem, B. W., ... Kleinman, C. S. (2003). Autoregulation of cerebral blood flow in fetuses with congenital heart disease: The brain sparing effect. *Pediatric Cardiology, 24*(5), 436–443. doi:10.100700246-002-0404-0 PMID:14627309

Donovan, L., Green, T. D., & Mason, C. (2014). Examining the 21st century classroom: Developing an innovation configuration map. *Journal of Educational Computing Research, 50*(2), 161–178. doi:10.2190/EC.50.2.a

Douglas, S. N. (2012). Teaching para educators to support communication of individuals who use augmentative and alternative communication: A literature review. *Current Issues in Education, 15*(1), 1–12.

Doumas, M., McKenna, R., & Murphy, B. (2015). Postural Control Deficits in Autism Spectrum Disorder: The Role of Sensory Integration. *Journal of Autism and Developmental Disorders, 46*(3), 853–861. doi:10.100710803-015-2621-4 PMID:26446773

Drewes, H. (2010). *Eye Gaze Tracking for Human Computer Interaction* (PhD dissertation). www.ndltd.org

Duchowski, A. T. (2007). Eye tracking methodology. *Theory into Practice, 328*(614), 2–3.

Duda, M., Ma, R., Haber, N., & Wall, D. P. (2016). Use of machine learning for behavioral distinction of autism and ADHD. *Translational Psychiatry, 6*(2), 732. doi:10.1038/tp.2015.221 PMID:26859815

Duffy, F. H., Hughes, J. R., Miranda, F., Bernard, P., & Cook, P. (1994). Status of quantitative EEG (QEEG) in clinical practice: 1994. *Clinical Electroencephalography.*

Dunst, C. J. (2002). Family-centered practices: Birth through high school. *The Journal of Special Education, 36*(3), 141–149. doi:10.1177/00224669020360030401

Duvekot, van der Ende, Verhulst, Slappendel, van Daalen, Maras, & Greaves-Lord. (2016). Factors influencing the probability of a diagnosis of autism spectrum disorder in girls versus boys. *SAGE Journals, 21*(6), 646 – 658.

Du, Y., Fu, Z., & Calhoun, V. D. (2018). Classification and prediction of brain disorders using functional connectivity: Promising but challenging. *Frontiers in Neuroscience, 12*, 1–29. doi:10.3389/fnins.2018.00525 PMID:30127711

Dvornek, N. C., Ventola, P., & Duncan, J. S. (2018). Combining Phenotypic and Resting-State fMRI Data For Autism Classification with Recurrent Neural Networks. *2018 IEEE 15th International Symposium on Biomedical Imaging (ISBI 2018)*, 725–728.

Dworzynski, K., Ronald, A., Bolton, P., & Happé, F. (2012). How different are girls and boys above and below the diagnostic threshold for autism spectrum disorders. *Journal of the American Academy of Child and Adolescent Psychiatry, 51*(8), 788–797. doi:10.1016/j.jaac.2012.05.018 PMID:22840550

Effort, M. (2019). 618 - பொறியின்மை யார்க்கும் பழியன்று அறிவறிந்து ஆள்வினை இன்மை பழி. *Manly Effort - Wealth - Thirukkural*. Available at: https://www.thirukkural.net/en/kural/kural-0618.html

Ekinci, O., Arman, A. R., Işık, U., Bez, Y., & Berkem, M. (2010). EEG abnormalities and epilepsy in autistic spectrum disorders: Clinical and familial correlates. *Epilepsy & Behavior*, *17*(2), 178–182. doi:10.1016/j.yebeh.2009.11.014 PMID:20042370

Elmquist, M., Simacek, J., Dimian, A. F., & Reichle, J. (2019). Impact of aided AAC interventions on speech comprehension of children with neurodevelopmental disabilities: A critically appraised topic. *Evidence-Based Communication Assessment and Intervention*, *13*(1-2), 67–84. published online16Apr2019. doi:10.1080/17489539.2019.1598011

Elsabbagh, M., Mercure, E., Hudry, K., Chandler, S., Pasco, G., Charman, T., … Johnson, M. H. (2012). *Infant neural sensitivity to dynamic eye gaze is associated with later emerging autism*. Academic Press.

Engelke, C., & Higginbotham, J. (2013). Looking to speak: On the temporality of misalignment in interaction involving an augmented communicator using eye-gaze technology. *Journal of Interactional Research in Communication Disorders*, *4*(1), 95–122. doi:10.1558/jircd.v4i1.95

Eshraghi, A. A., Liu, G., Kay, S. I. S., Eshraghi, R. S., Mittal, J., Moshiree, B., & Mittal, R. (2018). Epigenetics and Autism Spectrum Disorder: Is There a Correlation? *Frontiers in Cellular Neuroscience*, *12*, 78. doi:10.3389/fncel.2018.00078 PMID:29636664

Eslami, T., Mirjalili, V., Fong, A., Laird, A., & Saeed, F. (2019). *ASD-DiagNet : A hybrid learning approach for detection of Autism Spectrum Disorder using fMRI data*. ArXiv Preprint ArXiv:1904.07577

Estepa, A., Piriz, S. S., Albornoz, E., & Martínez, C. (2016, April). Development of a Kinect-based exergaming system for motor rehabilitation in neurological disorders. *Journal of Physics: Conference Series*, *705*(1), 012060. doi:10.1088/1742-6596/705/1/012060

Evans, D. W., Uljarević, M., Lusk, L. G., Loth, E., & Frazier, T. (2017). Development of two dimensional measures of restricted and repetitive behavior in parents and children. *Journal of the American Academy of Child and Adolescent Psychiatry*, *56*(1), 51–58. doi:10.1016/j.jaac.2016.10.014 PMID:27993229

Ewald, W., & Lightfoot, A. (2001). *I wanna take me a picture: Teaching photography and writing to children*. Boston: Beacon Press.

Fabri, M., Andrews, P. C. S., & Pukki, H. (2016). Using Design Thinking to engage autistic students in participatory design of an online toolkit to help with transition into higher education. *Journal of Assistive Technologies, 10*(2).

Fage, C., Consel, C. Y., Balland, E., Etchegoyhen, K., Amestoy, A., Bouvard, M., & Sauzéon, H. (2018). Tablet apps to support first school inclusion of children with autism spectrum disorders (ASD) in mainstream classrooms: A pilot study. *Frontiers in Psychology*, *9*. PMID:30405498

Fage, C., Consel, C., Etchegoyhen, K., Amestoy, A., Bouvard, M., Mazon, C., & Sauzéon, H. (2019). An emotion regulation app for school inclusion of children with ASD: Design principles and evaluation. *Computers & Education*, *131*, 1–21. doi:10.1016/j.compedu.2018.12.003

Faghri, F., Hashemi, S. H., Babaeizadeh, M., Nalls, M. A., Sinha, S., & Campbell, R. H. (2017). *Toward Scalable Machine Learning and Data Mining: the Bioinformatics Case*. arXiv preprint arXiv:1710.00112

Fallon, K. A., & Katz, L. A. (2008, May). Augmentative and alternative communication and literacy teams: Facing the challenges, forging ahead. *Seminars in Speech and Language*, *29*(02), 112–119. doi:10.1055-2008-1079125 PMID:18645913

Fan, H., Li, L., Gilbert, R., O'Callaghan, F., & Wijlaars, L. (2018). A machine learning approach to identify cases of cerebral palsy using the UK primary care database. *Lancet*, *392*, S33. doi:10.1016/S0140-6736(18)32077-4

Fan, J., Wade, J. W., Key, A. P., Warren, Z. E., & Sarkar, N. (2018). EEG-based affect and workload recognition in a virtual driving environment for ASD intervention. *IEEE Transactions on Biomedical Engineering*, *65*(1), 43–51. doi:10.1109/TBME.2017.2693157 PMID:28422647

Fauci, A. S., Braunwald, E., & Isselbacher, K. J. (1998). *Harrison's Principles of Internal Medicine*. New York: McGraw Hill.

Fedotchev, A. I., Parin, S. B., Polevaya, S. A., & Velikova, S. D. (2017). Brain-computer interface and neurofeedback technologies: current state, problems and clinical prospects (review). *Sovremennye tehnologii v medicine, 9*(1), 175-184.

Fedotchev, A. I., Parin, S. B., Polevaya, S. A., & Velikova, S. D. (2017). Brain–computer interface and neurofeedback technologies: current state, problems and clinical prospects. *Современные технологии в медицине, 9*(1).

Felce, D., & Perry, J. (1995). Quality of life: Its definition and measurement. *Research in Developmental Disabilities*, *16*(1), 51–74. doi:10.1016/0891-4222(94)00028-8 PMID:7701092

Feldman, B., Martin, E. M., & Skotnes, T. (2012). Big data in healthcare hype and hope. *October 2012. Dr. Bonnie, 360.*

Felten, P. (2008). Resource review: Visual literacy. *Change Magazine,* 60-63.

Fey, M., Warren, S., Brady, N., Finestack, L., Brejin-Oja, S., Fairchild, M., ... Yoder, P. (2006). Early e.ffects of responsivity education/prelinguistic milieu teaching for children with developmental delays and their parents. *International Journal of Speech-Language Pathology*, *49*(3), 526–547. PMID:16787894

Filipek, P.A., Accardo, P.J., & Baranek, G.T. (1999). The screening and diagnosis of autistic spectrum disorders. *Journal of Autism Developmental Disorder, 29*(6), 439–84.

Filipek, P. A., Accardo, P. J., Ashwal, S., Baranek, G. T., Cook, E. H. Jr, Dawson, G., ... Volkmar, F. R. (2000). Practice parameter: Screening and diagnosis of autism: Report of the Quality Standards Subcommittee of the American Academy of Neurology and the Child Neurology Society. *Neurology*, *55*(4), 468–479. doi:10.1212/WNL.55.4.468 PMID:10953176

Finke, E., Davis, J., Benedict, M., Goga, L., Kelly, J., Palumbo, L., ... Waters, S. (2017). Eff ects of a least-to-most prompting procedure on multi-symbol message production in children with autism spectrum disorder who use augmentative and alternative communication. *American Journal of Speech-Language Pathology*, *26*(1), 81–98. doi:10.1044/2016_AJSLP-14-0187 PMID:28056153

Fisher, D., & Frey, N. (2016). Making learning visible: Reflecting on John Hattie's ideology, new book, and upcoming conference session. International Literacy Association, 33(5).

Fisher, D., Frey, N., & Lapp, D. (2012). Building and activating students' background knowledge: It's what they already know that counts. *Middle School Journal*, *43*(3), 22–31. doi:10.1080/00940771.2012.11461808

Flippin, M. & Reszka, S. & Watson, L. (2010). Effectiveness of the Picture Exchange Communication System (PECS) on Communication and Speech for Children with Autism Spectrum Disorders: A Meta-Analysis. *American Journal of Speech-Language Pathology, 19,* 178-95. . doi:10.1044/1058-0360(2010/09-0022)

Flores, M. M., Hill, D. A., Faciane, L. B., Edwards, M. A., Tapley, S. C., & Dowling, S. J. (2014). The apple iPad as assistive technology for story-based interventions. *Journal of Special Education Technology*, *29*(2), 27–37. doi:10.1177/016264341402900203

Foley, B. E., & Staples, A. H. (2003). Developing augmentative and alternative communication (AAC) and literacy interventions in a supported employment setting. *Topics in Language Disorders*, *23*(4), 325–343. doi:10.1097/00011363-200310000-00007

Folstein, S. E., & Rosen-Sheidley, B. (2001). Genetics of autism: Complex aetiology for a heterogeneous disorder. *Nature Reviews. Genetics*, *2*, 943–955. PMID:11733747

Fong, T., Nourbakhsh, I., & Dautenhahn, K. (2003). A survey of socially interactive robots. *Robotics and Autonomous Systems*, *42*(3-4), 143–166. doi:10.1016/S0921-8890(02)00372-X

Ford, D. Y. (2014). Why education must be multicultural. *Gifted Child Today*, *37*(1), 59–62. doi:10.1177/1076217513512304

Fraise, N., & Brooks, J. S. (2015). Toward a theory of culturally relevant leadership for school-community culture. *International Journal of Multicultural Education*, *17*(1), 6–21. doi:10.18251/ijme.v17i1.983

Freeman, J., Vladimirov, N., Kawashima, T., Mu, Y., Sofroniew, N. J., Bennett, D. V., ... Ahrens, M. B. (2014). Mapping brain activity at scale with cluster computing. *Nature Methods*, *11*(9), 941–950. doi:10.1038/nmeth.3041 PMID:25068736

French, N. P., Hagan, R., Evans, S. F., Godfrey, M., & Newnham, J. P. (1999). Repeated antenatal corticosteroids: Size at birth and subsequent development. *American Journal of Obstetrics and Gynecology*, *180*(1), 114–121. doi:10.1016/S0002-9378(99)70160-2 PMID:9914589

Frey, B. B., Schmitt, V. L., & Allen, J. P. (2012). Defining authentic classroom assessment. *Practical Assessment, Research & Evaluation*, *17*(2), 1–18. Retrieved from https://pareonline.net/genpare.asp?wh=0&abt=17

Frey, N., & Fisher, D. (2010). Getting to quality: A meeting of the minds. *Principal Leadership*, *11*(1), 68–70. Retrieved from https://www.fisherandfrey.com/journal-publications

Fukuyama, H., Kumagaya, S. I., Asada, K., Ayaya, S., & Kato, M. (2017). Autonomic versus perceptual accounts for tactile hypersensitivity in autism spectrum disorder. *Scientific Reports*, *7*(1), 8259. doi:10.103841598-017-08730-3 PMID:28811601

Galgani, F., Sun, Y., Lanzi, P. L., & Leigh, J. (2009). Automatic analysis of eye tracking data for medical diagnosis. In *2009 IEEE Symposium on Computational Intelligence and Data Mining* (pp. 195–202). IEEE. 10.1109/CIDM.2009.4938649

Ganz, J. B., Davis, J. L., Lund, E. M., Goodwyn, F. D., & Simpson, R. L. (2012). Meta-analysis of PECS with individuals with ASD: Investigation of targeted versus non-targeted outcomes, participant characteristics, and implementation phase. *Research in Developmental Disabilities*, *33*, 406–418. PMID:22119688

Ganz, J. B., Earles-Vollrath, T. L., Heath, A. K., Parker, R. I., Rispoli, M. J., & Duran, J. B. (2012). A meta-analysis of single case research studies on aided augmentative and alternative communication systems with individuals with autism spectrum disorders. *Journal of Autism and Developmental Disabilities*, *42*, 60–74. doi:10.100710803-011-1212-2 PMID:21380612

Ganz, J. B., Earles-Vollrath, T. L., Mason, R. A., Rispoli, M. J., Heath, A. K., & Parker, R. I. (2011). An aggregate study of single-case research involving aided AAC: Participant characteristics of individuals with autism spectrum disorders. *Research in Autism Spectrum Disorders*, *5*(4), 1500–1509. doi:10.1016/j.rasd.2011.02.011

Ganz, J. B., Hong, E. R., Goodwyn, F., Kite, E., & Gilliland, W. (2015). Impact of PECS tablet computer app on receptive identification of pictures given a verbal stimulus. *Developmental Neurorehabilitation*, *18*(2), 82–87. doi:10.3109/17518423.2013.821539 PMID:23957298

Ganz, J. B., Lashley, E., & Rispoli, M. J. (2010). Non-responsiveness to intervention. Children with autism spectrum disorders who do not rapidly respond to communication interventions. *Developmental Neurorehabilitation*, *13*, 399–407.

Ganz, J. B., Morin, K. L., Foster, M. J., Vannest, K. J., Genç Tosun, D., Gregori, E. V., & Gerow, S. L. (2017). High-technology augmentative and alternative communication for individuals with intellectual and developmental disabilities and complex communication needs: A meta-analysis. *Augmentative and Alternative Communication*, *33*(4), 224–238. doi:10.1080/07434618.2017.1373855 PMID:28922953

Ganz, J. B., Rispoli, M. J., Mason, R. A., & Hong, E. R. (2014). Moderation of effects of AAC based on setting and types of aided AAC on outcome variables: An aggregate study of single-case research with individuals with ASD. *Developmental Neurorehabilitation*, *17*(3), 184–192. doi:10.3109/17518423.2012.748097 PMID:24102440

Gardner, H. (2000). Project zero: Nelson Goodman's legacy in arts education. *The Journal of Aesthetics and Art Criticism*, *245*(3), 245. doi:10.2307/432107

Geetha, B., Sukumar, C., Dhivyadeepa, E., Reddy, J. K., & Balachandar, V. (2018). Autism in India: A case–control study to understand the association between socio-economic and environmental risk factors. *Acta Neurologica Belgica*, *119*(3), 393–401. doi:10.100713760-018-01057-4 PMID:30554347

Gemmell, H. G., & Staff, R. T. (2005). Single Photon Emission Computed Tomography (SPECT). In Practical Nuclear Medicine (pp. 21–33). London: Springer. doi:10.1007/1-84628-018-4_2

Gepner, B., Mestre, D., Masson, G., & De Schonen, S. (1995). Postural effects of motion vision in young autistic children. *Neuroreport*, *6*(8), 1211–1214. doi:10.1097/00001756-199505300-00034 PMID:7662910

Gernsbacher, M. A., Sauer, E. A., Geye, H. M., Schweigert, E. K., & Goldsmith, H. H. (2008). Infant and toddler oral- and manual-motor skills predict later speech fluency in autism. *Journal of Child Psychology and Psychiatry, and Allied Disciplines*, *49*, 43–50.

Gevarter, C., & Zamora, C. (2018). Naturalistic speech-generating device interventions for children with complex communication needs: A systematic review of single-subject studies. *American Journal of Speech-Language Pathology*, *27*(3), 1073–1090. doi:10.1044/2018_AJSLP-17-0128 PMID:29971336

Geytenbeek, J. J., Vermeulen, R. J., Becher, J. G., & Oostrom, K. J. (2015). Comprehension of spoken language in non-speaking children with severe cerebral palsy: An explorative study on associations with motor type and disabilities. *Developmental Medicine and Child Neurology*, *57*(3), 294–300. doi:10.1111/dmcn.12619 PMID:25349105

Ghiassian, S., Greiner, R., Jin, P., & Brown, M. R. G. (2013). *Learning to Classify Psychiatric Disorders based on fMR Images: Autism vs Healthy and ADHD vs Healthy*. Academic Press.

Gilroy, S. P., Leader, G., & McCleery, J. P. (2018). A pilot community-based randomized comparison of speech generating devices and the picture exchange communication system for children diagnosed with autism spectrum disorder. *Autism Research*, *11*(12), 1701–1711. doi:10.1002/aur.2025 PMID:30475454

Gimeno, H., & Lin, J. P. (2017). The International Classification of Functioning (ICF) to evaluate deep brain stimulation neuromodulation in childhood dystonia-hyperkinesia informs future clinical & research priorities in a multidisciplinary model of care. *European Journal of Paediatric Neurology, 21*(1), 147-167.

Gitananda Giri Swami. (1976). *Yoga: Step-by-Step*. Pondicherry, India: Satya Press.

Gnouma, M., Ladjailia, A., Ejbali, R., & Zaied, M. (2019). Stacked sparse auto encoder and history of binary motion image for human activity recognition. *Multimedia Tools and Applications*, *78*(2), 2157–2179. doi:10.100711042-018-6273-1

Goff, D. A., Luan, X., Gerdes, M., Bernbaum, J., D'Agostino, J. A., Rychik, J., ... Gaynor, J. W. (2012). Younger gestational age is associated with worse neurodevelopmental outcomes after cardiac surgery in infancy. *The Journal of Thoracic and Cardiovascular Surgery*, *143*(3), 535–542. doi:10.1016/j.jtcvs.2011.11.029 PMID:22340027

Goldberg, J. H., & Kotval, X. P. (1999). Computer interface evaluation using eye movements: Methods and constructs. *International Journal of Industrial Ergonomics*, *24*(6), 631–645. doi:10.1016/S0169-8141(98)00068-7

Goldberg, J. H., Stimson, M. J., Lewenstein, M., Scott, N., & Wichansky, A. M. (2002, March). Eye tracking in web search tasks: design implications. In *Proceedings of the 2002 symposium on Eye tracking research & applications* (pp. 51-58). 10.1145/507072.507082

Goldstein, S., & Schwebach, A. J. (2004). The comorbidity of pervasive developmental disorders and attention deficit hyperactivity disorder: Results of a fretrospective chart review. *Journal of Autism and Developmental Disorders*, *34*(3), 323–339. PMID:15264500

González-Ortega, D., Díaz-Pernas, F. J., Martínez-Zarzuela, M., & Antón-Rodríguez, M. (2014). A Kinect-based system for cognitive rehabilitation exercises monitoring. *Computer Methods and Programs in Biomedicine*, *113*(2), 620–631. doi:10.1016/j.cmpb.2013.10.014 PMID:24263055

Gopaul, B. (2011). Distinction in doctoral education: Using Bourdieu's tools to assess the socialization of doctoral students. *Equity & Excellence in Education*, *44*(1), 10–21. doi:10.1080/10665684.2011.539468

Gorrindo P. (2013). *Gastrointestinal dysfunction in Autism.* Academic Press.

Gorrindo, P., Williams, K. C., Lee, E. B., Walker, L. S., McGrew, S. G., & Levitt, P. (2012). Gastrointestinal dysfunction in autism: Parental report, clinical evaluation, and associated factors. *Autism Research*, *5*(2), 101–108. doi:10.1002/aur.237 PMID:22511450

Gowen, E., & Hamilton, A. (2013). Motor abilities in autism: Are view using a computational context. *Journal of Autism and Developmental Disorders*, *43*(2), 323–344. doi:10.100710803-012-1574-0 PMID:22723127

Grandin, T. (1995). How People with Autism Think. In E. Schopler & G. B. Mesibov (Eds.), *Learning and Cognition in Autism. Current Issues in Autism.* Boston, MA: Springer.

Green, D., Charman, T., Pickles, A., Chandler, S., Loucas, T., Simonoff, E., & Baird, G. (2009). Impairment in movement skills of children with autistic spectrum disorders. *Developmental Medicine and Child Neurology*, *51*(4), 311–316. doi:10.1111/j.1469-8749.2008.03242.x PMID:19207298

Greene, H. H., & Rayner, K. (2001). Eye movements and familiarity effects in visual search. *Vision Research*, *41*(27), 3763–3773. doi:10.1016/S0042-6989(01)00154-7 PMID:11712988

Green, J., Charman, T., McConachie, H., Aldred, C., Slonims, V., Howlin, P., ... Pickles, A. (2010). Parent-mediated communication-focused treatment in children with autism (PACT): A randomised controlled trial. *Lancet*, *375*(9732), 2152–2160. doi:10.1016/S0140-6736(10)60587-9 PMID:20494434

Grensman, A., Acharya, B. D., Wändell, P., Nilsson, G. H., Falkenberg, T., Sundin, O., & Werner, S. (2018). Effect of traditional yoga, mindfulness–based cognitive therapy, and cognitive behavioral therapy, on health related quality of life: A randomized controlled trial on patients on sick leave because of burnout. *BMC Complementary and Alternative Medicine*, *18*(1), 80. doi:10.118612906-018-2141-9 PMID:29510704

Grillon, H., Riquier, F., Herbelin, B., & Thalmann, D. (2006). Use of Virtual Reality as Therapeutic Tool for Behavioural Exposure in the Ambit of Social. *International Conference Series on Disability, Virtual Reality and Associated Technologies (ICDVRAT).*

Grossard, C., Grynspan, O., Sylvie Serret, S., Jouen, A.-L., Bailly, K., & Cohen, D. (2017). Serious games to teach social interactions and emotions to individuals with autism spectrum disorders. *Computers & Education*, *113*, 195–211. doi:10.1016/j.compedu.2017.05.002

Grossman, R. B. (2015). Judgments of social awkwardness from brief exposure to children with and without high-functioning autism. *Autism, 19*(5), 580–587. doi:10.1177/1362361314536937 PMID:24923894

Grundmann, O., & Yoon, S. L. (2010). Irritable bowel syndrome: epidemiology, diagnosis and treatment: an update for healthcare practitioners. *Journal of Gastroenterology and Hepatology, 25*(4), 691–699. doi:10.1111/j.1440-1746.2009.06120.x PMID:20074154

Grynszpan, O., & Nadel, J. (2015). An eye-tracking method to reveal the link between gazing patterns and pragmatic abilities in high functioning autism spectrum disorders. *Frontiers in Human Neuroscience, 8*, 1067. doi:10.3389/fnhum.2014.01067 PMID:25642182

Gulati, K., Loganathan, N., Mooventhan, A., Lahiri, A., & Telles, S. (2018). Effect of yoga therapy on the symptoms of sensory processing disorder in autistic individuals. *Yoga Mimamsa, 50*(2), 60–61. doi:10.4103/ym.ym_9_18

Guo, C., Luo, M., Wang, X., Huang, S., Meng, Z., Shao, J., & Zhang, X. (2018). Reliability and Validity of the Chinese Version of Modified Checklist for Autism in Toddlers, Revised, with Follow-Up (M-CHAT-R / F). *Journal of Autism and Developmental Disorders*. doi:10.100710803-018-3682-y PMID:30047095

Guskey, T. R. (2009). Getting curriculum reform right. *School Administrator, 66*(11), 38.

Gwynette, M. F., Sidhu, S. S., & Ceranoglu, T. A. (2018). Electronic Screen Media Use in Youth With Autism Spectrum Disorder. *Child and Adolescent Psychiatric Clinics of North America, 27*(2), 203–219. doi:10.1016/j.chc.2017.11.013 PMID:29502747

Haglund, N., Dahlgren, S., Källén, K., Gustafsson, P., & Råstam, M. (2016). The Observation Scale for Autism (OSA): A New Screening Method to Detect Autism Spectrum Disorder before Age Three Years. *Journal of Intellectual Disability-Diagnosis and Treatment, 3*(4), 230–237. doi:10.6000/2292-2598.2015.03.04.9

Halcrow, K. (2018). Imitation and innovation: Harnessing the principles of music pedagogy for the writing classroom. *Literacy Learning: The Middle Years, 26*(3), 48–57.

Hall, D., Huerta, M. F., McAuliffe, M. J., & Farber, G. K. (2012). Sharing heterogeneous data: The national database for autism research. *Neuroinformatics, 10*(4), 331–339. doi:10.100712021-012-9151-4 PMID:22622767

Hall, L. (2013). *Autism spectrum disorders: From theory to practice* (2nd ed.). Boston, MA: Pearson.

Handen, B. L., Johnson, C. R., & Lubetsky, M. (2000). Efficacy of methylphenidate among children with autism and symptoms of attention-deficit hyperactivity disorder. *Journal of Autism and Developmental Disorders, 30*, 245–255. PMID:11055460

Hanna, K., & Rodger, S. (2002). Towards family-centered practice in pediatric occupational therapy: A review of the literature on parent–therapist collaboration. *Australian Occupational Therapy Journal, 49*(1), 14–24. doi:10.1046/j.0045-0766.2001.00273.x

Hanney, N. M., Jostad, C. M., LeBlanc, L. A., Carr, J. E., & Castile, A. J. (2012). Intensive behavioral treatment of urinary incontinence of Children with Autism Spectrum Disorders: An archival analysis of procedures and outcomes from an outpatient clinic. *Focus on Autism and Other Developmental Disabilities, 28*(1), 26–31. doi:10.1177/1088357612457987

Haputhanthri, D., Brihadiswaran, G., Gunathilaka, S., Meedeniya, D., Jayarathna, S., Jaime, M., & Jayawardena, Y. (2019). An EEG based Channel Optimized Classification Approach for Autism Spectrum Disorder. In *Moratuwa Engineering Research Conference (MerCon),* (pp. 123-128). IEEE. 10.1109/MERCon.2019.8818814

Harris, M. D., & Reichle, J. (2004). The impact of aided language stimulation on symbol comprehension and production in children with moderate cognitive disabilities. *American Journal of Speech-Language Pathology*, *13*(2), 155–167. doi:10.1044/1058-0360(2004/016) PMID:15198634

Harris, S. L., & Handleman, J. S. (2000). Age and IQ at intake as predictors of placement for young children with autism: A four-to six-year follow-up. *Journal of Autism and Developmental Disorders*, *30*(2), 137–142. PMID:10832778

Hart, S., & Banda, D. (2010). Picture Exchange Communication System with individuals with developmental disabilities: A meta-analysis of single subject studies. *Remedial and Special Education*, *31*, 463–477.

Ha, S., Sohn, I.-J., Kim, N., Sim, H. J., & Cheon, K.-A. (2015). Characteristics of Brains in Autism Spectrum Disorder: Structure, Function and Connectivity across the Lifespan. *Experimental Neurobiology*, *24*(4), 273–284. doi:10.5607/en.2015.24.4.273 PMID:26713076

Hazlett, H. C., Poe, M. D., Gerig, G., Smith, R. G., & Piven, J. (2006). *Cortical grey and white brain tissue volume in adolescents and adults with autism*. Academic Press.

Hazlett, H. C., Gu, H., McKinstry, R. C., Shaw, D. W. W., Botteron, K. N., Dager, S. R., & ... . (2012). Brain volume findings in 6-month-old infants at high familial risk for autism. *The American Journal of Psychiatry*, *169*, 601–608. PMID:22684595

Heide, W., Koenig, E., Trillenberg, P., Kömpf, D., & Zee, D. S. (1999). Electrooculography: Technical standards and applications. *Electroencephalography and Clinical Neurophysiology. Supplement*, *52*, 223–240. PMID:10590990

Heinsfeld, A. S., Franco, A. R., Craddock, R. C., Buchweitz, A., & Meneguzzi, F. (2018). Identification of autism spectrum disorder using deep learning and the ABIDE dataset. *NeuroImage. Clinical*, *17*, 16–23. doi:10.1016/j.nicl.2017.08.017 PMID:29034163

Helmi Adly, M. N., Faaizah, S., & Naim, C. P. (2012). Serious Game for Autism Children: Review of Literature. *International Conference on Computer Games, Multimedia, and Allied Technology*, 647-652.

Hemmingsson, H., Gustavsson, A., & Townsend, E. (2007). Students with disabilities participating in mainstream schools: Policies that promote and limit teacher and therapist cooperation. *Disability & Society*, *22*(4), 383–398. doi:10.1080/09687590701337892

Henriksen, D., Mishra, P., & Fisser, P. (2016). Infusing creativity and technology in 21st century education: A systemic view for change. *Journal of Educational Technology & Society*, *19*(3), 27–37. Retrieved from http://danah-henriksen.com/wp-content/uploads/2016/10/creativity-systemic-view.pdf

Henry, J., von Hippel, W., Molenberghs, P., Lee, T., & Sachdev, P. S. (2016). Clinical assessment of social cognitive function in neurological disorders. *Nature Reviews. Neurology*, *12*(1), 28–39. doi:10.1038/nrneurol.2015.229 PMID:26670297

Hewitt, G., Jurk, D., Marques, F. D., Correia-Melo, C., Hardy, T., Gackowska, A., ... Passos, J. F. (2012). Telomeres are favoured targets of a persistent DNA damage response in ageing and stress-induced senescence. *Nature Communications*, *28*(3), 1–9. PMID:22426229

Himmelmann, K., Hagberg, G., & Uvebrant, P. (2010). The changing panorama of cerebral palsy in Sweden. X. Prevalence and origin in the birth-year period 1999–2002. *Acta Paediatrica (Oslo, Norway)*, *99*(9), 1337–1343. doi:10.1111/j.1651-2227.2010.01819.x PMID:20377538

Hinds, O., Wighton, P., Dylan Tisdall, M., Hess, A., Breiter, H., & Van Der Kouwe, A. (2014). Neurofeedback using functional spectroscopy. *International Journal of Imaging Systems and Technology*, *24*(2), 138–148. doi:10.1002/ima.22088 PMID:24999293

Hinzen, H. (2013). Lifelong learning for all – A potential global goal for the post 2015 education and development agendas! *Adult Education and Development, 80*, 4–9. Retrieved from https://www.dvv-international.de/en/adult-education-and-development/editions/aed-802013-post-2015/articles/lifelong-learning-for-all-a-potential-global-goal-for-the-post-2015-education-and-development-agendas/

Hochstein, D. D., McDaniel, M. A., Nettleton, S., & Neufeld, K. H. (2003). The fruitfulness of a nomothetic approach to investigating AAC: Comparing 2 speech encoding schemes across cerebral palsied and nondisabled children. *American Journal of Speech-Language Pathology, 12*(1), 110–120. doi:10.1044/1058-0360(2003/057) PMID:12680818

Hodapp, R. M., Sanderson, K. A., Meskis, S. A., & Casale, E. G. (2017). Adult siblings of persons with intellectual disabilities: Past, present, and future. *International Review of Research in Developmental Disabilities, 53*, 163–202. doi:10.1016/bs.irrdd.2017.08.001

Hodge, S. (2007). Why is the potential of augmentative and alternative communication not being realized? Exploring the experiences of people who use communication aids. *Disability & Society, 22*(5), 457–471. doi:10.1080/09687590701427552

Höfer, J., Hoffmann, F., & Bachmann, C. (2017). Use of complementary and alternative medicine in children and adolescents with autism spectrum disorder: A systematic review. *Autism, 21*(4), 387–402. doi:10.1177/1362361316646559 PMID:27231337

Hollocks, M. J., Ozsivadjian, A., Matthews, C. E., Howlin, P., & Simonoff, E. (2013). The relationship between attentional bias and anxiety in children and adolescents with autism spectrum disorders. *Autism Research, 6*(4), 237–247. doi:10.1002/aur.1285 PMID:23907924

Holt-Lunstad, J., Smith, T. B., & Layton, B. (n.d.). Social relationships and mortality risk: A meta-analytic review. *PLoS Medicine, 7*(7), e1316. doi:1.1371/journal.pmed.1316

Hörmeyer, I., & Renner, G. (2013). Confirming and denying in co-construction processes: A case study of an adult with cerebral palsy and two familiar partners. *Augmentative and Alternative Communication, 29*(3), 259–271. doi:10.3109/07434618.2013.813968 PMID:23952567

Howes, O. D., Rogdaki, M., Findon, J. L., Wichers, R. H., Charman, T., King, B. H., ... Murphy, D. G. (2018). Autism Spectrum Disorder: Consensus guidelines on assessment, treatment and research from the British Association for Psychopharmacology. *Journal of Psychopharmacology (Oxford, England), 32*(1), 3–29. doi:10.1177/0269881117741766 PMID:29237331

Huang, I. C., Sugden, D., & Beveridge, S. (2009). Children's perceptions of their use of assistive devices in home and school settings. *Disability and Rehabilitation. Assistive Technology, 4*(2), 95–105. doi:10.1080/17483100802613701 PMID:19253098

Hughes, E. M., & Yakubova, G. (2016). Developing handheld video intervention for students with autism spectrum disorder. *Intervention in School and Clinic, 52*(2), 115–121. doi:10.1177/1053451216636059

Hughes, J. R. (2007). Autism: The first firm finding = under connectivity? *Epilepsy & Behavior, 11*(1), 20–24. doi:10.1016/j.yebeh.2007.03.010 PMID:17531541

Hunt, M. W. (2013). [APP]ETITE for instruction: 21st-century learners in a video and audio production classroom. *Techniques, 88*(8), 36-40. Retrieved from https://www.questia.com/magazine/1G1-349490089/app-etite-for-instruction-21st-century-learners

Hussain, A., Mkpojiogu, E. O. C., & Hassan, F. (2016). Systematic review of mobile learning applications for children. *Proceedings of the 2nd International Conference on Information and Communication Technology for Transformation*. 5-7.

Hustad, K. C., Gorton, K., & Lee, J. (2010). Classification of speech and language profiles in 4-year-old children with cerebral palsy: A prospective preliminary study. *Journal of Speech, Language, and Hearing Research: JSLHR*, *53*(6), 1496–1513. doi:10.1044/1092-4388(2010/09-0176) PMID:20643795

Hutchins, T. L., & Prelock, P. A. (2014). Using communication to reduce challenging behaviors in individuals with autism spectrum disorders and intellectual disability. *Child and Adolescent Psychiatric Clinics of North America*, *23*(1), 41–55. doi:10.1016/j.chc.2013.07.003 PMID:24231166

Hviid, A., Hansen, J. V., Frisch, M., & Melbye, M. (2019). Measles, Mumps, Rubella vaccination and autism: A nationwide cohort study. *Annals of Internal Medicine*, *170*(8), 513–520. doi:10.7326/M18-2101 PMID:30831578

Hyde, K. K., Novack, M. N., Lahaye, N., Parlett-pelleriti, C., Anden, R., Dixon, D. R., & Linstead, E. (2019). Applications of Supervised Machine Learning in Autism Spectrum Disorder Research : A Review. *Review Journal of Autism and Developmental Disorders*, *6*(2), 128–146. doi:10.100740489-019-00158-x

Iacono, T., & Duncum, J. (1995). Comparison of sign alone and in combination with an electronic communication device in early language intervention: Case study. *Augmentative and Alternative Communication*, *11*(4), 249–259. doi:10.1080/07434619512331277389

Ibrahim, S., Djemal, R., & Alsuwailem, A. (2018). Electroencephalography (EEG) signal processing for epilepsy and autism spectrum disorder diagnosis. *Biocybernetics and Biomedical Engineering*, *38*(1), 16–26. doi:10.1016/j.bbe.2017.08.006

Inclusive Practices Africa. (2019). *Disability Inclusion Drives Change.* Access at Inclusivepractices.co.za

Individuals with Disability Education Act Amendments of 1997 (IDEA). (1997). Retrieved from http://www.congress.gov/105/plaws/publ17/PLAW-105publ17.pdf

Inuth. (2019). *Three Differently-Abled youngsters welcome you with a warm smile at this Kerala restaurant.* Retrieved October 5, 2019 from https://m.dailyhunt.in/news/india/english/inuth-epaper-inuth/three+differently+abled+youngsters+welcome+you+with+a+warm+smile+at+this+kerala+restaurant-newsid-112330821

Ismaili, J., & Ibrahimi, E. H. O. (2017). Mobile learning as alternative to assistive technology devices for special needs students. *Education and Information Technologies*, *22*(3), 883–899. doi:10.100710639-015-9462-9

Jack, C. R. Jr, Lowe, V. J., Senjem, M. L., Weigand, S. D., Kemp, B. J., Shiung, M. M., ... Petersen, R. C. (2008). 11C PiB and structural MRI provide complementary information in imaging of Alzheimer's disease and amnestic mild cognitive impairment. *Brain*, *131*(3), 665–680. doi:10.1093/brain/awm336 PMID:18263627

Jacob, R. J. (1990, March). What you look at is what you get: eye movement-based interaction techniques. In *Proceedings of the SIGCHI conference on Human factors in computing systems* (pp. 11-18). 10.1145/97243.97246

Jaime, M., McMahon, C. M., Davidson, B. C., Newell, L. C., Mundy, P. C., & Henderson, H. A. (2016). Brief report: Reduced temporal-central EEG alpha coherence during joint attention perception in adolescents with autism spectrum disorder. *Journal of Autism and Developmental Disorders*, *46*(4), 1477–1489. doi:10.100710803-015-2667-3 PMID:26659813

Jain, S. M. (2018). *Detection of Autism using Magnetic Resonance Imaging data and Graph Convolutional Neural Networks Detection of Autism using Magnetic Resonance Imaging data and Graph Convolutional Neural Networks* (Master Dissertation). Rochester Institute of Technology.

Jamal, W., Das, S., Oprescu, I. A., Maharatna, K., Apicella, F., & Sicca, F. (2014). Classification of autism spectrum disorder using supervised learning of brain connectivity measures extracted from synchrostates. *Journal of Neural Engineering*, *11*(4), 046019. doi:10.1088/1741-2560/11/4/046019 PMID:24981017

Jang, H., Plis, S. M., Calhoun, V. D., & Lee, J. H. (2017). Task-specific feature extraction and classification of fMRI volumes using a deep neural network initialized with a deep belief network: Evaluation using sensorimotor tasks. *NeuroImage*, *145*, 314–328. doi:10.1016/j.neuroimage.2016.04.003 PMID:27079534

Jan, J. E., Lyons, C. J., Heaven, R. K., & Matsuba, C. (2001). Visual impairment due to a dyskinetic eye movement disorder in children with dyskinetic cerebral palsy. *Developmental Medicine and Child Neurology*, *43*(2), 108–112. doi:10.1017/S0012162201000184 PMID:11221897

Jin, Y., Wee, C. Y., Shi, F., Thung, K. H., Ni, D., Yap, P. T., & Shen, D. (2015). Identification of infants at high-risk for autism spectrum disorder using multiparameter multiscale white matter connectivity networks. *Human Brain Mapping*, *36*(12), 4880–4896. doi:10.1002/hbm.22957 PMID:26368659

John, N. (2017). The Early Origins of Autism. *Child and Adolescent Psychiatric Clinics of North America*, *26*(3), 555–570. doi:10.1016/j.chc.2017.02.008 PMID:28577609

Johnson, C. P., & Myers, S. M. (2007). Identification and evaluation of children with autism spectrum disorders. *Pediatrics*, *120*(5), 1183–1215. doi:10.1542/peds.2007-2361 PMID:17967920

Johnson, K. P., Giannotti, F., & Cortesi, F. (2009). Sleep patterns in autism spectrum disorders. *Child and Adolescent Psychiatric Clinics of North America*, *18*, 917–928. PMID:19836696

Johnston, D., Egermann, H. W., & Kearney, G. C. (2018). Innovative Computer Technology in music based interventions for individuals with autism - Moving beyond traditional interactive music therapy techniques. *Cognitive Psychology*, *5*, 1554773.

Jones, E. J. H., Gliga, T., Bedford, R., Charman, T., & Johnson, M. H. (2014). Developmental pathways to autism: A review of prospective studies of infants at risk. *Neuroscience and Biobehavioral Reviews*, *39*, 1–33. doi:10.1016/j.neubiorev.2013.12.001 PMID:24361967

Jones, J., & Stewart, H. (2004). A description of how three occupational therapists train children in using the scanning access technique. *Australian Occupational Therapy Journal*, *51*(3), 155–165. doi:10.1111/j.1440-1630.2004.00445.x

Jones, W., Carr, K., & Klin, A. (2008). Absence of preferential looking to the eyes of approaching adults predicts level of social disability in 2-year-old toddlers with autism spectrum disorder. *Achieves of general. Psychiatry.*, *65*(8), 946–954. PMID:18678799

Jones, W., & Klin, A. (2013). Attention to eyes is present but in decline in 2–6-month-old infants later diagnosed with autism. *Nature*, *504*, 427–431. PMID:24196715

Jong, D. M., Punt, M., Groot, D. E., Minderaa, R. B., & Hadders, A. M. (2011). Minor neurological dysfunction in children with autism spectrum disorder. *Developmental Medicine and Child Neurology*, *53*(7), 641–646. doi:10.1111/j.1469-8749.2011.03971.x PMID:21569013

Joseph, R. M., Tager-Flusberg, H., & Lord, C. (2002). Cognitive profiles and social-communicative functioning in children with autism spectrum disorder. *Journal of Child Psychology and Psychiatry, and Allied Disciplines*, *43*(6), 807–821. doi:10.1111/1469-7610.00092 PMID:12236615

Judd, D. B. (1975). Wys zeckiG. Color in Business, Science and Industry. *Wiiey*, *19*, 420–461.

Judge, S., & Friday, M. (2011). Ambiguous keyboards for AAC. *Journal of Assistive Technologies*, *5*(4), 249–256. doi:10.1108/17549451111190650

Kagohara, D., van der Meer, L., Ramdoss, S., O'Reilly, M., Lancioni, G., Davis, T. N., ... Sigafoos, J. (2013). Using iPods and iPads in teaching programs for individuals with developmental disabilities: A systematic review. *Research in Developmental Disabilities, 34*(1), 147–156. doi:10.1016/j.ridd.2012.07.027 PMID:22940168

Kakkar, D. (2018, February). Accounting For Order-Frame Length Tradeoff of Savitzky-Golay Smoothing Filters. In *2018 5th International Conference on Signal Processing and Integrated Networks (SPIN)* (pp. 805-810). IEEE.

Kakkar, D. (2018, January). A Study on Machine Learning Based Generalized Automated Seizure Detection System. In *2018 8th International Conference on Cloud Computing, Data Science & Engineering (Confluence)* (pp. 769-774). IEEE.

Kakkar, D. (2019, March). Automatic Detection of Autism Spectrum Disorder by Tracing the Disorder Co-morbidities. In *2019 9th Annual Information Technology, Electromechanical Engineering and Microelectronics Conference (IEMECON)* (pp. 132-136). IEEE.

Kakkar, D. (2019). Diagnostic Assessment Techniques and Non-Invasive Biomarkers for Autism Spectrum Disorder. *International Journal of E-Health and Medical Communications, 10*(3), 79–95. doi:10.4018/IJEHMC.2019070105

Kaltman, J. R., Di, H., Tian, Z., & Rychik, J. (2005). Impact of congenital heart disease on cerebrovascular blood flow dynamics in the fetus. *Ultrasound in Obstetrics & Gynecology, 25*(1), 32–36. doi:10.1002/uog.1785 PMID:15593334

Kamaruzaman, M. F., Rani, N. M., Nor, H. M., & Azahari, M. H. H. (2016). Developing user interface design application for children with autism. *Procedia: Social and Behavioral Sciences, 217*, 887–894. doi:10.1016/j.sbspro.2016.02.022

Kanner, L. (1943). Autistic disturbances of affective contact. *Nervous Child, 2*, 217–250.

Karimi, P., Kamali, E., Mousavi, S. M., & Karahmadi, M. (2017). Environmental factors influencing the risk of autism. *Journal of Research in Medical Sciences, 22*.

Kassraian-Fard, P., Matthis, C., Balsters, J. H., Maathuis, M. H., & Wenderoth, N. (2016). Promises, pitfalls, and basic guidelines for applying machine learning classifiers to psychiatric imaging data, with autism as an example. *Frontiers in Psychiatry, 7*(Dec). doi:10.3389/fpsyt.2016.00177 PMID:27990125

Katuwal, G. J., Cahill, N. D., Baum, S. A., & Michael, A. M. (2015). The predictive power of structural MRI in Autism diagnosis. In *Engineering in Medicine and Biology Society (EMBC), 2015 37th Annual International Conference of the IE.* 10.1109/EMBC.2015.7319338

Kaye, H.S., Yeager, P., & Reed, M. (2008). Disparities in usage of assistive technology among people with disabilities. *Assist Technol., 20*, 194-203.

Kazdin, A. E. (2001). *Behavior modification in applied settings* (6th ed.). New York: Wadsworth.

Keehn, B., Nair, A., Lincoln, A. J., Townsend, J., & Müller, R. A. (2016). Under-reactive but easily distracted: An fMRI investigation of attentional capture in autism spectrum disorder. *Developmental Cognitive Neuroscience, 17*, 46–56. doi:10.1016/j.dcn.2015.12.002 PMID:26708773

Kennedy, C. (2005). *Single case designs for educational research.* New York: Allyn & Bacon.

Kenny, M. S. (2002). Integrated Movement Therapy™: Yoga-Based Therapy as a Viable and Effective Intervention for Autism Spectrum and Related Disorders. *International Journal of Yoga Therapy, 12*, 71.

Kent, J. M., Kushner, S., Ning, X., Karcher, K., Ness, S., Aman, M., ... Hough, D. (2013). Risperidone dosing in children and adolescents with autism spectrum disorder: A double-blind placebo-controlled study. *Journal of Autism and Developmental Disorders, 43*(8), 1773–1783. doi:10.100710803-012-1723-5 PMID:23212807

Kent-Walsh, J., Binger, C., & Buchanan, C. (2015). Teaching children who use augmentative and alternative communication to ask inverted yes/no questions using aided modeling. *American Journal of Speech-Language Pathology*, *24*(2), 222–236. doi:10.1044/2015_AJSLP-14-0066 PMID:25650561

Kent-Walsh, J., Binger, C., & Hasham, Z. (2010). Effects of parent instruction on the symbolic communication of children using augmentative and alternative communication during storybook reading. *American Journal of Speech-Language Pathology*, *19*, 97–107. PMID:20181850

Kent-Walsh, J., Binger, C., & Malani, M. (2010). Teaching partners to support the communication skills of young children who use AAC: Lessons from the ImPAACT program. *Early Childhood Services (San Diego, Calif.)*, *4*(3), 210–226.

Kent-Walsh, J., & Light, J. (2003). General education teachers' experiences with inclusion of students who use augmentative and alternative communication. *Augmentative and Alternative Communication*, *19*(2), 104–124. doi:10.1080/0743461031000112043

Kent-Walsh, J., & McNaughton, D. (2005). Communication partner instruction in AAC: Present practices and future directions. *Augmentative and Alternative Communication*, *21*, 195–204.

Kent-Walsh, J., Murza, K. A., Malani, M. D., & Binger, C. (2015). Effects of communication partner instruction on the communication of individuals using AAC: A meta-analysis. *Augmentative and Alternative Communication*, *31*(4), 271–284. PMID:26059542

Ker, J., Wang, L., Rao, J., & Lim, T. (2017). Deep Learning Applications in Medical Image Analysis. *IEEE Access : Practical Innovations, Open Solutions*, *6*, 9375–9379. doi:10.1109/ACCESS.2017.2788044

Kerkhof, Y. J., Graff, M. J., Bergsma, A., de Vocht, H. H., & Dröes, R. M. (2016). Better self-management and meaningful activities thanks to tablets? Development of a person-centered program to support people with mild dementia and their carers through use of hand-held touch screen devices. *International Psychogeriatrics*, *28*(11), 1917–1929. doi:10.1017/S1041610216001071 PMID:27425002

Khalsa, D. S., Amen, D., Hanks, C., Money, N., & Newberg, A. (2009). Cerebral blood flow changes during chanting meditation. *Nuclear Medicine Communications*, *30*(12), 956–961. doi:10.1097/MNM.0b013e32832fa26c PMID:19773673

Khalsa, D. S., Ray, L. E., Levine, S., Gallen, C. C., Schwartz, B. J., & Sidorowich, J. J. (1999). Randomized controlled trial of yogic meditation techniques for patients with obsessive-compulsive disorder. *CNS Spectrums*, *4*(12), 34–47. doi:10.1017/S1092852900006805 PMID:18311106

Khedher, L., Illán, I. A., Górriz, J. M., Ramírez, J., Brahim, A., & Meyer-Baese, A. (2017). Independent Component Analysis-Support Vector Machine-Based Computer-Aided Diagnosis System for Alzheimer's with Visual Support. *International Journal of Neural Systems*, *27*(03), 1650050. doi:10.1142/S0129065716500507 PMID:27776438

Khetarpal, A. (2014). Information and communication technology (ICT) and disability. *Review of Market Integration*, *6*(1), 96-113.

Khosla, M., Jamison, K., Kuceyeski, A., & Mert, R. (2018). *3D Convolutional Neural Networks for Classification of Functional Connectomes. In Deep Learning in Medical Image Analysis and Multimodal Learning for Clinical Decision Support* (pp. 137–145). Cham: Springer.

KletteR. (2014). *Image Processing*. doi:10.1007/978-1-4471-6320-6_2

Klock, J. (2010). Building novel connections in an increasingly standardized world. *Teacher Librarian*, *38*(2), 15–18.

Klukowski, M., Wasilewska, J., & Lebensztejn, D. (2015). Sleep and gastrointestinal disturbances. *Dev Period Med*, *19*(2), 157–161. PMID:26384115

Koenig, K. P., Buckley-Reen, A., & Garg, S. (2012). Efficacy of the Get Ready to learn yoga program among children with autism spectrum disorders: A pretest–posttest control group design. *The American Journal of Occupational Therapy*, *66*(5), 538–546. doi:10.5014/ajot.2012.004390 PMID:22917120

Kok, E. M., & Jarodzka, H. (2017). Before your very eyes: The value and limitations of eye tracking in medical education. *Medical Education*, *51*(1), 114–122. doi:10.1111/medu.13066 PMID:27580633

Kolevzon, A., Gross, R., & Reichenberg, A. (2007). Prenatal and perinatal risk factors for autism: A review and integration of findings. *Archives of Pediatrics & Adolescent Medicine*, *1*(4), 326–333. PMID:17404128

Koller, M., Salzberger, T., Brenner, G., & Walla, P. (2012). Broadening the range of applications of eye-tracking in business research. *Analise, Porto Alegre*, *23*(1), 71–77.

Kondo, T., & Raff, M. (2000). Oligodendrocyte precursor cells reprogrammed to become multipotential CNS stem cells. *Science*, *289*(5485), 1754–1757. doi:10.1126cience.289.5485.1754 PMID:10976069

Kong, Y., Gao, J., Xu, Y., Pan, Y., Wang, J., & Liu, J. (2018). Classification of Autism Spectrum Disorder by Combining Brain Connectivity and Deep Neural Network Classifier. *Neurocomputing*. doi:10.1016/j.neucom.2018.04.080

Konst, M. J., & Matson, J. L. (2014). Temporal and diagnostic influences on the expression of comorbid psychopathology symptoms in infants and toddlers with autism spectrum disorder. *Research in Autism Spectrum Disorders*, *8*(3), 200–208. doi:10.1016/j.rasd.2013.11.009

Koppenhaver, D., & Williams, A. (2010). A conceptual review of writing research in augmentative and alternative communication. *Augmentative and Alternative Communication*, *26*(3), 158–176. doi:10.3109/07434618.2010.505608 PMID:20874079

Koshino, H., Carpenter, P. A., Minshew, N. J., Cherkassky, V. L., Keller, T. A., & Just, M. A. (2005). Functional connectivity in an fMRI working memory task in high-functioning autism. *NeuroImage*, *24*(3), 810–821. PMID:15652316

Koumpouros, Y., & Kafazis, T. (2019). Wearable and mobile technologies in Autism Spectrum Disorder interventions: A systematic literature review. *Research in Autism Spectrum Disorders*, *66*, 101405. doi:10.1016/j.rasd.2019.05.005

Kraemer, H. C., Measelle, J. R., Ablow, J. C., Essex, M. J., Boyce, W. T., & Kupfer, D. J. (2003). A New Approach to Integrating Data From Multiple Informants in Psychiatric Assessment and Research: Mixing and Matching Contexts and Perspectives. *The American Journal of Psychiatry*, *160*(9), 1566–1577. doi:10.1176/appi.ajp.160.9.1566 PMID:12944328

Krägeloh-Mann, I., & Cans, C. (2009). Cerebral palsy update. *Brain & Development*, *31*(7), 537–544. doi:10.1016/j.braindev.2009.03.009 PMID:19386453

Krakowiak, P., Goodlin-Jones, B., Hertz-Picciotto, I., Croen, L. A., & Hansen, R. L. (2012). Sleep problems in children with autism spectrum disorders, developmental delays, and typical development: A population-based study. *Journal of Sleep Research*, *21*(2), 231. PMID:23176607

Krauzlis, R. J., Goffart, L., & Hafed, Z. M. (2017). Neuronal control of fixation and fixational eye movements. *Philosophical Transactions of the Royal Society B: Biological Sciences, 372*(1718), 20160205.

Krigger, K. W. (2006). Cerebral palsy: An overview. *American Family Physician*, *73*(1), 91–100. PMID:16417071

Kroncke, Willard, & Huckabee. (2014). Assessment of Autism Spectrum Disorder: Critical Issues in Clinical, Forensic and School Settings. Springer Publications.

Kuang, D., Guo, X., An, X., Zhao, Y., & He, L. (2014). *Discrimination of ADHD Based on fMRI Data with Deep Belief Network*. Cham: Springer. doi:10.1007/978-3-319-09330-7_27

Kuddo, T., & Nelson, K. B. (2003). How common are gastrointestinal disorders in children with autism? *Current Opinion in Pediatrics*, *15*, 339–343. PMID:12806268

Kuo, M. H., Orsmond, G. I., Coster, W. J., & Cohn, E. S. (2014). Media use among adolescents with autism spectrum disorder. *Autism*, *18*, 914–923. PMID:24142797

L'Heureux, Grolinger, Elyamany, & Capretz. (2017). *Machine Learning With Big Data: Challenges and Approaches.* Academic Press.

Lahiri, U., Bekele, E., Dohrmann, E., Warren, Z., & Sarkar, N. (2013). Design of a virtual reality based adaptive response technology for children with autism. *IEEE Transactions on Neural Systems and Rehabilitation Engineering*, *21*(1), 55–64. doi:10.1109/TNSRE.2012.2218618 PMID:23033333

Lahiri, U., Warren, Z., & Sarkar, N. (2011c). Dynamic gaze measurement with adaptive response technology in virtual reality based social communication for autism. *2011 International Conference on Virtual Rehabilitation, ICVR 2011*, 10.1109/ICVR.2011.5971840

Lancioni, G. E., Bosco, A., Olivetti Belardinelli, M., Singh, N. N., O'Reilly, M. F., Sigafoos, J., & Oliva, D. (2014). Technology-based intervention programs to promote stimulation control and communication in post-coma persons with different levels of disability. *Frontiers in Human Neuroscience*, *8*, 48. doi:10.3389/fnhum.2014.00048 PMID:24574992

Lancioni, G. E., Comes, M. L., Stasolla, F., Manfredi, F., O'Reilly, M. F., & Singh, N. N. (2005). A microswitch cluster to enhance arm-lifting responses without dystonic head tilting by a child with multiple disabilities. *Perceptual and Motor Skills*, *100*(3), 892–894. doi:10.2466/pms.100.3.892-894 PMID:16060461

Lancioni, G. E., O'Reilly, M. F., Sigafoos, J., Campodonico, F., Perilli, V., Alberti, G., ... Miglino, O. (2018a). A modified smartphone-based program to support leisure and communication activities in people with multiple disabilities. *Advances in Neurodevelopmental Disabilities*, *2*. doi:10.100741252-017-0047-z

Lancioni, G. E., O'Reilly, M. F., Sigafoos, J., D'Amico, F., Buonocunto, F., Devalle, G., ... Lanzilotti, C. (2018b). A further evaluation of microswitch-aided intervention for fostering responding and stimulation control in persons in a minimally conscious state. *Advances in Neurodevelopmental Disorders*, *2*(3), 322–331. doi:10.100741252-018-0064-6

Lancioni, G. E., O'Reilly, M. F., Singh, N. N., Groeneweg, J., Bosco, A., Tota, A., ... Pidala, S. (2006). A social validation assessment of microswitch-based programs for persons with multiple disabilities employing teacher trainees and parents as raters. *Journal of Developmental and Physical Disabilities*, *18*(4), 383–391. doi:10.100710882-006-9024-6

Lancioni, G. E., O'Reilly, M. F., Singh, N. N., Sigafoos, J., Didden, R., Oliva, D., ... Groeneweg, J. (2009). Persons with multiple disabilities accessing stimulation and requesting social contact via microswitch and VOCA devices: New research evaluation and social validation. *Research in Developmental Disabilities*, *30*(5), 1084–1094. doi:10.1016/j.ridd.2009.03.004 PMID:19361954

Lancioni, G. E., Sigafoos, J., O'Reilly, M. F., & Singh, N. N. (2012). *Assistive technology: Interventions for individuals with severe/profound and multiple disabilities*. New York: Springer.

Lancioni, G. E., & Singh, N. N. (2014). *Assistive technologies for people with diverse abilities*. New York: Springer. doi:10.1007/978-1-4899-8029-8

Lancioni, G. E., Singh, N. N., O'Reilly, M. F., Oliva, D., Smaldone, A., Tota, A., ... Groeneweg, J. (2006). Assessing the effects of stimulation versus microswitch-based programmes on indices of happiness of students with multiple disabilities. *Journal of Intellectual Disability Research*, *50*(10), 739–747. doi:10.1111/j.1365-2788.2006.00839.x PMID:16961703

Lancioni, G. E., Singh, N. N., O'Reilly, M. F., Sigafoos, J., D'Amico, F., Pinto, K., ... Caffò, A. O. (2018d). Promoting supported ambulation in persons with advanced Alzheimer's disease: A pilot study. *Disability and Rehabilitation. Assistive Technology*, *13*(1), 101–106. doi:10.1080/17483107.2017.1297856 PMID:28287045

Lancioni, G., Singh, N., O'Reilly, M., Sigafoos, J., Alberti, G., Chiariello, V., ... Campodonico, F. (2018c). A smartphone-based technology package to support independent activity in people with intellectual disability and blindness. *Internet Technology Letters*, *2018*(5), e34. doi:10.1002/itl2.34

Lancioni, G., Singh, N., O'Reilly, M., Sigafoos, J., D'Amico, F., Pinto, K., ... Caffò, A. (2017). A technology-aided program for helping persons with Alzheimer's disease perform daily activities. *Journal of Enabling Technologies*, *11*(3), 85–91. doi:10.1108/JET-03-2017-0011

Landa, R. J., & Kalb, L. G. (2012). Long-term outcomes of toddlers with autism spectrum disorders exposed to short-term intervention. *Pediatrics*, *130*(2), 186–190. PMID:23118250

Landrigan, P. J., Lambertini, L., & Birnbaum, L. S. (2012). A research strategy to discover the environmental causes of autism and neurodevelopmental disabilities. *Environmental Health Perspectives*, *120*, 258–260. PMID:22543002

Larobina, M., & Murino, L. (2014). Medical image file formats. *Journal of Digital Imaging*, *27*(2), 200–206. doi:10.100710278-013-9657-9 PMID:24338090

Lau, H. M., Smit, J. H., Fleming, T., & Riper, H. (2017). Serious sames for mental health: Are they accessible, feasible, and effective? A systematic review and meta-analysis. *Frontiers in Psychiatry*, *7*, 209. doi:10.3389/fpsyt.2016.00209 PMID:28149281

Lawler, C. P., Croen, L. A., Grether, J. K., & Van de Water, J. (2004). Identifying environmental contributions to autism: Provocative clues and false leads. *Mental Retardation and Developmental Disabilities Research Reviews*, *10*, 292–302. PMID:15666339

LeBarton, E., & Iverson, J. M. (2013). Fine motor skill predicts expressive language in infant siblings of children with autism. *Developmental Science*, *16*(6), 815–827. PMID:24118709

Ledford, J. R., Barton, E. E., Hardy, J. K., Elam, K., Seabolt, J., Shanks, M., ... Kaiser, A. (2016). What equivocal data from single case comparison studies reveal about evidence-based practices in early childhood special education. *Journal of Early Intervention*, *38*(2), 79–91. doi:10.1177/1053815116648000

Lee, M. C., & Tsai, T. R. (2010). What drives people to continue to play online games? An extension of technology model and theory of planned behavior. *Intl. Journal of Human–Computer Interaction, 26*(6), 601-620.

Lee, B. H., Smith, T., & Paciorkowski, A. R. (2015). Autism spectrum disorder and epilepsy: Disorders with a shared biology. *Epilepsy & Behavior*, *47*, 191–201. doi:10.1016/j.yebeh.2015.03.017 PMID:25900226

Lee, C. E., Burke, M. M., & Stelter, C. R. (2019). Exploring the Perspectives of Parents and Siblings Toward Future Planning for Individuals With Intellectual and Developmental Disabilities. *Intellectual and Developmental Disabilities*, *57*(3), 198–211. doi:10.1352/1934-9556-57.3.198 PMID:31120401

Lesar, I. (2015). The role of the arts in Tagore's concept of schooling. *CEPS Journal, 5*(3), 111-128. Retrieved from https://www.researchgate.net/publication/283659456_The_Role_of_the_Arts_in_Tagore's_Concept_of_Schooling

Levy, S. E., & Hyman, S. L. (2015). Complementary and alternative medicine treatments for children with autism spectrum disorders. *Child and Adolescent Psychiatric Clinics of North America*, *24*(1), 117–143. doi:10.1016/j.chc.2014.09.004 PMID:25455579

Li, L. E., Chen, E., Hermann, J., Zhang, P., & Wang, L. (2017, July). Scaling machine learning as a service. In *International Conference on Predictive Applications and APIs* (pp. 14-29). Academic Press.

Liaw, A., & Wiener, M. (2002). Classification and regression by randomForest. *R News*, *2*, 18–22.

Li, B., Sharma, A., Meng, J., Purushwalkam, S., & Gowen, E. (2017). Applying machine learning to identify autistic adults using imitation: An exploratory study. *PLoS One*, *12*(8), e0182652. doi:10.1371/journal.pone.0182652 PMID:28813454

Lidström, H., Almqvist, L., & Hemmingsson, H. (2012). Computer-based assistive technology device for use by children with physical disabilities: A cross-sectional study. *Disability and Rehabilitation. Assistive Technology*, *7*(4), 287–293. doi:10.3109/17483107.2011.635332 PMID:22612787

Light, J., Binger, C., Agate, T., & Ramsay, K. (1999). Teaching partner-focused questions to individuals who use augmentative and alternative communication to enhance their communicative competence. *Journal of Speech and Hearing Research*, *42*, 241–255. PMID:10025558

Light, J., Collier, B., & Parnes, P. (1985). Communicative interaction between young nonspeaking physically disabled children and their primary caregivers: Part II— Communicative function. *Augmentative and Alternative Communication*, *1*(3), 98–107. doi:10.1080/07434618512331273591

Light, J., & Drager, K. (2007). AAC technologies for young children with complex communication needs: State of the science and future research directions. *Augmentative and Alternative Communication*, *23*(3), 204–216. doi:10.1080/07434610701553635 PMID:17701740

Light, J., & McNaughton, D. (2012). Supporting the communication, language, and literacy development of children with complex communication needs: State of the science and future research priorities. *Assistive Technology*, *24*(1), 34–44. doi:10.1080/10400435.2011.648717 PMID:22590798

Light, J., McNaughton, D., Beukelman, D., Fager, S. K., Melanie Fried-Okenc, M., Jakobs, T., & Jakobs, E. (2019). Challenges and opportunities in augmentative and alternative communication: Research and technology development to enhance communication and participation for individuals with complex communication needs. *Augmentative and Alternative Communication*, *35*(1), 1–12. doi:10.1080/07434618.2018.1556732 PMID:30648903

Lindahl, J., Stollon, N., Wu, K., Liang, A., Changolkar, S., Steinway, C., ... Jan, S. (2019). Domains of planning for future long-term care of adults with intellectual and developmental disabilities: Parent and sibling perspectives. *Journal of Applied Research in Intellectual Disabilities*, jar.12600. doi:10.1111/jar.12600 PMID:31012229

Lin, H. C. K., Su, S. H., Chao, C. J., Hsieh, C. Y., & Tsai, S. C. (2016). Construction of Multi-Mode Affective Learning System: Taking Affective Design as an Example. *Journal of Educational Technology & Society*, *19*(2), 132–147.

Li, S., Yang, Y., & Liu, C. (2018). Anomaly Detection based on two global grid motion templates. *Signal Processing Image Communication*, *60*, 6–12. doi:10.1016/j.image.2017.09.002

Li, S., Zhou, W., Yuan, Q., Geng, S., & Cai, D. (2013). Feature extraction and recognition of ictal EEG using EMD and SVM. *Computers in Biology and Medicine*, *43*(7), 807–816. doi:10.1016/j.compbiomed.2013.04.002 PMID:23746721

Litjens, G., Kooi, T., Bejnordi, B. E., Arindra, A., Setio, A., Ciompi, F., ... Clara, I. S. (2017). A Survey on Deep Learning in Medical Image Analysis. *Medical Image Analysis*, *42*, 60–88. doi:10.1016/j.media.2017.07.005 PMID:28778026

Liu, F., Guo, W., Fouche, J.-P., Wang, Y., Wang, W., Ding, J., ... Chen, H. (2015). Multivariate classification of social anxiety disorder using whole brain functional connectivity. *Brain Structure & Function*, *220*(1), 101–115. doi:10.100700429-013-0641-4 PMID:24072164

Lloyd, L. L., Fuller, D. R., & Arvidson, H. H. (1997). *Augmentative and alternative communication: A handbook of principles and practices*. Allyn and Bacon.

Loke, Y. J., Hannan, A. J., & Craig, J. M. (2015). The role of epigenetic change in autism spectrum disorders. *Frontiers in Neurology*, *6*, 107. doi:10.3389/fneur.2015.00107 PMID:26074864

Lombardo, M. V., Lai, M. C., & Baron-Cohen, S. (2018). Big data approaches to decomposing heterogeneity across the autism spectrum. *bioRxiv*, 278788.

Lorah, E. R., Parnell, A., Whitby, P. S., & Hantula, D. (2014). A systematic review of tablet computers and portable media players as speech generating devices for individuals with autism spectrum disorder. *Journal of Autism and Developmental Disorders*, *45*, 3792–3804. doi:10.100710803-014-2314-4 PMID:25413144

Lord, C., Elsabbagh, M., Baird, G., & Veenstra-Vanderweele, J. (2018). Autism Spectrum Disorder. *Lancet*, *392*(10146), 508–520. doi:10.1016/S0140-6736(18)31129-2 PMID:30078460

Lord, C., Risi, S., Lambrecht, L., Cook, J., Edwin, H., Leventhal, B. L., ... Rutter, M. (2000). The autism diagnostic observation schedule generic: A standard measure of social and communication deficits associated with the spectrum of autism. *Journal of Autism and Developmental Disability*, *24*, 659–685. doi:10.1007/BF02172145 PMID:11055457

Lovaas, O. I. (1987). Behavioural treatment and normal educational and intellectual functioning in young autistic children. *Journal of Consulting and Clinical Psychology*, *55*, 3–9. PMID:3571656

Ludi, S. (2007). Introducing Accessibility Requirements through External Stakeholder Utilization in an Undergraduate Requirements Engineering Course. *Proc. Soft. Eng.*, *07*, 736–743. doi:10.1109/ICSE.2007.46

Lukander, K. (2003). *Mobile usability-Measuring gaze point on handheld devices*. Master's thesis.

Lupu, R. G., & Ungureanu, F. (2013). A survey of eye tracking methods and applications. *Buletinul Institutului Politehnic din Iasi. Automatic Control and Computer Science Section*, *3*, 72–86.

Luyster, R. J., Kadlec, M. B., Carter, A., & Tager-Flusberg, H. (2008). Language assessment and development in toddlers with autism spectrum disorders. *Journal of Autism and Developmental Disorders*, *38*(8), 1426–1438. PMID:18188685

Lyall, K., Croen, L., Daniels, J., Fallin, M. D., Ladd-Acosta, C., Lee, B. K., ... Newschaffer, C. (2017). The changing epidemiology of Autism Spectrum Disorders. *Annual Review of Public Health*, *38*(1), 81–102. doi:10.1146/annurev-publhealth-031816-044318 PMID:28068486

Lynch, C. J., Uddin, L. Q., Supekar, K., Khouzam, A., Phillips, J., & Menon, V. (2013). Default mode network in childhood autism: Posteromedial cortex heterogeneity and relationship with social deficits. *Biological Psychiatry*, *74*(3), 212–219. doi:10.1016/j.biopsych.2012.12.013 PMID:23375976

Lynch, K., Chin, M., & Blazar, D. (2017). Relationships between observations of elementary mathematics instruction and student achievement: Exploring variability across districts. *American Journal of Education*, *123*(4), 615–646. doi:10.1086/692662

Madanmohan, T., Lakshmi, J., Udupa, K., & Bhavanani, A. B. (2003). Effect of yoga training on handgrip, respiratory Pressures and pulmonary function. *Indian Journal of Physiology and Pharmacology*, *47*(4), 387–392. PMID:15266949

Maguire, M. (2001). Methods to support human-centred design. *International Journal of Human-Computer Studies*, *55*(4), 587–634. doi:10.1006/ijhc.2001.0503

Majaranta, P., MacKenzie, I. S., Aula, A., & Räihä, K. J. (2003, April). Auditory and visual feedback during eye typing. In *Conference on Human Factors in Computing Systems: CHI'03 extended abstracts on Human factors in computing systems* (Vol. 5, No. 10, pp. 766-767). 10.1145/765891.765979

Majaranta, P., & Räihä, K. J. (2002, March). Twenty years of eye typing: systems and design issues. In *Proceedings of the 2002 symposium on Eye tracking research & applications* (pp. 15-22). 10.1145/507072.507076

Mallin, S. S. V., & de Carvalho, H. G. (2015). Assistive technology and user-centred design: Emotion as element for innovation. *Procedia Manufacturing*, *3*, 5570–5578.

Malmivuo, P., Malmivuo, J., & Plonsey, R. (1995). *Bioelectromagnetism: principles and applications of bioelectric and biomagnetic fields*. Oxford University Press. doi:10.1093/acprof:oso/9780195058239.001.0001

Mani, G., Berkovich, S., & Liao, D. (2014, August). Adaptive and Interactive Design Based on Big Data Computational Model for Treating Autism. In *Computing for Geospatial Research and Application (COM. Geo), 2014 Fifth International Conference on* (pp. 121-122). IEEE. 10.1109/COM.Geo.2014.7

Mannfolk, P., Wirestam, R., Nilsson, M., Ståhlberg, F., & Olsrud, J. (2010). Dimensionality reduction of fMRI time series data using locally linear embedding. *Magma (New York, N.Y.)*, *23*(5–6), 327–338. doi:10.100710334-010-0204-0 PMID:20229085

Mannini, A., & Sabatini, A. M. (2010). Machine learning methods for classifying human physical activity from on-body accelerometers. *Sensors (Basel)*, *10*(2), 1154–1175. doi:10.3390100201154 PMID:22205862

Marcano, J. L., Bell, M. A., & Beex, A. A. (2018). Classification of ADHD and non-ADHD subjects using a universal background model. *Biomedical Signal Processing and Control*, *39*, 204–212. doi:10.1016/j.bspc.2017.07.023 PMID:31186670

Marcoux, E. (2011). Turning the standards toward the student – A metacognition aspect. *Teacher Librarian*, *38*(3), 67–68.

Mariotti, V., Marconi, A., & Pardi, G. (2004). Undesired effects of steroids during pregnancy. *The Journal of Maternal-Fetal & Neonatal Medicine*, *16*(2), 5–7. doi:10.1080/jmf.16.2.5.7 PMID:15590425

Markram, K., & Markram, H. (2010). The intense world theory—A unifying theory of the neurobiology of autism. *Frontiers in Human Neuroscience*, *4*, 224. doi:10.3389/fnhum.2010.00224 PMID:21191475

Marlin, B. M., Kale, D. C., Khemani, R. G., & Wetzel, R. C. (2012, January). Unsupervised pattern discovery in electronic health care data using probabilistic clustering models. In *Proceedings of the 2nd ACM SIGHIT international health informatics symposium* (pp. 389-398) 10.1145/2110363.2110408

Masson, G. S., Yang, D. S., & Miles, F. A. (2002). Version and vergence eye movements in humans: Open-loop dynamics determined by monocular rather than binocular image speed. *Vision Research*, *42*(26), 2853–2867. doi:10.1016/S0042-6989(02)00334-6 PMID:12450510

Mastrovito, D., Hanson, C., & Hanson, S. J. (2018). NeuroImage : Clinical Differences in atypical resting-state effective connectivity distinguish autism from schizophrenia. *NeuroImage. Clinical*, *18*(February), 367–376. doi:10.1016/j.nicl.2018.01.014 PMID:29487793

Matson, J. L., & Jang, J. (2014). Treating aggression in persons with autism spectrum disorders: A review. *Research in Developmental Disabilities*, *35*(12), 3386–3391. doi:10.1016/j.ridd.2014.08.025 PMID:25194514

Matson, J. L., & Sturmey, P. (2011). *International handbook of autism and pervasive developmental disorders*. New York: Springer. doi:10.1007/978-1-4419-8065-6

Matson, L. J., Dempsey, T., & LoVullo, A. V. (2009). Characteristics of social skills for adult with intellectual disability, Autism and PDD-NOS. *Research in Autism Spectrum Disorders*, *3*, 207–213.

Mazurek, M. O., & Wenstrup, C. (2013). Television, video game and social media use among children with ASD and typically developing siblings. *Journal of Autism and Developmental Disorders*, *43*(6), 1258–1271. PMID:23001767

McBride, D. (2011). AAC evaluations and new mobile technologies: Asking and answering the right questions. *Perspectives on Augmentative and Alternative Communication*, *20*(1), 9–16. doi:10.1044/aac20.1.9

McCleery, J. P., Akshoomoff, N., Dobkins, K. R., & Carver, L. J. (2009). Atypical face versus object processing and hemispheric asymmetries in 10-month-old infants at risk for autism. *Biological Psychiatry*, *66*(10), 950–957. PMID:19765688

McConachie, H., & Pennington, L. (1997). In-service training for schools on augmentative and alternative communication. *European Journal of Disorders of Communication*, *32*(s3), 277–288. doi:10.1080/13682829709177101 PMID:9474293

McDonagh, D. and Thomas, J. (2010) Rethinking Design Thinking: Empathy Supporting Innovation. *Australasian Medical Journal - Health and Design 1, 3*(8), 458-464.

McLellan, A., Cipparone, C., Giancola, D., Armstrong, D., & Bartlett, D. (2012). Medical and surgical procedures experienced by young children with cerebral palsy. *Pediatric Physical Therapy*, *24*(3), 268–277. doi:10.1097/PEP.0b013e31825be2f6 PMID:22735479

McNaughton, D., & Light, J. (2013). The iPad and mobile technology revolution: Benefits and challenges for individuals who require augmentative and alternative communication. *Augmentative and Alternative Communication*, *29*(2), 107–116. doi:10.3109/07434618.2013.784930 PMID:23705813

McNaughton, D., Rackensperger, T., Benedek-Wood, E., Krezman, C., Williams, M. B., & Light, J. (2008). "A child needs to be given a chance to succeed": Parents of individuals who use AAC describe the benefits and challenges of learning AAC technologies. *Augmentative and Alternative Communication*, *24*(1), 43–55. doi:10.1080/07434610701421007 PMID:18256963

McWilliams, S. A. (2016). Cultivating constructivism: Inspiring intuition and promoting process and pragmatism. *Journal of Constructivist Psychology*, *29*(1), 1–29. doi:10.1080/10720537.2014.980871

Mead, G. H. (1962). *Mind, self, and society from the standpoint of a social behaviorist*. Univ. of Chicago Press.

Meng, X., Bradley, J., Yavuz, B., Sparks, E., Venkataraman, S., Liu, D., ... Xin, D. (2016). Mllib: Machine learning in apache spark. *Journal of Machine Learning Research*, *17*(1), 1235–1241.

Menon, P. (2015). *How Yoga Could Help 'Rewire' The Brains Of Mentally Disabled Children*. Retrieved from http://www.huffingtonpost.in/dr-praseeda-menon/how-yoga-could-helprewir_b_8336520.html#

Mertz, L. (2017). Sharing data to solve the autism riddle: An interview with Adriana Di Martino and Michael Milham of ABIDE. *IEEE Pulse*, *8*(6), 6–9. doi:10.1109/MPUL.2017.2750819 PMID:29155370

Meyer, C. F., & Rhoades, E. K. (2006). Multiculturalism: Beyond food, festival, folklore, and fashion. *Kappa Delta Pi Record*, *42*(2), 82–87. doi:10.1080/00228958.2006.10516439

Michel, P. (2004). *The use of technology in the study, diagnosis and treatment of autism*. Final term Paper for CSC350: Autism and Associated Developmental Disorders.

Miles, J. H. (2015). Complex autism spectrum disorders and cutting-edge molecular diagnostic tests. *Journal of the American Medical Association*, *314*(9), 879–880.

Millar, D. C., Light, J. C., & Schlosser, R. W. (2006). The impact of augmentative and alternative communication intervention on the speech production of individuals with developmental disabilities: A research review. *Journal of Speech, Language, and Hearing Research: JSLHR*, *49*, 248–264. PMID:16671842

Ming, K. (2012). 10 Content-area literacy strategies for art, mathematics, music, and physical education. *The Clearing House: A Journal of Educational Strategies, Issues and Ideas*, *85*(6), 213–220. doi:10.1080/00098655.2012.691568

Ming, X., Brimacombe, M., & Wagner, G. C. (2007). Prevalence of motor impairment in autism spectrum disorders. *Brain & Development*, *29*, 565–570.

Minshew, N. J., Sung, K., Jones, B. L., & Furman, J. M. (2004). Underdevelopment of the postural control system in autism. *Neurology*, *63*(11), 2056–2061. doi:10.1212/01.WNL.0000145771.98657.62 PMID:15596750

Mirenda, P., & Iacono, T. (2009). *Autism spectrum disorders and AAC*. Baltimore: Paul H. Brookes.

Mirenda, P., & Mathy-Laikko, P. (1989). Augmentative and alternative communication applications for persons with severe congenital communication disorders: An introduction. *Augmentative and Alternative Communication*, *5*(1), 3–13. doi:10.1080/07434618912331274916

Mirenda, P., & Schuler, A. L. (1988). Augmenting communication for persons with autism: Issues and strategies. *Topics in Language Disorders*, *9*, 24–43.

Miron, O., Ari-Even Roth, D., Gabis, L. V., Henkin, Y., Shefer, S., Dinstein, I., & Geva, R. (2015). Prolonged auditory brainstem responses in infants with autism. *Autism Research*, *9*(6), 689–695. doi:10.1002/aur.1561 PMID:26477791

Mishra, P., Fahnoe, C., & Henriksen, D. (2013). Creativity, self-directed learning and the architecture of technology rich environments. *TechTrends*, *57*(1), 10–13. doi:10.100711528-012-0623-z

Mitra, S. (2005). *Disability and Social Safety Nets in Developing Countries*. Social Protection Discussion Paper No. 0509. World Bank.

Mitra, S., Posarac, A., & Vick, B. (2013). Disability and poverty in developing countries: A multidimensional study. *World Development*, *41*, 1–18. doi:10.1016/j.worlddev.2012.05.024

Mizunoya, S., & Mitra, S. (2013). Is there a disability gap in employment rates in developing countries? *World Development*, *42*, 28–43. doi:10.1016/j.worlddev.2012.05.037

Mohan Shriya. (2018). *A bridge to planet Autism*. Retrieved October 5, 2019 from https://www.thehindubusinessline.com/blink/cover/a-bridge-to-planet-autism/article23772834.ece

Mohan, V., Kunnath, S. K., Philip, V. S., Mohan, L. S., & Thampi, N. (2019). Capitalizing on technology for developing communication skills in autism spectrum disorder: A single case study. *Disability and Rehabilitation. Assistive Technology*, *14*(1), 75–81. doi:10.1080/17483107.2017.1413144 PMID:29241371

Morimoto, C. H., & Mimica, M. R. (2005). Eye gaze tracking techniques for interactive applications. *Computer Vision and Image Understanding*, *98*(1), 4–24. doi:10.1016/j.cviu.2004.07.010

Morin, K. L., Ganz, J. B., Gregori, E. V., Foster, M. J., Gerow, S. L., Genç-Tosun, D., & Hong, E. R. (2018). A systematic quality review of high-tech AAC interventions as an evidence-based practice. *Augmentative and Alternative Communication*, *34*(2), 104–117. doi:10.1080/07434618.2018.1458900 PMID:29697288

Morrow, E. M., Yoo, S. Y., Flavell, S. W., Kim, T. K., Lin, Y., Hill, R. S., & … . (2008). Identifying autism loci and genes by tracing recent shared ancestry. *Science*, *321*, 218–223. PMID:18621663

Mubashir, M., Shao, L., & Seed, L. (2015). A survey on fall detection principles and approaches. *Neurocomputing, 100*, 144–152. doi:10.1016/j.neucom.2011.09.037

Mukherjee, M. m. (2017). Global design and local histories: Culturally embedded meaning-making for inclusive education. International Education Journal: *Comparative Perspectives, 16*(3), 32-48. Retrieved from https://www.academia.edu/37807740/Global_Design_and_Local_Histories_Culturally_embedded_meaning-making_for_Inclusive_Education?auto=download

Mulak, A., Tache, Y., & Larauche, M. (2014). Sex hormones in the modulation of irritable bowel syndrome. *World Journal of Gastroenterology*, *20*(10), 2433–2448. doi:10.3748/wjg.v20.i10.2433 PMID:24627581

Mullin, A. P., Gokhale, A., Moreno-De-Luca, A., Sanyal, S., Waddington, J. L. V., & Faundez, V. (2013). Neurodevelopmental disorders: Mechanisms and boundary definitions from genomes, interactomes and proteomes. *Translational Psychiatry*, *3*(12), e329. doi:10.1038/tp.2013.108 PMID:24301647

Mulroy, S., Robertson, L., Aiberti, K., Leonard, H., & Bower, C. (2008). The impact of having a sibling with an intellectual disability: Parental perspectives in two disorders. *Journal of Intellectual Disability Research*, *52*(3), 216–229. doi:10.1111/j.1365-2788.2007.01005.x PMID:18261021

Mumford, L., Lam, R., Wright, V., & Chau, T. (2014). An access technology delivery protocol for children with severe and multiple disabilities: A case demonstration. *Developmental Neurorehabilitation*, *17*(4), 232–242. doi:10.3109/17518423.2013.776125 PMID:23869969

Munakata, M., & Vaidya, A. (2012). Encouraging creativity in mathematics and science through photography. Teaching Mathematics and Its Applications: *An International. The Journal of IMA / Islamic Medical Association of North America*, *31*(3), 121–132.

Murphy, J., Marková, I., Moodie, E., Scott, J., & Boa, S. (1995). Augmentative and alternative communication systems used by people with cerebral palsy in Scotland: Demographic survey. *Augmentative and Alternative Communication*, *11*(1), 26–36. doi:10.1080/07434619512331277119

Murphy, M. D., Guggenmos, D. J., Bundy, D. T., & Nudo, R. J. (2016). Current challenges facing the translation of brain computer interfaces from preclinical trials to use in human patients. *Frontiers in Cellular Neuroscience*, *9*, 497. doi:10.3389/fncel.2015.00497 PMID:26778962

Murray, J., & Goldbart, J. (2009). Cognitive and language acquisition in typical and aided language learning: A review of recent evidence from an aided communication perspective. *Child Language Teaching and Therapy*, *25*(1), 31–58. doi:10.1177/0265659008098660

Mutch, L., Leyland, A., & McGee, A. (1993). Patterns of neuropsychological function in a low-birthweight population. *Developmental Medicine and Child Neurology*, *35*(11), 943–956. doi:10.1111/j.1469-8749.1993.tb11576.x PMID:8224562

Myers, T. (2010). *Housing options for Adults with Autism Spectrum Disorder*. Bureau of Autism Services, Pennsylvania Department of Public Welfare. Retrieved October 5, 2019 from http://www.dhs.pa.gov/cs/groups/webcontent/documents/report/p_012904.pdf

Myers, S. M., & Johnson, C. P. (2007). Management of children with autism spectrum disorders. *Pediatrics, 120*, 1162–1182. PMID:17967921

Myers, S. M., & Johnson, C. P. (2007). The Council on Children with Disabilities. Management of Children with Autism Spectrum Disorders. *Pediatrics*, *120*(5), 1162–1182. doi:10.1542/peds.2007-2362 PMID:17967921

Nakamura, K., Newell, A., Alm, N., & Waller, A. (1998). How do members of different language communities compose sentences with a picture-based communication system?—A cross–cultural study of picture–based sentences constructed by English and Japanese speakers. *Augmentative and Alternative Communication, 14*(2), 71–80. doi:10.1080/07434619812331278226

Narasingharao, K., Pradhan, B., & Navaneetham, J. (2016). Sleep Disorder, Gastrointestinal Problems and Behaviour Problems Seen in Autism Spectrum Disorder Children and Yoga as Therapy: A Descriptive Review. *Journal of Clinical and Diagnostic Research : JCDR, 10*(11), VE01–VE03. doi:10.7860/JCDR/2016/24175.8922 PMID:28050484

Narasingharao, K., Pradhan, B., & Navaneetham, J. (2017). Efficacy of Structured Yoga Intervention for Sleep, Gastrointestinal and Behaviour Problems of ASD Children: An Exploratory Study. *Journal of Clinical and Diagnostic Research : JCDR, 11*(3), VC01–VC06. doi:10.7860/JCDR/2017/25894.9502 PMID:28511484

Nascimento, N., Alencar, P., Lucena, C., & Cowan, D. (2018, October). A context-aware machine learning-based approach. In *Proceedings of the 28th Annual International Conference on Computer Science and Software Engineering* (pp. 40-47). IBM Corp.

Natarajan, B. (2002). *Thirumandiram - A Tamil Scriptural Classic of Thirumoolar* [English Translation]. Chennai, India: Sri Ramakrishna Math Publications.

Newberg, A. B., Wintering, N., Khalsa, D. S., Roggenkamp, H., & Waldman, M. R. (2010). Meditation effects on cognitive function and cerebral blood flow in subjects with memory loss: A preliminary study. *Journal of Alzheimer's Disease, 20*(2), 517–526. doi:10.3233/JAD-2010-1391 PMID:20164557

Newell, A. F., & Gregor, P. (2000). User sensitive inclusive design—in search of a new paradigm. In *Proceedings on the 2000 conference on Universal Usability* (pp. 39-44). ACM. 10.1145/355460.355470

News Hook. (2018). *SENS: A special show for special minds.* Retrieved October 5, 2019 from https://newzhook.com/story/19420

Nicolaidis, C., Kripke, C. C., & Raymaker, D. (2014). Primary care for adults on the autism spectrum. *The Medical Clinics of North America, 98*(5), 1169–1191. doi:10.1016/j.mcna.2014.06.011 PMID:25134878

Nielsen, J. A., Zielinski, B. A., Fletcher, P. T., Alexander, A. L., Lange, N., Bigler, E. D., ... Anderson, J. S. (2013). Multisite functional connectivity MRI classification of autism: ABIDE results. *Frontiers in Human Neuroscience, 7*(SEP), 1–12. doi:10.3389/fnhum.2013.00599 PMID:24093016

Nikolov, R. N., Bearss, K. E., Lettinga, J., Erickson, C., Rodowski, M., Aman, M. G., ... Scahill, L. (2009). Gastrointestinal symptoms in a sample of children with pervasive developmental disorders. *Journal of Autism and Developmental Disorders, 30*, 405–413. PMID:18791817

NIMH Depression. (2018). Retrieved December 4, 2018, from https://www.nimh.nih.gov/health/topics/depression/index.shtml

Northrup, C. M., Lantz, J., & Hamlin, T. (2016). Wearable stress sensors for children with autism spectrum disorder with in situ alerts to caregivers via a mobile phone. *Proceedings, 2*(1), e9.

Novak, I., Hines, M., Goldsmith, S., & Barclay, R. (2012). Clinical prognostic messages from a systematic review on cerebral palsy. *Pediatrics, 130*(5), e1285–e1312. doi:10.1542/peds.2012-0924 PMID:23045562

Nunes, D. (2008). AAC interventions for autism: A research summary. *International Journal of Special Education, 23*(2), 17–25.

Nybo, K. (2015). *Dimensionality reduction methods for fMRI analysis and visualization* (Thesis). Aslto University.

O'Neill, T., Light, J., & Pope, L. (2018). Effects of interventions that include aided augmentative and alternative communication input on the communication of individuals with complex communication needs: A meta-analysis. *Journal of Speech, Language, and Hearing Research: JSLHR*, *61*(7), 1743–1765. doi:10.1044/2018_JSLHR-L-17-0132 PMID:29931287

Odding, E., Roebroeck, M. E., & Stam, H. J. (2006). The epidemiology of cerebral palsy: Incidence, impairments and risk factors. *Disability and Rehabilitation*, *28*(4), 183–191. doi:10.1080/09638280500158422 PMID:16467053

Ohno, T., & Mukawa, N. (2004, March). A free-head, simple calibration, gaze tracking system that enables gaze-based interaction. In *Proceedings of the 2004 symposium on Eye tracking research & applications* (pp. 115-122). 10.1145/968363.968387

Oliver, D. J., Borasio, G. D., Caraceni, A., de Visser, M., Grisold, W., Lorenzl, S., ... Voltz, R. (2016). A consensus review on the development of palliative care for patients with chronic and progressive neurological disease. *European Journal of Neurology*, *23*(1), 30–38. doi:10.1111/ene.12889 PMID:26423203

O'Neill, S., Smyth, S., Smeaton, A. F., & O'Connor, N. E. (2019). Assistive technology: Understanding the needs and experiences of individuals with Autism Spectrum Disorder and/or Intellectual Disability in Ireland and the UK. *Assistive Technology: The Official Journal of RESNA*. doi:10.1080/10400435.2018.1535526

Oono, I. P., Honey, E. J., & McConachie, H. (2013). Parent-mediated early intervention for young children with autism spectrum disorders (ASD). *Cochrane Database of Systematic Reviews*, CD009774. PMID:23633377

Orme-Johnson, D. (2006). Evidence that the transcendental meditation program prevents or decreases diseases of the nervous system and is specifically beneficial for epilepsy. *Medical Hypotheses*, *67*(2), 240–246. doi:10.1016/j.mehy.2006.03.034 PMID:16723189

Orme-Johnson, D. W., Schneider, R. H., Son, Y. D., Nidich, S., & Cho, Z. H. (2006). Neuroimaging of meditation's effect on brain reactivity to pain. *Neuroreport*, *17*(12), 1359–1363. doi:10.1097/01.wnr.0000233094.67289.a8 PMID:16951585

Osterling, J., & Dawson, G. (1994). Early recognition of children with autism: A study of first birthday home videotapes. *Journal of Autism and Developmental Disorders*, *24*, 247–257. PMID:8050980

Ostryn, C., Wolfe, P., & Rusch, F. (2008). A Review and Analysis of the Picture Exchange Communication System (PECS) for Individuals with Autism Spectrum Disorders Using a Paradigm of Communication Competence. *Research and Practice for Persons with Severe Disabilities*, *33*, 13–24.

Owen, R., Sikich, L., Marcus, R. N., Corey-Lisle, P., Manos, G., McQuade, R. D., ... Findling, R. L. (2009). Aripiprazole in the treatment of irritability and in children and adolescents with autism disorder. *Pediatrics*, *124*(6), 1533–1640. doi:10.1542/peds.2008-3782 PMID:19948625

Ozcan, M.O., Doyuran, T., & Beynek, B. (2017). *A Survey on the Use of Microsoft Kinect for Physical Rehabilitation*. Academic Press.

Ozonoff, S., Young, G. S., Carter, A., Messinger, D., Yirmiya, N., Zwaigenbaum, L., ... Stone, W. L. (2011). Recurrence risk for autism spectrum disorders: A Baby Siblings Research Consortium study. *Pediatrics*, *128*, e488–e495. PMID:21844053

Palisano, R. J., Begnoche, D. M., Chiarello, L. A., Bartlett, D. J., McCoy, S. W., & Chang, H. J. (2012). Amount and focus of physical therapy and occupational therapy for young children with cerebral palsy. *Physical & Occupational Therapy in Pediatrics*, *32*(4), 368–382. doi:10.3109/01942638.2012.715620 PMID:22954372

Palmen, S. J., Hulshoff Pol, H. E., Kemner, C., Schnack, H. G., Durston, S., Lahuis, B. E., & ... . (2005). Increased gray-matter volume in medication-naive high-functioning children with autism spectrum disorder. *Psychological Medicine*, *35*(4), 561–570. PMID:15856726

Pang, R., Lansdell, B. J., & Fairhall, A. L. (2016). Dimensionality reduction in neuroscience. *Current Biology*, *26*(14), R656–R660. doi:10.1016/j.cub.2016.05.029 PMID:27458907

Pareekh. (2015). *Sai Bakery: A Mother's sweet gift to her Autistic son and his differently abled friends*. Retrieved October 5, 2019 from https://www.thebetterindia.com/22773/sai-bakery-chennai-adults-with-special-needs/

Park, M. J., Yoo, Y. J., Chung, C. Y., & Hwang, J. M. (2016). Ocular findings in patients with spastic type cerebral palsy. *BMC Ophthalmology*, *16*(1), 195. doi:10.118612886-016-0367-1 PMID:27821110

Parsons, S. (2016). Authenticity in *virtual reality* for assessment and intervention in Autism: A conceptual review. *Educational Research Review*, *19*, 138–157. doi:10.1016/j.edurev.2016.08.001

Pastor, P. N., & Reuben, C. A. (2008). Diagnosed attention deficit hyperactivity disorder and learning disability: United States, 2004-2006. *Vital and Health Statistics*, *10*, 237. PMID:18998276

Paszke, A., Chanan, G., Lin, Z., Gross, S., Yang, E., Antiga, L., & Devito, Z. (2017). Automatic differentiation in PyTorch. *31st Conference on Neural Information Processing Systems*, 1–4. 10.1017/CBO9781107707221.009

Paul, R. (2005). *Language Disorders from Infancy through Adolescence: Assessment & Intervention* (2nd ed.). Mosby, Inc.

Pellegrino, J. W. (2014). Assessment as a positive influence on 21st century teaching and learning. *Psicologia dell'Educazione*, *20*(2), 65–77. doi:10.1016/j.pse.2014.11.002

Pennington, B. F. (2008). *Diagnosing learning disorders: A neuropsychological framework*. Guilford Press.

Pennington, L., Goldbart, J., & Marshall, J. (2004). Speech and language therapy to improve the communication skills of children with cerebral palsy. *Cochrane Database of Systematic Reviews*, (2): CD003466. PMID:15106204

Pennington, L., & Mcconachie, H. (1999). Mother-child interaction revisited: Communication with non-speaking physically disabled children. *International Journal of Language & Communication Disorders*, *34*(4), 391–416. doi:10.1080/136828299247351 PMID:10884908

Pennington, M. C. (1999). Computer-aided pronunciation pedagogy: Promise, limitations, directions. *Computer Assisted Language Learning*, *12*(5), 427–440. doi:10.1076/call.12.5.427.5693

Pereira, F., Mitchell, T., & Botvinick, M. (2009). NeuroImage Machine learning classifiers and fMRI : A tutorial overview. *NeuroImage*, *45*(1), S199–S209. doi:10.1016/j.neuroimage.2008.11.007 PMID:19070668

Perilli, V., Lancioni, G. E., Hoogeveen, F., Caffó, A., Singh, N., O'Reilly, M., ... Oliva, D. (2013a). Video prompting versus other instruction strategies for persons with Alzheimer's disease. *American Journal of Alzheimer's Disease and Other Dementias*, *28*(4), 393–402. doi:10.1177/1533317513488913 PMID:23687181

Perilli, V., Lancioni, G. E., Laporta, D., Paparella, A., Caffò, A. O., Singh, N. N., ... Oliva, D. (2013b). A computer-aided telephone system to enable five persons with Alzheimer's disease to make phone calls independently. *Research in Developmental Disabilities*, *34*(6), 1991–1997. doi:10.1016/j.ridd.2013.03.016 PMID:23584179

Peterman, N. E., & Kennedy, J. (2003). Enterprise Education: Influencing Students' Perceptions of Entrepreneurship. *Entrepreneurship Theory and Practice*, *28*, 129–144.

Petersen, S., Baalsrud, J., Eds, H., & Hutchison, D. (2014). *Serious Games Development and Applications*. Springer International Publishing.

Peterson, P., Barrows, S., & Gift, T. (2016). After Common Core, states set rigorous standards. *Education Next, 16*(3), 9–15.

Petersson, S., Pedersen, N.L., Schalling, M., & Lavebratt, C. (1999). *Primary megalencephaly at birth and low intelligence level.* Academic Press.

Picot, A., Charbonnier, S., & Caplier, A. (2010, May). Drowsiness detection based on visual signs: blinking analysis based on high frame rate video. In *2010 IEEE Instrumentation & Measurement Technology Conference Proceedings* (pp. 801-804). IEEE. 10.1109/IMTC.2010.5488257

Pirila, S., van der Meere, J., Pentikainen, T., Ruusu-Niemi, P., Korpela, R., Kilpinen, J., & Nieminen, P. (2007). Language and motor speech skills in children with cerebral palsy. *Journal of Communication Disorders, 40*(2), 116–128. doi:10.1016/j.jcomdis.2006.06.002 PMID:16860820

Plitt, M., Anne, K., & Martin, A. (2015). NeuroImage : Clinical Functional connectivity classification of autism identifies highly predictive brain features but falls short of biomarker standards. *NeuroImage. Clinical, 7*, 359–366. doi:10.1016/j.nicl.2014.12.013 PMID:25685703

Płoński, P., Gradkowski, W., Altarelli, I., Monzalvo, K., van Ermingen-Marbach, M., Grande, M., ... Jednoróg, K. (2017). Multi-parameter machine learning approach to the neuroanatomical basis of developmental dyslexia. *Human Brain Mapping, 38*(2), 900–908. doi:10.1002/hbm.23426 PMID:27712002

Ploog, B. O., Scharf, A., Nelson, D. S., & Brooks, P. J. (2013). Use of Computer-Assisted Technologies (CAT) to Enhance Social, Communicative, and Language. Development in Children with Autism Spectrum Disorders. *Journal of Autism and Developmental Disorders, 43*(2), 301–322. doi:10.100710803-012-1571-3 PMID:22706582

Politte, L. C., Howe, Y., Nowinski, L., Palumbo, M., & McDougle, C. J. (2015). Evidence-Based Treatments for Autism Spectrum Disorder. *Current Treatment Options in Psychiatry, 2*(1), 38–56. doi:10.100740501-015-0031-z

Pousada García, T., Pereira Loureiro, J., Groba González, B., Nieto Riveiro, L., & Pazos Sierra, A. (2011). The use of computers and augmentative and alternative communication devices by children and young with cerebral palsy. *Assistive Technology, 23*(3), 135–149. doi:10.1080/10400435.2011.588988

Pratap, A., & Kanimozhiselvi, C. S. (2014). Predictive assessment of autism using unsupervised machine learning models. *International Journal of Advanced Intelligence Paradigms, 6*(2), 113–121. doi:10.1504/IJAIP.2014.062174

Preston, D., & Carter, M. (2009). A review of the efficacy of the Picture Exchange Communication System Intervention. *Journal of Autism and Developmental Disabilities, 39*, 1471–1486. PMID:19495952

Pridmore, J. (2009). The poet's school and the parrot's cage: The educational spirituality of Rabindranath Tagore. *International Journal of Children's Spirituality, 14*(4), 355–367. doi:10.1080/13644360903293572

Prizant, B. M., Wetherby, A. M., Rubin, E., & Laurent, A. C. (2003). The SCERTS Model: A Transactional, Family-Centered Approach to Enhancing Communication and Socioemotional Abilities of Children with Autism Spectrum Disorder. *Infants and Young Children, 16*, 296–316.

Provost, B., Heimerl, S., & Lopez, B. R. (2007). Levels of gross and fine motor development in young children with autism spectrum disorder. *Physical & Occupational Therapy in Pediatrics, 27*(3), 21–36. doi:10.1080/J006v27n03_03 PMID:17613454

Pua, E. P. K., Barton, S., Williams, K., Craig, J. M., & Seal, M. (2018). Individualised MRI training for paediatric neuroimaging in autism spectrum disorders: A child-focused approach. *bioRxiv, 61*(03), 462234.

Purves, D., Augustine, G. J., Fitzpatrick, D., Katz, L. C., LaMantia, A. S., McNamara, J. O., & Williams, S. M. (2001). Circuits within the basal ganglia system. In Neuroscience (2nd ed.). Sinauer Associates.

Putman, J. A., & Othmer, S. (2006). Phase sensitivity of bipolar EEG training protocols. *Journal of Neurotherapy*, *10*(1), 73–79. doi:10.1300/J184v10n01_06

Quinn, B.S., Behrmann, M., Mastropieri, M., Bausch, M.E., Ault, M.J., & Chung, Y. (2009). Who is using assistive technology in school? *J Spec Educ Technol.*, *24*, 1-13.

Radhakrishna, S., Nagarathna, R., & Nagendra, H. R. (2010). Integrated approach to yoga therapy and autism spectrum disorders. *Journal of Ayurveda and Integrative Medicine*, *1*(2), 120–124. doi:10.4103/0975-9476.65089 PMID:21836799

Radomski, M. V., & Latham, C. A. T. (Eds.). (2008). *Occupational therapy for physical dysfunction*. Lippincott Williams & Wilkins.

Raghavendra, P., Olsson, C., Sampson, J., Mcinerney, R., & Connell, T. (2012). School participation and social networks of children with complex communication needs, physical disabilities, and typically developing peers. *Augmentative and Alternative Communication*, *28*(1), 33–43. doi:10.3109/07434618.2011.653604 PMID:22364536

Raghupathi, W., & Raghupathi, V. (2014). Big data analytics in healthcare: Promise and potential. *Health Information Science and Systems*, *2*(1), 3. doi:10.1186/2047-2501-2-3 PMID:25825667

Rajagopalan, Dhall, & Goecke. (2013). *Self-Stimulatory Behaviours in the Wild for Autism Diagnosis*. IEEE Explore.

Rajagopalan, S. S., Dhall, A., & Goecke, R. (2013). Self-Stimulatory Behaviours in the Wild for Autism Diagnosis. *Proceedings of the IEEE International Conference on Computer Vision Workshops*, 755–761. 10.1109/ICCVW.2013.103

Ramanathan, M., & Bhavanani, A. B. (2017). *Yoga for Children with Special Needs*. Ministry of Ayush. Available from: https://moayush.wordpress.com/2017/05/09/yoga-for-children-with-specialneeds/

Ramanathan, M., & Bhavanani, A. B. (2018). Addressing Autism Spectrum Disorder through Yoga as a Complementary Therapy. *J Basic ClinAppl Health Sci*, *2*(2), 3–7. doi:10.5005/jp-journals-10082-01123

Ramani, S. A., & Sankar, A. (2016). "ISpeak"- Augmentative and Alternative Communication for children with Communication Disorders. *Sri Ramachandra Journal of Medicine*, *9*(1), 1–4.

Ratcliff, A., & Little, M. (1996). A conversation based barrier task approach to teach sight- word vocabulary to a young augmentative communication system user. *Child Language Teaching and Therapy*, *12*(2), 128–135. doi:10.1177/026565909601200203

Rayner, K. (1998). Eye movements in reading and information processing: 20 years of research. *Psychological Bulletin*, *124*(3), 372–422. doi:10.1037/0033-2909.124.3.372 PMID:9849112

Rayner, K., Rotello, C. M., Stewart, A. J., Keir, J., & Duffy, S. A. (2001). Integrating text and pictorial information: Eye movements when looking at print advertisements. *Journal of Experimental Psychology. Applied*, *7*(3), 219–226. doi:10.1037/1076-898X.7.3.219 PMID:11676100

Razzak, M. I., Naz, S., & Zaib, A. (2018). Deep learning for medical image processing: Overview, challenges and the future. *Lecture Notes in Computational Vision and Biomechanics*, *26*, 323–350. doi:10.1007/978-3-319-65981-7_12

Reber, M. E. (2009). *The autism spectrum: Scientific foundations and treatment* Doi:10.1017/CBO9780511978616

Reddihough, D. (2011). Cerebral palsy in childhood. *Australian Family Physician*, *40*(4), 192. PMID:21597527

Rehg, J. M., Abowd, G. D., Rozga, A. A., Romero, M., Clements, M. A., & Sclaroff, S. (2013). Decoding children's social behavior. IEEE CVPR.

Reichow, B., Barton, E. E., Boyd, B. A., & Hume, K. (2012). Early intensive behavioral intervention (EIBI) for young children with autism spectrum disorders (ASD). *Cochrane Database of Systematic Reviews*, CD009260. PMID:23076956

Renard, Y., Lotte, F., Gibert, G., Congedo, M., Maby, E., Delannoy, V., ... Lécuyer, A. (2010). Openvibe: An open-source software platform to design, test, and use brain–computer interfaces in real and virtual environments. *Presence (Cambridge, Mass.), 19*(1), 35–53. doi:10.1162/pres.19.1.35

Renton, A. I., Mattingley, J. B., & Painter, D. R. (2018). An open interface system for non-invasive brain-to-brain free communication between naive human participants. *bioRxiv*, 488825.

Rikert, T. D., & Jones, M. J. (1998, April). Gaze estimation using morphable models. In *Proceedings Third IEEE International Conference on Automatic Face and Gesture Recognition* (pp. 436-441). IEEE. 10.1109/AFGR.1998.670987

Riksen-Walraven, J. M. (1978). Effects of caregiver behavior on habituation and self-efficacy in infants. *International Journal of Behavioral Development, 1*, 105–130.

Rinaldi, C., Averill, O. H., & Stuart, S. (2011). Response to intervention: Educators' perceptions of a three-year RTI collaborative reform effort in an urban elementary school. *Journal of Education-Boston University School of Education,* (2), 43.

Rispoli, M. J., Franco, J. H., Van Der Meer, L., Lang, R., & Camargo, S. P. H. (2010). The use of speech generating devices in communication interventions for individuals with developmental disabilities: A review of the literature. *Developmental Neurorehabilitation, 13*(4), 276–293. doi:10.3109/17518421003636794 PMID:20629594

Rittel, H., & Webber, M. (1973). Dilemmas in a General Theory of Planning. *Policy Sciences, 4*(2), 155–179. doi:10.1007/BF01405730

Rochat, M. J., Veroni, V., Bruschweiler-stern, N., Pieraccini, C., Bonnet-brilhault, F., Barthélémy, C., ... Rizzolatti, G. (2013). Neuropsychologia Impaired vitality form recognition in autism. *Neuropsychologia, 51*(10), 1918–1924. doi:10.1016/j.neuropsychologia.2013.06.002 PMID:23792328

Roche, L., Sigafoos, J., Lancioni, G. E., O'Reilly, M. F., & Green, V. A. (2015). Microswitch technology for enabling self-determined responding in children with profound and multiple disabilities: A systematic review. *Augmentative and Alternative Communication, 31*(3), 246–258. doi:10.3109/07434618.2015.1024888 PMID:25791421

Rockstroh, B., Elbert, T., Birbaumer, N., & Lutzenberger, W. (1990). Biofeedback-produced hemispheric asymmetry of slow cortical potentials and its behavioural effects. *International Journal of Psychophysiology, 9*(2), 151–165. doi:10.1016/0167-8760(90)90069-P PMID:2228749

Rogala, J., Jurewicz, K., Paluch, K., Kublik, E., Cetnarski, R., & Wróbel, A. (2016). The do's and don'ts of neurofeedback training: A review of the controlled studies using healthy adults. *Frontiers in Human Neuroscience, 10*, 301. doi:10.3389/fnhum.2016.00301 PMID:27378892

Rogge, N., & Janssen, J. (2019). The economic costs of autism spectrum disorder: A literature review. *Journal of Autism and Developmental Disorders, 49*(7), 2873–2900. doi:10.100710803-019-04014-z PMID:30976961

Rohanachandra, Y. M., Dahanayake, D. M. A., Rohanachandra, L. T., & Wijetunge, G. S. (2017). Knowledge about diagnostic features and comorbidities of childhood autism among doctors in a tertiary care hospital. *Sri Lanka Journal of Child Health, 46*(1), 29. doi:10.4038ljch.v46i1.8093

Rohwerder, B. (2018). *Disability stigma in developing countries*. Academic Press.

Rojahn, J., Matson, J. L., Lott, D., Esbensen, A. J., & Smalls, Y. (2001). The Behavior Problems Inventory: An instrument for the assessment of self-injury, stereotyped behavior, and aggression/destruction in individuals with developmental disabilities. *Journal of Autism and Developmental Disorders*, *31*(6), 577–588. doi:10.1023/A:1013299028321 PMID:11814269

Rolfs, M. (2009). Microsaccades: Small steps on a long way. *Vision Research*, *49*(20), 2415–2441. doi:10.1016/j.visres.2009.08.010 PMID:19683016

Romanski, L. M. (2012). Integration of faces and vocalizations in ventral prefrontal cortex: Implications for the evolution of audiovisual speech. *Proceedings of the National Academy of Sciences of the United States of America*, *109*(Supplement 1), 10717–10724. doi:10.1073/pnas.1204335109 PMID:22723356

Romski, M. A., & Sevcik, R. A. (1996). Breaking the speech barrier: Language development through augmented means. Brookes Publishing Company.

Romski, M., & Sevcik, R. (2005). Augmentative communication and early intervention: Myths and realities. *Infants and Young Children*, *18*, 174–185.

Romski, M., Sevcik, R. A., Adamson, L. B., Smith, A., Cheslock, M., & Bakeman, R. (2011). Parent perceptions of the language development of toddlers with developmental delays before and after participation in parent-coached language interventions. *American Journal of Speech-Language Pathology*, *20*(2), 111–118. doi:10.1044/1058-0360(2011/09-0087) PMID:21330651

Rosa-Lugo, L. I., & Kent-Walsh, J. (2008). Effects of parent instruction on communicative turns of Latino children using augmentative and alternative communication during storybook reading. *Communication Disorders Quarterly*, *30*(1), 49–61.

Rosa, M. J., Portugal, L., Hahn, T., Fallgatter, A. J., Garrido, M. I., Shawe-Taylor, J., & Mourao-Miranda, J. (2015). Sparse network-based models for patient classification using fMRI. *NeuroImage*, *105*, 493–506. doi:10.1016/j.neuroimage.2014.11.021 PMID:25463459

Rosenbaum, P. (2003). Cerebral palsy: What parents and doctors want to know. *BMJ (Clinical Research Ed.)*, *326*(7396), 970–974. doi:10.1136/bmj.326.7396.970 PMID:12727772

Rosenbaum, P., King, S., Law, M., King, G., & Evans, J. (1998). Family-centred service: A conceptual framework and research review. *Physical & Occupational Therapy in Pediatrics*, *18*(1), 1–20.

Rosenbaum, P., Paneth, N., Leviton, A., Goldstein, M., Bax, M., Damiano, D., ... Jacobsson, B. (2007). A report: The definition and classification of cerebral palsy April 2006. *Developmental Medicine and Child Neurology. Supplement*, *109*, 8–14. PMID:17370477

Ross, M. K., Wei, W., & Ohno-Machado, L. (2014). "Big data" and the electronic health record. *Yearbook of Medical Informatics*, *9*(1), 97–104. doi:10.15265/IY-2014-0003 PMID:25123728

Royal Society. (2019). iHuman: blurring lines between mind and machine. Royal Society.

Rubasinghe, I. D., & Meedeniya, D. A. (2020). Automated Neuroscience Decision Support Framework. In Deep Learning Techniques for Biomedical and Health Informatics. Academic Press. doi:10.1016/B978-0-12-819061-6.00013-6

Ruppar, A., Roberts, C., & Olson, A. (2017). Perceptions about expert teaching for students with severe disabilities among teachers identified as experts. *Research and Practice for Persons with Severe Disabilities*, *42*(2), 121–135. doi:10.1177/1540796917697311

Ryan, Schachat, Wilkinson, Hinton, & Sadda. (2012). *Retina*. Elsevier Health Sciences.

Sabokrou, M., Fayyaz, M., Fathy, M., Moayed, Z., & Klette, R. (2018). Deep-anomaly: Fully convolution neural network for fast anomaly detection in crowded scenes. *Computer Vision and Image Understanding*, *172*, 88–97. doi:10.1016/j.cviu.2018.02.006

Sacchet, M. D., Prasad, G., Foland-Ross, L. C., Thompson, P. M., & Gotlib, I. H. (2015). Support Vector Machine Classification of Major Depressive Disorder Using Diffusion-Weighted Neuroimaging and Graph Theory. *Frontiers in Psychiatry*, *6*, 21. doi:10.3389/fpsyt.2015.00021 PMID:25762941

Sage, G. (1895). *The Gheranda Samhita: A Treatise on Hatha Yoga* (S. C. Vasu, Trans. & Ed.). Bombay, India: Theosophical.

Sagiv, S. K., Thurston, S. W., Bellinger, D. C., Tolbert, P. E., Altshul, L. M., & Korrick, S. A. (2010). Prenatal organochlorine exposure and behaviors associated with attention deficit hyperactivity disorder in school-aged children. *American Journal of Epidemiology*, *171*(5), 593–601. doi:10.1093/aje/kwp427 PMID:20106937

Saleh, M. S., Aljaam, J. M., Karime, A., & El Saddik, A. (2013). An edutainment system for assisting qatari children with moderate intellectual and learning disability through exerting physical activities. *IEEE Global Engineering Education Conference (EDUCON)*, 886–892.

Salvatore, C., Cerasa, A., Castiglioni, I., Gallivanone, F., Augimeri, A., Lopez, M., ... Quattrone, A. (2014). Machine learning on brain MRI data for differential diagnosis of Parkinson's disease and Progressive Supranuclear Palsy. *Journal of Neuroscience Methods*, *222*, 230–237. doi:10.1016/j.jneumeth.2013.11.016 PMID:24286700

Samhita, S. (2010a). Nibandha Samgraha commentary chikitsa, 15/3, ed: 2010. Chaukhambha Sanskrit sansthan. Varanasi.

Samhita, S. (2010b). Nibandha Samgraha commentary sutra, 35/27, ed:2010. Chaukhambha Sanskrit sansthan. Varanasi.

Sanchack, K. E., & Thomas, C. A. (2016). Autism spectrum disorders: Primary care principles. *American Family Physician*, *94*, 972–979. PMID:28075089

Sanders, E., & Stappers, P. J. (2008). Co-Creation and the New Landscapes of Design. *CoDesign*, *4*(1), 5–18. doi:10.1080/15710880701875068

Sandin, S., Lichtenstein, P., Kuja-Holkola, R., Larsson, H., Hultman, C. M., & Reichenberg, A. (2014). The familial risk of autism. *Journal of the American Medical Association*, *311*(17), 1770–1777. doi:10.1001/jama.2014.4144 PMID:24794370

Sangare, M., Toure, H. B., Toure, A., Karembe, A., Dolo, H., Coulibaly, Y. I., ... Geschwind, D. H. (2019). Validation of two parent-reported autism spectrum disorders screening tools M-CHAT-R and SCQ in Bamako, Mali. *eNeurologicalSci*, *15*(March), 1–5. doi:10.1016/j.ensci.2019.100188 PMID:30923752

Sarkar, B. K. (2017). Big data for secure healthcare system: A conceptual design. *Complex & Intelligent Systems*, *3*(2), 133–151. doi:10.100740747-017-0040-1

Sarraf, S., & Tofighi, G. (2016). *Classification of Alzheimer's Disease using fMRI Data and Deep Learning Convolutional Neural Networks*. arXiv:1603.0863

Sartipi, S., Shayesteh, M. G., & Kalbkhani, H. (2018). Diagnosing of Autism Spectrum Disorder based on GARCH Variance Series for rs-fMRI data. *2018 9th International Symposium on Telecommunications (IST)*, 86–90.

Sasson, N. J., & Elison, J. T. (2012). Eye tracking young children with autism. *Journal of Visualized Experiments*, *§§§*, 61. PMID:22491039

Sato, J. R., Moll, J., Green, S., Deakin, J. F. W., Thomaz, C. E., & Zahn, R. (2015). Machine learning algorithm accurately detects fMRI signature of vulnerability to major depression. *Psychiatry Research: Neuroimaging*, *233*(2), 289–291. doi:10.1016/j.pscychresns.2015.07.001 PMID:26187550

Savino, P. J., & Danesh-Meyer, H. V. (Eds.). (2012). *Color Atlas and Synopsis of Clinical Ophthalmology--Wills Eye Institute--Neuro-Ophthalmology*. Lippincott Williams & Wilkins.

Sayorwan, W., Phianchana, N., Permpoonputtana, K., & Siripornpanich, V. (2018). A Study of the Correlation between VEP and Clinical Severity in Children with Autism Spectrum Disorder. *Autism Research and Treatment*, *2018*, 2018. doi:10.1155/2018/5093016 PMID:29568651

Schaefer, G. B. (2008). Genetics considerations in cerebral palsy. *Seminars in Pediatric Neurology*, *15*(1), 21–26. doi:10.1016/j.spen.2008.01.004 PMID:18342257

Schaefer, G. B., & Mendelsohn, N. J.Professional Practice Guidelines Committee. (2008). Clinical genetics evaluation in identifying the etiology of autism spectrum disorders. *Genetics in Medicine*, *10*(4), 301–305. doi:10.1097/GIM.0b013e31816b5cc9 PMID:18414214

Schlosser, R. W., & Koul, R. (2015). Speech Output Technologies in Interventions for Individuals with Autism Spectrum Disorders: A Scoping Review. *Augmentative and Alternative Communication*, *31*(4), 1–25. PMID:26170252

Schlosser, R. W., & Wendt, O. (2008). Effects of augmentative and alternative communication intervention on speech production in children with autism: A systematic review. *American Journal of Speech-Language Pathology*, *17*, 212–230. PMID:18663107

Schlosser, R., & Koul, R. (2015). Speech output technologies in Interventions for individuals with autism spectrum disorders: A scoping review. *Augmentative and Alternative Communication*, *31*(4), 285–309. doi:10.3109/07434618.2015.1063689 PMID:26170252

Schmidt, L. A., Trainor, L. J., & Santesso, D. L. (2003). Development of frontal electroencephalogram (EEG) and heart rate (ECG) responses to affective musical stimuli during the first 12 months of post-natal life. *Brain and Cognition*, *52*(1), 27–32. doi:10.1016/S0278-2626(03)00006-X PMID:12812802

Schreck, K. A., Mulick, J. A., & Smith, A. F. (2004). Sleep problems as possible predictors of intensified symptoms of autism. *Research in Developmental Disabilities*, *25*(1), 57–66. doi:10.1016/j.ridd.2003.04.007 PMID:14733976

Scott, L., & Temple, P. (2017). A conceptual framework for building UDL in a special education distance education course. *Journal of Educators Online*, *14*(1), 48–59. Retrieved from https://eric.ed.gov/?id=EJ1133749

Sealey, L. A., Hughes, B. W., Sriskanda, A. N., Guest, J. R., Gibson, A. D., Johnson-Williams, L., ... Bagasra, O. (2016). Environmental factors in the development of autism spectrum disorders. *Environment International*, *88*, 288–298. doi:10.1016/j.envint.2015.12.021 PMID:26826339

Sebat, J., Lakshmi, B., Malhotra, D., Troge, J., Lese-Martin, C., Walsh, T., & ... . (2007). Strong association of *de novo* copy number mutations with autism. *Science*, *316*, 445–449. PMID:17363630

Sedden, M. L., & Clark, K. R. (2016). Motivating Students in the 21st Century. *Radiologic Technology*, *87*(6), 609–616. PMID:27390228

Segal, Z. V., Bieling, P., Young, T., MacQueen, G., Cooke, R., Martin, L., ... Levitan, R. D. (2010). Antidepressant monotherapy vs sequential pharmacotherapy and mindfulness based cognitive therapy, or placebo, for relapse prophylaxis in recurrent depression. *Archives of General Psychiatry*, *67*(12), 1256–1264. doi:10.1001/archgenpsychiatry.2010.168 PMID:21135325

Sen, B., Borle, N. C., Greiner, R., & Brown, M. R. G. (2018). A general prediction model for the detection of ADHD and Autism using structural and functional MRI. *PLoS One*, *13*(4), e0194856. doi:10.1371/journal.pone.0194856 PMID:29664902

Sennott, S. C., Light, J. C., & McNaughton, D. (2016). AAC modeling intervention research review. *Research and Practice for Persons with Severe Disabilities*, *41*(2), 101–115. doi:10.1177/1540796916638822

Sequeira, S., & Ahmed, M. (2012). Meditation as a Potential Therapy for Autism: A Review. Autism Research and Treatment. doi:10.1155/2012/835847

Shane, S. (2012). Reflections on the 2010 AMR decade award: Delivering on the promise of entrepreneurship as a field of research. *Academy of Management Review*, *37*(1), 10–20. doi:10.5465/amr.2011.0078

Shannahoff-Khalsa, D. S. (2010). *Kundalini Yoga Meditation for Complex Psychiatric Disorders: Techniques Specific for Treating the Psychoses, Personality, and Pervasive Developmental Disorders*. New York: WW Norton & Company.

Sharp, H., Rogers, Y., & Preece, J. (2007). *Interaction design: beyond human-computer interaction*. Wiley.

Shaw, L., Zaichkowsky, L., & Wilson, V. (2012). Setting the balance: Using biofeedback and neurofeedback with gymnasts. *Journal of Clinical Sport Psychology*, *6*(1), 47–66. doi:10.1123/jcsp.6.1.47

Sheikhani, A., Behnam, H., Mohammadi, M. R., Noroozian, M., & Golabi, P. (2008) Connectivity analysis of quantitative electroencephalogram background activity in autism disorders with short time fourier transform and coherence values. Congress on image and signal processing, 207–212. doi:10.1109/CISP.2008.595

Shelton, J. F., Hertz-Picciotto, I., & Pessah, I. N. (2012). Tipping the balance of autism risk: Potential mechanisms linking pesticides and autism. *Environmental Health Perspectives*, *120*, 944–951. PMID:22534084

Shih, S. W., & Liu, J. (2004). A novel approach to 3-D gaze tracking using stereo cameras. *IEEE Transactions on Systems, Man, and Cybernetics. Part B, Cybernetics*, *34*(1), 234–245. doi:10.1109/TSMCB.2003.811128 PMID:15369066

Shinohara, K., Bennett, C. L., Pratt, W., & Wobbrock, J. O. (2018). Tenets for Social Accessibility: Towards Humanizing Disabled People in Design. *ACM Transactions on Accessible Computing*, *11*(1), 6. doi:10.1145/3178855

Shinohara, K., Bennett, C. L., & Wobbrock, J. O. (2016). How designing for people with and without disabilities shapes student design thinking. In *Proceedings of the 18th International ACM SIGACCESS Conference on Computers and Accessibility*, (pp. 229-237). ACM. 10.1145/2982142.2982158

Shire, S. Y., & Jones, N. (2015). Communication partners supporting children with complex communication needs who use AAC. *Communication Disorders Quarterly*, *37*(1), 3.

Shriberg, L., Paul, R., McSweeney, J., Klin, A., Cohen, D., & Volkmar, F. (2001). Speech and prosody characteristics of adolescents and adults with high functioning autism and Asperger syndrome. *Journal of Speech, Language, and Hearing Research: JSLHR*, *44*, 1097–1115. PMID:11708530

Shuhaida, Y., Azuan, N., & Osman, A. (2007). *Prosthetic hand for the brain-computer interface system*. Academic Press.

Siegel, E. B., & Cress, C. J. (2002). Overview of the Emergence of Early AAC Behaviors: Progression from Communicative to Symbolic Skills. *Exemplary Practicies for Beginning Communicators: Implications for AAC.*

Sigafoos, J., Drasgow, E., Halle, J. W., O'reilly, M., Seely-York, S., Edrisinha, C., & Andrews, A. (2004). Teaching VOCA use as a communicative repair strategy. *Journal of Autism and Developmental Disorders*, *34*(4), 411–422. doi:10.1023/B:JADD.0000037417.04356.9c PMID:15449516

Sigafoos, J., Drasgow, E., & Schlosser, R. W. (2003). Strategies for beginning communicators. In R. W. Schlosser (Ed.), *The efficacy of augmentative and alternative communication: Toward evidence-based practice* (pp. 323–346). Boston, MA: Academic Press.

Sigafoos, J., Lancioni, G. E., O'Reilly, M. F., Achmadi, D., Stevens, M., Roche, L., ... Green, V. A. (2013). Teaching two boys with autism spectrum disorders to request the continuation of toy play using an iPad®-based speech-generating device. *Research in Autism Spectrum Disorders*, *7*(8), 923–930. doi:10.1016/j.rasd.2013.04.002

Sigafoos, J., O'Reilly, M. F., Ledbetter-Cho, K., Lim, N., Lancioni, G. E., & Marschik, P. B. (2019). Addressing sequelae of developmental regression associated with developmental disabilities: A systematic review of behavioral and educational intervention studies. *Neuroscience and Biobehavioral Reviews*, *96*, 56–71. doi:10.1016/j.neubiorev.2018.11.014 PMID:30481529

Sigurdardottir, S., Eiriksdottir, A., Gunnarsdottir, E., Meintema, M., Arnadottir, U., & Vik, T. (2008). Cognitive profile in young Icelandic children with cerebral palsy. *Developmental Medicine and Child Neurology*, *50*(5), 357–362. doi:10.1111/j.1469-8749.2008.02046.x PMID:18355334

Silk, T. J., Rinehart, N., Bradshaw, J. L., Tonge, B., Egan, G., O'Boyle, M. W., & Cunnington, R. (2006). Article. *The American Journal of Psychiatry*, *163*(8), 1440–1443. PMID:16877661

Simons, VIP Consortium. (2012). Simons Variation in Individuals Project (Simons VIP): A genetics-first approach to studying autism spectrum and related neurodevelopmental disorders. *Neuron*, *73*(6), 10631067. PMID:22445335

Singh, Marks, Jones, Tuzel, & Shao. (2016). A multistream bidirectional recurrent neural network for fine grained action detection. *The IEEE Conference on Computer Vision and Pattern Recognition (CVPR)*, 1961-1970.

Singh, H., & Singh, J. (2012). Human eye tracking and related issues: A review. *International Journal of Scientific and Research Publications*, *2*(9), 1–9.

Sinha, P., Kjelgaard, M. M., Gandhi, T. K., Tsourides, K., Cardinaux, A. L., Pantazis, D., ... Held, R. M. (2014). Autism as a disorder of prediction. *Proceedings of the National Academy of Sciences, 111*(42), 15220-15225.

Siuly, S., & Zhang, Y. (2016). Medical Big Data: Neurological Diseases Diagnosis Through Medical Data Analysis. *Data Science and Engineering.*, *1*(2), 54–64. doi:10.100741019-016-0011-3

Sivertsen, B., Posserud, M.-B., Gillberg, C., Lundervold, A. J., & Hysing, M. (2012). Sleep problems in children with autism spectrum disorder. A longitudinal population-based study. *Autism*, *16*(2), 139–150. doi:10.1177/1362361311404255 PMID:21478225

Skotko, B. G., Macklin, E. A., Muselli, M., Voelz, L., McDonough, M. E., Davidson, E., ... Rosen, D. (2017). A predictive model for obstructive sleep apnea and Down syndrome. *American Journal of Medical Genetics. Part A*, *173*(4), 889–896. doi:10.1002/ajmg.a.38137 PMID:28124477

Slotkin, T. A., & Seidler, F. J. (2013). Terbutaline impairs the development of peripheral noradrenergic projections: Potential implications for autism spectrum disorders and pharmacotherapy of preterm labor. *Neurotoxicology and Teratology*, *36*, 91–96. doi:10.1016/j.ntt.2012.07.003 PMID:22813780

Smalley, S. L. (1998). Autism and tuberous sclerosis. *Journal of Autism and Developmental Disorders*, *28*(5), 407–414. PMID:9813776

Smith, D. L., Atmatzidis, K., Capogreco, M., Lloyd-Randolfi, D., & Seman, V. (2017). Evidence-based interventions for increasing work participation for persons with various disabilities: A systematic review. *OTJR: Occupation, Participation, and Health*, *37*, 3–13.

Smith, M., Sandberg, A. D., & Larsson, M. (2009). Reading and spelling in children with severe speech and physical impairments: A comparative study. *International Journal of Language & Communication Disorders*, *44*(6), 864–882. doi:10.1080/13682820802389873 PMID:19105069

Smith, S. (2016). (Re)counting meaningful learning experiences: Using student-created reflective videos to make invisible learning visible during PjBL experiences. *Interdisciplinary Journal of Problem-based Learning, 10*(1). doi:10.7771/1541-5015.1541

Snodderly, D. M., Kagan, I., & Gur, M. (2001). Selective activation of visual cortex neurons by fixational eye movements: Implications for neural coding. *Visual Neuroscience, 18*(2), 259–277. doi:10.1017/S0952523801182118 PMID:11417801

Soderstrom, M., Jeding, K., Ekstedt, M., Perski, A., & Akerstedt, T. (2012). Insufficient sleep predicts clinical burnout. *Journal of Occupational Health Psychology, 17*(2), 175–183. doi:10.1037/a0027518 PMID:22449013

Solomon-Rice, P. L., & Soto, G. (2014). Facilitating vocabulary in toddlers using AAC: A preliminary study comparing focused stimulation and augmented input. *Communication Disorders Quarterly, 35*(4), 204–215. doi:10.1177/1525740114522856

Somogyia, E. (2016). Visual feedback increases postural stability in children with autism spectrum disorder. *Research in Autism Spectrum Disorders, 29*, 48–56. doi:10.1016/j.rasd.2016.06.001

Song, R., Liu, J., & Kong, X. J. (2016). Autonomic Dysfunction and Autism: Subtypes and Clinical Perspectives. *North American Journal of Medicine & Science, 9*(4).

Sorte, Patil, & Bhamare. (2016). Motion Detection Using Optical Flow And Standard Deviation. *IEEE International Conference on Automatic Control and Dynamic Optimization Techniques*, 295-300.

Soto, G., & Clarke, M. T. (2017). Effects of a conversation-based intervention on the linguistic skills of children with motor speech disorders who use augmentative and alternative communication. *Journal of Speech, Language, and Hearing Research, 60*(7), 1980–1998. doi:10.1044/2016_JSLHR-L-15-0246 PMID:28672283

Soto, G., Müller, E., Hunt, P., & Goetz, L. (2001). Critical issues in the inclusion of students who use augmentative and alternative communication: An educational team perspective. *Augmentative and Alternative Communication, 17*(2), 62–72. doi:10.1080/aac.17.2.62.72

Soto, G., Müller, E., Hunt, P., & Goetz, L. (2001). Professional skills for serving students who use AAC in general education classrooms. *Language, Speech, and Hearing Services in Schools, 32*(1), 51–56. doi:10.1044/0161-1461(2001/005) PMID:27764437

Soto, S. (2015). An analysis of curriculum development. *Theory and Practice in Language Studies, 5*(6), 1129–1139. doi:10.17507/tpls.0506.02

Spasov, S. E., Passamonti, L., Duggento, A., Lio, P., & Toschi, N. (2018). A Multi-modal Convolutional Neural Network Framework for the Prediction of Alzheimer's Disease. In *2018 40th Annual International Conference of the IEEE Engineering in Medicine and Biology Society (EMBC)* (pp. 1271–1274). IEEE. 10.1109/EMBC.2018.8512468

Spence-Cochran, K., & Pearl, C. (2012). *Assistive technology to support people with autism spectrum disorders.* Doi:10.4324/9780203848180

Sreeja, S. R., Rabha, J., Samanta, D., Mitra, P., & Sarma, M. (2017, December). Classification of moator imagery based EEG signals using sparsity approach. In *International Conference on Intelligent Human Computer Interaction* (pp. 47-59). Springer.

Stagg, S., Slavny, R., Hand, C., Cardoso, A., & Smith, P. (2013). Does facial expressivity count? How typically developing children respond initially to children with autism. *Autism*, 704–711. PMID:24121180

Starble, A., Hutchins, T., Favro, M. A., Prelock, P., & Bitner, B. (2005). Family-centered intervention and satisfaction with AAC device training. *Communication Disorders Quarterly, 27*(1), 47–54.

Stasolla, F., Boccasini, A., & Perilli, V. (2017). Assistive technology-based programs to support adaptive behaviors by children with autism spectrum disorders: A literature overview. In Y. Kats (Ed.), *Supporting the education of children with autism spectrum disorders* (pp. 140–159). Hershey, PA: IGI Global. doi:10.4018/978-1-5225-0816-8.ch008

Stasolla, F., Caffò, A. O., Damiani, R., Perilli, V., Di Leone, A., & Albano, V. (2015). Assistive technology-based programs to promote communication and leisure activities by three children emerged from a minimal conscious state. *Cognitive Processing*, *16*(1), 69–78. doi:10.100710339-014-0625-1 PMID:25077461

Stasolla, F., Caffò, A. O., Perilli, V., Boccasini, A., Damiani, R., Albano, V., & Albano, A. (2017). Comparing self-monitoring and differential reinforcement of an alternative behavior to promote on-task behavior by three children with cerebral palsy: A pilot study. *Life Span and Disability*, *20*, 63–92.

Stasolla, F., Caffò, A. O., Perilli, V., Boccasini, A., Damiani, R., & D'Amico, F. (2019). Assistive technology for promoting adaptive skills of children with cerebral palsy: Ten cases evaluation. *Disability and Rehabilitation. Assistive Technology*, *14*(5), 489–502. doi:10.1080/17483107.2018.1467972 PMID:29732901

Stasolla, F., Caffò, A. O., Picucci, L., & Bosco, A. (2013). Assistive technology for promoting choice behaviors in three children with cerebral palsy and severe communication impairments. *Research in Developmental Disabilities*, *34*(9), 2694–2700. doi:10.1016/j.ridd.2013.05.029 PMID:23770888

Stasolla, F., Damiani, R., & Caffò, A. O. (2014). Promoting constructive engagement by two boys with autism spectrum disorders and high functioning through behavioral interventions. *Research in Autism Spectrum Disorders*, *8*(4), 376–380. doi:10.1016/j.rasd.2013.12.020

Stasolla, F., Damiani, R., Perilli, V., D'Amico, F., Caffò, A. O., Stella, A., ... Leone, A. D. (2015). Computer and micro-switch-based programs to improve academic activities by six children with cerebral palsy. *Research in Developmental Disabilities*, *45-46*, 1–13. doi:10.1016/j.ridd.2015.07.005 PMID:26196086

Stasolla, F., Perilli, V., & Boccasini, A. (2016). Assistive technologies for persons with severe-profound intellectual and developmental disabilities. In J. K. Luiselli & A. J. Fischer (Eds.), *Computer-assisted and web-based innovations in psychology, special education, and health* (pp. 287–310). New York: Springer. doi:10.1016/B978-0-12-802075-3.00011-5

Stasolla, F., Perilli, V., Boccasini, A., Caffò, A. O., Damiani, R., & Albano, V. (2016). Enhancing academic performance of three boys with autism spectrum disorders and intellectual disabilities through a computer-based program. *Life Span and Disability*, *19*, 153–183.

Stasolla, F., Perilli, V., Caffò, A. O., Boccasini, A., Stella, A., Damiani, R., ... Albano, A. (2017). Extending micro-switch-cluster programs for promoting occupational activities and reducing mouthing by six children with autism spectrum disorders and intellectual disabilities. *Journal of Developmental and Physical Disabilities*, *29*(2), 307–324. doi:10.100710882-016-9525-x

Stasolla, F., Perilli, V., & Damiani, R. (2014). Self monitoring to promote on-task behavior by two high functioning boys with autism spectrum disorders and symptoms of ADHD. *Research in Autism Spectrum Disorders*, *8*(5), 472–479. doi:10.1016/j.rasd.2014.01.007

Stasolla, F., Perilli, V., Damiani, R., Caffò, A. O., Di Leone, A., Albano, V., ... Damato, C. (2014c). A microswitch-cluster program to enhance object manipulation and to reduce hand mouthing by three boys with autism spectrum disorders and intellectual disabilities. *Research in Autism Spectrum Disorders*, *9*(9), 1071–1078. doi:10.1016/j.rasd.2014.05.016

Steenbergen, B., & Gordon, A. M. (2006). Activity limitation in hemiplegic cerebral palsy: Evidence for disorders in motor planning. *Developmental Medicine and Child Neurology*, *48*(9), 780–783. doi:10.1017/S0012162206001666 PMID:16904028

Sterman, M. B., & Egner, T. (2006). Foundation and practice of neurofeedback for the treatment of epilepsy. *Applied Psychophysiology and Biofeedback*, *31*(1), 21–35. doi:10.100710484-006-9002-x PMID:16614940

Stewart, C., & Varner, L. (2012). Common Core and the rural student. *National Teacher Education Journal*, *5*(4), 67–73.

Stiebel, D. (1999). Promoting augmentative communication during daily routines: A parent problem-solving intervention. *Journal of Positive Behavior Interventions*, *1*(3), 159–169. doi:10.1177/109830079900100304

Still, K., Rehfeldt, R. A., Whelan, R., May, R., & Dymond, S. (2014). Facilitating requesting skills using high-tech augmentative and alternative communication devices with individuals with autism spectrum disorders: A systematic review. *Research in Autism Spectrum Disorders*, *8*(9), 1184–1199.

Streeter, C. C., Gerbarg, P. L., Saper, R. B., Ciraulo, D. A., & Brown, R. P. (2012). Effects of yoga on the autonomic nervous system, gamma-aminobutyric-acid, and allostasis in epilepsy, depression, and post-traumatic stress disorder. *Medical Hypotheses*, *78*(5), 571–579. doi:10.1016/j.mehy.2012.01.021 PMID:22365651

Stromland. (1994). Autism in thalidomide embryopathy: a population study. *Developmental Medicine & Child Neurology, 36,* 351.

Sturman, N., Deckx, L., & van Driel, M. L. (2017). Methylphenidate for children and adolescents with autism spectrum disorder. *Cochrane Database of Systematic Reviews*, CD0011144. PMID:29159857

Sturm, D., Peppe, E., & Ploog, B. (2016). EMot-iCan: Design of an assessment game for emotion recognition in players with autism. *2016 IEEE International Conference on Serious Games and Applications for Health, SeGAH 2016,* 10.1109/SeGAH.2016.7586228

Sudirman, R., Saidin, S., & Safri, N. M. (2010). Study of electroencephalography signal of Autism and down syndrome children using FFT. In *IEEE symposium on industrial electronics and applications* (pp. 401–406). ISIEA. doi:10.1109/ISIEA.2010.5679434

Sun, J., & Reddy, C. K. (2013, August). Big data analytics for healthcare. In *Proceedings of the 19th ACM SIGKDD international conference on Knowledge discovery and data mining* (pp. 1525-1525). ACM.

Suresh, P. A. (2018). Global prevalence of autism: A mini-review. *SciFed Journal of Autism*, *2*, 1.

Sutherland, D. E., Gillon, G. G., & Yoder, D. E. (2005). AAC use and service provision: A survey of New Zealand speech-language therapists. *Augmentative and Alternative Communication*, *21*(4), 295–307. doi:10.1080/07434610500103483

Swaminathan, A. (2015). Transition Planning in adolescents with Low Functioning Autism. *The Indian Journal of Occupational Therapy*, *47*(3), 67–71.

Sylvan, L. J., & Christodoulou, J. A. (2010). Understanding the role of neuroscience in brain based products: A guide for educators and consumers. *Mind, Brain and Education : the Official Journal of the International Mind, Brain, and Education Society*, *4*(1), 1–7. doi:10.1111/j.1751-228X.2009.01077.x

Tager-Flusberg, H., & Kasari, C. (2013). Minimally verbal school-aged children with autism spectrum disorder: The neglected end of the spectrum. *Autism Research*, *6*, 468–478. PMID:24124067

Tamboer, P., Vorst, H. C. M., Ghebreab, S., & Scholte, H. S. (2016). Machine learning and dyslexia: Classification of individual structural neuro-imaging scans of students with and without dyslexia. *NeuroImage. Clinical*, *11*, 508–514. doi:10.1016/j.nicl.2016.03.014 PMID:27114899

Tammimies, K., Marshall, C. R., Walker, S., Kaur, G., Thiruvahindrapuram, B., Lionel, A. C., ... Woodbury-Smith, M. (2015). Molecular diagnostic yield of chromosomal microarray analysis and wholeexome sequencing in children with autism spectrum disorder. *Journal of the American Medical Association, 314*(9), 895–903. doi:10.1001/jama.2015.10078 PMID:26325558

Tanu, D. K. (2018). Drift Diffusion Model Parameters Underlying Cognitive Mechanism and Perceptual Learning in Autism Spectrum Disorder. In *SoCTA-2018: 3rd International Conference: with theme:Soft Computing: Theories and Applications*. NIT Jalandhar.

Tanu, D. K. (2019). Analysis of Weighted Visibility Graphs in Evaluation of Austim Spectrum Disorder and Epilepsy Relationship. *ICTESM-2019: 1st International Conference: with theme International Conference on Current Trends in Engineering, Sciences and Management*, 37-43.

Tanu, K. D. (2018). A Study on Machine Learning Based Generalized Automated Seizure Detection System. In *2018 8th International Conference on Cloud Computing, Data Science and Engineering (Confluence)* (pp. 769-774). IEEE.

Tanu, K. D. (2018). Eye Tracker: An Assistive Tool in Diagnosis of Autism Spectrum Disorder. In *Emerging Trends in the Diagnosis and Intervention of Neurodevelopmental Disorders*. IGI.

Tanu, K. D. (2018). Pre-Clinical ASD Screening Using Multi-Biometrics-Based System. In *Design and Implementation of Healthcare Biometric Systems*. IGI.

Tanu, K. D. (2018). Strengthening risk prediction using statistical learning in children with autism spectrum disorder. *Advances in Autism*.

Tanu, K., D. (2018). Accounting For Order-Frame Length Tradeoff of Savitzky-Golay Smoothing Filters. In *5th International Conference on Signal Processing and Integrated Networks (SPIN)* (pp. 805-810). IEEE. 10.1109/SPIN.2018.8474194

Tanu, K., & Kakkar, D. (2019). D. Influence of Emotional Imagery on Risk Perception and Decision Making in Autism Spectrum Disorder. *Neurophysiology, 51*(4), 281–292. doi:10.100711062-019-09822-8

Tanu, T., & Kakkar, D. (2018). *Strengthening risk prediction using statistical learning in children with autism spectrum disorder*. Advances in Autism.

Taube-Schiff, M., Suvak, M. K., Antony, M. M., Bieling, P. J., & McCabe, R. E. (2007). Group cohesion in cognitive-behavioral group therapy for social phobia. *Behaviour Research and Therapy, 45*(4), 687–698. doi:10.1016/j.brat.2006.06.004 PMID:16928359

Taylor, B., Miller, E., Lingam, R., Andrews, N., Simmons, A., & Stowe, J. (2002). MMR vaccination and bowel problems or developmental regression in children with autism: Population study. *British Medical Journal, 324*, 393–396. PMID:11850369

Taylor, R., & Iacono, T. (2003). AAC and scripting activities to facilitate communication and play. *Advances in Speech Language Pathology, 5*(2), 79–93. doi:10.1080/14417040510001669111

Telles, S., Joseph, C., Venkatesh, S., & Desiraju, T. (1993). Alterations of auditory middle latency evoked potentials during yogic consciously regulated breathing and alternative states of the mind. *International Journal of Psychophysiology, 14*(3), 189–198. doi:10.1016/0167-8760(93)90033-L PMID:8340237

Telles, S., & Naveen, K. V. (1997). Yoga for rehabilitation: An overview. *Indian Journal of Medical Sciences, 51*, 123–127. PMID:9355699

Tenev, A., Markovska-Simoska, S., Kocarev, L., Pop-Jordanov, J., Müller, A., & Candrian, G. (2014). Machine learning approach for classification of ADHD adults. *International Journal of Psychophysiology*, *93*(1), 162–166. doi:10.1016/j.ijpsycho.2013.01.008 PMID:23361114

Thabtah, F. (2017). Autism Spectrum Disorder Screening : Machine Learning Adaptation and DSM-5 Fulfillment. *Proceedings of the 1st International Conference on Medical and Health Informatics 2017*, 1–6.

Thabtah, F. (2018). Machine learning in autistic spectrum disorder behavioral research : A review and ways forward. *Informatics for Health & Social Care*, *00*(00), 1–20. doi:10.1080/17538157.2017.1399132 PMID:29436887

The Apache Software Foundation. (2015). *Apache Spark*. Available online at: https://spark.apache.org/

Therrien, M. C. S., & Light, J. C. (2018). Promoting peer interaction for preschool children with complex communication needs and autism spectrum disorder. *American Journal of Speech-Language Pathology*, *27*, 207–221. doi:10.1044/2017_AJSLP-17-0104 PMID:29383382

Thiemann-Bourque, K. S., McGuff, S., & Goldstein, H. (2017). Training peer partners to use a speech-generating device with classmates with autism spectrum disorder: Exploring communication outcomes across preschool contexts. *Journal of Speech, Language, and Hearing Research: JSLHR*, *60*, 2648. doi:10.1044/2017_JSLHR-L-17-0049 PMID:28854313

Thiemann-Bourque, K., Brady, N., McGuff, S., Stump, K., & Naylor, A. (2016). Picture exchange communication system and pals: A peer-mediated augmentative and alternative communication intervention for minimally verbal preschoolers with autism. *Journal of Speech, Language, and Hearing Research: JSLHR*, *59*(5), 1133–1145. doi:10.1044/2016_JSLHR-L-15-0313 PMID:27679841

Think Change India. (2019). *This Kolkata Café has a unique offering besides cupcakes and cookies*. Retrieved October 5, 2019 from https://yourstory.com/socialstory/2019/05/kolkata-cafe-sip-n-bite-specially-abled-team

Thomas, S., Hovinga, M. E., Rai, D., & Lee, B. K. (2017). Brief report: prevalence of co-occurring epilepsy and autism spectrum disorder: the US national Survey of Children's Health 2011-2012. *Journal of Autism and Developmental Disorders*, *47*(1), 224–229. doi:10.100710803-016-2938-7 PMID:27752862

Thompson, T. W., Hinds, O., Ghosh, S., Lala, N., Triantafyllou, C., Gabrieli, S., & Gabrieli, J. (2009). Training selective auditory attention with real-time fmri feedback. *NeuroImage*, *47*, 22. doi:10.1016/S1053-8119(09)70339-8

Tick, B., Bolton, P., Happe, F., Rutter, M., & Rijsdijk, F. (2016). Heritability of autism spectrum disorders: A metanalysis of twin studies. *Journal of Child Psychology and Psychiatry, and Allied Disciplines*, *57*(5), 585–595. doi:10.1111/jcpp.12499 PMID:26709141

Tincani, M., & Devis, K. (2011). Quantitative synthesis and component analysis of single- participant studies on the picture exchange communication system. *Remedial and Special Education*, *32*, 458–470. doi:10.1177/0741932510362494

Toennies, K. D. (2017b). *Registration and Normalization*. doi:10.1007/978-1-4471-7320-5_10

Toennies, K. D. (2017a). *Guide to Medical Image Analysis*. London: Springer London; doi:10.1007/978-1-4471-7320-5

Tönsing, K. M., Alant, E., & Lloyd, L. L. (2005). Augmentative and alternative communication. *Augmentative and alternative communication and severe disabilities: Beyond poverty*, 30-67.

Tonsing, K. M., Alant, E., & Lloyd, L. I. (2005). Intervention issues. In E. Alant & L. Lloyd (Eds.), *Augmentative and Alternative Communication and Severe Disabilities: Beyond Poverty* (pp. 30–67). London, UK: Whurr Publishers.

Torrado, J. C., Gomez, J., & Montoro, G. (2017). Emotional self-regulation of individuals with autism spectrum disorders: Smartwatches for monitoring and interaction. *Sensors (Switzerland)*, *17*(6), 1359. doi:10.339017061359 PMID:28604607

Tran, D., Hoffman, M. D., Saurous, R. A., Brevdo, E., Murphy, K., & Blei, D. M. (2017). Deep Probabilistic Programming. *International Conference on Learning Representations.*

Trattler, W. B., Kaiser, P. K., & Friedman, N. J. (2012). *Review of Ophthalmology: Expert Consult – Online and Print.* Elsevier Health Sciences.

Treviranus, J., & Roberts, V. (2003). Supporting competent motor control of AAC systems. *Communicative competence for individuals who use AAC*, 199-240.

Tripathi, R. K., Jalal, A. S., & Agrawal, S. C. (2018). Suspicious human activity recognition: A review. *Artificial Intelligence Review*, *50*(2), 283–339. doi:10.100710462-017-9545-7

Trivette, C. M., Dunst, C. J., & Hamby, D. W. (1996). Factors associated with perceived control appraisals in a family-centered early intervention program. *Journal of Early Intervention*, *20*(2), 165–178. doi:10.1177/105381519602000207

Trottier, N., Kamp, L., & Mirenda, P. (2011). Effects of peer-mediated instruction to teach use of speech-generating devices to students with autism in social game routines. *Augmentative and Alternative Communication*, *27*, 26–39. doi:10.3109/07434618.2010.546810 PMID:21284561

Tsangouri, C., Li, W., Zhu, Z., Abtahi, F., & Ro, T. (2018). An interactive facial-expression training platform for individuals with autism spectrum disorder. *2016 IEEE MIT Undergraduate Research Technology Conference, URTC 2016*, 1-4. doi:10.1109/URTC.2016.8284067

Tsikinas, S., & Xinogalos, S. (2018). Studying the effects of computer serious games on people with intellectual disabilities or autism spectrum disorder: A systematic literature review. *Journal of Computer Assisted Learning*, *35*(1), 61–73. doi:10.1111/jcal.12311

Tsui, K. M., Feil-Seifer, D. J., Matarić, M. J., & Yanco, H. A. (2009). *Performance evaluation methods for assistive robotic technology.* Doi:10.1007/978-1-4419-0492-8_3

Uchino, B. N. (2006). Social support and health: A review of physiological processes potentially underlying links to disease outcomes. *Journal of Behavioral Medicine*, *29*(4), 377–387. doi:10.100710865-006-9056-5 PMID:16758315

Urigüen, J. A., & Garcia-Zapirain, B. (2015). EEG artefact removal-state-of-the-art and guidelines. *Journal of Neural Engineering*, *12*(3), 031001. doi:10.1088/1741-2560/12/3/031001 PMID:25834104

Vadiraja, H. S., Raghavendra, R. M., Nagarathna, R., Nagendra, H. R., Rekha, M., Vanitha, N., & … . (2009). Effects of a yoga program on cortisol rhythm and mood states in early breast cancer patients undergoing adjuvant radiotherapy: A randomized controlled trial. *Integrative Cancer Therapies*, *8*(1), 37–46. doi:10.1177/1534735409331456 PMID:19190034

Vahabzadeh, A., Keshav, N. U., Abdus-Sabur, R., Huey, K., Liu, R., & Sahin, N. T. (2018). Improved socio-emotional and behavioral functioning in students with autism following school-based smartglasses intervention: Multi-stage feasibility and controlled efficacy study. *Behavioral Science*, *8*(10). doi:10.3390/bs8100085 PMID:30241313

Vaidya, S. (2016). *Autism and the family in urban India: Looking back, looking forward.* Springer. doi:10.1007/978-81-322-3607-8

Valadão, C. T., Goulart, C., Rivera, H., Caldeira, E., Bastos Filho, T. F., Frizera-Neto, A., & Carelli, R. (2016). Analysis of the use of a robot to improve social skills in children with autism spectrum disorder. *Revista Brasileira de Engenharia Biomédica*, *32*, 161–175.

Valvano, J., & Newell, K. M. (1998). Practice of a precision isometric grip-force task by children with spastic cerebral palsy. *Developmental Medicine and Child Neurology*, *40*(7), 464–473. doi:10.1111/j.1469-8749.1998.tb15397.x PMID:9698060 van der Meer, L. A., & Rispoli, M. (2010). Communication interventions involving speech-generating devices for children with autism: A review of the literature. *Developmental Neurorehabilitation, 13,* 294–306. 0367149413 doi:10.3109/175184210

Van der Meer, L. A. J., & Rispoli, M. (2010). Communication interventions involving speech-generating devices for children with autism: A review of the literature. *Developmental Neurorehabilitation, 13*(4), 294–306. doi:10.3109/17518421003671494 PMID:20629595

Van der Meer, L., Sigafoos, J., O'Reilly, M. F., & Lancioni, G. E. (2011). Assessing preferences for AAC options in communication interventions for individuals with developmental disabilities: A review of the literature. *Research in Developmental Disabilities, 32*(5), 1422–1431. doi:10.1016/j.ridd.2011.02.003 PMID:21377833

van Geijn, H. P., Lenglet, J. E., & Botte, A. C. (2005). Nifedipine trials: Effectiveness and safety aspects. *BJOG, 112*(1), 79–83. doi:10.1111/j.1471-0528.2005.00591.x PMID:15715601

Venkataramanan, S., Prabhat, P., Choudhury, S. R., Nemade, H. B., & Sahambi, J. S. (2005, January). Biomedical instrumentation based on electrooculogram (EOG) signal processing and application to a hospital alarm system. In *Proceedings of 2005 International Conference on Intelligent Sensing and Information Processing* (pp. 535-540). IEEE. 10.1109/ICISIP.2005.1529512

Venkateswaran, S., & Shevell, M. I. (2008). Comorbidities and clinical determinants of outcome in children with spastic quadriplegic cerebral palsy. *Developmental Medicine and Child Neurology, 50*(3), 216–222. doi:10.1111/j.1469-8749.2008.02033.x PMID:18248493

Vermillion, S. T., Soper, D. E., & Chasedunn-Roark, J. (1999). Neonatal sepsis after betamethasone administration to patients with preterm premature rupture of membranes. *American Journal of Obstetrics and Gynecology, 181*(2), 320–322. doi:10.1016/S0002-9378(99)70555-7 PMID:10454676

Verrall, C. E., Blue, G. M., Loughran-Fowlds, A., Kasparian, N., Gecz, J., Walker, K., ... Winlaw, D. (2019). 'Big issues' in neurodevelopment for children and adults with congenital heart disease. *Open Heart, 6*(2), e000998. doi:10.1136/openhrt-2018-000998 PMID:31354955

Vidal, M., Turner, J., Bulling, A., & Gellersen, H. (2012). Wearable eye tracking for mental health monitoring. *Computer Communications, 35*(11), 1306–1311. doi:10.1016/j.comcom.2011.11.002

Volioti, C., Tsiatsos, T., Mavropoulou, S., & Karagiannidis, C. (2016). VLEs, Social Stories and Children with Autism: A Prototype Implementation and Evaluation. *Education and Information Technologies, 21*(6), 1679–1697.

Volkmar, F. R., Lord, C., Bailey, A., Schultz, R. T., & Klin, A. (2004). Autism and pervasive developmental disorders. *Journal of Child Psychology and Psychiatry, and Allied Disciplines, 45*(1), 135–170. PMID:14959806

Volkmar, F. R., & Nelson, D. S. (1990). Seizure disorder in autism. *Journal of the American Academy of Child and Adolescent Psychiatry, 29*, 127–129. PMID:2295565

von Tetzchner, S., Brekke, K. M., Sjøthun, B., & Grindheim, E. (2005). Constructing preschool communities of learners that afford alternative language development. *Augmentative and Alternative Communication, 21*(2), 82–100. doi:10.1080/07434610500103541

Vostanis, P., Smith, B., Chung, M. C., & Corbett, J. (1994). Early detection of childhood autism: A review of screening instruments and rating scales. *Child: Care, Health and Development, 6*(3), 165–177. doi:10.1111/j.1365-2214.1994.tb00378.x PMID:8062410

Waddington, D. I., & Weeth Feinstein, N. (2016). Beyond the search for truth: Dewey's humble and humanistic vision of science education. *Educational Theory*, *66*(1/2), 111–126. doi:10.1111/edth.12157

Waddington, H. (2018). Meta-analysis provides support for the use of high tech speech-generating devices for teaching a range of communication skills to children with autism spectrum disorders. *Evidence-Based Communication Assessment and Intervention*, *12*(1-2), 7–11. doi:10.1080/17489539.2018.1472903

Wade, N. J. (2010). Pioneers of eye movement research. *Perception*, *1*(2), 33–68. doi:10.1068/i0389 PMID:23396982

Wadhera, T., & Kakkar, D. (2019). Eye Tracker: An Assistive Tool in Diagnosis of Autism Spectrum Disorder. In Emerging Trends in the Diagnosis and Intervention of Neurodevelopmental Disorders (pp. 125-152). IGI Global.

Wadhera, T., Kakkar, D., Kaur, G., & Menia, V. (2019). Pre-Clinical ASD Screening Using Multi-Biometrics-Based Systems. In *Design and Implementation of Healthcare Biometric Systems* (pp. 185–211). IGI Global. doi:10.4018/978-1-5225-7525-2.ch008

Wadhera, T., Kakkar, D., Wadhwa, G., & Raj, B. (2019). Recent Advances and Progress in Development of the Field Effect Transistor Biosensor: A Review. *Journal of Electronic Materials*, *48*(12), 7635–7646. doi:10.100711664-019-07705-6

Wallace, G. L., Dankner, L., Kenworthy, L., Giedd, J. N., & Martin, A. (2010). Age-related temporal and parietal cortical thinning in autism spectrum disorders. *Brain*, *133*(12), 3745–3754. doi:10.1093/brain/awq279 PMID:20926367

Wall, D. P., Dally, R., Luyster, R., Jung, J.-Y., & DeLuca, T. F. (2012). Use of artificial intelligence to shorten the behavioral diagnosis of autism. *PLoS One*, *7*(8), 1–8. doi:10.1371/journal.pone.0043855 PMID:22952789

Wall, D. P., Kosmicki, J., Deluca, T. F., Harstad, E., & Fusaro, V. A. (2012). Use of machine learning to shorten observation-based screening and diagnosis of autism. *Translational Psychiatry*, *2*(4), e100. doi:10.1038/tp.2012.10 PMID:22832900

Waller, A., Hanson, V. L., & Sloan, D. (2009). Including accessibility within and beyond undergraduate computing courses. *Proc. ASSETS '09*, 155–162. 10.1145/1639642.1639670

Walter, K. O., Baller, S. L., & Kuntz, A. M. (2012). Two Approaches for Using Web Sharing and Photography Assignments to Increase Critical Thinking in the Health Sciences. *International Journal on Teaching and Learning in Higher Education*, *24*(3), 383–394.

Walton, K. M., & Ingersoll, B. R. (2015). Psychosocial adjustment and sibling relationships in siblings of children with autism spectrum disorder: Risk and protective factors. *Journal of Autism and Developmental Disorders*, *45*(9), 2764–2778. doi:10.100710803-015-2440-7 PMID:25847756

Wang, L., Chen, D., Ranjan, R., Khan, S. U., KolOdziej, J., & Wang, J. (2012, December). Parallel processing of massive EEG data with MapReduce. In *Parallel and Distributed Systems (ICPADS), 2012 IEEE 18th International Conference on* (pp. 164-171). IEEE.

Wang, R. H., Sudhama, A., Begum, M., Huq, R., & Mihailidis, A. (2017). Robots to assist daily activities: Views of older adults with Alzheimer's disease and their caregivers. *International Psychogeriatrics*, *29*(1), 67–79. doi:10.1017/S1041610216001435 PMID:27660047

Wang, Y., Kung, L., & Byrd, T. A. (2018). Big data analytics: Understanding its capabilities and potential benefits for healthcare organizations. *Technological Forecasting and Social Change*, *126*, 3–13. doi:10.1016/j.techfore.2015.12.019

Watling, R., Deitz, J., Kanny, E. M., & McLaughlin, J. F. (1999). Current practice of occupational therapy for children with autism. *The American Journal of Occupational Therapy*, *53*(5), 498–505. doi:10.5014/ajot.53.5.498 PMID:10500858

Watson, L. R., Crais, E. R., Baranek, G. T., Dykstra, J. R., Wilson, K. P., Hammer, C. S., & Woods, J. (2013). Communicative gesture use in infants with and without autism: A retrospective home video study. *American Journal of Speech-Language Pathology*, *22*(1), 25–39. PMID:22846878

Wehmeyer, M.L. (1998). National survey of use of assistive technology by adults with mental retardation. *Ment Retard.*, *36*(1), 44-51.

Weil, A. R. (2014). *Big data in health: a new era for research and patient care*. Academic Press.

Werner, E., & Dawson, G. (2005). Validation of the phenomenon of autistic regression using home videotapes. *Archives of General Psychiatry*, *62*(8), 889–895. PMID:16061766

Whitehead, W. E., Palsson, O., & Jones, K. R. (2002). Systematic review of the comorbidity of irritable bowel syndrome with other disorders: What are the causes and implications? *Gastroenterology*, *122*(4), 1140–1156. doi:10.1053/gast.2002.32392 PMID:11910364

WHO. (2016). *World Health Organization Report, Neurological Disorders: Public Health Challenges*. https://www.who.int/mental_health/neurology/neurological_disorders_report_web.pdf

Wilhelm, F. H., Schneider, S., & Friedman, B. H. (2006). Psychophysiological Assessment. Clinician's Handbook of Child Behavioral Assessment, 201–231. doi:10.1016/B978-012343014-4/50010-1

Wilkinson, K. M., & Hennig, S. (2007). The state of research and practice in augmentative and alternative communication for children with developmental/intellectual disabilities. *Mental Retardation and Developmental Disabilities Research Reviews*, *13*(1), 58–69. doi:10.1002/mrdd.20133 PMID:17326111

Williams, D. (2012). *Neurological basis for autism: Implications for speech-language pathologists*. Mini-seminar presented at the Ohio Speech-Language-Hearing Association, Columbus, OH.

Williams, I.A., Fifer, C., Jaeggi, E., Levine, J.C., Michelfelder, E.C., & Szwast, A.L. (2013). The association of fetal cerebrovascular resistance with early neurodevelopment in single ventricle congenital heart disease. *Am Heart J, 165,* 544. doi:10.1016/j.ahj.2012.11.013

Williams, B. L., Hornig, M., Parekh, T., & Lipkin, W. I. (2012). Application of novel PCR-based methods for detection, quantitation, and phylogenetic characterization of Sutterella Species in intestinal biopsy samples from Children with Autism and gastrointestinal disturbances. *mBio*, *3*(1), 1–11. doi:10.1128/mBio.00261-11 PMID:22233678

Withell, A., & Heigh, N. (2013). Developing Design Thinking Expertise in Higher Education. *2nd International Conference for Design Education Researchers*, Oslo, Norway.

Wolfers, T., Arenas, A. L., Onnink, A. M. H., Dammers, J., Hoogman, M., Zwiers, M. P., ... Beckmann, C. F. (2017). Refinement by integration: Aggregated effects of multimodal imaging markers on adult ADHD. *Journal of Psychiatry & Neuroscience*, *42*(6), 386–394. doi:10.1503/jpn.160240 PMID:28832320

World Health Organisation. (n.d.). *International Classification of Functioning, Disability and Health (ICF)*. Accessed at https://www.who.int/classifications/icf/en/

World Health Organization. (2004). *International statistical classification of diseases and related health problems: instruction manual* (Vol. 2). World Health Organization.

Wu, Zaheer, Hu, Manmatha, Alexander, Smola, & Krahenbuhl. (2016). Compressed video action recognition. *The IEEE Conference on Computer Vision and Pattern Recognition (CVPR)*, 6026-6035.

Xiao, X., Fang, H., Wu, J., Xiao, C., Xiao, T., Qian, L., ... Xiao, Z. (2017). Diagnostic Model Generated by MRI-Derived Brain Features in Toddlers With Autism Spectrum Disorder. *Autism Research, 10*(4), 620–630. doi:10.1002/aur.1711 PMID:27874271

Xin, Y., Hunt, J., Thouless, H., & Tzur, R. (2018). Special Education and Mathematics Working Group. *Conference Papers -- Psychology of Mathematics & Education of North America*, 1515–1525.

Xu, G., Zhang, Z., & Ma, Y. (2006, July). Improving the performance of iris recogniton system using eyelids and eyelashes detection and iris image enhancement. In *2006 5th IEEE International Conference on Cognitive Informatics* (Vol. 2, pp. 871-876). IEEE. 10.1109/COGINF.2006.365606

Yahud, S., & Osman, N. A. (2007). Prosthetic hand for the brain-computer interface system. In *3rd Kuala Lumpur International Conference on Biomedical Engineering 2006* (pp. 643-646). Springer. 10.1007/978-3-540-68017-8_162

Yang, X., Sarraf, S., & Zhang, N. (2018). Deep Learning-based framework for Autism functional MRI Image Classification. *Journal of the Arkansas Academy of Science, 72*(1), 47–52.

Yasin, H., Gibson, W. T., Langlois, S., Stowe, R. M., Tsang, E. S., & Lee, L. (2018). A distinct neurodevelopmental syndrome with intellectual disability, autism spectrum disorder, characteristic facies, and macrocephaly is caused by defects in CHD8. *Journal of Human Genetics*. doi:10.103810038-019-0561-0 PMID:30670789

Yau, W. Y. W., Tudorascu, D. L., McDade, E. M., Ikonomovic, S., James, J. A., Minhas, D., ... Klunk, W. E. (2015). Longitudinal assessment of neuroimaging and clinical markers in autosomal dominant Alzheimer's disease: A prospective cohort study. *Lancet Neurology, 14*(8), 804–813. doi:10.1016/S1474-4422(15)00135-0 PMID:26139022

Yeh, G., Wang, C., Wayne, P., & Phillips, R. (2009). Tai chi exercise for patients with cardiovascular conditions and risk factors: A systematic review. *Journal of Cardiopulmonary Rehabilitation and Prevention, 29*(3), 152–160. doi:10.1097/HCR.0b013e3181a33379 PMID:19471133

Yoder, P., McCathern, R., Warren, S., & Watson, A. (2001). Important distinctions in measuring maternal responses to communication in pre-linguistic children with disabilities. *Communication Disorders Quarterly, 22*(3), 135–147.

Yoo, D. H., & Chung, M. J. (2005). A novel non-intrusive eye gaze estimation using cross-ratio under large head motion. *Computer Vision and Image Understanding, 98*(1), 25–51. doi:10.1016/j.cviu.2004.07.011

Young, R. L., Brewer, N., & Pattison, C. (2003). Parental identification of early behavioural abnormalities in children with autistic disorder. *Autism, 7*(2), 125–143. doi:10.1177/1362361303007002002 PMID:12846383

Yuen, R. K., Merico, D., Bookman, M., Howe, J. L., Thiruvahindrapuram, B., Patel, R. V., ... Pellecchia, G. (2017). Whole genome sequencing resource identifies 18 new candidate genes for autism spectrum disorder. *Nature Neuroscience, 20*(4), 602–611. doi:10.1038/nn.4524 PMID:28263302

Yuen, R. K., Thiruvahindrapuram, B., Merico, D., Walker, S., Tammimies, K., Hoang, N., ... Gazzellone, M. J. (2015). Whole-genome sequencing of quartet families with autism spectrum disorder. *Nature Medicine, 21*(2), 185–191. doi:10.1038/nm.3792 PMID:25621899

Zafeiriou, D. I., Ververi, A., & Vargiami, E. (2007). Childhood autism and associated comorbidities. *Brain & Development, 29*, 257–272. PMID:17084999

Zander, E., Willfors, C., Berggren, S., Coco, C., Holm, A., Jifält, I., ... Bölte, S. (2017). The Interrater Reliability of the Autism Diagnostic Interview-Revised (ADI-R) in Clinical Settings. *Psychopathology, 50*(3), 219–227. doi:10.1159/000474949 PMID:28528329

Zeidan, F., Martucci, K. T., Kraft, R. A., Gordon, N. S., Mchaffie, J. G., & Coghill, R. C. (2011). Brain mechanisms supporting the modulation of pain by mindfulness meditation. *The Journal of Neuroscience : The Official Journal of the Society for Neuroscience, 31*(14), 5540–5548. doi:10.1523/JNEUROSCI.5791-10.2011 PMID:21471390

Zhang, F., Savadjiev, P., Cai, W., Song, Y., Verma, R., Westin, C. F., & O'Donnell, L. J. (2016). Fiber clustering based white matter connectivity analysis for prediction of Autism Spectrum Disorder using diffusion tensor imaging. *Proceedings - International Symposium on Biomedical Imaging,* 564–567. 10.1109/ISBI.2016.7493331

Zhang, K., Zhao, X., Ma, Z., & Man, Y. (2010, November). A simplified 3D gaze tracking technology with stereo vision. In *2010 International Conference on Optoelectronics and Image Processing* (Vol. 1, pp. 131-134). IEEE. 10.1109/ICOIP.2010.346

Zhang, Z. (2012). Microsoft kinect sensor and its effect. *IEEE MultiMedia, 19*(2), 4–10. doi:10.1109/MMUL.2012.24

Zhao, Y., Chen, H., Li, Y., Lv, J., Jiang, X., Ge, F., ... Zhao, S. (2016). Connectome-scale group-wise consistent resting-state network analysis in autism spectrum disorder. *NeuroImage. Clinical, 12*, 23–33. doi:10.1016/j.nicl.2016.06.004 PMID:27358766

Zhou, Y., Yu, F., & Duong, T. (2014). Multiparametric MRI Characterization and Prediction in Autism Spectrum Disorder Using Graph Theory and Machine Learning. *PLoS One, 9*(6), 1–10. doi:10.1371/journal.pone.0090405 PMID:24922325

Zhu, Z., Ji, Q., & Bennett, K. P. (2006, August). Nonlinear eye gaze mapping function estimation via support vector regression. In *18th International Conference on Pattern Recognition (ICPR'06)* (Vol. 1, pp. 1132-1135). IEEE.

Zimmer, C. (2012). Our strange, important, subconscious light detectors. *Discover Magazine.*

Zwaigenbaum, L., Bauman, M. L., Choueiri, R., Fein, D., Kasari, C., Pierce, K., ... Wetherby, A. (2015a). Early identification and intervention for autism spectrum disorder. Executive Summary. *Pediatrics, 136*(Supplement), S1–S9. doi:10.1542/peds.2014-3667B PMID:26430167

Zwaigenbaum, L., Bauman, M. L., Choueiri, R., Kasari, C., Carter, A., Granpeesheh, D., ... Natowicz, M. R. (2015). Early intervention for children with autism spectrum disorder under 3 years of age: Recommendations for practice and research. *Pediatrics, 136*(Suppl 1), 60–81. doi:10.1542/peds.2014-3667E PMID:26430170

Zwaigenbaum, L., Bauman, M. L., Stone, W. L., Yirmiya, N., Estes, A., Hansen, R. L., ... Wetherby, A. (2015b). Early identification for autism spectrum disorder: Recommendation for Practice and Research. *Pediatrics, 136*(Supplement), S10–S40. doi:10.1542/peds.2014-3667C PMID:26430168

Zwaigenbaum, L., Bryson, S., Rogers, T., Roberts, W., Brian, J., & Szatmari, P. (2005). Behavioural manifestations of autism in the first year of life. *International Journal of Developmental Neuroscience, 23*(2–3), 143–152. PMID:15749241

About the Contributors

Tanu Wadhera received the B.tech degree in Electronics and Communication from Guru Nanak Engineering college, Ludhiana, India and M.tech degree in Eletronics & Communication from Punjabi University, Patiala, India. Currently, she is a Research Scholar in National institute of Technology, Jalandhar, India. Her research interests are cognitive neuroscience, behavioral understanding, technology in Autism Spectrum Disorder, biomedical signal processing, signal classification and prediction of neurodevelopmental disorders.

Deepti Kakkar was born in 1982, in Jalandhar, Punjab, India. She did her Bachelor of Technology in Electronics and Communication Engineering from Himachal Pradesh University, India in 2003 and Masters of Engineering in electronics product design and technology from Punjab University, Chandigarh. Deepti did her PhD in Cognitive Radios from Dr. B.R. Ambedkar National Institute of Technology, Jalandhar, India. She has a total academic experience of 15 years and at present she is ASSISTANT PROFESSOR in Electronics and Communication department with Dr. B. R. Ambedkar National Institute of Technology, Jalandhar, India. Earlier, she had worked as lecturer in Electronics and Communication department with DAV Institute of Engineering and Technology, Jalandhar, Punjab. She has guided more than 40 post graduate engineering dissertations and several projects. She is currently guiding 3 PhD thesis. She has more than 30 papers in the proceedings of various International Journals and Conferences. Her recent research interests include cognitive neuroscience, neuro-developmental disorder, dynamic spectrum allocation, spectrum sensing, and Cognitive Radios.

* * *

S. P. Abirami received the Bachelor's degree in Computer Science and Engineering from K.S.Rangasamy College of Technology, Tiruchengode and Master's degree in Computer Science and Engineering from PSG College of Technology, Coimbatore. Currently pursuing the research in Anna University, Chennai carrying a teaching experience of seven years in Coimbatore Institute of Technology. Some of the area of interests include cloud computing, virtualization, big data analytics, machine learning and computer vision for healthcare applications.

S. Artchoudane is currently working as a Yoga Therapist-cum-Teacher at Center for Yogic Sciences, Aarupadai Veedu Medical College and Hospital, Vinayaka Mission's Research Foundation (DU), Pondicherry. He has published 4 papers, compilations and abstracts on chronic obstructive pulmonary disorder, autism spectrum disorder, yoga, and yoga research in National and International Journals. He has authored a chapter, Stethograpy, in Handbook of Practical Physiology, Paras Medical Books. He has received several honors for "Jury" and award for "Best Yoga Teacher". He is a yoga professional member of Indian Yoga Association, member of jury board of Pondicherry Yogasana Association, and member of Pondicherry Yoga Teachers Development Association.

P. Balakrishnan presently working as Associate Professor in School of Computer Science and Engineering, VIT, Vellore. He completed his PhD in Madras Institute of Technology, Chennai. After that, he had completed first PostDoctoral Fellowship in National University of Singapore in the area of Mobile cloud computing. Then he completed his second PostDoc from Qatar University,Doha,Qatar in the area of Cloud Infrastructure for BioInformatics workflows. He authored a book entitled "Automated workflow scheduling in self adaptive clouds" in Springer publications. Also, he published nearly 30 research papers in reputed journals and conferences. His major research areas are cloud computing, IoT, IIoT, Machine learning and Blockchain technologies.

Sheetal Bhatia is currently Software engineer in IT industry, graduated from NIT jalandhar. Its techincal college located in punjab region. she is working on software product based Multinational company. she works of BP management tools. She has a keen interest in Biomedical possesion. She has a hobby of writing and travelling to new places.

Ananda Balayogi Bhavanani, MBBS, ADY, DPC, DSM, PGDFH, PGDY, FIAY, MD (Alt.Med), C-IAYT, DSc (Yoga), is Director of the Centre for Yoga Therapy Education and Research (CYTER), and Professor of Yoga Therapy at the Sri Balaji Vidyapeeth, Pondicherry (www.sbvu.ac.in). A recipient of the prestigious DSc (Yoga) from SVYASA Yoga University in January 2019, he is a Gold Medalist in Medical Studies (MBBS) with postgraduate diplomas in both Family Health (PGDFH) as well as Yoga (PGDY) and the Advanced Diploma in Yoga under his illustrious parents in 1991-93. A Fellow of the Indian Academy of Yoga, he has authored 19 DVDs and 23 books on Yoga as well as published nearly 300 papers, compilations and abstracts on Yoga and Yoga research in National and International Journals. His literary works have more than 2100 Citations, with a h-Index of 23 and an i10-Index of 40.

Adheesh Budree holds an MSc in Financial Economics from the University of London, UK and a Ph.D. degree in Information Systems from the University of the Western Cape, South Africa. He is currently a Senior Lecturer in Information Systems at the University of Cape Town, South Africa. His main research interests are in the Socio-Economics of Technology, eCommerce and Data Analytics.

Harpreet Kaur Dhir received her BA in multiple subjects from University of Redlands, CA, USA and MA in Curriculum and Instruction with an emphasis on Design-Based Learning from California Polytechnic University, Pomona, CA, USA. Teaching for the past 27 years, her teaching career began at the Ontario-Montclair Unified School District. Presently, she teaches at Hacienda La Puente Unified School District in CA, USA. Harpreet has served as an advisory board member and a faculty member at the Art Center College of Design and a lecturer for the MA courses in the Department of Integrative Studies at California Polytechnic University, Pomona. Currently, a doctoral candidate at the American College of Education, her dissertation is centered around the problem of educators not prepared to teach the 21st-Century Competencies as enshrined in the P21 framework. She has a broad range of field experience serving on school and district level committees. Member of the international honor society,

Kappa Delta Pi, Teacher of the Year for the Los Angeles Sherriff Youth Organization and a Teacher of the Year at a school, Leadership in Education awardee from California Polytechnic University, Pomona, and a nominee for the Disney Teacher of the Year award, her classroom research continues to examine the compatible teaching and curriculum planning methods for 21st-century classrooms including experiential learning methods through curriculum integration. Besides writing as one of her interests, Harpreet enjoys spending creative time in her art studio designing and making jewelry, writing fiction novels, and academic poetry to develop vocabulary and comprehension.

Jatinder Singh Goraya is currently Associate Professor in the Division of Pediatric Neurology, Department of Pediatrics, Dayanand Medical College & Hospital (DMCH), Ludhiana, Punjab, India. He obtained his MBBS, and MD (Postgraduation in Pediatrics) from Dayanand Medical College. Later he worked at Postgraduate Institute of Medical Education and Research, Chandigarh (PGIMER) as Senior Resident. He joined Government Medical College Chandigarh as Assistant Professor in Pediatrics and was later promoted as Associate Professor. In 2005, he went to US for further training in Pediatric Neurology. He returned in 2009. He joined DMCH in 2010, where he established Pediatric Neurology services for the patients of the region. In 2011, he was awarded the prestigious fellowship of Royal College of Physicians of Canada (FCRPC). He has published more than 90 papers in peer-reviewed national and international journals of repute. He has presented his papers in various national and international conferences. He has delivered several talks in the field of Pediatric Neurology.

Harsha Kathard co-leads Inclusive Practices Africa (IPA) at University of Cape Town (UCT). She has held leadership positions as Head of Department in Health and Rehabilitation Sciences and Health Sciences Education. She has also participated in curriculum change leadership at UCT. IPA is a transdisciplinary project which translates research into disability inclusive practices. She supported the development of a critical, inclusive approach in the Disability Studies postgraduate programmes. She is an NRF rated scientist who conducts research into disability inclusion in higher education, economy and health systems. She has a special interest in communication disability and inclusion.

Amarjot Kaur is currently working as Data Scientist with Alert Enterprise, Chandigarh which is a Fremont, CA based enterprise Software Company. She is currently developing AI based software to mitigate insider threat at enterprise level. She received her Bachelors in Technology with focus on Computer Science and Engineering from Guru Nanak Dev Engineering College, Ludhiana. She has worked closely with many SMEs and Start-ups in retail industry to setup their data platforms and processes. She is one of the initiators at GNDEC Data Science where she has mentored many budding data scientists. She has an analytical approach to solve business problems and has experience in different organizational functions as she works across multiple functions in the organization.

Pavneet Kaur is a Research scholar in Indian Institute of Technology, Delhi. She completed M.Tech. in Electronics and Communication Engineering from NIT, Jalandhar.

Rajandeep Kaur completed her M.Tech at Sant Baba Bhag Institute of Engineering & Technology in the field of Digital Image Processing. At present, she is Research Scholar at NIT Jalandhar. She has worked as Assistant Professor in various Engineering Institutes. She authored 10 research papers in journals and conferences.

Pallavi Khanna is currently working as a counsellor in NIT Jalandhar. She is pursuing her PhD in the field of Human Value and Professional Ethics and her subject is Happiness where she is exploring the eastern and western concepts and notions of happiness and finding a universal theory of Happiness. She has a Masters degree in Medical and psychiatric social Work from Tata Institute of Social Sciences, Mumbai. Also, she is a trained special educator. She is a graduate in psychology from Osmania university, Hyderabad. She actively supports families with children who have special needs by offering them training support and guidance. Her area of interests are mental health, rehabilitation of special children, social work and community service.

Arun Khosla is presently working as Professor in the Department of Electronics and Communication Engineering, Dr B R Ambedkar National Institute of Technology, Jalandhar, India. His areas of interest are fuzzy modeling, biologically inspired computing, high performance computing, autism & assisted technologies and emerging technologies. He is a reviewer for various IEEE and other National and International conferences and journals. He also serves on the editorial board of International Journal of Swarm Intelligence Research. He has conducted a number of tutorials in the domain of soft computing at various national & international conferences.

G. Kousalya, Professor and Head, Department of Computer Science and Engineering, Coimbatore Institute of Technology, Coimbatore has completed her B.E. Electronics and Communication Engineering in the year 1991, M.E. Computer Science and Engineering in the year 2000 and completed her PhD in the area on Cloud Interoperability in the year 2007. Her research areas includes Cloud Computing, Edge Computing, Data Analytics, Network Security, Cyber Physical Systems, Block chain technology, etc., She has got various funding for laboratory setups like Cloud laboratory, IoT laboratory and for working with Cyber Physical systems. She has numerous conference and journal publications in the highly prescribed journal list and has also written a book based on workflow scheduling.

Gayathri Krishnan is a Speech- Language Pathologist by qualification and practise. She is pursuing her doctoral degree in rehabilitation of persons with swallowing disorders from the All India Institute of Speech and Hearing, Mysore. She has published approximately 13 research papers in national and international journals. She has received research grants and have completed three research projects in the field of speech-language pathology. Apart from these, many conference presentations, two resource books and a book chapter is in her credit.

Dulani Meedeniya is a Senior Lecturer in the Department of Computer Science and Engineering at the University of Moratuwa, Sri Lanka. She holds a PhD in Computer Science from the University of St Andrews, United Kingdom. Her main research interests are Software modelling and design, Workflow tool support for bioinformatics, Data Visualization and Recommender systems. Dr. Meedeniya is a Fellow of HEA(UK), MIET, MIEEE, and a Charted Engineer registered at EC (UK).

Meena is Associate Professor and Deputy Director of CYTER, the Centre for Yoga Therapy Education and Research at Sri Balaji Vidyapeeth. She has completed numerous undergraduate and postgraduate degrees and diplomas in Yoga, Science and English has completed her PhD in Yoga through Tamil Nadu Physical Education and Sports University (TNPESU). She is a recognized IAYT Certified Yoga Therapist by the International Association of Yoga Therapists, USA. She has been recognized as PhD

Guide (Yoga Therapy and Interdisciplinary Research) by Sri Balaji Vidyapeeth, Pondicherry in March 2016, appointed as Lead Examiner for Yoga Certification Board (YCB) through Indian Yoga Association, recognized by AYUSH, Central Ministry of Health, and New Delhi in Sep 2016. She has been nominated as "Subject Expert" in the Selection Committee of the Govt of Puducherry, Directorate of Indian Systems of Medicine and Homeopathy; under National Health Mission. She recently received the Achiever's Award for "Best Yoga Therapist 2016". She is currently a Professional and Executive Committee member of Indian Yoga Association representing Pondicherry. She has authored and co-authored a dozen books and more than three dozen papers on Yoga in English and Tamil in various journals. She is currently carrying on many Research/Pilot Studies at CYTER of SBV at MGMCRI as a guide and co-guide for PhD and MPhil in Yoga Therapy, and has published 40 scientific papers, 11 compilations and a dozen abstracts in leading Scientific Journals.

Piyush Mishra has a younger brother Punit (23-years-old now) with autism and severe intellectual disability. Piyush graduated with M.Tech (Mechanical Engineering) from National Institute of Technology, Rourkela in June, 2019. He is the co-founder of VARTA (Nov,2019), a startup working for building online and offline platforms for sex education for persons with intellectual and developmental disabilities (IDD). He is majorly interested in research in future planning for adults with autism, particularly in residential planning after parents/primary care-givers become incapable of providing further care or in case of demise of parents/primary care-givers. His other research interests include sex education for persons with IDD, sibling studies, health assessments for persons with IDD. He is currently looking for research positions in these fields.

Anna Passaro, MA, Psychologist is an e-tutor at "Giustino Fortunato" University of Benevento (Italy). She deals with cognitive-behavioral interventions and assistive technology-based programs for promoting self-determination and independence of individuals with developmental disabilities. Her interests are focused on the aided-alternative and augmentative strategies and rehabilitative solutions aimed at promoting the on-task behavior among children and adolescents with ADHD.

Hiten Rajpurohit is pursuing his doctorate from Dr B. R. Ambedkar National Institute of Technology, Jalandhar in Electronics and Communication Engineering. He is M.Tech from Dr B. R. Ambedkar National Institute of Technology, Jalandhar and B.Tech from Sai Vidya Institute of Technology, Bengaluru in Electronics and Communication Engineering. He has 2 years of total experience as a Software Engineer. He has good teaching experience at under graduate and post graduate level. His areas of interest are autism & assisted technologies, deep learning, machine learning and emerging technologies.

Rajneesh Rani has received the B.Tech and M.Tech degrees, both in Computer Science and Engineering from Punjab Technical University, Jalandhar, India in 2001 and Punjabi University Patiala, India in 2003 respectively. She has done her Ph.D.in Computer Science and Engineering from NIT Jalandhar in 2015. From 2003 to 2005, she was a lecturer in Guru Nanak Dev Engineering College, Ludhiana. Currently, she has been working as an Assistant Professor in NIT Jalandhar since 2007. Her teaching and research include areas like Image Processing, Pattern Recognition, Machine Learning, Computer Programming and Document Analysis and Recognition.

Iresha Rubasinghe is a postgraduate student at the Department of Computer Science and Engineering, University of Moratuwa, Sri Lanka. She has research experience in Software Engineering, bioinformatics, Embedded Systems, Information Security, Image Processing and Computer Vision.

Gajendra Singh is a Research scholar in the field of Electronics and Communication Engineering at NIT Jalandhar.

Navjot Singh is working as a Data Scientist in AlertEnterprise which is headquartered in Fremont, with Indian development Centre in Chandigarh. He has done his Bachelors in Information Technology from Guru Nanak Dev Engineering College, Ludhiana. He takes care of AI based application development for his current employer and responsible for building a Security Platform leveraging deep learning and neural networks to mitigate enterprise security challenges. He has also worked in different industries such as Aviation and Entertainment helping India's biggest Airlines and a TV Channel to incorporate data driven solutions in their business and wore different hats such as an Engineer, Analyst and consultant. He uses psychometrics and AI based applications to solve day to day challenges and has a strong hold in these areas.

Fabrizio Stasolla, PhD, has a post-doctoral degree. He is an Associate Professor at Giustino Fortunato University of Benevento (Italy). His topic concerns the assistive technologies for children with multiple disabilities, developmental disabilities, autism spectrum disorders, ADHD, Rett and Down syndromes, cerebral palsy, congenital encephalopathy, fragile X syndrome, post-coma patients who are in a vegetative state either in a minimally conscious state or are emerging/emerged from it. His interest deals with cognitive-behavioral interventions and aided-alternative and augmentative communication strategies for non verbal individuals, and/or for persons who are estimated within a normal intellectual functioning but who present pervasive motor disabilities. He teaches developmental psychology to educational sciences and psychology students. Furthermore, he works on technological supports, PECS, VOCA, SGD, literacy process, ambulation responses, self-monitoring and self management of instruction cues to promote on-task behavior of students with learning disabilities. Finally, his framework is focused on behavioral strategies and technological aids for pursuing the dual goal of enhancing adaptive responses and reducing challenging behaviors by children with severe to profound developmental disabilities. From 2013 up to present, he is ad-hoc reviewer for 25 peer-reviewed journals, he serves on the editorial board of 5 more peer-reviewed journals. Additionally, he is an associate editor of the International Journal of Behavioral Research & Psychology, and an Editor Review of Frontiers in Psychology (Section of Neuropsychology). He is the sole selected Editor for the forthcoming Nova Publishers volume entitled "Understanding Children with Cerebral Palsy" (2020).

Yashomathi is a Speech-Language Pathologist (SLP) by qualification and practise. She is presently working as 'Lecturer in Speech Pathology' in Department of Speech-Language Pathology, All India institute of Speech and Hearing (AIISH), Mysuru, India. She has received her Doctoral degree (Speech-Language Pathology) from All India institute of Speech and Hearing (AIISH) (University of Mysore), with specialization in "Comparison of Syntax of Indian Sign Language between two dialects". She is a member of Indian Speech and Hearing Association (ISHA) which is a National Association of Speech, Language and Hearing Professionals. She has published few research papers in national and international journals and have also delivered talks in conference presentations.

Index

H

I

L

M

N

O

P

Q

R

S

T

V

www.ingramcontent.com/pod-product-compliance
Lightning Source LLC
LaVergne TN
LVHW060301011026
849161LV00011B/2751
* 9 7 8 1 7 9 9 8 3 0 6 9 6 *